Lung Cancer

A Comprehensive Treatise

Lung Cancer
A Comprehensive Treatise

Edited by

Jacob D. Bitran, M.D.
Associate Professor of Medicine
Pritzker School of Medicine
Director, Clinical Research Development
Joint Section of Hematology/Oncology
University of Chicago Medical Center
Michael Reese Medical Center
Chicago, Illinois

Harvey M. Golomb, M.D.
Professor of Medicine
Pritzker School of Medicine
Director, Joint Section of Hematology/Oncology
University of Chicago Medical Center
Michael Reese Medical Center
Chicago, Illinois

Alex G. Little, M.D.
Associate Professor of Surgery
Pritzker School of Medicine
Chief, Section of Thoracic Surgery
Department of Surgery
University of Chicago Medical Center
Chicago, Illinois

Ralph R. Weichselbaum, M.D.
Professor and Chairman
Department of Radiation Oncology
Pritzker School of Medicine
Michael Reese/University of Chicago Center for Radiation Therapy
Chicago, Illinois

Grune & Stratton, Inc.
Harcourt Brace Jovanovich, Publishers
Orlando   New York   San Diego   London
San Francisco   Tokyo   Sydney   Toronto

Library of Congress Cataloging-in-Publication Data

Lung cancer.

   Includes index.
   1. Lungs—Cancer.   I. Bitran, Jacob D.   II. Golomb,
Harvey M. (Harvey Morris), 1943-   [DNLM: 1. Lung
Neoplasms. WF 658 L9607]
RC280.L8L767   1988   616.99′424   87-14874
ISBN 0-8089-1876-1

Grune & Stratton, Inc.
Orlando, Florida 32887

Distributed in the United Kingdom by
Grune & Stratton, Ltd.
24/28 Oval Road
London NW 1 70X

Library of Congress Catalog Number 87-14874
International Standard Book Number 0-8089-1876-1
Printed in the United States of America
87 88 89 90   10 9 8 7 6 5 4 3 2 1

To Linda, Lauren, and Dina
for all their love and support.

_____ Contents _____

Editorial Method   *xi*

Contributors   *xiii*

PART I   BASIC PRINCIPLES

1. The Multimodality Approach to Lung Cancer   3
    Jacob D. Bitran, Harvey M. Golomb, Alex G. Little,
    and Ralph R. Weichselbaum

2. Pathology of Lung Cancer—An Update   5
    Mary J. Matthews and R. Ilona Linnoila

3. Biology of Lung Cancer   35
    Steven T. Rosen and James A. Radosevich

4. Principles of Surgical Oncology   55
    Alex G. Little

5. Principles of Radiation Oncology   61
    Ralph R. Weichselbaum and Azhar M. Awan

6. Principles of Medical Oncology   71
    Jacob D. Bitran and Harvey M. Golomb

7. Diagnostic Methods in Lung Cancer   87
    Heber MacMahon, Stephen R. Ell, and Mark K. Ferguson

8.   Noninvasive and Invasive Staging of Lung Cancer   *113*
     Mark K. Ferguson, Heber MacMahon, Carlos Bekerman,
     and James W. Ryan

PART II   STAGE I NON-SMALL CELL LUNG CANCER

9.   Surgical Therapy   *135*
     Tom R. DeMeester and Mario Albertucci

10. Radiation Therapy   *149*
     Azhar M. Awan, Ralph R. Weichselbaum, and George T. Y. Chen

PART III   STAGE II NON-SMALL CELL LUNG CANCER

11. Surgical Therapy of Patients with Modified Stage II
     ($T_1N_1M_0$ and $T_2N_1M_0$) Non-Small Cell Lung Cancer   *161*
     Alex G. Little, Mark K. Ferguson, and David B. Skinner

12. Adjuvant Radiotherapy and Its Role in the Treatment of
     Stage II Lung Cancer   *165*
     Thomas J. Fitzgerald and Joel S. Greenberger

13. Adjuvant Therapy of Stage II Non-Small Cell Lung Cancer   *173*
     Thomas Lad

PART IV   STAGE III$_{M_0}$ NON-SMALL CELL LUNG CANCER

14. Management of $T_3N_0 - T_3N_1$ Non-Small Cell Carcinoma of
     the Lung   *185*
     Douglas J. Mathisen and Hermes C. Grillo

15. Surgical Therapy of Mediastinal (N_2) Disease   *201*
     F. Griffith Pearson

16. Radiation Treatment for Locally Advanced Stage III$_{M_0}$
     Non-Small Cell Carcinoma of the Lung   *207*
     Thomas J. Fitzgerald and Joel S. Greenberger

17. Chemotherapy as an Adjuvant to Surgery or Radiotherapy in
     Stage III_{M_0} Non-Small Cell Lung Carcinoma   221
     Renee H. Jacobs and Jacob D. Bitran

**PART V   STAGE III_{M_1}/STAGE IV NON-SMALL CELL LUNG
           CANCER**

18. Chemotherapy of Disseminated Non-Small Cell Lung Cancer   233
     John C. Ruckdeschel

19. The Role of Radiation Therapy in Stage III_{M_1} Non-Small Cell
     Lung Cancer   243
     Azhar M. Awan and Ralph R. Weichselbaum

PART VI   SMALL CELL LUNG CANCER

20. Small Cell Lung Cancer: A Distinct Clinicopathologic Entity   257
     Eric J. Seifter and Daniel C. Ihde

21. Biomarkers in Small Cell Lung Cancer   281
     David H. Johnson and F. Anthony Greco

22. Chemotherapy for Small Cell Carcinoma of the Lung   307
     Joseph Aisner

23. The Role of Radiation Therapy in the Treatment of Small Cell
     Lung Cancer   329
     Allen S. Lichter and Daniel C. Ihde

24. The Role of Surgical Resection in the Management of Small
     Cell Carcinoma of the Lung   359
     Philip C. Hoffman

25. Patterns of Relapse in Small Cell Lung Cancer—Implications
     for Future Studies   369
     David G. Dienhart and Paul A. Bunn, Jr.

PART VII   SUPPORTIVE CARE

26.   Endobronchial Therapy for Unresectable Lung Cancer   401
         James B. D. Mark and John C. Baldwin

27.   Diagnosis and Management of Medical and Surgical Problems
       in the Patient with Lung Cancer   411
         Martin D. Abeloff and David S. Ettinger

       Index   439

Editorial Method

We have attempted to incorporate the proposed new staging system into our book with the editors' comments at the end of each chapter. In addition, the chapter on staging describes both the previous and new staging system. In fact, the proposed system appears to be similar to the previous staging system in terms of stage grouping. That is, $T_1N_0M_0$ and $T_2N_0M_0$ tumors constitute stage I under the new system, and we regarded them in this fashion under the old system. Similarly, stage II consists of $T_1N_1M_0$ and $T_2N_0M_0$ lung cancers

The major impact of the new staging system is that locally extensive primary tumors are classified as either T_3 or T_4, and metastases to regional lymph nodes can be classified as either N_2 or N_3. Patients with T_4 tumors or involvement of N_3 nodes constitute a stage IIIB group, and patients with distant organ metastases are in stage IV.

JACOB D. BITRAN, HARVEY M. GOLOMB
ALEX G. LITTLE, RALPH R. WEICHSELBAUM

Contributors

Martin D. Abeloff, M.D.
Chief, Medical Oncology, The Johns Hopkins Oncology Center; Professor of Oncology, The Johns Hopkins University School of Medicine, Baltimore, Maryland

Joseph Aisner, M.D., F.A.C.P.
Professor of Medicine, Oncology, Pharmacology, and Experimental Therapeutics, Department of Medicine, University of Maryland School of Medicine; Deputy Director for Clinical Affairs, University of Maryland Cancer Center; University of Maryland Medical Systems, Baltimore, Maryland

Mario Albertucci, M.D.
Department of Surgery, Creighton University School of Medicine, Omaha, Nebraska

Azhar M. Awan, M.D.
Assistant Professor, Department of Radiation Oncology, University of Chicago Medical Center, Chicago, Illinois

John C. Baldwin, M.D.
Assistant Professor of Cardiovascular Surgery, Department of Cardiovascular Surgery, Stanford University School of Medicine, Stanford, California

Carlos Bekerman, M.D.
Associate Professor, Department of Radiology, Michael Reese Hospital and Medical Center, Chicago, Illinois

Jacob D. Bitran, M.D.
Associate Professor of Medicine, Pritzker School of Medicine; Director, Clinical Research Development, Joint Section of Hematology/Oncology, University of Chicago Medical Center, Michael Reese Medical Center, Chicago, Illinois

Paul A. Bunn, Jr., M.D.
Professor of Medicine and Head, Division of Medical Oncology, Department of Medicine, University of Colorado Health Sciences Center, Denver, Colorado

George T. Y. Chen, Ph.D.
Professor and Director, Medical Physics, Department of Radiation Oncology, University of Chicago, Chicago, Illinois

Tom R. DeMeester, M.D.
Professor and Chairman, Department of Surgery, Creighton University School of Medicine, Omaha, Nebraska

David G. Dienhart, M.D.
Instructor, Division of Medical Oncology, University of Colorado Health Sciences Center, Denver, Colorado

Stephen R. Ell, M.D., Ph.D., F.A.C.P.
Associate Professor, Department of Radiology, University of Chicago Medical
Center, Chicago, Illinois

David S. Ettinger, M.D., F.A.C.P.
Associate Professor of Oncology and Medicine, The Johns Hopkins Oncology
Center, The Johns Hopkins University School of Medicine, Baltimore, Maryland

Mark K. Ferguson, M.D.
Assistant Professor, Department of Surgery, University of Chicago Medical
Center, Chicago, Illinois

Thomas J. Fitzgerald, M.D.
Assistant Professor, Department of Radiation Oncology, University of
Massachusetts Medical Center, Worcester, Massachusetts

Harvey M. Golomb, M.D.
Professor of Medicine, Pritzker School of Medicine; Director, Joint Section of
Hematology/Oncology, University of Chicago Medical Center, Michael Reese
Medical Center, Chicago, Illinois

F. Anthony Greco, M.D.
Director and Professor of Medicine, Division of Oncology, Department of
Medicine, Vanderbilt University, Nashville, Tennessee

Joel S. Greenberger, M.D.
Professor and Chairman, Department of Radiation Oncology, University of
Massachusetts Medical Center, Worcester, Massachusetts

Hermes C. Grillo, M.D.
Chief, General Thoracic Surgery, Massachusetts General Hospital; Professor of
Surgery, Harvard Medical School, Boston, Massachusetts

Philip C. Hoffman, M.D.
Associate Professor of Clinical Medicine, Joint Section of Hematology/
Oncology, Department of Medicine, The University of Chicago Medical Center,
Chicago, Illinois

Daniel C. Ihde, M.D.
Head, Clinical Investigations Section, NCI-Navy Medical Oncology Branch,
National Cancer Institute and Naval Hospital; Professor of Medicine,
Department of Medicine, Uniformed Services University of the Health Sciences,
Bethesda, Maryland

Renee H. Jacobs, M.D.
Clinical Instructor, Section of Hematology/Oncology, Department of Medicine,
University of Chicago and Michael Reese Medical Center, Chicago, Illinois

David H. Johnson, M.D.
Assistant Professor of Medicine, Division of Oncology, Department of Medicine,
Vanderbilt University, Nashville, Tennessee

Thomas Lad, M.D.
Associate Professor of Clinical Medicine, University of Illinois College of
Medicine; Chief, Medical Oncology Section, Veterans Administration West Side
Medical Center, Chicago, Illinois

Allen S. Lichter, M.D.
Professor and Chairman, Department of Radiation Oncology, University of
Michigan Medical Center, Ann Arbor, Michigan

R. Ilona Linnoila, M.D.
Pathologist, Human Tumor Biology Section, NCI-Navy Medical Oncology
Branch, Naval Hospital, Bethesda, Maryland

Alex G. Little, M.D.
Associate Professor of Surgery, Pritzker School of Medicine; Chief, Section of
Thoracic Surgery, Department of Surgery, University of Chicago Medical Center,
Chicago, Illinois

Heber MacMahon, M.D.
Associate Professor, Department of Radiology, University of Chicago Medical
Center, Chicago, Illinois

James B. D. Mark, M.D.
Johnson & Johnson Professor of Surgery; Head, Division of Thoracic Surgery,
Stanford University School of Medicine, Stanford, California

Douglas J. Mathisen, M.D.
General Thoracic Surgical Unit, Massachusetts General Hospital; Assistant
Professor of Surgery, Harvard Medical School, Boston, Massachusetts

Mary J. Matthews, M.D. (deceased)
Pathologist, Department of Anatomic Pathology and NCI-Navy Medical
Oncology Branch, Naval Hospital, Bethesda, Maryland

F. Griffith Pearson, M.D., F.R.C.S (C), F.A.C.S.
Professor of Surgery, University of Toronto; Surgeon-in-Chief, Toronto General
Hospital, Toronto, Ontario, Canada

James A. Radosevich, Ph.D.
Assistant Professor of Medicine, Section of Hematology/Oncology, Department
of Medicine, Northwestern University; Staff Research Scientist, Veterans
Administration Lakeside Medical Center, Chicago, Illinois

Steven T. Rosen, M.D., F.A.C.P.
Associate Professor of Medicine, Section of Hematology/Oncology, Department
of Medicine, Northwestern University, Veterans Administration Lakeside Medical
Center, Chicago, Illinois

John C. Ruckdeschel, M.D.
Professor of Medicine and Head, Division of Medical Oncology, Albany Medical
College; Executive Officer, Lung Cancer Study Group, Albany, New York

James W. Ryan, M.D.
Associate Professor, Department of Radiology, Nuclear Medicine Division,
University of Chicago Medical Center, Chicago, Illinois

Eric J. Seifter, M.D.
Assistant Professor of Medicine, Department of Medicine, Uniformed Services
University of the Health Sciences; Investigator, NCI-Navy Medical Oncology
Branch, National Cancer Institute, Bethesda, Maryland

David B. Skinner, M.D., F.A.C.S.
Dallas B. Phemister Professor and Chairman, Department of Surgery, Pritzker
School of Medicine, University of Chicago, Chicago, Illinois

Ralph R. Weichselbaum, M.D.
Professor and Chairman, Department of Radiation Oncology, Pritzker School of
Medicine; Michael Reese/University of Chicago Center for Radiation Therapy,
Chicago, Illinois

Lung Cancer

A Comprehensive Treatise

Basic Principles

Jacob D. Bitran, Harvey M. Golomb
Alex G. Little, Ralph R. Weichselbaum

——— 1 ———

The Multimodality Approach to Lung Cancer

The title of this book reflects its goals: to be both reasonably comprehensive and serve as a textbook. With regard to the first goal, we have attempted to address the important issues of lung cancer biology, diagnosis, staging, and treatment by all three therapeutic modality groups. Regarding the second goal, our aim is to present the state of the art regarding lung cancer in a fashion that is useful to residents, fellows, and practicing physicians. Where there is controversy or an important difference of opinion, we have attempted to present all sides. Authors have been selected from many places, but the editorial board is from the Chest Oncology Group at The University of Chicago Medical Center. We stress throughout the philosophy that has emerged from our joint endeavors over the decade that this group has been in existence.

In particular, we want to emphasize the value of a prospective, multimodality approach to patients with lung cancer. The stress is on the word "approach." All physicians involved in the care of lung cancer patients in any institution should take part in the important decision-making steps involved in diagnosis, staging, and long-term follow-up of these patients, as well as therapy. In addition, there should be a disease- and patient-oriented approach, not a procedure-oriented approach for surgical and radiation therapy oncologists or a chemotherapy-oriented approach for medical oncologists. These desiderata can best be achieved through a group, multimodality approach such as has been utilized by the Chest Oncology Group at The University of Chicago Medical Center. We would like to offer a description of our group's interactions as an archetype to be used in considering the benefits, practicalities, and logistics of this approach.

Our weekly Chest Oncology conference is attended by representatives from the Medical Oncology, Thoracic Surgery, and Radiation Oncology sections who combine to form the Chest Oncology Group. Also present is a radiologist for interpretation of radiologic examinations, a nuclear medicine representative for nuclear scan readings, and a pathologist who reviews material pertinent to the patients to be discussed. Three groups of patients are reviewed and discussed. First, new patients with suspected or newly diagnosed lung cancer are presented in detail and clinical information is re-

LUNG CANCER: A COMPREHENSIVE TREATISE
ISBN 0-8089-1876-1

viewed. Diagnostic and staging alternatives are discussed with the referring physician and appropriate strategies developed. Treatment strategies based on the potential outcomes of diagnostic and staging plans are also evaluated at that time. The referring physician leaves the conference knowing the recommended plan and having contributed to its formulation. The second group of patients presented are those in the hospital who have been previously discussed by the Chest Oncology Group. New results of diagnostic or staging evaluations are reviewed, as well as results or complications of ongoing treatment. A group plan is formulated for further evaluation or therapy and alternatives are developed. Feedback to the responsible physicians is instantaneous as most of the patients are on the Medical Oncology or Thoracic Surgery Services; physicians treating patients on other services are present and participate in discussions and decisions. The third group of patients discussed are those being followed in the outpatient clinic for whose care a decision must be made or for whom a change in management needs to be considered. The responsible physician can succinctly present the pertinent information and immediately receive multimodality consultation in an integrated fashion.

This group approach can be threatening to an individual physician who fears the potential loss of control over his or her patients. It is always clear, however, that when patients are presented by a physician outside the Chest Oncology Group that the group is acting in a consultative capacity. It is only by utilizing this approach, with experienced physicians representing the three modalities presently used to treat lung cancer, that decisions can be made and strategies planned that afford the patient the optimal approach. For example, a referring physician is able to hear and participate in an open discussion of therapeutic options and the rationales for their selection. Discussions can take place regarding a patient's physiologic status and ability to withstand surgery or tolerate chemotherapy or radiation therapy. Only in this fashion can the three modalities be integrated to achieve their maximum benefits for therapy; the full treatment plan is decided together and a coordinated therapeutic schedule devised. It is a system of checks and balances; with an open discussion among representatives of three therapeutic modalities, diagnostic, staging, and therapeutic plans are developed in a balanced manner to the patient's benefit. Patients referred to any member of the Chest Oncology Group are presented and discussed by the group, except for occasional patients requiring urgent intervention prior to any therapy. This prevents the possibility of patients referred to one specialty automatically receiving that particular modality prior to consideration of other options. The prospective and group approach encourages the development of an integrated plan in which the three modalities are combined to maximize their joint efforts.

Another important benefit from this organized multimodality approach is that of the ability to jointly develop therapeutic and/or investigative protocols and subsequently to maintain control over patients entered into them. With the opportunity to participate prospectively in the design of clinical protocols, the odds of adherence to protocol aspects by each therapeutic group are maximized. The "tunnel vision" that can result when any one therapeutic modality group alone treats a patient is prevented by prior agreement between groups, and this is supported by the joint discussion and review of patients in the weekly conference.

Mary J. Matthews
R. Ilona Linnoila

2

Pathology of Lung Cancer—An Update

DEFINITION AND PROBLEMS

Lung tumors include a wide spectrum of benign and malignant neoplasms, predominantly of epithelial type and entodermal derivation. This chapter is limited to discussion of the major types of epithelial tumors (squamous cell, small cell, adenocarcinoma, and large cell carcinoma) and carcinoids, which constitute over 90-95 percent of all primary pulmonary neoplasms.

It is paradoxical and possibly prophetic that many concepts concerning lung cancer proferred 10 years ago as gospel have been challenged and found inappropriate. Simple, relatively benign techniques such as fiberoptic bronchoscopy and guided fine-needle aspirates have permitted diagnoses of central, peripheral, and apical lung tumors.[73,82] Cytology has been raised to a fine art in the interpretation of these aspirates.[36,42,45,74,105] Staging procedures to define regional or extensive disease have been profoundly altered by computed tomographic (CT) scans and by magnetic resonance (MR) imaging. Restaging procedures utilizing these techniques have altered impressions concerning the complete or partial response of the tumor to therapy. Operability of small cell lung cancer (SCLC), once considered an excercise in futility, has become feasible for the small number (5 percent) of these patients who present with a $T^1N^0M^0$ pulmonary mass.[97] Treatment policies and protocols based on older concepts thus become problematic.

CHALLENGE TO LIGHT-MICROSCOPIC CONCEPTS

Electron microscopy (EM), immunohistochemistry (IHC), and basic experimental research techniques have profoundly altered and immensely improved our understanding of the embryogenesis, histogenesis, and morphogenesis of all lung cancers. The entodermal rather than neural crest origin of SCLC is currently accepted by almost all serious students of the disease.[27] It is likewise recognized from a number of reports that some non-small cell lung cancers (NSCLC) demonstrate, by one or all of the techniques mentioned above, distinct neuroendocrine (NE) features.[5,8,29,46,54,67,114] Because of the relative paucity of data to date, there is no clear indication of the extent of this problem, whether NSCLC with NE features respond to radiation or chemotherapy, and/or whether they are associated with relatively long or shortened host survivals.

These research techniques, unfortunately, have engendered a plethora of new lung cancer classifications and terminologies that confuse both clinicians and pathologists.[66,79,98,110] Some classifications require EM for the diagnosis of SCLC. Others identify cell type by the various hormones or proteins elaborated by the tumor. Research pathologists have devised terminologies to describe SCLC, including a classic and a variant subtype, according to the altered biochemical or morphologic profile of tumors studied in continuous cell culture lines.[10,28] The real concern perceived from these classifications is that they will evoke the same confusion in diagnoses of lung cancer that was prevalent in the 1960s and 1970s. Instead of promoting a greater consensus in the diagnosis of lung cancers, there is a danger that diagnoses based on research procedures rather than light microscopy (LM) will permit no validation or review and that cooperative clinical protocols between various institutions, as they are designed to date, will become inoperative.

PURPOSE OF WORLD HEALTH ORGANIZATION LUNG CANCER CLASSIFICATION

It was and has been the purpose of the World Health Organization (WHO) Lung Cancer Classifications[51,100] to provide LM criteria for the various types of lung cancer. It was hoped that acceptance of these criteria on a worldwide basis would permit uniform diagnoses, which would become the common denominators of treatment protocols. Such classifications, imperfect as they must be and are, have to be based on the talents, personnel, and resources of all hospitals on an international basis. Additional concerns of the WHO Lung Cancer Classifications have been to (1) assure consistency and reliability of lung cancer diagnoses on an international basis, (2) contribute to the better understanding of the behavior of all lung cancer cell types, (3) identify risk factors associated with these neoplasms, and (4) allow evaluation of treatment protocols and response to therapy.

In 1967 the first WHO Lung Cancer Classification identified 14 categories of tumors and tumor-like lesions.[51] Although specific criteria were given for the major cell types, criteria for subtypes frequently were minimal or misleading. The second WHO Lung Cancer Classification, formulated in 1977, attempted to update and simplify the original classification.[100] Cytology was recognized as a significant diagnostic tool in the interpretation of dysplastic, in situ, and frankly invasive malignancies.

CHAPTER CONTENTS

This chapter briefly discusses the morphogenesis and pathogenesis of lung tumors. Current statistical studies relating to lung cancers are summarized. Gross, LM, and research data available on the major lung cancer cell types and carcinoids are emphasized. The significance and value of EM, IHC, and research pathology are stressed. Monoclonal antibodies developed against various lung cancers are beyond the scope of this chapter. The interrelationships of lung cancers are discussed.

MORPHOGENESIS AND PATHOGENESIS OF LUNG CANCERS

Morphogenesis

An impressive amount of information has accrued in the past decade concerning the histogenesis and morphogenesis of lung tumors. It has long been appreciated that the epithelial cells of the tracheobronchial tree share an entodermal derivation with the foregut. It was speculated but unproved in the 1960s and 1970s that endocrine cells of the lung were of neural crest origin.[83]

The tracheobronchial tree, down to and including the terminal bronchioles, is lined by pseudostratified reserve cells (basal cells admixed with rare NE-type cells indentifiable only by special techniques) and ciliated or goblet (mucus-secreting) columnar cells. Bronchial submucous glands are lined by serous and mucus producing cells, similar to those identified in salivary glands. NE cells and myoepithelial cells cuff these glands. By EM, mucus-secreting and ciliated columnar cells contain an abundance of organelles, including mitochondria, Golgi complexes, and free ribosomes. Numerous microvilli project from the free or luminal surfaces of the cells. Secretory vacuoles filled with globular material and ciliary basal bodies are markers of these cells.[58] Reserve basal cells contain tonofilamentous elements, predicting their potential to form squamous as well as columnar cells in response to chronic injury. Metaplastic squamous cells are identified by LM as stratifying cells apposed to each other by periodic intercellular bridges. By EM, these cells are bound by similar periodic prominent desmosomes. Tonofilamentous parallel bundles may abut on the desmosomes. Dense lamellar cytoplasmic aggregates, representing keratohyaline granules, may be present.

In the mid-1960s and early 1970s, bronchial mucosal epithelial cells containing membrane-bound dense core (neurosecretory) granules, measuring from 800 to 1700 Å, were identified by EM throughout the tracheobronchial tree.[6,104] These cells, called endocrine or NE cells, are sparse, are in contact with the basement membrane and interdigitate with adjacent columnar cells in dendritic fashion (Fig. 2-1). With few exceptions, they are not identified by routine hematoxylin and eosin stain by LM. Abundant NE cells have been found dispersed throughout the bronchial and bronchiolar mucosa in both fetal and newborn human and animal species.[19,38,53] In contrast, NE cells are sparse and less readily identified in normal adult lung but do proliferate in response to chronic lung injury.[34] The cells may aggregate to form so-called neuroepithelial bodies.[52] Cells fluoresce on exposure to formaldehyde vapors after incubation with 5-hydroxytryptophan or L-dopa, confirming the presence of dopa decarboxylase and the amine precursor uptake and decarboxylation (APUD) nature of the cells.[19] Amines and/or polypeptide hormones such as bombesin, calcitonin, and leu-enkephalin have been identified in NE cells by immunohistochemical techniques.[18] These cells have been considered the putative progenitors for SCLC and bronchial carcinoids.[7]

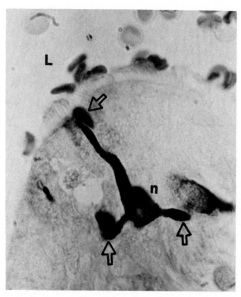

Fig. 2-1. Photomicrograph of a human pulmonary neuroendocrine cell containing serotonin in adult lung. Note the basally located nucleus (n), cell processes (arrows), and contact with bronchial lumen (L) lined by ciliated cells. Immunoperoxidase staining, original magnification ×1400.

Respiratory bronchioles are lined by low cuboidal ciliated epithelial cells, granular and basal-type reserve cells, and secretory Clara cells. The latter cells project as knob-like processes between the ciliated cuboidal cells. Mucin-secreting cells are not normally observed in bronchioles. On the contrary, reserve or Clara cells are capable of undergoing metaplasia to a mucin-producing cell in response to chronic injury. Lining cells of alveolar walls are rarely identified in the normal lung by usual light microscopic technics. On EM, Clara cells contain apical small dense secretory granules.[20] It is speculated that lipoproteins or glycoproteins produced by these cells may contribute to airway patency.[85] These cells are also rich in drug-metabolizing enzymes such as cytochrome p-450.[95]

Alveolar septa are lined by two types of cells: the type I pneumocytes, which cover over 90 percent of the surface of the alveolar walls, and type II pneumocytes, which contain osmiophilic bodies producing surfactant. Epithelial cells are adjoined by desmosomes to protect and maintain the integrity of alveolar septa.

Pathogenesis

The pathogenesis of lung cancer has been investigated by a number of authors concerned with mechanisms of carcinogenesis, cancer epidemiology, and early cytologic and tissue diagnoses of these tumors. It has been stressed that at sites of segmental bronchial bifurcations, airflow and mucus production are altered and bronchial epithelium becomes particularly susceptible to injury.[57] Carcinogenic agents are likely to be deposited and absorbed in these zones. Saccomanno followed uranium miners closely with repeated sputum examinations over many years.[88] He demonstrated that metaplastic squamous cells were replaced in a progressive manner over time by dysplastic, in situ, and frankly invasive neoplastic cells. It was and remains perplexing that a number of these closely monitored patients, thought to be candidates for squamous cell carcinoma of the lung, developed infiltrating small cell carcinoma. In the early lung cancer study, to the contrary, Melamed found that basal cell hyperplasia, squamous metaplasia, or atypia are independent smoke-related phenomena that did not necessarily predict dysplastic or neoplastic change.[69,70] He was unable to document the progression of metaplasia, dysplasia, and in situ malignancy noted by Saccomanno. In situ carcinoma frequently was seen without adjacent preneoplastic lesions.

Neoplasias in the lungs are produced by exposure to a host of exogenous as well as endogenous risk factors.[76] Familial and genetic disorders have also been associated with lung cancer.[32] The single most important risk factor in lung cancer is tobacco smoke, with its inherent nicotine and tar content. This factor, synergistic with other exogenous or endogenous risks, is probably the cause of the majority of lung cancers, whether central or peripheral in origin.

Environmental or occupational risk factors associated with lung cancer include (1) carcinogenic agents, such as benzopyrene and radon particles associated with uranium mining, radiation, and nuclear bombs; (2) procarcinogens, such as polycyclic aromatic hydrocarbons (PAH); and (3) cocarcinogens, such as arsenicals, asbestos fibers (crocidolite), chloromethyl methyl ether, chromates, diesel exhaust, nitrogen mustard gasses, nickel, silica, and vinyl chloride. Air pollution, coal, and iron mining exposure are also considered risk factors.

Endogenous risk factors associated with lung cancers include almost any disease that may induce pulmonary fibrosis: scars secondary to infarcts, abscesses, mycobacterial or fungal granulomata, scleroderma, bronchiectasis, pneumoconiosis, and interstitial pulmonary fibrosis.

Genetic and familial factors associated with idiopathic interstitial fibrosis have been reported in siblings with lung cancer.[32] The role of increased levels of aryl hydrocarbon hydroxylase, an enzyme responsible for conversion of the procarcinogens (PAH), to active compunds associated with carcinogenesis has not been resolved. However, increased levels of this enzyme have been identified in smokers and associated with an increased incidence of lung, laryngeal, and oral cavity neoplasms.[50]

STATISTICS

It has been estimated that 144,000 new lung cancer cases will be identified in 1985.[99] The current male: female ratio is 2.1:1, as compared with a ratio of 5:1 in 1977. In males, lung cancers constitute 22 percent of all malignancies, followed by prostatic malignancies (19 percent). In females, breast cancers constitute 26 percent of all malignancies, followed by colorectal cancer (16 percent) and lung cancer (10 percent). It is estimated that approximately 125,000 persons will die with lung cancer in 1985, with a male:female ratio of 2.3:1. Strikingly, lung cancer remains the chief cause of death in males (35 percent as compared to 10 percent for prostate), and, for the first time, deaths due to breast and lung cancers in the female are essentially equivalent (18 percent).

A small glimmer of optimism relates to two facts: (1) for the first time in almost 20 years, there has been an actual significant reduction (3.4 percent) in the incidence of lung cancer in white males, noted in the years 1982 and 1983; and (2) a 20 percent 5-year survival rate has been achieved in patients presenting with local disease.

Less optimistic is the fact that there is now a higher probability of black males developing lung cancer than white males. There has been a 6 percent increase in the incidence of lung cancer over the past 10 years in females. Finally, there has been very minimal improval in the 5-year survival rate of males in the past 20 years (8-13 percent) despite heroic efforts to improve these numbers.

PATHOLOGY

Squamous Cell Carcinoma

In the United States, squamous cell carcinomas constitute between 30 and 35 percent of all lung cancers, representing a striking decline in incidence in the past two decades. Two decades ago, this tumor was reported to have a 49 percent incidence, based on biopsy specimens.[115] Less than a decade later, the same author reported that the incidence of these tumors had dropped to 36 percent.[116]

It is estimated that over two-thirds of squamous cell tumors are central in origin. Up to 10 percent of peripheral squamous tumors may be cavitary and well differentiated. It is also estimated that over 80 percent of all cavitary pulmonary neoplasms are squamous in type.[12] Likewise, almost one-half of superior sulcus (Pancoast tumors) or tumors invading chest wall have been reported to be of this cell type.[64,81]

Gross

Occult squamous cell tumors, whether in situ or superficially invasive, have been identified predominantly by cytologic techniques, particularly by members of the early lung cancer study.[11,69,112,113] Lesions occasionally are difficult to visualize grossly. More often, the mucosa appears thickened and opaque, with obliteration of the usual longitudinal ridges. On occasion, the mucosa may appear red, granular, and friable. Lesions are particularly identified at sites of bronchial bifurcation and tend to extend toward the proximal portion of the bronchial tree.[11]

In frankly infiltrating malignancies, the tumors tend to present as bulky fungating gray-white intraluminal masses that partially occlude the bronchial lumina. The tumor, as with in situ malignancies, tends to grow centrally toward the main stem bronchus; invades bronchial walls; lung parenchyma; and bronchial, hilar, and/or mediastinal lymph nodes and soft tissues. As luminal obstruction progresses, organizing pneumonia and abscess formation may be identified in the distal lung parenchyma.

Microscopic

In situ squamous malignancies involve predominantly the bronchial mucosal lining but may also extend to involve bronchial ducts and mucous glands with which the mucosa communicates.[11] The mucosa is replaced by a disorganized proliferation of neoplastic reserve or squamous cells that show variability in nuclear size and staining reaction. Atypical mitoses may be identified throughout the thickness of the membrane. The mucosa, ducts, and glands are demarcated from the surrounding tissues by a bsasement membrane. As long as the tumor is restricted by this membrane, no invasion is present, even though the process may extend within bronchial glands almost to the level of the underlying cartilage.

Squamous tumors are classified according to whether they are well, moderately,

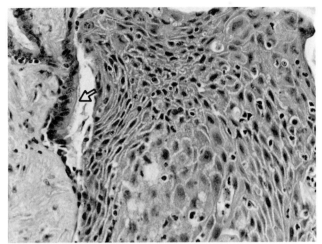

Fig. 2-2 Photomicrograph of a squamous cell carcinoma of the lung bulging into a bronchus. Note intercellular bridges in the tumor and normal ciliated bronchial epithelium (arrow). Hematoxylin eosin stain, original magnification ×330.

or poorly differentiated. Except for cavitary peripheral tumors, which may be well differentiated, most squamous malignancies of the lung are pleomorphic and vary from well to poorly differentiated in any single tumor. Criteria for LM diagnosis of squamous malignancies are fairly straightforward. Cells usually are arranged in nests or pseudoductal pattern, are stratified, and show intercellular bridge formation, the "sine qua non" of squamous malignancies, regardless of site (Fig. 2-2). Individual cells may have variable enlarged, irregular hyperchromatic nuclei and abundant or scanty cytoplasm. Individual cell keratinization, cell nesting, whorling, and keratin pearl formation are seen in moderately and well-differentiated tumors. An abundant amount of necrotic neoplastic keratotic debris may be seen in the center of the cell nests. In poorly differentiated tumors, the bulk of the tumor may be so anaplastic that LM features of differentiation may not be identified. In this group of tumors, nuclei may be vesicular and nucleoli prominent. Numerous tumor giant cells also may be seen, a factor that connotes a poor prognosis.[47,56,62]

In cytologic specimens, neoplastic cells tend to be large, shed singly, and are identified by the variable pattern of their nuclear hyperchromasia, irregularity of nuclear membrane, and orangeophilia of their cytoplasm. Poorly differentiated squamous cells have dense basophilic cytoplasm; their nuclei may be vesicular and contain prominent nucleoli.

By EM, neoplastic squamous cells share characteristics of their mature counterpart; in moderately and well differentiated tumors, plasma membranes are distinct, and cells are bound to each other by numerous desmosomes.[58] Dense tonofilamentous bundles may be seen abutting on desmosomes or may be dispersed diffusely throughout the cytoplasm. In poorly differentiated tumors or in poorly differentiated zones of a moderately differentiated tumor, the desmosomes and tonofilaments may be sparse and difficult to identify. Some tumors show ultrastructural evidence of squamous and glandular differentiation.[14,58]

Research Efforts

All lung cancer types contain one or, more frequently, several molecular species of cytokeratin, with molecular weights ranging from 44,000 to 67,000 Da. In 1984 Banks-Schlegel et al. identified 44,000-Da keratin in all squamous cell tumors regardless of differentiation and abundant higher-molecular-weight (57,000–59,000 Da) keratins in well and moderately differentiated tumors.[4] By IHC, keratin staining in general is strongly positive in squamous cell malignancies, regardless of the degree of differentiation (Fig. 2-3). Moreover, staining with antibodies to high-molecular-weight keratins (63,000 Da) is restricted to well-differentiated areas of squamous cell carcinomas and is negative in adenocarcinomas.[90] Although antibodies to cytokeratin are not

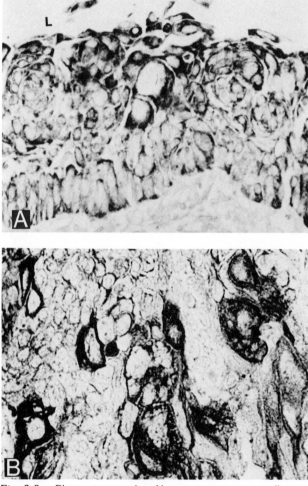

Fig. 2-3. Photomicrographs of keratin in squamous cell carcinoma of the lung. Note heavily stained pleomorphic cells of carcinoma in situ (*A*). Only the large, keratinizing cells are positive for high-molecular-weight keratin in invasive tumor (*B*) (L = bronchial lumen). Immunoperoxidase staining, original magnification ×500.

tumor-specific, they do serve well to distinguish epithelial tumors from sarcomas, lymphomas, and melanomas. All stratified squamous epithelia, regardless of whether they possess a stratum corneum, contain involucrin, which is chemically and immuno-chemically distinct from keratins, and can be induced to form cross-linked envelopes; non-squamous epithelia do not express these features.[86] Localization of involucrin by IHC constitutes a specific marker for squamous differentiation in lung tumors.[91]

Nearly all epithelial tumors produce carcinoembryonic antigen (CEA) as well. Mesothelial cells lack this antigen but are positive for keratin and negative for involu-crin. CEA positivity becomes a tool in distinguishing various types of epithelial neo-plasms from mesotheliomas.[30,59,89]

Comments

Little difficulty exists in the diagnoses of well or moderately differentiated squa-mous cell cancers. The predominant anaplastic nature of poorly differentiated squa-mous cell tumors may create problems in interpretation. It is not clear, however, from studies of surgically resected patients, that cell subtype has any influence on survival. Tumor, nodal, metastases (TNM) stage appears to be more significant.[96] Cytology is an immensely valuable tool in the diagnosis of this tumor in primary or metastatic sites. Cytologic diagnoses are probably as valid as tissue diagnoses in most instances.

Both EM and IHC are helpful when positive. These techniques are useful for verification of the epithelial nature of metastatic poorly differentiated or anaplastic tumors or for distinction between lung cancers and mesotheliomas. Both EM and IHC are subject to the same problems as LM, that is quality of material biopsied; tissue fixation; processing; and, in IHC, the type of antibody used. Polyclonal antibodies, in particular, are often poorly characterized and less selective, and thus cross reactivities may cause problems. Formalin fixation with routine processing renders many lower-molecular-weight keratin antigens difficult to identify.

Small Cell Carcinoma

SCLC constitutes up to 25 percent of all lung cancers.[21] It is estimated that most of these tumors are central in origin.[61,87] In Rilke and co-workers' experience, 11 out of 13 (almost 85 percent) surgically resected SCLC tumors were central in origin. In a larger series, 19 out of 33 (almost 60 percent) SCLC tumors identified in surgically resected patients entered into the Veterans Administration Surgical Oncology Group (VASOG) Lung Cancer Study were central in origin. On rare occasions, superior sulcus and Pancoast tumors invading chest wall are also of a SCLC type.[44]

Gross

The gross characteristics of early SCLC have been defined mostly by bronchosco-pists involved in the diagnosis and treatment of lung cancer. The bronchi contain single or multiple white friable nodules. The bronchial lumina may be narrowed or stenosed as a result of submucosal infiltration or extrinsic compression by involved bronchohilar lymph nodes. Over 75 percent of these tumors are located in the upper lobes.

In the VASOG study, the 19 centrally located tumors measured 1–9 cm in diameter and were associated with thickening of the bronchial walls.[61] The mucosa was eroded or ulcerated in only a few cases, and no intraluminal bulky mass was observed. In contrast, the bronchial lumina were partially or totally stenosed or obstructed in 7 cases. In 14 out of 19 cases, metastatic tumor was identified in regional lymph nodes. The primary tumor measured 2 cm or less in 3 out of 5 cases in which lymph node metastases were not observed. The cut surfaces of the tumors were glossy, granular, friable, focally hemorrhagic, and/or necrotic. In 6 out of 19 cases, the tumors had well-defined borders. The majority of the 14 peripheral tumors were circumscribed and measured 1–4 cm in diameter. Eight tumors measuring 3 cm or less showed no lymph node metastases. Only 12 percent of the entire 33 cases showed evidence of pleural invasion.

Combining the 46 cases in the two surgical studies, over 65 percent of SCLC tumors were central in origin and over 75 percent involved the upper lobes. There appears to be no significant difference between involvement of right or left lung. The mean size of the excised small cell tumors ranged from 3 to 4.8 cm. Pleural invasion (13 percent) was related to the peripheral location of the tumor. Regional lymph node metastases related to the location and size of the tumors; thus almost 75 percent of central tumors showed lymph node involvement, whereas only 33 percent of peripheral tumors were associated with nodal metastases.

At autopsy, SCLC often has a mucoid glossy appearance on cut surface, suggesting a mucinous adenocarcinoma. Following chemotherapy and/or radiation therapy, residual tumors often are represented by discrete hemorrhagic necrotic nodules. In fields of irradiation, a primary or metastatic tumor may be represented by an ill-defined zone of fibrosis. In some instances the primary lesion may be difficult to identify at autopsy.

Microscopic

In situ SCLCs rarely, if ever, have been identified. In some instances SCLC has been associated with an intrabronchial mucosal reserve cell hyperplasia and/or atypia, which might be interpreted as an associated preneoplastic or frankly in situ neoplastic phenomenon by some. Similarly, reserve cell tumorlets, which proliferate about respiratory bronchioles in response to injury, may be considered preneoplastic precursors of carcinoids or SCLC.

Classic SCLC tumors are characterized by cells arranged in cords, nests, or trabeculae, separated by a thin fibrous or fibrovascular stroma. Well-preserved neoplastic cells have nuclei that measure 2–3 times the size of lymphocytes. Nuclei may be oval, polygonal, or fusiform. Nuclear chromatin is distributed diffusely throughout the nucleus in fine or coarse pattern (Fig. 2-4A). Nucleoli generally are absent or indistinct; however, in B5 fixed material small but distinct intranuclear bodies, suggestive of nucleoli, may be appreciated. In areas of necrosis or in some crushed bronchial biopsy specimens, the nuclei may be small, round, and hyperchromatic (Fig. 2-4B). Neoplastic cells, for the most part, appear devoid of cytoplasm, grow in clusters, and show evidence of molding. Occasional SCLC tumors may have distinct cytoplasmic structures. At autopsy, these tumors have classic SCLC features. In tumors showing extensive zones of necrosis, DNA material frequently is seen deposited on and outlining elastic fibers of preexisting necrotic vessels.

In some SCLC tumors (5–6 percent), small clusters of cells with prominent nucleoli may be identified dispersed throughout the tumor.[63,84,108] Tumors with this component have been classified as mixed small cell/ large cell carcinomas by NCI-Navy Medical Oncology Branch (MOB) personnel (Fig. 2-4C). An even smaller group of tumors (less than 1 percent by LM) contain distinct discrete squamous nests or show

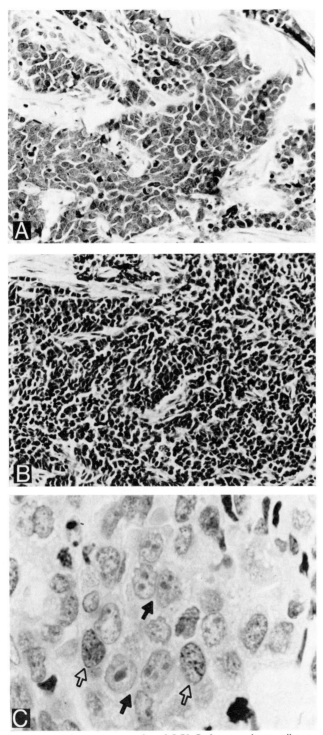

Fig. 2-4. Photomicrographs of SCLC. Intermediate cell type (A), oat cell type (B). Original magnification ×330. Mixed small cell/large cell carcinoma (C). Note typical larger cell morphology with nucleoli (black arrows) mixed with typical SCLC cells (open arrows). Original magnification ×1440. Hematoxylin eosin stain.

evidence of tubular or glandular formation in primary biopsies. Another very small percentage (probably less than 1 percent by LM) show evidence of SCLC combined with a significant squamous or glandular component. These tumors are usually identified in surgical lung resections and are interpreted as combined SCLC, by the WHO Lung Cancer Classification.[100]

The cytology of SCLC is remarkably similar to biopsy specimens. Neoplastic cells cluster, appear to mold, have variable-shaped nuclei, show diffuse distribution of chromatin material, and have indistinct nucleoli and minimal cytoplasm.

By EM, SCLC neoplasms have ultrastructural characteristics resembling those of pulmonary NE cells described in the morphogenesis section earlier. Neurosecretory granules are usually small and sparse, however, and are identified in only a few neoplastic cells. In contrast to the dendritic nature of their normal counterparts in the bronchial mucosa, neoplastic cells tend to be joined by small desmosomes and may have inconspicuous cytoplasmic organelles and scanty cytoplasm.[58] Nuclei are often ovoid, with smooth nuclear membranes, and have evenly and diffusely dispersed chromatin granules and inconspicuous nucleoli.

By EM, distinct evidence of tripartite differentiation of SCLC have been observed in both fresh tissue specimens and following cell culture.[68] In a given tumor some cells contain neurosecretory granules; while others contain glandular and/or squamous ultrastructural components.[15] On rare occasions all three components may be identified in a single cell.[25,68]

Research Efforts

SCLC is currently recognized as a NE tumor characterized by the presence of dense core or neurosecretory granules, L-dopa decarboxylase, a key amine handling enzyme, high levels of neuron specific enolase, a glycolytic isoenzyme characteristic of the diffuse endocrine system, high levels of creatine kinase brain isoenzyme, and the production of peptide hormones.[25] The establishment of numerous continuous cell lines from SCLC has enchanced our knowledge on the biology of SCLC. Following the in vitro studies, two types of SCLC have emerged: a classic subtype expressing the full range of NE characteristics, and a variant subtype that demonstrates a selective loss of NE characteristics, decreased population doubling time, and c-myc amplification.[28] The morphology of the variant subtype often resembles that of small cell–large cell carcinoma. The clinical implications of these two subtypes, classic and variant, are not fully understood.[108] It appears that amplification and expression of members of myc proto-oncogene family in SCLC may be associated with shorter survival and prior treatment of patients.[43] By applying sensitive in situ hybridization techniques it is possible to study the expression of myc proto-oncogenes in diagnostic patient specimens[37] (Fig. 2-5). Hopefully the results will permit better correlation of the LM morphology to the outcome of a patient's disease.

Bombesin, a tetradecapeptide originally isolated from anuran skin, has been demonstrated in the human pulmonary NE cells,[111] SCLC,[23,75] and carcinoids and appears to be a unique autocrine growth factor for SCLC.[17] Bombesin-like immunoreactivity is almost invariably present in classic SCLC cell lines.[26] In fresh SCLC tumors, however it is demonstrable in only 45–69 percent of the specimens by IHC, which reduces its value as a diagnostic marker for SCLC.[54,92] Currently it is not known whether the presence or absence of bombesin in surgical or cytological tumor specimens has any prognostic implications.

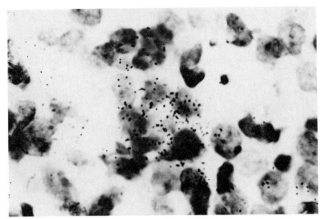

Fig. 2-5 Photomicrograph of a SCLC expressing N-*myc*. Note numerous grains following autoradiography after RNA-RNA in situ hybridization on metastatic SCLC in a lymph node. Hematoxylin counterstain, original magnification × 1440.

Comments

Confusion has arisen in the diagnosis of SCLC because of various non-WHO classifications that have been proferred in the past several years.[33,79,110] The term *neuroendocrine carcinoma* has been employed to designate both atypical carcinoids as well as SCLC. Unfortunately, the distinctions between malignant or atypical carcinoids and intermediate NE carcinomas are not clear to all pathologists. It is also not known whether there is any difference in behavior or response to therapy of the various forms of NE carcinomas. In some instances, the WHO criteria for the intermediate form of SCLC have been used to describe and diagnose atypical carcinoids.[71,72]

EM and IHC, using antibodies to chromogranin, which is a structural protein in dense core or neurosecretory granules, and neuron-specific enolase, are adjunct methods that may affirm the diagnosis of SCLC. Because of the paucity of granules in SCLC, particularly in fiberoptic bronchial biopsies, negative findings by EM or anti-chromogranin do not rule out the diagnosis of SCLC.[98] Moreover, positive staining of NSCLC by antineuron-specific enolase has also been reported, which reduces the value of this marker as a diagnostic aid.[54,92]

It has been well documented that SCLC may be associated with NSCLC elements following chemotherapy and/or radiotherapy.[1,60] It is thought that such differentiation reflects the inherent multipotentiality of the basal (reserve) cells of the bronchial mucosa. The presence of keratin in SCLC as assessed by IHC has not been associated with more adverse prognosis.[93]

Adenocarcinoma

Adenocarcinomas constitute between 25 and 30 percent of lung cancers diagnosed in the United States. In 1965 Yesner et al. estimated the incidence of adenocarcinomas as 16 percent based on biopsy and surgical material studied by the Veterans Administration Lung Group (VALG).[115] In 1974 the incidence based on equivalent material was reported as 29 percent by the same authors.[116] Similar findings have been documented in other reports.[106,107] In contrast to squamous malignancies, the majority of adenocarcinomas are peripheral in origin and usually related to bronchi only by local invasion or submucosal lymphatic spread. Occasional tumors may be identified as arising from the surface epithelium or from bronchial mucous glands of segmental bronchi. The majority of adenocarcinomas are peripheral scar carcinomas, solid adenocarcinomas, or the occasional classic bronchioloalveolar adenocarcinoma (BAC). Spencer estimates that scar carcinomas constitute approximately 50 percent of all adenocarcinomas.[102] Almost inevitably, some degree of chronic pulmonary disease is associated with these neoplasms. It is estimated that the classic BAC constitutes less than 3 percent of lung tumors.[11] The term *classic* is used to describe those tumors that use alveolar septa to support their growth and show no significant desmoplasia or gland formation.

Gross

In situ adenocarcinomas probably do not exist unless one wishes to interpret the classic well-differentiated BAC as such a phenomenon. The majority of adenocarcinomas present as subpleural fairly circumscribed masses, associated with thickening and puckering of the overlying pleura. The tumors may stimulate a desmoplastic response, be small and overlooked, or be misinterpreted at autopsy as an unimpressive scar. The majority of tumors have firm gray-white, occasionally mucoid, cut surfaces. Scar carcinomas ofter have a central desmoplastic pigmented core and may show villiform processes extending into the adjacent parenchyma. In a very small percentage of cases, the tumors may invade the pleura, converting this structure into a thick fibrous coat, difficult to distinguish grossly or even microscopically from mesotheliomas. Classic BAC usually present as single ill-defined masses with indistinct borders. In advanced cases, the tumor may be multicentric, lobar, or even bilateral. The cut surfaces of the tumor at autopsy may suggest a bronchopneumonia, lobar pneumonia, or even sclerosing hemangioma. In the United States, a small percentage of adenocarcinomas are thought to be derived from the bronchial surface epithelium or bronchial mucous glands. These bronchial tumors usually project into the bronchial lumina in polypoid fashion. Rarely such tumors may present without a mass lesion and at autopsy appear as "pipe-stemmed" thickened bronchi, with narrowed lumina. Metastases from the breast, gastrointestinal tract and pancreas may also present in this fashion.

Microscopic

Adenocarcinomas are identified on LM by the formation of glands, papillary structures, and/or production of significant amounts of mucin (Fig. 2-6A). The tumors tend to be pleomorphic, varying in degrees of differentiation from field to field. Individual neoplastic cells tend to be cuboidal to columnar in shape and form simple or complicated glandular or cribriform structures. Papillary tumors form intraluminal or intra-alveolar excrescences. In scar-related tumors, the core of the tumor usually is composed of an anthracotic scar. Less commonly, an organized thromboembolus or fibrocaseous granulomata may be observed in the center of the scar. At the periphery of the scar, neoplastic glands proliferate. The adjoining recognizable alveoli are lined by neoplastic cells similar to those described in the classic BAC described below. It is not possible to distinguish these tumors from the classic BAC in metastatic sites. The classic well-differentiated BAC is composed of mucin secreting cuboidal to tall columnar epithelial cells that migrate over alveolar walls in lepidic fashion (Fig. 2-6B).

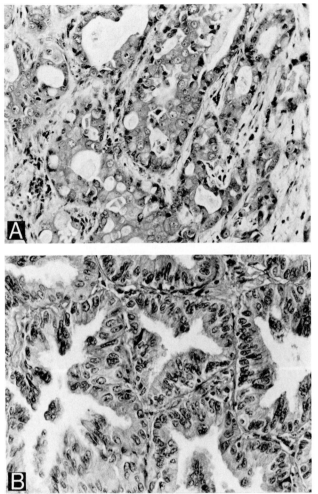

Fig. 2-6. Photomicrographs of adenocarcinoma of the lung. typical adenocarcinoma with gland formation (*A*); original magnification ×220 and bronchioloalveolar carcinoma with lepidic growth (*B*); original magnification ×330. Hematoxylin eosin stain.

Papillary lesions composed of fibrous stalks lined by similar epithelial cells project into alveolar lumina. Mitoses may be scanty, and nuclei may be bland. A number of these tumors may have anaplastic nuclei.

The Japanese literature documents a number of tumors in that country arising from bronchogenic surface epithelium or bronchial mucous glands.[49] Although these tumors seldom are seen in the United States, an aggressive mucoepidermoid carcinoma and classic signet ring adenocarcinoma have been studied at the NCI-Navy Medical Oncology Service. Both tumors are growing in tissue culture. It is presumed that these tumors arise from bronchial mucous glands. The signet ring tumor was identified prior to death in pleural fluid, sputum, and cervical lymph nodes. No pulmonary mass lesion was identified during life, and it was presumed that the primary tumor was located in the gastrointestinal tract. At autopsy, no bulky pulmonary tumor was identified, but the lumina of all major bronchi of the right upper lobe were narrowed and cuffed by a 2-3-mm band of tumor. There was no evidence of any other primary site.

A small percentage of lung cancers show little or no evidence of glandular or squamous differentiation. Intracytoplasmic vacuoles or microacini may be identified in some of these cells. With special stains, such as mucicarmine or Periodic Acid Schiff (PAS) with or without diastase, many of these cells contain mucin vacuoles. These tumors were interpreted as a large cell carcinoma in the 1967 Lung Cancer Classification[51] but are considered poorly differentiated adenocarcinomas in the 1981 Lung Cancer Classification.[100]

Cytologically, adenocarcinomas are fairly distinctive. Often exfoliative cytology is more diagnostic than a random bronchial biopsy, which contains only a few clusters of neoplastic cells.[13] Cells tend to be more uniform in nuclear and cytoplasmic detail than do squamous malignancies; they tend to cohere, have "community" cell borders, finely granular chromatin, prominent nucleoli, and variable occasionally vacuolated or mucin-producing cytoplasm. The papillary nature of these tumors is confirmed by the presence of multiple clusters of cells with common cell borders arranged in three-dimensional pattern.

By EM, distinctive features of adenocarcinoma include the presence of microvilli on surface epithelium or within small intracytoplasmic microacini. As with other lung cancers, it is not uncommon to identify ultrastructural evidence of squamous or NE differentiation. Mucin production, Clara cells, and type II pneumocytes have been identified in all types of adenocarcinomas.[24,35,58,78]

Research Efforts

Adenocarcinomas, like other pulmonary epithelial neoplasms, produce cyto-keratin, and distinctive bundles of tonofilaments can be seen by EM. The majority of tumors are thought to be of Clara or reserve cell origin. By EM, a few bronchioloalveolar tumors contain characteristic type II pneumocytes in primary and metastatic sites.[24] Langerhans cells with tennis racket or rod-shaped ultrastructural structures have been identified in almost 20 percent of bronchioloalveolar tumors.[40] The significance of these cells is not understood at present. By IHC, adenocarcinomas demonstrate generally positive staining with keratin antibodies, although they are negative for high-molecular-weight keratin (63,000 Da).[89] Adenocarcinomas are also positive for CEA (Fig. 2-7). Since mesotheliomas do not demonstrate this antigen, this test is particularly helpful in distinguishing adenocarcinomas from mesotheliomas.[30] Monoclonal antibodies against adenocarcinomas and other NSCLC may be particularly useful for identifying the presence of these tumors in cytological specimens including pleural fluid.[77] Approximately 10-20 percent of ordinary adenocarcinomas demonstrate a considerable population of cells positive for multiple NE markers and are discussed further in the section of carcinoids and NSCLS with NE. Many more adeno-carcinomas[54] may contain occasional rare cells that are positive for various antibodies against NE markers such as chromogranin, the structural matter of dense core or neurosecretory granules, serotonin, or various polypeptide hormones. This reflects the heterogeneity and common origin of various lung tumors.

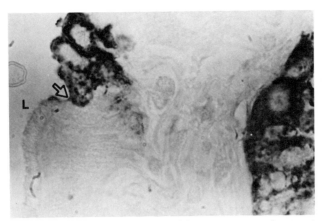

Fig. 2-7. Photomicrograph of CEA containing adenocarcinoma of the lung. Note the sharp border (arrow) between darkly staining tumor and normal, unstained ciliated bronchial epithelium (L = bronchial lumen). Also note the darkly staining tumor mass on the right. Immunoperoxidase staining; original magnification ×1440.

Comments

Adenocarcinomas in the United States are considered basically peripheral lung tumors, with unusual presentation as a primary central bronchial surface or mucous gland origin. Debates concerning the cell type of origin or designation of ultrastructural tumor type seem academic and philosophic at this time.

Regardless of size or cell derivation, adenocarcinomas often penetrate pleural lymphatics and metastasize to distant sites prior to identification of the primary tumor. The clinical silence of this tumor in its primary site contrasts significantly with central obstructive pulmonary neoplasms, which produce a multiplicity of symptoms.

There is poor consensus or uniformity in the diagnosis of BAC tumors. Although scar adenocarcinomas are considered basically papillary and bronchioloalveolar in origin, there is significant reason to segregate these tumors from the classic BAC. If a single focus of classic BAC is identified and resected, and no pleural invasion or lymph node metastases are found, the patient may anticipate a prolonged survival. Most BAC tumors, contrary to scar carcinomas, have an indolent course and invade lymphatics and pleura late in the course of the disease.

As with other pulmonary malignancies, the TNM staging system to date seems the most reliable predictor of survival, regardless of cell subtype or cell of origin. Response of these tumors to chemotherapy and/or radiotherapy has improved very modestly over the past 10 years.[73]

Adenosquamous Carcinoma

It has been estimated that adenosquamous carcinomas constitute 1-2 percent of surgically resected lung cancers. The tumors tend to be peripheral in origin and form bulky masses. Within a single high-power field, sheets of stratifying neoplastic squamous cells and proliferating neoplastic glandular structures may be observed. Intercellular bridge formation, whorling, and/or keratin formation may be observed in the squamous areas; mucin formation may be identified in the glandular components.

The tumors tend to behave as adenocarcinomas. The cytology of these tumors may be interpreted as either squamous or glandular in type. In the same or different specimens, both elements may be appreciated.

Large Cell Carcinoma

The concept of large cell carcinoma of the lung was introduced in the 1950s by pathologists and surgeons at the Mayo Clinic who were concerned by the variability of survival of lung cancer patients who were considered good surgical candidates.[80] The term implies no LM evidence of glandular or squamous differentiation. SCLC was considered such a distinct pathologic entity that little difficulty was anticipated in distinguishing SCLC from large cell undifferentiated carcinomas. Approximately 10–20 percent of lung tumors fall into the category of large cell carcinomas. The majority of these tumors share the exogenous and endogenous risks of adenocarcinomas.

Gross

Large cell carcinomas present as large silent bulky hemorrhagic or necrotic circumscribed masses. The tumors are almost inevitably located in the periphery of the lungs and usually are unrelated to segmental bronchi, except by contiguous invasion or lymphatic spread.

Microscopic

Large cell carcinomas are composed of sheets and nests of neoplastic epithelial cells, arranged in lobules. Cells usually have abundant cytoplasm, distinct cytoplasmic borders, and enlarged nuclei with prominent nucleoli (Fig. 2-8). The cell nests or sheets are supported by a fibrovascular stroma infiltrated by lymphocytes and plasma

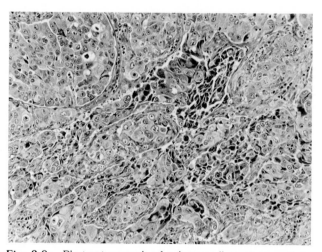

Fig. 2-8. Photomicrograph of a large cell carcinoma of the lung. Note sheets of undifferentiated cells without evidence of glandular formation or keratinization. Hematoxylin eosin stain, original magnification ×130.

cells. In some tumors, there may be an abunance of multinucleated giant cells. The cytoplasm of some of these cells may show phagocytosis of leukocytes, red blood cells, and/or nuclear debris. Mucin frequently is identified in this subtype. A clear cell subtype of large cell carcinoma is included in the WHO Lung Cancer Classifications. Such tumors have water clear cytoplasm, distinct cytoplasmic membranes, and neoplastic nuclei.[48] Although almost all types of lung cancer may show this water-clear phenomenon, it usually is presumed that these changes are artifactual and degenerative in origin. It is extremely unusual to identify a tumor composed solely of clear cells. Stains for glycogen, mucin, or fat are frequently negative. Renal cell tumors are considered in the differential diagnosis of any lung cancer with this clear cell component.

The diagnosis of large cell carcinoma in cytologic specimens is made predominantly by exclusion of other cell types. Cells often occur singly or may rarely occur in small clusters or sheets. Individual cells may be quite large to giant in size with prominent nuclei and nucleoli and abundant cytoplasm. Binucleation and multinucleation may be apparent. Mistakes can be made in the cytologic interpretation of these single neoplastic cells. In two cases within the past 2 years, single cells were identified as large cell carcinoma on fine-needle aspiration. Because of the the peculiar clinical presentations, surgical biopsies were performed and correct diagnoses of Hodgkin's disease were made. Although Reed-Sternberg cells were readily apparent on touch preps of the biopsied lymph nodes, even in retrospect these were not obvious or diagnostic on the aspirated specimens. As has been previously mentioned, regardless of the LM interpretation of large cell carcinoma, features of glandular, squamous, or even NE differentiation may be identified by EM. Only a small number of tumors are devoid of these ultrastructural characteristics. It is not clear whether such ultrastructural differentiation can be correlated with differences in behavior, response to therapy, or survival.

Research Efforts

There is little research data available to support the LM concept of large cell carcinoma. To the contrary, epithelial tumors with little or no differentiation by LM show evidence of cytokeratin and CEA antigenicity verifying, at least, their epithelial nature.

Comments

The LM diagnosis of large cell carcinoma, particularly in small bronchial biopsy specimens, does not preclude the diagnosis of poorly differentiated squamous cell or adenocarcinoma. There should be no difficulty in distinguishing this tumor from SCLC. A caveat must be given: single enlarged neoplastic cells cannot be presumed to be large cell or epithelial in nature in cytologic specimens.

It is of interest that in the WHO Lung Cancer Classification of 1967, solid carcinomas with mucin production were classified into the large cell carcinoma category, but they have been placed in the adenocarcinoma category in the current WHO Classification of Lung Cancer.

EM performed on these tumors often identifies ultrastructural structures, suggesting other non-small cell malignancies. It has not been proved to date that these characteristics have any clinical relevance.[2,41]

Carcinoids

Bronchopulmonary carcinoids are uncommon tumors that constitute approximately 2 percent of lung tumors. They are low-grade malignant neoplasms whose cells show the biochemical and ultrastructural features characteristic of both normal NE cells and tumors of the APUD or diffuse endocrine system.[83] These tumors are not related to cigarette smoking or to other known pulmonary carcinogenic factors. Carcinoids occur over a wide age range, but most patients are considerably younger than most patients with bronchogenic carcinoma.[11,22]

Approximately 90 percent of bronchial carcinoid tumors occur centrally, but 10 percent arise peripherally as asymptomatic pulmonary nodules detected only on chest x-ray. It is estimated that 10-20 percent of the bronchopulmonary carcinoids will have regional or distant metastases.[31] Invasiveness and large size of bronchial carcinoids are associated with a high incidence of metastatic disease and are considered reliable prognostic indicators.[39,65]

Gross

The centrally located carcinoid tumor is a fleshy, smooth, bosselated, polypoid mass covered by intact mucosa and projecting into the bronchial lumen. Endobronchial biopsy of the lesion may produce brisk hemorrhage as a result of the abundant vascularity. In addition to the exophytic component, the tumor extends below the level of the bronchial cartilage to involve the bronchial wall and surrounding lung parenchyma. The peripheral carcinoid tumors are nonencapsulated nodules within the parenchyma of the lung, often without apparent relationship to the bronchial tree. Multiple such tumors have been reported in individual patients.

On sectioning, carcinoids appear fleshy and gray or pale tan to dark red in color, rarely with foci of hemorrhage. The tumors range in size from a few millimeters up to 10 cm in diameter, with most measuring 2-4 cm. Moreover, tiny asymptomatic nodules measuring not more than 3 or 4 mm in greatest diameter can be found incidentally in lungs studied at autopsy or surgically removed for other reasons. These represent tumorlet type bronchial carcinoid tumors.

Microscopic

By LM, the cells commonly grow in solid sheets or as combinations of sheets, cords, nests, trabeculae, and ribbons similar to the patterns of carcinoid tumors elsewhere (Fig. 2-9). Numerous delicate capillaries are present throughout the tumor, which is typical of endocrine neoplasms. The cells have abundant clear or lightly eosinophilic cytoplasm and regular, centrally placed nuclei, most of which have uniform dispersal of the chromatin. Mitoses are absent or very rare; mucin production can occur.

The histologic appearance of the peripheral carcinoid often is more variable than that of the central carcinoid. In addition to the patterns described, a spindle-cell component or disorganized areas frequently are noted in the peripheral carcinoid, which as a rule is also devoid of mucin.

Approximately 10 percent of carcinoid tumors show more disturbing histologic features such as increased cellular pleomorphism, frequent mitotic figures, hyperchromatic nuclei, and reduced amount of cytoplasm as well as necrosis and hemorrhage.

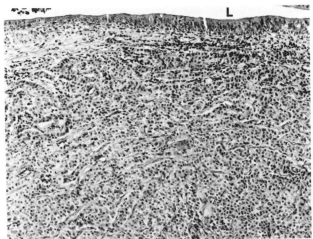

Fig. 2-9.   Photomicrograph of a typical central carcinoid. Note intact epithelium of bronchial lumen (L) and trabecular growth pattern of the tumor underneath. Hematoxylin eosin stain, original magnification ×130.

This particular group of carcinoids has been called *atypical carcinoid tumors*, which are associated with worse prognosis than the other bronchopulmonary carcinoids.

As a result of the intact bronchial mucosa overlying the tumor (Fig. 2-9), it is rare to obtain a positive cytologic sputum specimen for a carcinoid. Small groups of carcinoid cells characterized by evenly dispersed nuclear chromatin or hyperchromatic nuclei with relatively abundant cytoplasm can be obtained after brushing at bronchoscopy.

EM of carcinoids reveals uniformly shaped cells in distinct clusters with frequent well-developed cell junctions. The cells are characterized by prominent dense core (neurosecretory) granules that are larger and more abundant than in SCLC. The granules within a given tumor and even within single cells can be markedly heterogeneous with respect to size, configuration, and electron density. Groups of granules are often admixed with abundant, haphazardly arranged cytoplasmic filaments of intermediate type. Atypical carcinoids contain fewer neurosecretory granules.

Research Efforts

By IHC, the overwhelming majority of bronchial carcinoids display reactivity for neuron specific enolase, serotonin, and various neuropeptides, and the majority are immunoreactive for more than one hormone.[33,34] The materials most frequently demonstrated are endogeneous to lung, including serotonin, bombesin, and leu-enkephalin. In addition, ectopic neuropeptides such as gastrin, melanin-stimulating hormone, vasoactive intestinal peptide, and pancreatic polypeptide are also found. Furthermore, there is evidence that NE substances can be synthesized in cells containing a typical epithelial cytoskeleton, specifically, cytokeratin filaments and desmosomes.[9] Despite the frequently identified neuropeptides in bronchial carcinoids, clinical hormonal syndromes are rare.

The fact that bronchial carcinoids provide a rich source of neuropeptides has led to successful cloning and characterization of cDNAs encoding human gastrin-releasing peptide, a peptide closely related to bombesin that is an important autocrine growth factor for human SCLC.[17,94,101]

Comments

Although typical bronchial carcinoids are associated with prolonged survival, it has been clearly documented that the atypical carcinoids that are histologically defined by increased mitotic activity, pleomorphism, prominent nucleoli, hyperchromatism, increased cellularity, disorganized architecture, and areas of tumor necrosis possess increased metastatic potential. In 1972 Arrigoni[3] reviewed 201 patients with bronchial carcinoids, and in his series 70 percent or 16 out of 23 atypical carcinoids developed metastases, as compared to 5.6 percent of tumors with typical histology for carcinoid. Furthermore, 30 percent of patients with histologically atypical carcinoids were dead at the time of follow-up, having survived for an average of only 27 months. Unfortunately, the criteria and nomenclature of atypical carcinoids may vary among different pathologists. The separation of this group of tumors from other carcinoids has so far only prognostic significance and does not imply that these tumors will be responsive to chemotherapy or have clinical similarities to SCLC.[22]

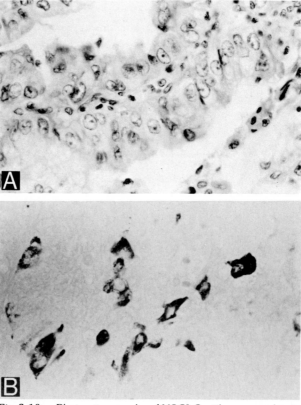

Fig.2-10. Photomicrographs of NSCLC with neuroendocrine features. Characteristic bronchioloalveolar pattern of an adenocarcinoma by hematoxylin eosin stain (A). Note numerous chromogranin containing tumor cells by immunoperoxidase staining (B); original magnification ×580.

RESPIRATORY MUCOSA: UNITARIAN THEORY OF ORIGIN

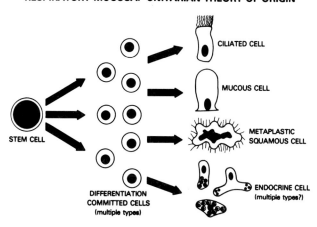

Fig.2-11. According to the unitarian theory of the origin of cells, the stem cell undergoes progressive differentiation through morphologically undifferentiated intermediate stages that are committed to certain pathways of differentiation (differentiation committed cells) to fully differentiated cells. The pulmonary NE cells are one type of differentiated cell. When exposed to carcinogens, the differentiation committed cells may simultaneously differentiate along more than one pathway or switch from one pathway to another. The stem cell concept explains the presence of tumors having more than one morphologic component and also the presence of NE features in NSCLCs. (Reproduced from Gazdar AF, Carney DN, Guccion JG, et al: Small cell carcinoma of the lung: Cellular origin and relationship to other tumors, in Greco FA, Oldham RK, Bunn PA Jr (eds): Small Cell Lung Cancer. Orlando, FL, Grune & Stratton, 1981, p 166. With permission.)

Bronchial carcinoids and SCLC are currently recognized as NE neoplasms characterized by the presence of dense core or neurosecretory granules and polypeptide hormones. There are other NE lung tumors that cannot be easily classified into these two categories. It appears that NE lung tumors constitute a morphologic and biologic spectrum from carcinoid to SCLC both in vivo and in long-term cell culture.[33,34,55,67] We feel that it is very important to further characterize the neoplasms at the midpoint of the spectrum, including their responses to various treatment modalities.

Non-Small Cell Lung Cancers with Neuroendocrine Features

A specific category of lung tumors has emerged as a result of biochemical and radioimmunological studies that have shown that the NE properties such as high levels of L-dopa decarboxylase activity or the presence of neuropeptides are not restricted to SCLC or carcinoids but are shared to a variable degree among all the histologic types.[8] A significant degree of NE differentiation in NSCLC (Fig. 2-10) is demonstrated by special studies in at least 10 percent of tumors.[46,54,109,114] This phenomenon is most often associated with adenocarcinomas followed by large cell carcinomas. These findings are in agreement with the theory that human lung cancers represent neoplastic changes within a common cell lineage (Fig. 2-11). At NCI-Navy we have designated the tumors with NSCLC morphology that demonstrate high levels of multiple NE markers as NSCLC with NE features. By definition, these tumors are indistinguishable from other NSCLC by conventional LM; however, by IHC, they contain numerous cells positive for general NE markers such as chromogranin (Fig.2-10B) and neuron specific enolase as well as individual neuropeptides. It remains to be seen whether partial NE differentiation in NSCLC is of clinical importance, which would warrant a new category in lung cancer classification.

INTERRELATIONSHIP OF LUNG TUMORS

There is a fairly precise understanding of the distinction between the clinical behavior and pathology of small cell and non-small cell lung cancers. At the same time, there has been renewed awareness of the pleomorphism of lung cancers. Electron microscopists have affirmed a multiplicity of ultrastructural elements that may exist in a single tumor. Immunohistochemists have identified a variety of markers that affirm the epithelial, mesenchymal, and/or neuroendocrine products of the cell. There is a group of tumors interpreted by LM as large cell carcinoma or adenocarcinoma that has been found to contain an abundance of neurosecretory granules. Similarly, by other research modalities, these tumors have been found to contain an enormous amount of dopa decarboxylase and other products considered as markers of SCLC and carcinoids. These tumors serve an extraordinary purpose at the present time: the documentation of the relationship of all lung cancers to each other. It is not possible at the present time to determine the incidence of these NSCLC tumors with NE properties or their natural behavior or response to therapy. The NCI-Navy MOB has begun treating these patients on SCLC protocols, but until the tumors are identified in a timely fashion and treatment begun shortly after diagnosis, little estimate can be made of the efficacy of treatment or the import of the NE properties in this variant of NSCLC. Correlation of clinical behavior with EM, IHC, and experimental research must be made and monitored by LM and the WHO Lung Cancer Classification.

NOTE

The opinions or assertions contained herein represent the private views of the authors and are not to be construed as official or as reflecting the views of the Department of the Navy or the Department of Defense.

REFERENCES

1. Abeloff MD, Eggleston JC, Mendelsohn G, et al: Changes in morphologic and biochemical characteristics of small cell carcinoma of the lung. Am J Med 66:757-764, 1979
2. Albain K, True L, Golomb H: Large cell carcinoma of the lung. Ultrastructural differentiation and clinicopathologic correlations. Proc AACR 25:48,1984
3. Arrigoni MG, Woolner LB, Bernatz PE: Atypical carcinoid tumors of the lung. J Thorac Cardiovasc Surg 64:413-421, 1972
4. Banks-Schlegel SP, McDowell EM, Wilson TS, et al: Keratin proteins in human lung carcinomas. Am J Pathol 114:237-286, 1984
5. Baylin SG, Mendelsohn G: Ectopic (inappropriate) hormone production by tumors. Mechanisms involved and clinical implications. Endocrinol Rev 1:45-56, 1980
6. Bensch KG, Gordon GB, Miller LR: Studies on the bronchial counterpart of the Kults-

chitzky (argentaffin) cells and innervation of bronchial glands. J Ultrastruct Res 12:668-674, 1965

7. Bensch KG, Corrin LB, Pariente R, et al: Oat cell carcinoma of the lung. Clinical and morphologic studies in relation to its histogenesis. Cancer 22:1163-1172, 1968

8. Berger CL, Goodwin G, Mendelsohn G, et al: Endocrine related biochemistry in the spectrum of human lung carcinoma. J Clin Endocr Metab 53:422-430, 1981

9. Blobel GA, Gould VE, Moll R, et al: Coexpression of neuroendocrine markers and epithelial cytoskeletal proteins in bronchopulmonary neuroendocrine neoplasms. Lab Invest 52:39-45, 1985

10. Carney DN, Gazdar AF, Bepler G, et al: Establishment and identification of small cell lung cancer cell lines having classic and variant features. Cancer Res 45:2913-2923, 1985

11. Carter D, Eggleston JC: Tumors of the lower respiratory tract. Atlas of Tumor Pathology, Second Series, Fascicle 17; Washington, D.C. Armed Forces Institute of Pathology, 1980

12. Chaudhuri MR: Primary pulmonary cavitary carcinomas. Thorax 28:354-366, 1973

13. Chuang P: Problems in the diagnosis of non-small cell lung cancer. Thorax 39:175-178, 1984

14. Churg A: The fine structure of large cell undifferentiated carcinoma of the lung. Evidence for its relationship to squamous cell carcinoma and adenocarcinoma. Human Pathol 9:143-156, 1978

15. Churg A, Johnston WH, Stulberg R: Small cell squamous and mixed small cell squamous/small cell anaplastic carcinoma of the lung. Am J Surg Pathol 4:255-263, 1980

16. Cuttitta F, Carney DN, Mulshine J, et al: Monoclonal antibodies against endocrine tumors of the human lung, in Becker KL, Gazdar AF (eds): The Endocrine Lung in Health and Disease. Philadelphia, Saunders, 1984, pp 488-500.

17. Cuttitta F, Carney DN, Mulshine J, et al: Bombesin-like peptides can function as autocrine growth factors in human small cell lung cancer. Nature 316:823-825, 1985

18. Cutz E, Chan W, Tracks NS: Bombesin, calcitonin and leu-enkephalin immunoreactivity in endocrine cells of human lung. Experientia 37:765-768, 1981

19. Cutz E, Chan W, Wong V, et al: Ultrastructure and fluorescence histochemistry of endocrine (APUD-type) cells in tracheal mucosa of human and various animal species. Cell Tissue Res 158:425-430, 1975

20. Cutz E, Conen PE: Ultrastructure and cytochemistry of Clara cells. Am J Pathol 62:127-134, 1971

21. Davis S, Wright PW, Schulman SF, et al: Long-term survival in small cell carcinoma of the lung: A population experience. J Clin Oncol 3:80-91, 1985

22. Eggleston JC: Bronchial carcinoids and their relationship to other pulmonary tumors with endocrine features, in Becker KL, Gazdar AF (eds): The Endocrine Lung in Health and Disease. Philadelphia, Saunders, 1984, pp 389-405

23. Erisman MD, Linnoila RI, Hernandez O, et al: Human lung small cell carcinoma contains bombesin. Proc Natl Acad Sci (USA) 79:2379-1283, 1982

24. Espinosa CG, Bolis JU, Saba SR: Ultrastructure and immunohistochemical studies of bronchioloalveolar carcinoma. Cancer 54:2182-2189, 1984

25. Gazdar A: The biology of endocrine tumors of the lung, in Becker KL, Gazdar AF (eds): The Endocrine Lung in Health and Disease. Philadelphia, Saunders, 1984, pp 448-457

26. Gazdar AF, Carney DN, Becker KL, et al: Expression of peptide and other markers in lung cancer cell lines, in Haveman K, Sorenson G, Gropp C, (eds): Peptide Hormones in Lung Cancer. Heidelberg, Springer-Verlag, 1985, pp 167-174

27. Gazdar AF, Carney DN, Guccion JG, et al: Small cell carcinoma of the lung: Cellular origin and relationship to other tumors, in Greco FA, Oldham RK, Bunn PA Jr (eds): Small Cell Lung Cancer. Orlando, FL, Grune & Stratton, 1981, pp 145-175

28. Gazdar AF, Carney DN, Nau MM, et al: Characterization of variant subclasses of cell lines derived from small cell lung cancer having distinctive biochemical, morphological and growth properties. Cancer Res 45:2924-2930, 1985

29. Gewirtz G, Yalow R: Ectopic ACTH production in carcinoma of the lung. J Clin Invest 53:1022-1025, 1974

30. Gibbs AR, Harach, R; Wagner JC, et al: Comparison of tumor markers in malignant mesotheliomas and pulmonary adenocarcinoma. Thorax 40:91-95, 1985

31. Godwin JD: Carcinoid tumors. An analysis of 2387 cases. Cancer 36:560-569, 1975

32. Goffman TE, Hassinger DD, Mulvihill JJ: Familial respiratory tract cancer. Opportunities for research and prevention. JAMA 247:1020-1023, 1982

33. Gould VE, Linnoila RI, Memoli VA, et al: Neuroendocrine cells and neuroendocrine neoplasms of the lung. Pathol Annu 18:287-330, 1983

34. Gould VE, Linnoila RI, Memoli VA, et al: Biology of disease. Neuroendocrine components of the bronchopulmonary tract: Hyperplasias, dysplasias and neoplasms. Lab Invest 49:519-530, 1983

35. Greenberg SD, Smith MN, Spjut HT: Bronchioloalveolar cell carcinoma: Cell of origin. Am J Clin Pathol 63:153-167, 1975

36. Greenberg SD: Recent advances in pulmonary cytopathology. Human Pathol 14:901-912, 1983

37. Gu J, Kirsch IR, Hollis GF, et al: Demonstration of *myc* oncogene in human tumor cell lines and xenografts by RNA-RNA in situ hybridization. Proc AACR 27:157, 1986

38. Hage E: Electron microscopic identification of several types of endocrine cells in the bronchial epithelium of human foetuses. Z Zellforsch Mikrosk Anat 124:532-536, 1972

39. Hajdu SI, Winawer SJ, and Myers WPL: Carcinoid tumors. A study of 204 cases. Am J Clin Pathol 61:521-528, 1974

40. Hammar SP, Bockus D, Remington F, et al: Langerhans cells and serum precipitating antibodies against fungal antigens in bronchioloalveolar cell carcinoma. Ultrastruct Pathol 1:19-37, 1980

41. Horie A, Ohta M: Ultrastructural features of large cell carcinoma of the lung, with reference to the prognosis of patients. Human Pathol 12:423-432, 1981

42. Horsley JR, Miller RE, Amy RW: Bronchial submucosal needle aspiration performed through fiberoptic bronchoscope. Acta Cytol 28:211-217, 1984

43. Johnson BE, Nau M, Gazdar AF, et al: Amplification of *myc* oncogenes is less common in small cell lung cancer (SCLC) patients than in SCLC cell lines. Proc ASCO 5:16, 1986

44. Johnson L, Hainsworth J, Greco AJ: Small cell carcinoma and pancoast tumors. Chest 82:602-606, 1982

45. Johnston WW: Percutaneous fine needle aspiration biopsy of the lung. A study of 1015 patients. Acta Cytol 28:218-224, 1984

46. Kameya T, Shimosato Y, Kodama T, et al: Peptide hormone production by adenocarcinomas of the lung: Its morphologic basis and histogenetic considerations. Virchows Arch (Pathol Anat) 400:245-257, 1983

47. Katlic M, Carter D: Prognostic inplications of histology, size and location of primary tumors, in Muggia F, Rozencweig M (eds): Treatment of Lung Cancer. New York, Raven Press, 1979, pp 143-150

48. Katzenstein A, Prioleau PG, Askin FB: The histologic spectrum and significance of clear cell change in lung carcinoma. Cancer 45:943-947, 1980

49. Kodama T, Shimosato Y, Kameya T: Histology and ultrastructure of bronchogenic and bronchial gland adenocarcinomas in relation to histogenesis, in Shimosato Y, Melamed M, Nettesheim P (eds): Morphogenesis of Lung Cancer, vol. I. Boca Raton, FL, CRC Press, 1982, pp 147-156

50. Korsgaard R, Trell E, Simonsson BG, et al: Aryl hydrocarbon hydroxylase. Induction

levels in patients with malignant tumors associated with smoking. J Cancer Res Clin Oncol 108:286–289, 1984

51. Kreyberg L: Histological typing of lung tumors, in International Histologic Classification of Tumours, Geneva, World Health Organization, 1967

52. Lauweryns JM, Peuskens JC: Neuroepithelial bodies (neuroreceptor or secretory organ?) in human infant bronchial and bronchiolar epithelium. Anat Rec 172:471–475, 1972

53. Lauweryns JM, Joddeeris P: Neuroepithelial bodies in the human child and adult lung. Am Rev Resp Dis 111:469–475, 1975

54. Linnoila RI, Funa K, Norton JC, et al: Immunohistochemical evidence for endocrine differentiation in various types of lung cancer. Proc IASLC 33, 1985

55. Linnoila RI, Schuller HM, Oie HK, et al: Establishment and characterization of cell lines from neuroendocrine (NE) tumors of lung. Identification of 5 subtypes. Proc ASCO 5:17, 1986

56. Lipford EG, Eggleston JG, Lillemore KD, et al: Prognostic factors in surgically resected limited stage non small cell lung cancer. Am J Surg Pathol 8:357–365, 1984

57. Macholda F: Bronchogenic carcinoma. A study of growth and evolutionary dynamics of bronchogenic carcinoma, its significance for early diagnosis. Acta Univ Carol (Med) (Praha) 41(suppl):39–62, 1970

58. Mackay B, Osborne BM, Wilson RA: Ultrastructure of lung neoplasms, in Straus MJ (ed); Lung Cancer, Clinical Diagnosis and Treatment. Orlando, FL, Grune & Stratton, 1983, pp 85–96

59. Marshall RJ, Herbert A, Braye SJ, et al: Use of antibodies to carcinoembryonic antigen and human milk fat globules to distinguish carcinoma, mesothelioma and reactive mesothelium. J Clin Pathol 37:1215–1221, 1984

60. Matthews MJ: Effects of therapy on the morphology and behavior of small cell carcinoma of the lung. A clinicopathologic study, in Lung Cancer: Progress in Therapeutic Research. New York, Raven Press, 1979, pp 155–170

61. Matthews MJ Gazdar AF: Small cell carcinoma of the lung. Its morphology, behavior and nature, in Shimosato Y, Melamed MR, Nettesheim P (eds): Morphogenesis of Lung Cancer. Boca Raton, FL, CRC Press, 1982, pp 1–14

62. Matthews MJ, Gordon PR: Morphology of pulmonary and pleural malignancies, in Straus MJ (ed): Lung Cancer, Clinical Diagnosis and Treatment, 2d ed. Orlando, FL, Grune & Stratton, 1983, pp 63–84

63. Matthews MJ, and Gazdar AF: Pathology of small cell carcinoma of the lung and its subtypes: A clinicopathologic correlation, in Livingston RB, (ed): Lung Cancer. The Hague, Martinus Nijhoff Publishers, 1981, pp 283–306

64. McCaughan BC, Martini N, Bains MS, et al: Chest wall invasion in carcinoma of the lung. Therapeutic and prognostic implications. J Thorac Cardiovasc Surg 89:836–841, 1985

65. McCaughan BC, Martini N, Bains MS, et al: Bronchial carcinoids. Review of 124 cases. J Thorac Cardiovasc Surg 89:8–17, 1985

66. McDowell EM, Becci P, Barrett LA, et al: Lung carcinomas. A new classification. Lab Invest 36:361, 1977

67. McDowell EM, Wilson TS, Trump BF: Atypical endocrine tumors of the lung. Arch Pathol Lab Med 105:20–35, 1981

68. McDowell EM, Trump BF: Pulmonary small cell carcinoma showing tripartite differentiation in individual cells. Human Pathol 12:286–294, 1981

69. Melamed MR, Zamen MP: Pathogenesis of epidermoid carcinoma of the lung, in Shimosato Y, Melamed MR, Nettesheim P (eds): Morphogenesis of Lung Cancer. Boca Ratan, FL, CRC Press, 1982, pp 37–64

70. Melamed MR, Flehinger BJ, Zaman MB, et al: Screening for early lung cancer. Results of the Memorial Sloan-Kettering Study in New York. Chest 86:44-53, 1984

71. Memoli VA, Maurer LH: Retrospective histologic reclassification of long term survivors with small cell carcinoma (SCC). Proc IASLC, 99, 1985

72. Mills SE, Cooper PH, Walker A, et al: Atypical carcinoid tumors of the lung. A clinico-pathologic study of 17 cases. Am J Surg Pathol 6:643-654, 1982

73. Minna JD, Higgins GA, Glatstein EJ: Cancer of the lung, in Devita VT, Hellman S, Rosenberg S (eds) Cancer, Principles and Practice of Oncology, 2nd ed. Philadelphia, Lippincott, 1984, pp 507-597

74. Mitchell BL, King DE, Bonfiglio TA, et al: Fine needle aspirate in 272 patients over a 5 year period. Acta Cytologica 28:72-76, 1984

75. Moody TW, Pert CB, Gazdar AF, et al: High levels of intracellular bombesin characterize human small cell lung carcinoma. Science 214:1246-1248, 1981

76. Morgan RW, Larson SR: Newer occupational lung carcinogens, in Gee JB, Morgan WK, Brooks SM, (eds): Occupational Lung Disease. New York, Raven Press, 1984, pp 69-77

77. Mulshine JL, Cuttitta F, Bibro M, et al: Monoclonal antibodies that distinguish non small cell from small cell lung cancer. J Immunol 131:497-502, 1983

78. Ogato T, Endo K: Clara cell granules of peripheral lung cancers. Cancer 54:1635-1644, 1984

79. Paladuga, RR, Benfield JR, Pak HY, et al: Bronchopulmonary Kulchitzky cell carcinomas. A new classification scheme for typical and atypical carcinoids. Cancer 55:1303-1311, 1985

80. Patton MM, McDonald JR, Moersch HJ: Bronchogenic large cell carcinoma. J Thorac Surg 22:88-93, 1951

81. Paulson DL: Superior sulcus tumors. Results of combined therapy. NY State J Med VII:2050-2057, 1971

82. Paulson DL, Weed TE, Rian RL: Cervical approach for percutaneous needle biopsy of Pancoast tumors. Ann Thorac Surg 39:586-587, 1985

83. Pearse AGE: The cytochemistry and ultrastructure of polypeptide hormone producing cells of the APUD series and the embryologic, physiologic and pathologic implications of this concept. J Histochem Cytochem 17:303-311, 1969

84. Radice P, Matthews MJ, Ihde DC, et al: The clinical behavior of mixed small cell/large cell bronchogenic carcinoma, compared to "pure" small cell subtypes. Cancer 50:2894-2899, 1982

85. Reid LM, Coles SJ: The bronchial epithelium of humans. Cytology, innervation and function, in Becker KL, Gazdar AF (eds): The Endocrine Lung in Health and Disease. Philadelphia, Saunders, 1984, pp 56-78

86. Rice RH, Green H: Presence in human epidermal cells of a soluble protein precursor of the cross-linked envelope: Activation of the cross-linking by calcium ions. Cell 18:681-694, 1979

87. Rilke F, Carbone A, Clemente C, et al: Surgical pathology of resected lung cancers, in Muggia FM, Rozenscweig M, (eds): Lung Cancer, Progress in Therapeutic Research. New York, Raven Press, 1979, pp 129-142

88. Saccomanno G, Archer VE, Auerbach O, et al: Histologic types of lung cancer among uranium miners. Cancer 27:515-523, 1971

89. Said JW, Nash G, Tepper LG, et al: Keratin proteins and CEA in lung carcinoma. An immunoperoxidase study of 54 cases with ultrastructural correlations. Human Pathol 14:70-76, 1983

90. Said JW, Nash G, Banks-Schlegel SP, et al: Keratin in human lung tumors. Patterns of localization of different molecular weight keratin proteins. Am J Pathol 113:27-32, 1983

91. Said JW, Nash G, Sassoon AF: Involucrin in lung tumors. A specific marker for squamous differentiation. Lab Invest 49:563-570, 1983

92. Said JW, Vimadalal S, Nash G, et al: Immunoreactive neuron specific enolase, bombesin and chromogranin as markers for neuroendocrine lung tumors. Hum Pathol 16:236-240, 1985

93. Sappino AP, Ellison ML, Gusterson BA: Immunohistochemical localization of keratin in small cell carcinoma of the lung. Correlation with response to combination chemotherapy. Eur J Cancer Clin Oncol 19:1365-1370, 1983

94. Sausville EA, Lebaccq-Verheyden A-M, Spindel ER, et al: Expression of the gastrin-releasing peptide gene in human small cell lung cancer. Evidence for alternative processing resulting in three distinct mRNAs. J Biol Chem 261:2451-2457, 1986

95. Serabjit-Singh CJ, Wolf CR, Philpot RM, et al: Cytochrome p-450: Localization in rabbit lung. Science 207:1469-1473, 1980

96. Shields TW, Humphrey EW, Matthews MJ, et al: Pathological stage grouping of patients with resected carcinoma of the lung. J Thorac Cardiovasc Surg 80:400-405, 1980

97. Shepherd FA, Ginsberg R, Evans WK, et al: Very limited small cell lung cancer. Results of non-surgical treatment. Proc. ASCO, 223, 1984

98. Sidhu GS: The ultrastructure of malignant epithelial neoplasms of the lung. Pathol Annu 17:235-266, 1982

99. Silverberg E: Cancer statistics, 1985. CA 35:19-35, 1985

100. Sobin LH, Yesner R: Histologic typing of lung tumors. International Histologic Classification of Tumors. Geneva, World Health Organization, 1981

101. Spindel ER, Chin WW, Price J, et al: Cloning and characterization of cDNAs encoding human gastrin-releasing peptide. Proc Natl Acad Sci (USA)81:5699-5703, 1984

102. Spencer H: Pathology of the Lung, 3d ed. London, Saunders, 1977, pp 773-860

103. Strauchen JA, Egbert BM, Kosek JC, et al: Morphologic and clinical determinants in small cell carcinoma of the lung. Cancer 52:1088-1092, 1983

104. Terzakis JA, Sommers SC, Anderson B: Neurosecretory appearing cells of human segmental bronchi. Lab Invest 26:127-132, 1972

105. Truong LD, Underwood RD, Greenberg SD, et al: Diagnosis and typing of lung carcinomas by cytopathological methods. A review of 108 cases. Acta Cytol 29:379-384, 1985

106. Valaitis J, Warren S, Gamble, D: Increasing incidence of adenocarcinoma of the lung. Cancer 47:1042-1046, 1981

107. Vincent RG, Pickren JW, Lane WW, et al: The changing histopathology of lung cancer. A review of 1682 cases. Cancer 39:1647-1655, 1977

108. Vollmer RT, Birch R, Ogden L, et al: Subclassification of small cell cancer of the lung. The Southeastern Cancer Study Group experience. Human Pathol 16:247-252, 1985

109. Warren WH, Memoli VA, Kittle CF, et al: Neuroendocrine features in non-small cell tumors. J Thorac Cardiovasc Surg 87(2):274-282, 1984

110. Warren WH, Gould VE, Faber LP, et al: Neuroendocrine neoplasms of the bronchopulmonary tract. A classification of the spectrum of carcinoid to small cell carcinoma and intervening variants. J Thorac Cardiovasc Surg 89:819-825, 1985

111. Wharton J, Polak JM, Bloom SR, et al: Bombesin-like immunoreactivity in the lung. Nature 273:769-770, 1978

112. Woolner LB, David E, Fontana LRS, et al: In situ and early invasive bronchogenic carcinomas. Report of 28 cases with postoperative survival data. J Thorac Cardiovasc Surg 60:275-290, 1970

113. Woolner LB, Fontana RS, Cortese DA, et al: Roentgenographically occult lung cancer: Pathologic findings and frequency of multicentricity during a 10 year period. Mayo Clinic Proc 59:453-466, 1984

114. Yamaguchi K, Abe K, Adachi I, et al: Peptide hormone production in primary lung

tumors, in Haveman K, Sorenson A, Gropp C, (eds): Peptide Hormones in Lung Cancer, vol 99. Heidelberg, Springer Verlag, 1985, pp 107-226

115. Yesner R, Gerstl B, Auerbach O: Application of the World Health Organization Classification of Lung Carcinoma to biopsy material. Ann Thorac Surg 1:33-49, 1965

116. Yesner R, Gelfman N, Feinstein A: A reappraisal of histopathology in lung cancer and correlation of cell types with antecedent cigarette smoking. Am Rev Resp Dis 107:790-797, 1973

Steven T. Rosen
James A. Radosevich

———— **3** ———————————————————————————————

Biology of Lung Cancer

Lung cancer accounted for greater than 100,000 deaths in the United States in 1986.[117] Despite warnings that emphasize the risk associated with tobacco abuse, the incidence of this malignancy continues to rise. Mass screening programs of target populations utilizing sputum cytology and periodic chest x-rays have not altered the low (10 percent) cure rate seen with this disease. New approaches for the early detection and for effective therapy are desperately needed.

The major histologic types of lung cancer include squamous cell, adenocarcinoma, large cell carcinoma, and small cell carcinoma (SCLC).[3,64,106,109,110,185] The first three histologies are collectively referred to as non-small cell lung carcinomas (NSCLC). They are distinguished from SCLC by clinical presentation, response to chemotherapy and radiation therapy, and biologic characteristics.[44,114,115] Dramatic advances in our knowledge of the basic cellular and molecular biology of these neoplasms have occurred in the last decade. It is anticipated that this information will ultimately be applied to the prevention, early detection, and treatment of human lung tumors.

DEVELOPMENT OF HUMAN LUNG CANCER CELL LINES

Improved tissue culture techniques and identification of growth factor requirements have allowed investigators to successfully grow lung cancer cells in vitro. More than 100 SCLC lines have been established. As a result, there has been an explosion of information concerning the biology of this tumor type. Although a substantial number of NSCLC lines exist, knowledge of the biology of these tumors is less comprehensive. Selective pressures are exerted in vitro; however, lung cancer lines usually retain many of the properties from the tumor of origin.

LUNG CANCER: A COMPREHENSIVE TREATISE
ISBN 0-8089-1876-1

CELL LINE CHARACTERISTICS

SCLC cell lines have been established from primary and metastatic lesions in newly diagnosed untreated and in previously treated patients.[30,63,68,71,73,135,136] No significant differences in biologic behavior has been witnessed in cell lines from different sites. SCLC cells grow as floating aggregates of tightly to loosely packed cells that frequently demonstrate areas of central necrosis (Fig. 3-1). A small percentage grow as adherent monolayer cultures as large overlapping polygonal cells. Cell line attachment to a substrate appears to be influenced by the culture medium. Most cell lines have been established in either RPMI-1640 or Waymouth's MB-7521 medium supplemented with 10-20 percent heat-inactivated fetal bovine serum. The majority of tumor specimens can be grown in vitro by using conditioned medium from other established cell lines or by using serum-free selective medium for SCLC. A chemically defined medium containing hydrocortisone, insulin, transferrin, 17-B-estradiol, and selenium (HITES) has been used with great success.[31,32,153] Benefits of serum-free chemically defined medium include (1) selective growth of SCLC with elimination of nonneoplastic stromal cells, (2) removal of growth-inhibiting factors from serum, (3) a system that allows for the easy evaluation of growth factors, and (4) the ability to identify and purify secreted SCLC metabolic products.[98] In addition, serum-free medias are less costly and reduce mycoplasma contamination.[10]

Cytologic features of the cell line, histology of athymic nude mouse xenografts, and electron microscopy studies demonstrate characteristics seen in the original tumor specimen. Of interest, the oat cell subtype morphology is not seen in cell cultures or in xenografts.[33] In general, SCLC lines have the appearance of the intermediate type. These cells appear as fusiform or polygonal cells with nuclei 2-3 times the size of mature lymphocytes. The chromatin is finely granular, and nucleoli are inconspicuous. Cytoplasm is scant or moderate. Nuclear molding can be seen in cytospin preparations. These observations and clinical data suggesting similar clinical behavior between these two subtypes have led some pathologists to theorize that the oat cell subtype is an artifact resulting from ischemia, crushing, and/or poor fixation.[38,85] Ultrastructure analysis of SCLC cell lines typically demonstrates dense core vesicles. The vesicles are pleomorphic and vary considerably in size. The nucleus is frequently cleft and contains

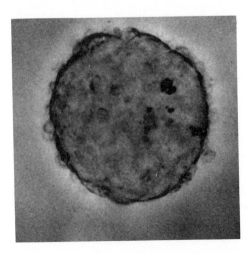

Fig. 3-1. SCLC cell line growing as floating aggregates of tightly packed cells.

prominent chromatin aggregations at the periphery, as well as dispensed throughout the nucleus. Often one or more prominent nucleoli are present. Specialized membrane junctions frequently are appreciated. Electron microscopy findings suggest both neuroendocrine and epithelial derivation. Intracranial and subcutaneous heterotransplants of SCLC in athymic nude mice retain the characteristic morphology and ultrastructure.[43] Tumors from subcutaneous injections (approximately 1×10^6 cells) typically have long latent periods (several weeks to months), seldom are invasive, and rarely metastasize. Intracranial heterotransplantation can be accomplished with a 10-100 times lower tumor inoculum, and there is a shorter latent period with frequent meningeal involvement, central nervous system invasion, and a lethal course.[72] These xenografts provide ideal models for the biologic and therapeutic investigation of SCLC.[96,108,131,187]

The in vitro growth rate of SCLC lines tends to be relatively slow. Doubling times are variable and range from 24 hours to several weeks. In one report, utilizing tritiated thymidine, labeling indices between 12.1 and 56.4 percent were calculated from nine separate SCLC lines.[149] No correlation between labeling indices and doubling times was seen. These data suggested that the SCLC lines have cell replication S-phase periods of variable duration or variable cell death rates. Cells from an individual SCLC line will demonstrate proliferative heterogeneity. Published results from analysis of patient specimens where tritiated thymidine was employed show an average labeling index of 14 percent for SCLC.[149] Studies utilizing flow cytometric (FCM) DNA content analysis have yielded similar results.[25,168,169] In vitro and in vivo data utilizing the percent labeled mitosis method suggest that the more rapidly proliferating SCLC cells have cell cycle times in the range of 24-72 hours. The initial impression that SCLC is a rapidly growing tumor has not been substantiated. Published mean or median clinical tumor doubling times are approximately 65-90 days, with a range of 17-264 days for individual patients.[122]

Approximately 20 percent of SCLC lines derived from patients with classic SCLC features have a "variant" morphology with features of large cell undifferentiated carcinoma.[33,70] These variant SCLC lines grow as loosely attached floating aggregates with relatively short doubling times. In addition to altered growth characteristics, these cell lines have a different biochemical profile, are less radiosensitive, and are associated with amplification of select oncogenes in the myc family. Of interest, at presentation approximately 5 percent of SCLC tumors contain a subpopulation of admixed cells with large cell features, and at autopsy the incidence is much greater (30-50 percent).[1,2] Patients with combined small cell-large cell histologies have a lower response rate to chemotherapy and a shorter median survival.[38,86,138]

In contrast to SCLC, there is considerable in vitro heterogeneity of NSCLC tumors.[65,69,104] There are also many shared properties, however, both within NSCLC types as well as between NSCLC and SCLC. For this reason, several investigators have speculated that there is a common stem cell or origin for all lung cancers.[69,112,143]

Most NSCLC lines attach to substrate and have an epithelioid morphology (Fig. 3-2). Some adenocarcinomas from malignant effusions may grow as floating aggregates. Although most NSCLC lines have been established with routine serum supplemented medium, chemically defined serum free media preparations are currently being employed.[65,69] Adenocarcinomas have been grown in RPMI-1640 medium supplemented by insulin, transferrin, sodium selenite, hydrocortisone, bovine serum albumin, epidermal growth factor (EGF), triiodothyronine, glutamine, and sodium

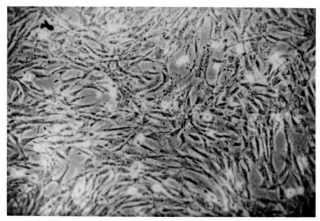

Fig. 3-2. Non-SCLC cell lines growing as adherent monolayer.

pyruvate, with collagen and fibronectin as attachment factors (ACL-3 medium).[23,24] The growth requirements for squamous cell cancer lines are complex, and only a few have been established with a partially defined medium containing Dulbecco's modified eagle medium and nutrient mixture F-12 plus 5 percent fetal calf serum, hydrocortisone, EGF, cholera toxin, and fibroblast feeder layers.[65,69] Terminal differentiation is often seen with differentiated squamous cell cultures, while continuous lines tend to become undifferentiated or simultaneously exhibit glandular and squamous differentiation.

Adenocarcinomas arising in the central or peripheral airways demonstrate mucin production and are gland forming in athymic nude mice. In some instances subcutaneous heterotransplants will demonstrate local invasion and systemic metastases. These lines will also grow as ascitic tumors. Bronchioloalveolar carcinoma cell lines originating from mucin-secreting bronchiolar cells, Clara cells, and type II alveolar pneumocytes have been propagated. These lines maintain features seen in the original tumor specimens. Squamous cell cultures will display bundles of keratin (tonofilaments) and well-formed desmosomes.[54]

The doubling time range of NSCLC lines is about 24-72 hours. The range and average values of tritiated thymidine labeling indices from patients with squamous or large cell lung cancers is similar to values seen with SCLC.[149] Adenocarcinomas have a lower average labeling index than do the other cell types. Published mean clinical tumor doubling times for squamous and large cell lung cancer are also similar to SCLC, while adenocarcinomas have a longer log mean doubling time of 134 days with a range of 17-960 days.

IN VITRO SOFT AGAROSE CLONING

In vitro soft agarose cloning can be utilized to assess the activity of chemotherapeutic or biologic agents against SCLC. The methodology for these assays is outlined in several reviews.[13,29,34,35,36,133,147] Fresh SCLC tumor specimens can be successfully cloned in most instances; however, the cloning efficiency is low (usually less than 0.1

percent). Confirmation of SCLC origin is accomplished by gross morphology, cytologic examination, DNA content analysis, and heterotransplantation in athymic nude mice. It is possible to enhance the yield of clonogenic tumor cells from biopsy specimens by discontinuous albumin gradient separation.[77] On rare occasions SCLC colony formation can be detected in cytologically negative specimens, thereby confirming metastatic disease.[137] To properly evaluate multiple drugs, established cell lines or short-term cultures from SCLC patients may be necessary. Results obtained from evaluation of established cell lines appear to mirror those obtained from the fresh specimen.

Cell lines established from previously untreated patients tend to be sensitive to drugs traditionally used to treat SCLC, while in vitro resistance is noted when lines from previously treated patients are investigated.[30] Cell lines can be utilized to study activity of new chemotherapeutic reagents and will allow for a better understanding of the mechanism of radiation and drug resistance.[39,40,75,121,173] Methotrexate resistance has been demonstrated in a SCLC cell line displaying amplification of the gene coding for dihydrofolate reductase and a large number of double minute chromosomes.[47] After serial passage in serum free medium fewer cells contained double minute chromosomes, amplification of dihydrofolate reductase activity was not observed, and sensitivity to methotrexate was noted.

Approximately two-thirds of NSCLC specimens can be cloned in soft agarose, with a colony-forming efficiency of 0.17 percent.[65,69] In vitro drug testing has confirmed that these tumors are often resistant to chemotherapeutic drugs de novo. Squamous cell cancer appears to be the most difficult to clone because of terminal differentiation and the absence of necessary growth factors for its propagation.

FLOW CYTOMETRIC DNA CONTENT ANALYSIS

Analysis of DNA content by FCM permits the rapid analysis of cellular DNA content of large numbers of cells independently of the proliferative state of the cells. SCLC clinical specimens demonstrate an aneuploid population of cells in approximately 75 percent of cases with DNA content of 1.1–2.3 times the diploid.[25,168] The remaining cases often have near-diploid DNA contents or too few tumor cells to be detected. Occult metastases in specimens microscopically free of tumor cells on rare occasions can be detected by the demonstration of an aneuploid population. Between 10 and 20 percent of SCLC samples are heterogenous and have multiple aneuploid cell lines. Survival of SCLC patients is similar for individuals with near-diploid and aneuploid tumors.[109] In several cases where tumor DNA content was analyzed on a serial basis, no change was witnessed on comparison of pretreatment samples with those obtained at time of relapse. The SCLC lines in general demonstrate a DNA content identical to that found in the clinical specimen. With subsequent passages, however, alterations may be noted secondary to tumor heterogeneity in the original culture and the development of new mutations.

In general, NSCLC tumors are aneuploid and have higher DNA contents than do SCLC tumors. Approximately 10 percent of the specimens are polyclonal. It appears that the DNA distribution in a NSCLC tumor correlates with prognosis.[170]

CYTOGENETICS

Cytogenetic analysis on fresh SCLC specimens is difficult because of the low number of metaphase tumor cells and the problem of contamination by admixed nonmalignant cells. A recurring rearrangement has been observed in established SCLC lines involving an interstitial deletion of the short arm of chromosome 3.[174-176] The chromosome breakpoints in the *del* (3p) may vary; however, bands p14 to p23 commonly are deleted. All metaphase cells demonstrate the deletion. This chromosome 3 abnormality is an acquired somatic cell defect, not present in autologous diploid peripheral blood or bone marrow cells. This deletion has been detected in cell lines established from previously untreated and treated patients and from different metastatic sites. Using short-term cultures with selective growth medium, this abnormality was identified in fresh clinical specimens of SCLC. This *del* (3p) has been confirmed utilizing molecular probes.[126] In addition, an enzyme aminoacylase-1 specific for the short arm of chromosome 3 has reduced or absent activity in SCLC lines.[113] The incidence of this defect has been disputed, however, and overall the data from several laboratories suggest that the *del* (3p) is not a universal finding.[28,60,182,183] In addition to this *del* (3p), nonrecurring abnormalities in chromosome number and/or structural aberrations have been detected in all SCLC lines studied. The most frequent structural changes involve chromosomes 1, 2, 9, 10, and 14. In many specimens double minute chromosomes or homogenous staining regions have been observed.

Multiple chromosomal abnormalities have been seen in NSCLC lines and specimens. A specific recurring chromosome defect has not been noted. Numerical and structural abnormalities most frequently involve chromosomes 1, 2, 3, 9, 11, and 12.

ONCOGENES

Members of the *myc* family of proto-oncogenes (C-*myc*, L-*myc*, and N-*myc*) frequently are amplified and overexpressed in SCLC lines.[90,105,124,125] Amplification has also been reported in SCLC biopsy specimens.[179] In particular, C-*myc* oncogene amplification and/or overexpression has been detected in SCLC variant lines with a more aggressive growth behavior. Transfection of the C-*myc* gene into a classic SCLC line can produce a more aggressive phenotype.[89] It appears that *myc* gene products may be important in the establishment, maintenance, or malignant behavior of SCLC.[80]

The DNAs from a variety of neoplasms, including NSCLC, contain activated transforming genes that efficiently induce transformation of NIH 3T3 mouse fibroblast cells on transfection.[45] A single transforming gene (*ras*^{k}) has been reported in six independent human adenocarcinomas of the lung.[53] The *ras* family of genes produce a protein product with a molecular weight of 21,000 Da, which has been found to have both GTP binding activity, as well as GTPase activity.[132] The *ras* p21 has been implicated as being associated with the inner surface of the plasma membrane and may play a role in signal transduction from extracellular stimuli. It appears that mutations that alter the structure of the *ras*^{k} gene product are responsible for the transforming activity. Enhanced expression of the p21 gene product can be seen in a large percentage of NSCLC tumors as detected by the RAP-5 monoclonal antibody

(MA).[101] The MA DWP produced against an amino acid sequence of p21 with a substitution of valine for glycine at position 12 recognizes a mutated form of the protein found in approximately 15 percent of NSCLC specimens.[140]

PEPTIDE HORMONE PRODUCTION, GROWTH FACTORS, AND RECEPTORS

SCLC is a neuroendocrine tumor that expresses amine precursor uptake and decarboxylation (APUD) properties, including L-dopa decarboxylase (DDC), dense core granules, formaldehyde-induced fluorescence, and production of chromogranin A (a structural protein in dense core granules).[11,128] This tumor type is frequently associated with polypeptide hormone production, and a number of paraneoplastic syndromes have been reported.* Peptide hormones that frequently are elevated in sera of patients with SCLC include adrenocorticotrophic hormone (ACTH), β-endorphin, lipotropin (LPH), the hypothalamic neurophysins, arginine vasopressin (AVP), oxytocin, and calcitonin. Production of ACTH, β-endorphin, LPH, and the less frequently detected β-melanocyte-stimulating hormone results from the intra- or extracellular proteolytic cleavage of the common precursor molecule pro-opiomelanocortin. Parathormone (PTH), B-human chorionic gonadotropin (β-HCG), gastrin, glucagon, insulin, secretin, substance P, and vasoactive intestinal peptide occasionally are detected, but typically at low levels. Secreted peptides could serve as valuable tumor markers because they often reflect tumor burden and can be utilized to monitor therapy. However, only calcitonin appears to have potential application in the management of patients with SCLC.[42,172] The fact that these ectopic hormones may be biologically inactive can account for the frequent discrepancy observed between the immunologic detection of marker elevation and the absence of a clinical paraneoplastic syndrome. Peptide production by SCLC line has been demonstrated in vitro and after heterotransplantation in athymic nude mice.[94]

A peptide immunologically related to the tetradecapeptide amphibian neuropeptide bombesin or its larger molecular weight mammalian homologue gastrin-releasing peptide[157] is present in almost all SCLC tumors and lines.[57,119,148,151,155,177,180,181] In mammals, bombesin-like immunoreactivity (BLI) has been found mainly in brain, gut, and lung. A common 7C-terminal amino acid sequence is essential for biologic activity of these molecules. Both bombesin and AVP have been shown to stimulate the cloning of SCLC in agarose. It has been speculated that bombesin is an autocrine growth factor in SCLC because the majority of SCLC line express high amounts (1–2 log values higher than other peptides) and have bombesin-like peptide receptors and because exogenous bombesin influences the growth of these cells.[48,159] A monoclonal antibody directed against bombesin has been shown to inhibit the growth of SCLC in vitro and cause regression of SCLC heterotransplants.[48] Although high bombesin concentrations are found in the media of SCLC lines, elevated levels infrequently are found in patient plasma. Possible explanations for this phenomenon include increased in vivo catabolism, selection for bombesin-producing cells in culture, and/or modulatory factors that inhibit in vivo synthesis and/or secretion. Another amphibian peptide

*References 5,13–16,66,67,79,81,83,127,129,134,152,156,162, and 184.

physalaemin has also been detected in SCLC by radioimmunoassay and by immuno-histochemistry.[97] This peptide belongs to the tachykinin family.

There are variant SCLC lines, including those demonstrating the large cell morphology with loss of APUD characteristics.[69,70] They have very low, often undetectable, levels of DDC and BLI. These cells obtained from patients with SCLC retain the 3p cytogenetic-deletion, however, confirming their SCLC lineage.

NSCLC lines also produce peptide hormones.[65,69] In general, these tumors lack APUD characteristics and do not express DDC and BLI; however, production of ACTH, calcitonin, and AVP have been reported. Of interest, non-APUD cell markers associated with NSCLC clinical specimens such as carcinoembryonic antigen (CEA) and β-HCG are seen more frequently on SCLC lines, possibly reflecting a state of cellular differentiation. The actual distribution of peptide hormones produced by these tumors remains controversial.

The clinical paraneoplastic syndrome of pulmonary osteoarthropathy is confined to patients with NSCLC histologies.[27] The hormonal substance responsible for this pathologic process has not been identified. Hypercalcemia is seen in approximately 10 percent of NSCLC patients without evidence of bone involvement and is in most instances mediated by a PTH-like factor, prostaglandins, vitamin-D-like sterols, or osteoclast activating factor.[27]

Most epithelial cells express EGF receptors and require EGF for growth. In vitro data suggest decreased or absent expression of EGF receptors on SCLC lines in comparison to NSCLC lines.[150] Analysis of clinical specimens suggests very high levels of expression of EGF receptors on squamous cell tumors.[84] Lower levels are seen on large cell and adenocarcinomas. EGF receptors were not detected on clinical SCLC specimens. In addition, EGF appears to be an important ingredient of chemically defined growth media for NSCLC.

ENZYME MARKERS

Neuron-specific enolase (NSE) is one of several isoenzymes of the glycolytic enzyme enolase (2-phospho-d-glycerate hydrolase, EC 4.2.1.1.).[88,120] It is a cytoplasmic enzyme that catalyzes the conversion of 2-phosphoglycerate to phosphoenolpyruvate and water. NSE has been identified in both central and peripheral nervous tissue and in tissues of the APUD network. Tumors originating in the APUD network contain significant amounts of NSE, including neuroblastoma, medullary thyroid carcinoma, islet cell carcinoma, pheochromocytoma, Merkel cell tumors, and SCLC.[163]

Elevated levels of NSE are noted in SCLC lines and in the sera of approximately 70 percent of SCLC patients.[4,37,58,91,105,107] Both mean levels and the percentage of patients with elevated levels correlate with extent of disease. Serial NSE measurements following treatment closely reflect clinical response to therapy. In addition, rising NSE levels will predate clinical evidence of relapse or progressive disease. SCLC variant lines have reduced expression of NSE. NSCLC lines and patient sera rarely have elevated levels of NSE.

Creatine kinase (CK) (ATP–creatine N-phosphotransferase; EC 2.7.3.2) occurs in the serum primarily as three isoenzymes.[166] There are three main types of CK: (1) CK-BB, which is found in large amounts in the brain, thyroid, lung, gastrointestinal tract, and genitourinary tract; (2) CK-MM, which is found in skeletal and cardiac muscle; and (3) the hybrid-MB, which is found primarily in cardiac muscle. The predominant serum isoenzyme in adults is the CK-MM, and the concentration of CK-BB is low.[166] Elevated serum CK-BB bioenzyme levels have been noted in a variety of human tumors.[188] It has been demonstrated that CK-BB measurements are of value in estimating tumor burden, assigning prognosis, and monitoring response the therapy in SCLC.[41] Elevated levels were noted in 41 percent of SCLC patients with extensive disease; however, only 1 out of 42 patients with limited disease had an elevated level. Sequential serum determinations revealed an excellent correlation between clinical response to therapy and serum CK-BB levels. In vitro production of CK-BB by established SCLC lines, including the morphologic variants, has also been demonstrated.[70,74]

Deoxythymidine kinase (TK) (ATP-thymidine 5'-phosphotransferase; EC 2.7.1.21) catalyzes the conversion of deoxythymidine to deoxythymidine-monophosphate.[78] The cytoplasmic TK is only expressed in dividing cells, and its activity indirectly relates to proliferative activity. Serum TX levels have been shown to correlate with stage of disease and prognosis in SCLC patients.[78]

CYTOSKELETAL PROTEINS

Differential expression of intermediate filament (IF) cytoskeletal proteins are features of tissues reflecting differentiation and lineage characteristics. Antibodies to keratin, vimentin, desmin, glial fibrillary acidic protein, and the neurofilament proteins can distinguish between cells of epithelial, mesenchymal, and neural origin. Tumors retain their tissue-specific IF proteins.[178] Utilizing antibody probes, IF typing can help to distinguish different tumor types, classify tumors, and improve the accuracy of diagnosis. Keratin, the most complex IF, which is composed of multiple molecular weight species, is present in all carcinomas.

The IF profile of SCLC remains controversial. To date, results have been inconsistent presumably because of the use of different antisera and detection methods. Investigators have reported the presence of keratin, neurofilament, or both in individual studies.[17,19] In general, SCLC contains the smaller keratins species (relative molecular weight 44,000–52,000 Da).[6,9] SCLC lines have been shown to express keratin and in some instances coexpress neurofilament.[6,102,103,165] In addition, vimentin has been detected in SCLC lines.[6] Other carcinoma cells have also been reported to coexpress vimentin in culture. A recent report suggests differential expression of IF proteins in classic and variant SCLC lines.[22] Classic lines contained keratin proteins, while variant lines contained neurofilament and vimentin.

All NSCLC lines and clinical specimens contain keratin.[†] Low-molecular-weight keratin proteins are present in adenocarcinomas and large cell cancers. Squamous cell cancers display a preponderance of keratins of a higher molecular weight (relative molecular weight 57,000 and 59,000 Da).[20,46] High-molecular-weight keratins are more abundant in squamous cell lines and tumors demonstrating terminal differentiation as suggested by the presence of involucrin, a precursor protein associated with cross-linked envelope formation.[7,146] In vitro expression of vimentin has also been

†References 6,8,20,46,56,61,118,142,145 and 177.

witnessed in NSCLC lines. It appears that hormones and growth factors may effect the expression of IFs.

MONOCLONAL ANTIBODIES AGAINST LUNG CANCER-ASSOCIATED ANTIGENS

MAs prepared by somatic cell hybridization techniques are ideal tools for the discrimination of cellular antigens and therefore have great potential for the immuno-diagnosis and immunotherapy of malignant disease.[93,116] These reagents can reveal qualitative and quantitative differences in the antigenic composition of normal and malignant cells. Light and electron microscopic evaluations of lung tumor at times fail to provide consistent categorization. Knowledge of the antigen profile of these cancers may allow for a more reproducible classification schema. Investigators have shown by two-dimensional gel electrophoresis of radiolabeled plasma membrane proteins that distinct phenotypes exist that distinguish SCLC from NSCLC lines.[12,76] In addition, the pattern of glycolipid antigen expression appears to differ between lung cancer types.[49,50,59,82,87,158,186] MAs against these components may be useful in distinguishing SCLC from NSCLC.

A large number of MAs directed against SCLC have been produced by immuni-zation with whole cells, or extracts of SCLC lines, and biopsy speci-mens.[18,26,51-53,59,130,144,160,164] However, only a small percentage have been ade-quately characterized. Representative examples include (1) SM1, an IgM mouse MA that binds to a cell-surface carbohydrate antigen present in both glycolipids and glyco-proteins that is effected by routine fixation and paraffin embedding;[18] (2) LAM-8, an IgM mouse MA that recognizes a major band of 135,000 Da by Western blot analysis and using routine formalin fixed paraffin embedded tissues stained 80 percent of SCLC tumors tested;[161] and (3) HNK-1, an IgM MA that detects a 110,000-Da glycoprotein also present on a subpopulation of large granular lymphocytes known to have natural killer cell function.[26]

A great number of MAs directed against NSCLC have been described that recog-nize antigens ranging from high-molecular-weight mucin-like molecules to small pro-teins.‡ Representative examples include (1) 44-3A6 on IgG_{2a} mouse MA that reacts with a 40,000-Da cell surface protein, which is preserved in routine formalin-fixed, paraffin-embedded tissue and present on adenocarcinomas, and a subset of large cell carcinomas (Figs. 3-3 and 3-4).[9,100,139] (This MA does not bind to squamous cell tumors or SCLC); (2) MA B72.3, an IgG_1 MA that recognizes a high-molecular-weight mucin-like molecule that is preserved in formalin fixed tissue (this antigen can be detected in patient sera and reacts with a subset of adenocarcinomas, large cell carcinomas, and a limited number of squamous cell tumors); (3) the MA 624A12 and CSLEX-1, MA that recognize the ceramide pentasaccharide that contains the lacto-N-fucopentaose III sequence of sugars, an isomere of the Lewis A blood group antigen, or its sialosylated derivative, respectively, which are preserved in formalin-fixed tissue, detected in patient sera, and present on a wide spectrum of lung cancer tumors but not on mesotheliomas[4,99]; and (4) LuCa3 and LuCa4 MA of the IgG isotype, which bind

‡References 9,21,24,85,92,95,99,111,123,139,141, and 167.

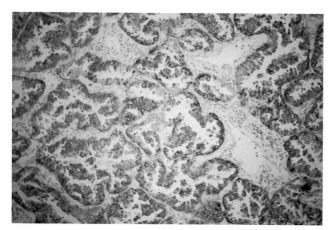

Fig. 3-3. Immunohistochemical staining of adenocarcinoma of the lung with monoclonal antibody 44-3A6.

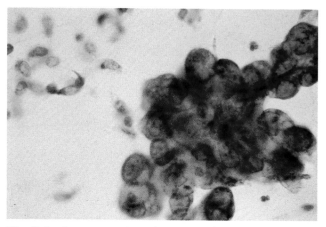

Fig. 3-4. Immunocytological staining of adenocarcinoma of the lung with monoclonal antibody 44-3A6.

protein antigens restricted to squamous cell histologies.[95] Their reactivity patterns were determined by staining of frozen tissues.

CEA is a β migrating glycoprotein with a molecular weight of about 10,000.[154] The antigen is synthesized by epithelial cells and is concentrated in the glycocalyx. Immunohistochemistry has demonstrated CEA production in all lung cancer cell types. Circulating antigen can be detected in patient plasma by use of commercially available MAs. A recent report evaluating 243 patients with untreated advanced lung cancer demonstrated elevated plasma levels (>5 ng/ml) in adenocarcinomas (54 percent), large cell lung carcinomas (38 percent), squamous cell carcinomas (53 percent), and SCLC (35 percent).[151] The authors noted a relationship between pre-treatment CEA level and extent of disease. Serial measurements of plasma CEA correlated with response to therapy in this study. These observations confirm the observation that CEA levels may be useful in monitoring treatment in lung cancer patients.[151,171]

Tumors may also demonstrate selective loss of normal cellular antigens. Investigators have shown a marked deficiency of HLA-A, B, and C antigens and β-2 microglobulin expression in the cell surface of SCLC cell lines using monoclonal antibody probes.[55] These studies demonstrated a deficit in synthesis of both HLA and β-2 microglobulin peptide chains resulting from an RNA transcription block. Clinical SCLC specimens also demonstrate this selective loss.[62] This phenonmenon is not seen with NSCLC tumors.

CONCLUSION

The establishment of SCLC and NSCLC lines has facilitated detailed biologic investigation of lung cancer. It is clear that the in vitro similarities and differences between these tumor types is also seen in clinical specimens. In addition, within each lung cancer cell type, morphologic, biochemical, and molecular heterogeneity is witnessed. These cell lines have contributed to our knowledge of the relationships among the varied histologic subtypes of human lung cancer.

ACKNOWLEDGEMENT

This work was supported in part by a Veterans Administration Merit Review Grant.

REFERENCES

1. Abeloff MD, Eggleston JC: Morphologic changes following therapy, in Greco A, Oldham R, Bunn PA (eds): Small Cell Cancer of the Lung. Orlando, FL, Grune & Stratton, 1981, pp 235-258
2. Abeloff MD, Eggleston JC, Mendelsohn G, et al: Changes in morphologic and biochemical characteristics of small cell carcinoma of the lung. Am J Med 66:757-764, 1979
3. Anon. The world health organization histological typing of lung tumors. Am J Clin Pathol 77:123-136, 1982
4. Ariyoshi Y, Kato K, Ishiguro Y, et al: Evaluation of serum neuron specific enolase as a tumor marker for carcinoma of the lung. Gann 74:219-225, 1983

5. Ayvazian LF, Schneider B, Gerwitz G, et al: Ectopic production of big ACTH in carcinoma of the lung. Am Rev Resp Dis 111:279-287, 1975

6. Banks-Schlegel SP, Gazdar AF, Harris CC: Intermediate filament and cross-linked envelop expression in human lung tumor cell lines. Cancer Res 45:1187-1197, 1985

7. Banks-Schlegel SP, Green H. Involucrin synthesis and tissue assembly by keratinocytes in natural and cultured human epithelia. J Cell Biol 90:732-737, 1981

8. Banks-Schlegel SP, Harris CC: Tissue-specific expression of keratin proteins in human esophageal and epidermal epithelium and their cultured keratinocytes. Exp Cell Res: 146:271-280, 1983

9. Banner BF, Gould VE, Radosevich JA, et al: Application of monoclonal antibody 44-3A6 in the cytodiagnosis and classification of pulmonary carcinomas. Diagn Cytopathol 1:300-307, 1985

10. Barnes D, Sato G: Serum-free cell culture: A unifying approach. Cell 22:649-55, 1980

11. Baylin SB, Abeloff MD, Goodwin G, et al: Activities of L-dopa decarboxylase and diamine oxidase (histaminase) in human lung cancers and decarboxylase as a marker for small (oat) cell cancer in cell culture. Cancer Res 40:1990-1994, 1980

12. Baylin SB, Gazdar AF, Minna JD, et al: A unique cell-surface protein phenotype distinguishes human small-cell from non-small cell lung cancer. Proc Natl Acad Sci (USA) 79:4650-4654, 1982

13. Baylin SB, Jackson RD, Goodwin G, et al: Neuroendocrine related biochemistry in the spectrum of human lung cancers. Exp Lung Res 3:209-233, 1982

14. Baylin SB, Weisbuager WR, Eggelston JC, et al: Variable content of histaminase, L-dopa decarboxylase and calcitonin in small cell carcinoma of the lung. New Engl J Med 299:105-110, 1978

15. Becker KL, Gazdar AF, Carney DN, et al: Calcitonin secretion by continuous cultures of small cell carcinoma of the lung: incidence and immunoheterogeneity studies. Cancer Lett 18:179-185, 1983

16. Berger CL, Goodwin G, Mendelsohn G, et al: Endocrine-related biochemistry in the spectrum of human lung carcinoma. J Clin Endocrinol Metab 53:422-429, 1981

17. Bernal SD, Baylin SB, Shaper JH, et al: Cytoskeleton-associated proteins of human lung cancer cells. Cancer Res 43:1798-1808, 1983

18. Bernal SD, Speak JA: Membrane antigen in small cell carcinoma of the lung defined by monoclonal antibody SM1. Cancer Res 44:265-270, 1984

19. Blobel GA, Gould VE, Moll R, et al: Coexpression of neuroendocrine markers and epithelial cytoskeletal proteins in bronchopulmonary neuroendocrine neoplasms. Lab Invest 52:39-51, 1985

20. Blobel GA, Moll R, Franke WW, et al: Cytokeratins in normal lung and lung carcinomas. Virchows Arch Cell Pathol, 45:407-429, 1984

21. Brenner BG, Jothy S, Shuster J: Monoclonal antibodies to human lung tumor antigens demonstrated by immunofluorescence and immunoprecipitation. Cancer Res 42:3187-3192, 1982

22. Broers JL, Carney DN, DeLey L: Differential expression of intermediate filament proteins distinguishes classic from variant small-cell lung cancer cell lines. Proc Natl Acad Sci (USA) 82:4409-4413, 1985

23. Brower M, Carney DN, Oie HK, et al: Growth of cell lines and clinical specimens of human non-small cell lung cancer in a serum-free defined medium. Cancer Res 46:798-806, 1986

24. Brown DT, Moore M: Monoclonal antibodies against two human lung carcinoma cell lines. Br J Cancer 46:794-801, 1982

25. Bunn PA, Carney DN, Gazdar AF, et al: Diagnostic and biological implications of flow cytometric DNA content analysis in lung cancer. Cancer Res 43:5026-5032, 1983

26. Bunn PA, Linnoila I, Minna JD, et al: Small cell lung cancer, endocrine cells of the fetal

bronchus, and other neuroendocrine cells express the Leu-7 antigenic determinant present on natural killer cells. Blood 65:764-768, 1985

27. Bunn PA, Minna JD: Paraneoplastic syndromes, in DeVita VT, Hellman S, Rosenberg SA (eds): Principles and Practice of Oncology. Philadelphia, Lippincott, 1985, pp 1797-1842

28. Buys CHCM, van der Veen AY, de Ley L: Chromosome analysis of three cell lines established from small cell carcinoma of the lung. 8th Internatl Chromosome Conference. Lubeck, 1983 (Abstr)

29. Callahan SK, Coltman CA, Kitten C, et al: Tumour cloning assay: Application and potential usefulness in lung cancer management, in Greco FA (ed): Biology and Management of Lung Cancer. Martinus, Nijhoff Publishers, 1983, 51-72

30. Carney DN, Broder L, Edelstein M, et al: Experimental studies of the biology of human cell lung cancer. Cancer Treat Rep 57:27-36, 1983

31. Carney DN, Brower M, Bertness V, et al: The selective growth of human small cell lung cancer lines and clinical specimens in serum-free medium, in Sato G, Barnes D (eds): Methods in Molecular and Cell Biology. New York, Alan R. Liss, 1984, pp 57-72

32. Carney DN, Bunn PA, Gazdar AF, et al: Selective growth in serum-free hormone supplemented medium of tumor cells obtained by biopsy from patients with small cell carcinoma of the lung. Proc Natl Acad Sci (USA) 78:3185-3189, 1981

33. Carney DN, Gazdar AF, Bepler G, et al: Establishment and identification of small cell lung cancer cell line having classic and variant features. Cancer Res 45:2913-2923, 1985

34. Carney DN, Gazdar AF, Bunn PA, et al: Demonstration of the stem cell nature of clonogenic cells in lung cancer specimens. Stem Cells 1:149-164, 1981

35. Carney DN, Gazdar AF, Bunn PA, et al: In vitro cloning of small cell carcinoma of the lung, in Greco FA, Bunn PA Jr, Oldham RK (eds): Small Cell Lung Cancer. New York, Grune & Stratton, 1981, pp 74-94

36. Carney DN, Gazdar AF, Minna JD: Positive correlation between histological tumour involvement and generation of tumour cell colonies in agarose in specimens taken directly from patients with small-cell carcinoma of the lung. Cancer Res 40:1820-1823, 1980

37. Carney DN, Marangos PJ, Ihde DC, et al: Neuron specific enolase: A marker for disease extent and response to therapy in patients with small cell lung cancer. Lancet 1:583-585, 1982

38. Carney DN, Matthews MJ, Ihde DC, et al: Influence of histologic subtype of small cell carcinoma of the lung on clinical presentation, response to therapy and survival. J Natl Cancer Inst 65:1225, 1980

39. Carney DN, Mitchell JB, Kinsella TJ: In vitro radiation and chemotherapy sensitivity of established cell lines of human small cell lung cancer and its large cell morphological variants. Cancer Res 43:2806-2811, 1983

40. Carney DN, Winkler CW: In vitro assays of chemotherapeutic sensitivity, in DeVita V, Hellman S, Rosenberg S (eds): Important Advances in Oncology. Philadelphia, JB Lippincott, 1985, pp 55-70

41. Carney DN, Zweig MH, Ihde DC, et al: Elevated serum creatinine kinase BB levels in patients with small cell lung cancer. Cancer Res 44:5399-5403, 1984

42. Cate CC, Douple EB, Andrews KM, et al: Calcitonin as an indicator of the response of human small cell carcinoma of the lung cells to drugs and radiation. Cancer Res 44:949-954, 1984

43. Chambers WF, Pettengill OS, Sorenson GD: Intracranial growth of pulmonary small cell carcinoma cells in nude athymic mice. Exp Cell Biol 49:90-97, 1981

44. Cohen MH, Matthews MJ: Small cell bronchogenic carcinoma: A distinct clinicopathologic entity. Sem Oncol 5:234-243, 1978

45. Cooper GM: Cellular transforming genes. Science 217:801–806, 1982

46. Cooper D, Schermer A, Sun T: Classification of human epithelia and their neoplasms using monoclonal antibodies to keratin: Strategies, applications, and limitations. Lab Invest 52:243–256, 1985

47. Curt GA, Carney DN, Cowan KH, et al: Unstable methotrexate resistance in human small cell carcinoma associated with double minute chromosomes. New Engl J Med 308:199–202, 1983

48. Cuttitta F, Carney DN, Mulshine J, et al: Bombesin-like peptides can function as autocrine growth factors in human small-cell lung cancer. Nature 316:823–826, 1985

49. Cuttitta F, Rosen S, Carney DN, et al: Monoclonal antibodies against human lung cancer: Potential diagnostic and therapeutic use, in Greco FA (ed): Biology and Management of Lung Cancer: Lung Cancer II. Boston, Martginus Nijhoff Publishers, 1983, pp 25–36

50. Cuttitta F, Rosen S, Fedorko J, et al: Monoclonal antibodies and cancer: Monoclonal antibodies to human cancer, in Wright GL (ed): Cancer and Disease. New York, Marcel Dekker, 1983, pp 161–180

51. Cuttitta F, Rosen S, Gazdar, AF, et al: Monoclonal antibodies which demonstrate specificity for several types of human lung cancer and neuroblastoma. Proc Natl Acad Sci (USA) 78:4591–4595, 1981

52. Cutz E, Chan W, Track NS: Bombesin, calcitonin and leuenkephalin immunoreactivity in endocrine cells of human lung. Experientia 37:765–766, 1981

53. Der CJ, Cooper GM: Altered gene products are associated with activation of cellular ras^k genes in human lung and colon carcinomas. Cell 32:201–208, 1983

54. Dingemans KP, Mooi WJ: Ultrastructure of squamous cell carcinoma of the lung. Pathol Ann 19:249–273, 1984

55. Doyle A, Martin WJ, Funa K, et al: Markedly decreased expression of class I histocompatability antigens, protein and mRNA in human small cell lung cancer. J Exp Med 161:1135–1151, 1985

56. Eichner R, Bonitz P, Sun TT: Classification of epidermal keratins according to their immunoreactivity, isoelectric point and mode of expression. J Cell Biol 98:1388–1396, 1984

57. Erisman MD, Linnoila RI, Hernandez O, et al: Human lung small cell carcinoma contains bombesin, Proc Natl Acad Sci (USA) 79:2379–2383, 1982

58. Esscher T, Steinholtz L, Bergh J, et al: Neuron specific enolase: A useful diagnostic serum marker for small cell carcinoma of the lung. Thorax 40:85–90, 1985

59. Fagion S, Carney D, Mulshine J, et al: Heterogeneity of cell surface antigen expression of human SCLC as detected by monoclonal antibodies. Cancer Res 46:2633–2638, 1986

60. Falor WH, Ward-Skinner R, Wegryn S: A 3p deletion in small cell lung carcinoma. Cancer Genet Cytogenet 16:175–177, 1985

61. Franke WW, Schiller DL, Moll R, et al: Differentiation-related pattern of expression of proteins of intermediate-sized filaments in tissues and cultured cells. Cold Spring Harbor Symp Quant. Biol 46: 431–453, 1982

62. Funa K, Gazdar AF, Minna JD, et al: Paucity of B_2-microglobulin expression on small cell lung cancer, bronchial carcinoids and certain other neuroendocrine tumors. Lab Invest 45:186–193, 1986

63. Gazdar AF: The biology of endocrine tumors of the lung, in Becker KL, Gazdar AF (eds): The Endocrine Lung in Health and Disease. Philadelphia, Saunders, 1984, pp 448–459

64. Gazdar AF: The pathology of endocrine tumors of the lung, in Becker KL, Gazdar AF (eds): The Endocrine Lung in Health and Disease. Philadelphia, Saunders, 1984, pp 364–372

65. Gazdar AF: Advances in the biology of non-small cell lung cancer. Chest 89:277s–283s, 1986

66. Gazdar AF, Carney DN: Endocrine properties of small cell carcinoma of the lung, in Becker KL, Gazdar AF (eds): The Endocrine Lung in Health and Disease. Philadelphia, Saunders, 1984, pp 501–508

67. Gazdar AF, Carney DN, Becker KL, et al: Expression of peptides and other markers in lung cancer cell lines. Recent Results Cancer Res., 99:167–174, 1985

68. Gazdar AF, Carney DN, Guccion JG, et al: Small cell carcinoma of the lung: Cellular origin and relationship to other pulmonary tumors, in Greco A, Bunn PA, Oldham R (eds): Small Cell Lung Cancer. New York; Grune & Stratton, 1981, pp 1145-1175.

69. Gazdar AF, Carney DN, Minna JD: The biology of non-small cell lung cancer. Semin Oncol 10:3–19, 1983

70. Gazdar AF, Carney DN, Nau MM, et al: Characteristics of variant subclasses of cell lines derived from small cell lung cancer having distinctive biochemical, morphological and growth properties. Cancer Res 45:2924–2930, 1985

71. Gazdar AF, Carney DN, Russell EK, et al: Establishment of continuous clonable cultures of small cell carcinoma of the lung which have amine precursor uptake and decarboxylation properties. Cancer Res 40:3502–3507, 1980

72. Gazdar AF, Carney DN, Sims HL, et al: Heterotransplantation of small cell carcinoma of the lung into nude mice: Comparison of intracranial and subcutaneous routes. Internatl J Cancer 28:777–783, 1981

73. Gazdar AF, Oie HK: Cell culture methods for human lung cancer. Cancer Genet Cytogenet 19:5–10, 1986

74. Gazdar AF, Zweig MH, Carney DN, et al: Levels of creatine kinase and its BB isoenzyme in lung cancer tumors and cultures. Cancer Res 41:2773–2777, 1981

75. Goodwin G, Baylin SB: Relationships between neuroendocrine differentiation and sensitivity to radiation in culture line OH-1 of human small cell lung carcinoma. Cancer Res 42:1361–1367, 1982

76. Goodwin G, Shaper HH, Abeloff MD, et al: Anaysis of cell surface proteins delineates a differentiation pathway linking endocrine and nonendocrine human lung cancers. Proc Natl Acad Sci (USA) 80:3807–3811, 1983

77. Gordon LT, Rosen ST, Vriesendorp HM, et al: Density separation of clonogenic tumor cells from small-cell lung cancer cell lines: Implications for autologous bone marrow transplantation. Cancer Res 44:5404–5408, 1984

78. Gronowitz JS, Steinholz L, Kallander CFR, et al: Serum deoxythymidine kinase in small cell carcinoma of the lung. Cancer 58:111–118, 1986

79. Greco FA, Hainsworth J, Sismani A, et al: Hormone production and paraneoplastic syndromes, in Greco FA, Bunn PA, Jr, Oldham RK (eds): Small Cell Lung Cancer. New York, Grune & Stratton, 1981, pp 177–225

80. Griffin CA, Nelkin BD, Baylin SB: c-myb transcripts in human small cell lung carcinoma cell lines. J Cell Biochem (Suppl), 8A, 1984

81. Gropp C, Havemann K, Scheuer A: Ectopic hormones in lung cancer patients at diagnosis and during therapy. Cancer 46:327–243, 1980

82. Hakomori S: Aberrant glycosylation in cancer cell membranes as focused on glycolipids: Overview and perspectives. Cancer Res 45:2405–2414, 1985

83. Hansen M, Hammer M, Hummer L: ACTH, ADH, and calcitonin concentrations as markers for response and relapse in small cell carcinoma of the lung. Cancer 46:2062–2067, 1980

84. Hendler FJ, Ozanne BW: Human squamous cell lung cancers express increased epidermal growth factor receptors. J Clin Invest 74:647–651, 1984

85. Hirota M, Fukushima K, Terasaki PI, et al: Detection of tumor-associated antigens in the

sera of lung cancer patients by three monoclonal antibodies. Cancer Res 45:6453–6456, 1985

86. Hirsch FR, Osterlind K, Hansen HH: The prognostic significance of histopathologic subtyping of small cell carcinoma of the lung according to the World Health Organization's classification. Cancer 52:2144–2160, 1983

87. Huang L, Brockhaus M, Magnani J: Many monoclonal antibodies with an apparent specificity for certain lung cancers are directed against a sugar sequence found in Lacto-N-fucopentaose III. Arch Biochem Biophys 220:317–320, 1983

88. Hullin DA, Brown K, Kynoch PAM, et al: Purification, radioimmunoassay, and distribution of human brain 14-3-2 protein (nervous system-specific enolase) in human tissues. Biochem Biophys Acta 628:98–108, 1980

89. Johnson BE, Battey J, Linnoila I, et al: Changes in the phenotype of human small cell lung cancer cell lines after transfection and expression of the c-myc proto-oncogene. J Clin Invest 78:525–532, 1986

90. Johnson BE, Nau MN, Gazdar AF, et al: Oncogene amplification of c-myc and N-myc in cell lines established from patients with small cell lung cancer is associated with shortened survival. Proc Am Assoc Clin Oncol 4:186, 1985

91. Johnson DH, Marangos PJ, Forbes JT, et al: Potential utility of serum neuron-specific enolase levels in small cell carcinoma of the lung. Cancer Res 44:5409–5419, 1984

92. Johnson WW, Szpak CA, Lottich SC, et al: Use of a monoclonal antibody (B72.3) as an immunocytochemical adjunct to diagnosis of adenocarcinoma in human effusions. Cancer Res 45:1894–1900, 1985

93. Kohler G, Milstein C: Continuous cultures of fused cells secreting antibody of predefined specificity. Nature 256:495–497, 1975

94. Kondo Y, Mizumoto Y, Katayama S, et al: Inappropriate secretion of antidiuretic hormone in nude mice bearing a human bronchogenic carcinoma. Cancer Res 41:1545–1548, 1981

95. Kyoizumi S, Akiyama M, Kuno N: Monoclonal antibodies to human squamous cell carcinoma of the lung and their application to tumor diagnosis. Cancer Res 45:3274–3281, 1985

96. Lambert EH, Lennon VA: Neuromuscular transmission in nude mice bearing oat-cell tumours from Lambert-Eaton myasthenic syndrome. Muscle & Nerve 5:539–545, 1982

97. Lazarus LH, DiAugustine RP, Jahnke GD, et al: Physalaemin: An amphibian tachykinin in human lung small-cell carcinoma. Science 19:79–81, 1983

98. Lechner JF, Haugen A, McClendon IA, et al: Clonal growth of normal adult human bronchial epithelial cells in a serum-free medium. In Vitro 18:633–642, 1982

99. Lee I, Radosevich JA, Ma Y, et al: Immunohistochemical demonstration of lacto-N-fucopentaose III in lung carcinomas with monoclonal antibody 624A12. Pathol Pract Res in press

100. Lee I, Radosevich JA, Rosen ST, et al: Immunohistochemical analysis of lung carcinomas using monoclonal antibody 44-3A6. Cancer Res 45:5808–5812, 1985

101. Lee I, Radosevich JA, Thor A, et al: Enhanced ras oncogene product immunoreactivity in pulmonary neoplasms, submitted for publication

102. Leff EL, Brooks JS, Trojanowski JQ: Expression of neurofilament and neuron-specific enolase in small cell tumors of skin using immunohistochemistry. Cancer 56:625–631, 1985

103. Lehto VP, Stenman S, Miettinen M, et al: Expression of a neural type of intermediate filament as a distinguishing feature between oat cell carcinoma and other lung cancers. Am J Pathol 110:113–118, 1983

104. Levitt ML, Oie HK, Sausville EA, et al: Biologic markers for squamous differentiation in human lung cancer cell lines. Proc Am Assoc Clin Oncol 5:17, 1986

105. Little CD, Nau MM, Carney DN, et al: Amplification and expression of the c-myc oncogene in human lung cancer cell lines. Nature 306:194-196, 1983

106. Mackay B, Osborne BM, Wilson RA: Ultrastructure of lung neoplasms, in Straus MJ (ed): Lung Cancer, Clinical Diagnosis and Treatment. New York, Grune & Stratton, 1977, pp 71-84

107. Marangos PJ, Gazdar AF, Carney DN: Neuron specific enolase in human cell carcinoma cultures. Cancer Lett 15:67-71, 1982

108. Mattern J, Haag D, Wayss K, et al: Growth kinetics of human lung tumors in nude mice. Exp Cell Biol 49:34-40, 1981

109. Matthews MJ, Gazdar AF: Pathology of small cell carcinoma of the lung and its subtypes. A clinico-pathologic correlation, in Livingston RB (ed): Lung Cancer. The Hague, Martinus Nijhoff, 1981, pp 283-306

110. Matthews MJ, Mackay B, Lukeman J: The pathology of non-small cell carcinoma of the lung. Sem Oncol 10:34-55, 1983

111. Mazauric T, Mitchell KF, Letchworth GJ, et al: Monoclonal antibody-defined human lung cell surface proteins antigens. Cancer Res 42:150-154, 1982

112. McDowell EM, Trump BF: Pulmonary small cell carcinoma showing tripartite differentiation in individual cells. Human Pathol 12:286-294, 1981

113. Miller YE, Sullivan N, Kao B, et al: Reduced or absent aminoacylase-1 activity in small cell lung cancer: Evidence for inactivation of genes encoded by chromosome 3p. Clin Res 34:568A, 1986

114. Minna JD, Bunn PA Jr, Carney DN, et al: Experience of the national cancer institute (USA) in the treatment and biology of small cell lung cancer. Bulletin du Cancer 69:83-93, 1982

115. Minna JD, Carney DN, Alverez R, et al: Heterogeneity and homogeneity of human small cell lung cancer, in Owens AH, Coffey DS, Baylin SB (eds): Tumor Cell Teterogeneity, Origin and Implications. New York, Academic Press, 1982, pp 29-52

116. Minna J, Cuttitta F, Rosen S, et al: Methods for producing monoclonal antibodies with specificity for human lung cancer cells. In Vitro 17:1058-1070, 1981

117. Minna JD, Higgins GA, Glatstein EJ: Cancer of the lung, in DeVita VT, Hellman S, Rosenberg SA (eds): Principles and Practice of Oncology. Philadelphia, Lippincott, 1985, pp 507-597

118. Moll R, Franke WW, Schiller DL: The catalog of human cytokeratins: Patterns of expression in normal epithelia, tumors and cultured cells. Cell 31:11-24, 1982

119. Moody TW, Pert CB, Gazdar AF, et al: High levels of intracellular bombesin characterize human small cell lung cancer. Science 214:1246-1248, 1981

120. Moore BW. Chemistry and biology of two proteins, S-100 and 14-3-2, specific to the nervous system, in Pfeiffer CC, Symthies JR (eds): International Review of Neurobiology, vol 15. New York, Academic Press, 1972, pp 215-225

121. Morstyn G, Russo A, Carney DN, et al: Heterogeneity in the radiation survival curves and biochemical properties of human lung cancer cell lines. J Natl Cancer Inst 73:801-807, 1984

122. Muggia FM, Krezoski SK, Hansen HH: Cell kinetic studies in patients with small cell lung cancer. Cancer 34:1683-1690, 1974

123. Mulshine JL, Cuttitta, F, Bibro M, et al: Monoclonal antibodies that distinguish non-small cell cancer from small cell cancer. J Immunol 131:497-502, 1983

124. Nau MM, Brooks BJ, Carney DN, et al: Human small cell lung cancers show amplification and expression of the n-myc gene. Proc Natl Acad Sci (USA) 83:1092-1096, 1986

125. Nau MM, Carney N, Battey J, et al: Amplification, expression and rearrangement of c-myc and n-myc oncogenes in human lung cancer. Curr Top Microbiol Immunol 113:172-177, 1984

126. Naylor S, Minna J, Johnson B, et al: DNA polymorphisms confirm the deletion in the short arm of chromosome 3 in small cell lung cancer. Am J Human Genet 36:35S, 1986

127. North WG, Maurer H, Valtin H, et al: Human neurophysins as potential markers for small cell carcinoma of the lung: Applications of specific radioimmunoassay. J Clin Endocrinol Metab 51:892-896, 1980

128. O'Connor DT, Deftos LF: Secretion of chromogranin A by peptide-producing endocrine neoplasms. New Engl J Med 314:1145-1151, 1986

129. Odell WD, Wolfsen AR, Bachelot I, et al: Ectopic production of lipotropin by cancer. Am J Med 66:631, 1979

130. Okabe T, Kaizu T, Ozawa K, et al: Elimination of small cell lung cancer cells in vitro from human bone marrow by a monoclonal antibody. Can Res 45:1930-1935, 1985

131. Ovejera AA, Houchens DP: Human tumor xenografts in athymic nude mice as a preclinical screen for anticancer agents. Semin Oncol 4:386-393, 1981

132. Papageorge A, Lowy D, Scolnick EM: Comparative biochemical properties of p21 ras molecules coded for by viral and cellular ras genes. J Virol 44:509-519, 1982

133. Pavelic ZP, Soleum HK, Rustum YM, et al: Growth of cell colonies in soft agar from biopsies of different human tumors. Cancer Res, 40:4151-4158, 1980

134. Pearse AG: The cytochemistry and ultrastructure of polypeptide hormone producing cells of the APUD series, and the embryologic, physiologic and pathologic implications of the concept. J Histochem Cytochem 17:303-313, 1969

135. Pettengill OS, Sorenson GD: Tissue culture and in vitro characteristics, in Greco FA, Oldham RK, Bunn PA (eds): Small Cell Lung Cancer. New York, Grune & Stratton, 1981, pp 51-77

136. Pettengill OS, Sorenson GD, Wurster-Hill DH, et al: Isolation and growth characteristics of continuous cell lines from small-cell carcinoma of the lung. Cancer 45:906-918, 1980

137. Pollard EB, Tio F, Myers JW, et al: Utilization of a human tumor cloning system to monitor for marrow involvement with small cell carcinoma of the lung. Cancer Res 41:1015-1020, 1981

138. Radice PA, Matthews MJ, Ihde DC, et al: The clinical behavior of mixed small cell/large cell bronchogenic carcinoma compared to pure small cell subtypes. Cancer 50:2894-2902, 1982

139. Radosevich JA, Ma Y, Lee I, et al: Monoclonal antibody 44-3A6 detects a novel antigen present in lung carcinomas with glandular differences. Cancer Res 45:5813-5817, 1985

140. Radosevich JA, Lee I, Ma Y, et al: Comparison of normal and altered ras oncogene p21 expression in lung cancer using monoclonal antibodies RAP-5 and DWP, submitted for publication

141. Reeve JG, Wulfank DA, Stewart J, et al: Monoclonal-antibody-defined human lung tumor cell-surface antigens. Internatl J Cancer 35:769-775, 1985

142. Rheinwald JG, Germain E, Beckett MA: Expression of keratins and cross-linked envelope proteins in normal and malignant human keratinocytes and mesothelial cells, in Harris CC, Autrup HN (eds): Human Carcinogenesis, vol 3. New York, Academic Press, 1983, pp 85-96

143. Roggli VL, Vollmer RT, Greenberg SD, et al: Lung cancer heterogeneity. Human Pathol 16:569-579, 1985

144. Rosen ST, Mulshine JL, Cuttitta F, et al: Analysis of small cell lung cancer differentiation antigens using a panel of rat monoclonal antibodies. Cancer Res 44:2052-2061, 1984

145. Said JW, Nash G, Banks-Schlegel S, et al: Keratin in human lung tumors. Pattern of localization of different molecular weight keratin proteins. Am J Pathol 113:27-32, 1983

146. Said JW, Nash G, Sasson AF, et al: Involucrin in lung tumors. A specific marker for squamous differentiation. Lab Invest 49:563-568, 1983

147. Salmon SE, Von Hoff DD: In vitro evaluation of anticancer drugs with the human tumor stem cell assay. Semin Oncol 4:377-385, 1986

148. Sausville EA, Lebacq-Verheyden AM, Spindel ER, et al: Expression of the gastrin-releasing peptide gene in human small cell lung cancer. J Biol Chem 261:2451-2457, 1986

149. Shackney SE, Straus NJ, Bunn PA: The growth characteristics of small cell carcinoma of the lung, in Greco FA, Oldham RK, Bunn PA (eds): Small Cell Lung Cancer. New York, Grune & Stratton, 1981, pp 225-234

150. Sherwin SA, Minna JD, Gazdar AF, et al: Expression of epidermal and nerve growth factor receptors and soft agar growth factor production by human lung cancer cells. Cancer Res 41:3538-3542, 1981

151. Shinkai T, Saijo N, Tominago K, et al: Serial plasma carcinoembryonic antigen measurement for monitoring patients with advanced lung cancer during chemotherapy. Cancer 57:1318-1323, 1986

152. Silva OL, Brode LE, Doppman JL, et al: Calcitonin as a marker for bronchogenic cancer. Cancer 44:680-684, 1979

153. Simms E, Gazdar AF, Abrams PG, Minna JD: Growth of human small cell (oat cell) carcinoma of the lung in serum-free growth factor-supplemented medium. Cancer Res 40:4356-4363, 1980

154. Slayter HS, Coligan JE: Electron microscopy and physical characterization of the carcinoembryonic antigen. Biochemistry 14:2323-2330, 1975

155. Sorenson GD, Bloom SR, Ghatei MA: Bombesin production by human small cell carcinoma of the lung. Regul Pept 4:59-66, 1982

156. Sorenson GD, Pettengill OS, Brinck-Johnsen T, et al: Hormone production by cultures of small cell carcinoma of the lung. Cancer 47:1289-1296, 1981

157. Spindel ER, Chin WW, Price J, et al: Cloning and characterization of cDNAs encoding human gastrin-releasing peptide. Proc Natl Acad Sci (USA) 81:5699-5703, 1984

158. Spitalnik SL, Spitalnik PF, Dubois C, et al: Glycolipid antigen expression in human lung cancer. Cancer Res 46:4751-4755, 1986

159. Sporn MB, Todaro GJ: Autocrine secretion and malignant transformation of cells. New Engl J Med 303:878-880, 1980

160. Stahel RA, Mabry M, Skarin A, et al: Detection of bone marrow metastasis in small cell carcinoma of the lung by monoclonal antibodies. J Clin Oncol 3:455-461, 1984

161. Stahel RA, O'Hara CJ, Mabry M, et al: Cytotoxic murine monoclonal antibody LAM8 with specificity for human small cell carcinoma of the lung. Cancer Res 46:2077-2084, 1986

162. Szabo M, Berecowitz M, Pettengill OS, et al: Ectopic production of somatostatin-like immuno and bioactivity by cultured human small cell carcinoma. J Clin Endocrinol Metab 51:978-987, 1980

163. Tapia FJ, Polak JM, Barbosa AJA, et al: Neuron-specific enolase is produced by neuroendocrine tumors. Lancet 1:808-811, 1981

164. Tong AW, Lee J, Stone MJ: Characterization of two human small cell lung carcinoma-reactive monoclonal antibodies generated by a novel immunization approach. Cancer Res 44:4987-4992, 1984

165. Van Muijen GN, Ruiter DJ, Van Leeuwen CV, et al. Cytokeratin and neurofilament in lung carcinomas. Am J Pathol 116:363-369, 1984

166. Van Steirteghem AC, Robertson EA, Zweig MH: Distribution of serum concentrations of creatine kinase MM and BB isoenzymes measured by radioimmunoassay. Clin Chim Acta 93:25-28, 1979

167. Varki NM, Reisfield RA, Walker LE: Antigens associated with human lung adenocarcinoma defined by monoclonal antibodies. Cancer Res 44:681-687, 1984

168. Vindelov LL, Hansen HH, Christensen IJ, et al: Clonal heterogeneity of small cell anaplastic carcinoma of the lung demonstrated by flow cytometric DNA analysis, Cancer Res 40:4295-4300, 1980

169. Vindelow LL, Hansen HH, Gersel A, et al: Treatment of small cell carcinoma of the lung monitored by sequential flow cytometric DNA analysis. Cancer Res 42:2499-2505, 1982

170. Volm M, Mattern J, Sonka J, et al: DNA distribution in non-small cell lung carcinomas and its relationship to clinical behavior. Cytometry 6:348-356, 1985

171. Walkes TP, Abeloff MA, Woo KB, et al: Carcinoembryonic antigen for monitoring patients with small cell carcinoma of the lung during treatment. Cancer Res 40:4420-4427, 1980

172. Wallach S, Royston I, Wohl H, et al: Plasma calcitonin as a marker of disease activity in patients with small cell carcinoma of the lung. J Clin Endocrinol Metab 53:602-606, 1981

173. Weisenthal LW: In vitro assays in preclinical anti-neoplastic drug screening. Semin Oncol 4:362-377, 1981

174. Whang-Peng J, Bunn PA, Kao-Shan CS, et al: A nonrandom chromosomal abnormality, del 3p (14-223), in human small cell lung cancer. Cancer Genet Cytogenet 6:119-134, 1982

175. Whang-Peng J, Kao-Shan CS, Lee EC, et al: A specific chromosome defect associated with human small cell lung cancer, del(3p) (14-23). Science 215:181-183, 1982

176. Whang-Peng J, Kao-Shun CS, Lee EC, et al: Human small cell lung cancer: Deletion 3p(14-23), double minute chromosomes and homogeneously staining regions in human small cell lung cancer, in Gene Amplification, The Banbury Report, Cold Spring Harbor, New York Lab Press, 1982, pp 107-114

177. Wharton J, Polak JM, Bloom SR et al: Bombesin-like immunoreactivity in the lung. Nature 273:769-770, 1978

178. Wilson TS, McDowell EM, Trump BF: Immunohistochemical studies of keratin in human bronchus and lung tumors. Arch Pathol Lab Med 109:621-628, 1985

179. Wong AJ, Ruppert JM, Eggleston J, et al: Gene amplification of C-myc in small cell carcinoma of the lung. Science 233:461-463, 1986

180. Wood SM, Wood JR, Ghatel MD, et al: Bombesin, somatostatin and neurotensin-like immunoreactivity in bronchial carcinoma. J Clin Endocrinol Metab 53:1310-1312, 1981

181. Wood SM, Wood J, Ghatel MD, et al: Is bombesin a tumour marker for small cell carcinoma. Lancet 1:610, 1982

182. Wurster-Hill DH, Cannizarro LA, Pettengill OS, et al: Cytogenetics of small cell carcinoma of the lung. Cancer Genet Cytogenet 13:303-330, 1984

183. Wurster-Hill DH, Maurer LH: Cytogenetic diagnosis of cancer, abnormalities of chromosomes and polyploid levels in the bone marrow of patients with small cell carcinoma of the lung. J Natl Cancer Inst 61:1065-1075, 1978

184. Yalow RS: Big ACTH and bronchogenic carcinoma. Ann Rev Med 30:241-248, 1979

185. Yesner R: Classification of lung cancer histology. New Engl J Med 312:652-653, 1985

186. Yoda Y, Gasa S, Makita A, et al: Glycolipids in human lung carcinoma of histologically different types. J Natl Cancer Inst 63:115-1160, 1979

187. Zimmer AM, Rosen ST, Spies SM, et al: Radioimmunoimaging of human small cell lung carcinoma with a I-131 tumor specific monoclonal antibody. Hybridoma 4:1-11, 1985

188. Zweig MH, Van Steirteghem AC: Assessment by radioimmunoassay of serum creatine kinase BB (CK-BB) as a tumor marker: Studies in patients with various cancers and a comparison of CK-BB concentrations to prostate acid phosphatase concentrations. J Natl Cancer Inst 66:859-862, 1981

Alex G. Little

4

Principles of Surgical Oncology

The specific principles of thoracic surgical oncology related to the treatment of lung cancer are derived from the general principles of surgical oncology. The major priority is a disease-oriented approach to patients with lung cancer rather than a technique-oriented approach. The surgeon must be familiar with and have access to the other modalities involved in lung cancer treatment; thus allowing consideration of all the therapeutic options that can be afforded the patient. Without this background the surgeon cannot function properly as a physician in relation to the patient.

DIAGNOSIS

Not all patients have a firm (i.e., histologic) diagnosis of lung cancer prior to thoracotomy. The patient's age and smoking history are relative factors to consider, as most, but not all, lung cancers occur in smokers and in patients over the age of 40. If the chest x-ray (CXR) appearance is compatible with carcinoma (particularly if it can be proven to be new or enlarging by comparison with previous films), however, our group proceeds with thoracotomy, even if results of sputum cytology and flexible bronchoscopy—which should be performed in all patients—are not diagnostic. We rarely use percutaneous needle biopsy, as a negative (i.e. noncancer) result does not deter us from operating if the clinical and radiographic data are compatible with a cancer diagnosis. Since a positive needle biopsy also leads to thoracotomy, this means that results will not influence treatment. We therefore reserve this technique for patients who demand that all attempts at securing a preoperative tissue diagnosis be made, to establish the cell type in patients with metastatic disease, and to distinguish between a lung primary and a metastasis from a previously treated cancer of another organ.

When operation is performed without a tissue diagnosis, gross findings are compatible with carcinoma, and a lobectomy will suffice to remove all evident disease, the surgeon should proceed with that operation. If the patient's pulmonary reserve is severely limited or the operative findings suggest a benign disorder, or if a pneumonec-

LUNG CANCER: A COMPREHENSIVE TREATISE
ISBN 0-8089-1876-1

tomy is technically required to remove all pathologic tissue, then a wedge resection or biopsy, needle or incisional, should be performed initially to establish a definite diagnosis by frozen section analysis. The appropriate resection can be carried out based on the result.

STAGING

The importance of both preoperative and intraoperative staging of patients is emphasized here. At present the American Joint Commission (AJC) staging definitions are employed. The principles of pretreatment staging are developed in greater detail in Chapter 8. The techniques and considerations involved must be familiar to and utilized by the surgeon in order to select patients most likely to benefit from surgery. Accurate staging, both clinical and pathological, is important for selection of therapeutic strategies, as prognosis is determined by the stage. Accurate and reliable staging is also the only way to ensure precise communication by guaranteeing that patients are comparable.

Clinical Staging

The obvious starting point is a careful history and physical examination. Further evaluation of the primary tumor requires a CXR and bronchoscopy in every patient. Computerized tomographic (CT) scanning is useful in patients suspected of having T3 tumors by better defining questionable chest wall or mediastinal invasion. It is most accurate in predicting the absence of involvement.[14] The additional information assists in planning the operation and in predicting the possibility of extended surgery for the patient.

Staging of N1 nodes is inaccurate, and results rarely affect surgical decisions.[3] One exception is an enlarged hilum, by CXR or CT scan, in a patient with marginal pulmonary reserve. This indicates the real possibility that a pneumonectomy will be required and signals the need for careful physiologic evaluation and intensive preoperative preparation of the patient. Several techniques for evaluation of N2 nodes are available, but the most useful are CT scanning and either cervical or parasternal mediastinoscopy. A CT scan is most reliable when all nodes identified are less than 1 cm in diameter; these small nodes are unlikely to contain metastases, and invasive staging does not seem warranted.[3] Enlargement does not necessarily mean involvement, however, and biopsy by mediastinoscopy is indicated when nodes larger than 1 cm are seen. The role of surgery in patients with involved N2 nodes is controversial (see Chapter 15). Regardless of one's feelings about the role of surgery in these patients, accurate staging is essential.

The best way to evaluate the patient for metastatic disease is unclear. The routine use of organ-specific radionuclide scans, such as brain and liver–spleen scans, has been shown to be of no value in the asymptomatic patient.[7] Wholesale organ scanning results in a large number of false-positive tests, which greatly complicates the situation, and few otherwise occult metastases are detected. Our group has had good results with ^{67}Ga scanning, in which the isotope is taken up by lung cancer cells. False-positive results are uncommon, and clinically occult metastases are found in approximately 10 percent of patients.[11] These results are contingent on the use of a high gallium dose, waiting 3 days after injection before scanning, and—perhaps most importantly—use of a Phocon scanner to obtain tomographic views. Two caveats to be mentioned are that this scan is insensitive to lesions smaller than 2 cm and that gallium is taken up by inflammatory cells and some other cancers such as melanoma. We employ other scans only when the history (e.g., bone pain), physical examination (e.g., a neurologic deficit), or a laboratory result (e.g., an elevated alkaline phosphatase) suggests metastatic involvement of a particular organ system and the gallium scan is normal.

Surgical–Pathologic Staging

Intraoperatively, the surgeon must routinely sample all accessible mediastinal nodal area and identify them separately prior to submission for pathologic analysis. This is a crucial aspect for ensuring the most accurate operative-pathological staging possible as there is a definite incidence of nodal involvement even when the nodes appear normal to the surgeon.[12] The nodes may either be identified by location (e.g., high or low paratracheal, subcarinal, subaortic, or inferior pulmonary ligament) or may be designated by using the American Thoracic Society classification system.[1] If this sampling is not consistently done, regardless of the gross appearance of the nodes, patients with occult involvement of N1 and N2 nodes will be understaged and will not receive potential benefits of appropriate adjuvant therapy. Further, for surgical treatment results to be unambiguous, all patients must be well staged both surgically and pathologically.

PHYSIOLOGIC EVALUATION

Many lung cancer patients have reduced pulmonary function because of their many years of cigarette smoking, chronic bronchitis, and chronic obstructive pulmonary disease and do not have the physiologic reserve to tolerate an extensive resection of functioning lung parenchyma. In addition to diagnostic and staging considerations, then, the preoperative period is also a time for physiologic assessment of the patient. Many techniques for evaluating preoperative lung function are available. Clinical assessment of the patient's ability to exercise or perform routine activities without respiratory limitation is probably a sufficient screen when there are no limitations. As a further screen, patients must have reasonable arterial blood gas values with a Po_2 in excess of 55 mm Hg and a Pco_2 of less than 50 mm Hg. These are extreme parameters and represent absolute cutoff limits. In addition, our group relies heavily on the forced expiratory volume in one second (FEV_1), which is determined by pulmonary function testing. It is our experience that patients must have a postoperative FEV_1 of 1 liter or more in order to perform normal life activities without respiratory compromise. This value may be varied slightly depending on the patient's size but is a reasonable figure to aim at. This means that a patient with a preoperative FEV_1 of 2.0 liters or more should be able to tolerate a pneumonectomy on grounds of pulmonary function alone. When the preoperative FEV_1 is less than 2 liters and a pneumonectomy is thought to be technically possible and potentially necessary, quantitative ventilation perfusion scans should be used as a further aid.[15] This quantitates function of both the involved lung, which is to be removed, and the uninvolved lung and can thus be used to predict the FEV_1 that will be present following resection. If this value is greater than 1 liter, then pneumonectomy is a reasonable consideration from this criterion. This approach is also applicable to assessment of the physiologic effect of a lesser operation such as lobectomy.

When the patient's pulmonary function is compromised, it usually can be improved by cessation of smoking, antibiotics if chronic bronchitis is present, bronchodilator therapy to treat bronchospasm, and intensive chest physiotherapy. A few weeks devoted to this type of enterprise can frequently improve a marginal patient sufficiently that resection becomes a valid consideration. The value of this is obvious as it offers the only realistic hope for a cure.

Pulmonary function alone, of course, is not the sole consideration when evaluating the patient's physiologic status, and the patient must be considered as a whole. The cardiovascular and all other organ systems must be thoughtfully evaluated. There are few absolute contraindications to surgical resection as advances in anesthetic management and postoperative support make surgical resection a reasonable consideration for most patients,[4] especially considering the certain outcome when resection is impossible.[2] Advanced age per se should certainly not be considered a contraindication to surgical intervention, as older patients can undergo pulmonary resection with good results and acceptable morbidity and mortality.[4]

OPERATIVE CONSIDERATIONS

Patients in clinical stage I or II have limited disease and should undergo potentially curative resection whenever possible; further discussions of these patients can be found in the appropriate book sections. Treatment of stage III patients is dependent on the reason for the patient's inclusion, a T_3 tumor, involvement of mediastinal (N_2) nodes, or the presence of metastases (M_1). The considerations used to select patients for or exclude them from surgical therapy are elaborated in the appropriate book sections. In summary, patients with M_1 disease are never candidates for surgical resection. Surgeons can play a useful role by biopsying sites of suspected metastasis, such as an abnormal area identified by a radionuclide bone scan.[10] If a metastasis is indefinite on the basis of noninvasive tests, a biopsy is mandatory to ensure potentially curative therapy is not withheld. Patients with $T_3N_0M_0$ or $T_3N_1M_0$ disease on the basis of chest wall invasion or the presence of primary tumor within 2 cm of the carina should always be considered for surgical resection as en bloc resection of a tumor and chest wall or carina results in a significant 5-year survival.[6,13] The present author believes that there is a role for surgery in some patients with metastasis to mediastinal nodes (N_2) but, as discussed in detail in Chapter 15, patient selection is critical and dependent on precise staging.

Although the principle of conservation of lung tissue is important, especially when operating on patients with marginal pulmonary reserve, all identifiable disease must be encompassed by the resection or the patient will not benefit; that is, the value of debulking operations is nil. The operating surgeon must therefore be familiar with the techniques of segmental lung resection, bronchial and carinal sleeve resection, and chest wall resection to ensure that a complete operation can be carried out even in patients with marginal reserve and/or locally advanced disease.

Operative morbidity and mortality have been decreased by advances in surgical technique, such as use of a stapling device on the bronchus, anesthetic management, and postoperative support. Morbidity is usually due to pulmonary complications so that postthoracotomy supportive efforts should be focused on the lung. Appropriate surgical mortality for the "average risk" patient, determined by review of multiple surgical experiences, should be about 3 percent following lobectomy and 7 percent for pneumonectomy.[4]

POSTOPERATIVE CONSIDERATIONS

The priority concern in the immediate postoperative period is the continuing function of the patient's remaining pulmonary tissue. Regardless of the starting point, some pulmonary reserve is lost and any further embarrassment of lung function may not be tolerated. Accordingly, early and continuing efforts are directed toward reexpanding bronchoalveolar units that have collapsed during the operation and maintaining their expansion. In physiologic terms, this means maintaining the functional residual capacity; this translates into less right-to-left shunt, better oxygenation, and less work of breathing. Techniques that maximize inspiratory efforts work best and include incentive spirometry and glottic and carinal stimulation with a transnasal catheter. Intravenous fluid therapy should be appropriate for the patient's cardiovascular and renal function; aggressive fluid restriction to "keep the patient dry" is inappropriate, as patients seem to be no more prone to interstitial fluid accumulation in the lung than at any other time, and this strategy may be harmful to other organ systems.[8] A Swan-Ganz catheter should be inserted into the pulmonary artery in patients with compromised cardiac function or in whom the clinical assessment of the intravascular volume status is unclear to ensure optimum monitoring of left heart filling pressures during fluid replacement.

Long-term follow-up includes monitoring for recurrence or development of second lung cancers and administration of adjuvant therapy to selected patients. The ideal setting for these endeavors is a joint clinic attended by surgical, medical, and radiation therapy oncologists. This, especially in conjunction with a prospective (i.e., pretherapy) multimodality group approach to therapy avoids the tendency to sequester patients by any one therapeutic group. The frequency with which patients should be followed is based on the fact that more than 75 percent of recurrences are within the first year and essentially all within 2 years.[9] Patients can develop second lung cancers, however, even if they stop smoking, as late as 10 years after their resection. These are important to detect in an early stage as many patients can undergo a curative re-resection. Follow-up should therefore be intensive for the first year and less frequent thereafter but should continue indefinitely on a yearly basis. In the absence of new symptoms or physical findings, a CXR is the only clearly necessary follow-up examination. CT and gallium scanning provide more information and occasionally can identify an early, presymptomatic recurrence,[5] but since treatment is likely to be ineffective until more efficacious chemotherapy agents are available, their benefit is of marginal importance.

REFERENCES

1. American Thoracic Society: Clinical staging of primary lung cancer. Am Rev Respir Dis 127:659-664, 1983
2. Cooper CD, Pearson FG, Todd TR, et al: Radiotherapy alone for patients with operable carcinoma of the lung. Chest 87:289-292, 1985
3. Ferguson MK, MacMahon H, Little AG, et al: The regional accuracy of computerized tomography of the mediastinum in lung cancer staging. J Thorac Cardiovasc Surg 91:498-504, 1986
4. Ginsberg RJ, Hill LD, Eagan RT, et al: Modern 30-day operative mortality for surgical resections in lung cancer. J Thorac Cardiovasc Surg 86:654-658, 1983
5. Hatfield MK, MacMahon H, Ryan JW, et al: Postoperative recurrence of lung cancer: Detection by whole-body gallium scintigraph. Am J Radiol 147:911-915, 1986
6. Jensik RJ, Faber LP, Kittle CF, et al: Survival in patients undergoing tracheal sleeve pneumonectomy for bronchogenic carcinoma. J Thorac Cardiovasc Surg 84:489-496, 1982
7. Kies MS, Baker AW, Kennedy PS: Radionuclide scans in staging of carcinoma of the lung. Surg Gynecol Obstet 147:175-176, 1978
8. Lee E, Little A, Hsu WH, et al: Effect of pneumonectomy on extravascular lung water in dogs. J Surg Res 38:568-573, 1985
9. Little AG, DeMeester TR, Ferguson MK, et al: Modified stage I ($T_1N_0M_0$, $T_2N_0M_0$) non-small cell lung cancer: Treatment results, recurrence patterns and adjuvant immunotherapy. Surgery 100:621-628, 1986
10. Little AG, DeMeester TR, Kirchner PT, et al: Guided biopsies of abnormalities on nuclear bone scans: Technique and indications. J Thorac Cardiovasc Surg 85:396-403, 1983
11. Little AG, DeMeester TR, MacMahon H: The staging of lung cancer. Semin Oncol 10:56-70, 1983
12. Martini N, Flehinger BJ, Zaman MB, et al: Results of resection in non-oat cell carcinoma of the lung with mediastinal lymph node metastases. Ann Thorac Surg 198:386-397, 1983
13. McGaughan BC, Martini N, Bains MS, et al: Chest wall invasion in carcinoma of the lung. Therapeutic and prognostic implications. J Thorac Cardiovasc Surg 89:836-841, 1985
14. Modini C, Passariello R, Iascone C, et al: TNM staging in lung cancer: Role of computed tomography. J Thorac Cardiovasc Surg 84:569-574, 1982
15. Wernly JA, DeMeester TR, Kirchner PT, et al: Clinical value of quantitative ventilation-perfusion lung scans in the surgical management of bronchogenic carcinoma. J Thorac Cardiovasc Surg 80:535-543, 1980

Ralph R. Weichselbaum
Azhar M. Awan

5

Principles of Radiation Oncology

In this chapter we delineate the principles of radiation physics and biology and discuss their importance in the management of lung cancer.

RADIATION PHYSICS

As the energy and penetrating power of ionizing radiation increases, the photon wave length decreases. Therefore, understanding the properties of varying energies of radiation is critical to optimal radiotherapy. Radiation dosages exceeding 500 kilovolts (kV) is designated as supervoltage. Important advantages are seen when radiation reaches 500 kV because there is reduced absorption in bone, less damage to skin at portal entry, and decreased scatter of radiation into adjacent tissues. The importance of using supravoltage radiation in the treatment of deep seated tumors such as lung cancer is that skin tolerance does not limit the dose delivered. The maximal ionization with supravoltage radiation occurs below the level of the epidermis. The percentage of radiation at a specific depth compared with the maximal electron buildup (0.5-2 cm below the skin) increases as energy increases. Radiation between 140 and 500 kV is termed *orthovoltage*, and radiation between 50 and 140 kV is designated as superficial radiation. These energies may be useful in the treatment of skin cancer or other superficial tumors. In the treatment of carcinoma of the lung, however, supervoltage radiation should be used exclusively.

Radiation may be closely applied to tumors by means of implanting radioactive material directly into and adjacent to the tumor. "Interstitial radiation" refers to the application of removable sources such as radium, ^{60}Co, and ^{192}Ir or of nonremovable sources such as radon or radioactive gold, which are inserted directly into the tumor. Interstitial implantation of radioactive gold has found use in unresectable lung cancer as well as lung cancer resected with microscopically positive margins.

Treatment planning is essential for radiotherapy and depends on anatomic guidelines for tumor localization. In lung cancer, this may include tomograms, computerized tomography (CT), and newer modalities such as nuclear magnetic resonance (NMR)

LUNG CANCER: A COMPREHENSIVE TREATISE
ISBN 0-8089-1876-1

imaging. Treatment planning insures that a tumor will receive an optimal radiation dose and that the normal tissue will receive as little dose as possible. Reproducibility of daily setup is necessary to assure accuracy of treatments. This is achieved by minute skin tatoos as well as weekly portal films that are compared to original planning films.

Interaction of Ionizing Radiation with Matter

Ionizing radiation interacts with molecules and causes ionization and excitation of atoms. In an excited atom, electrons are shifted to different orbits and become chemically reactive. In ionization, orbiting electrons are ejected from atoms, leaving free radicals that cause breakage of chemical bonds and biological effects. Charged particles such as electrons or protons are directly ionizing with sufficient energy to break chemical bonds, and x-rays and γ-rays are indirectly ionizing and produce a secondary electron with high kinetic energy that break chemical bonds. Neutrons do this by interacting with cellular nuclei and thereby create a direct biological effect.

Linear energy transfer (LET) refers to the energy that is transferred per unit length in the absorbing material. This is usually designed as kiloelectron volt (keV) per micron of unit density of the absorbing material. Typical LET values are as follows: ^{60}Co γ-rays, 0.3 keV per micrometer; 250-keV x-rays, 2 keV per micrometer; 14-MeV neutrons, 12 keV per micrometer. Differences in LET account for the fact that although various types of radiation generally produce qualitatively similar effects initially, there are marked quantitative differences as well as differences in biological effects. This is due to dissimilarity in proximity of ionization and the influence of secondary electrons. Equal doses of different types of ionizating radiation do not produce equal biological effects. It is customary to express the relative biological effectiveness (RBE) of some test radiation compared with 250-keV x-rays used as the standard. The relative biological effectiveness is the ratio of the dose of 250-keV x-rays to the test radiation for an equal biological effect.

Many of the ionization and excitation properties of radiation depend on molecular oxygen. Although the exact mechanism of oxygen as a dose modifying agent is not completely agreed on, it is thought to act at the level of free-radical formation. It has been noted by many investigators that many cells are resistant to radiation in the absence of oxygen. This is because when no oxygen is present, chemical reactions involving free radicals do not take place and many ionized target molecules can repair or recover from inability to function normally. The ratio of hypoxic to aerated doses needed to achieve the same biological effect is the same at all surviving levels because oxygen is said to be a dose-modifying agent. This ratio is called the *oxygen-enhancement ratio* (OER).[3]

BIOLOGICAL ASPECTS OF RADIATION ONCOLOGY

Radiosensitivity, Radiocurability and Radioresponsiveness

The term *radiosensitive* refers to the inverse of the slope of the radiation survival curve (D_0) when survival data are plotted as a logarithm of cell surviving fraction versus a linear plot of dose. The extrapolation number ($\bar{n}$) is a measure of the initial shoulder of the radiation survival curve and is obtained by back-extrapolation of the linear portion of the curve to the ordinate. The width of the shoulder is a measure of the ability of cells to accumulate and repair sublethal x-ray injury (Fig. 5-1).[3]

Radiocurability is a clinical term that refers to whether a tumor is locally controlled by a maximum tolerable dose of radiation. *Radioresponsiveness* refers to regression after radiation treatment, but not necessarily to whether a tumor is radiocurable. For example, carcinoma of the prostate regresses slowly, probably because it is characterized by a slowly proliferating cell renewal system. Local control rates for early-stage prostate cancer are high (over 75 percent); therefore, prostate cancer is considered a radiocurable tumor. Conversely, oat cell carcinoma of the lung may regress rapidly after delivery of relatively low doses of radiation, yet if inadequate doses are delivered, local control rates may be very poor. Therefore, oat cell carcinoma is a radioresponsive yet not necessarily radiocurable lesion. This must be taken into account when curative treatment regimens are proposed.

The radiobiological definition of death is inability to reproduce. Until cell division occurs, radiation induced lethality may not be expressed and some cells may appear to be morphologically viable. Cells destined to die may actually undergo several generations of progeny before the original cell as well as all daughter cells die. Therefore, clinicians should not be misled by positive biopsies obtained at inappropriately early time intervals after radiation therapy or by slow tumor regression.

Cell Cycle Effects

The lethal effects of radiation are cell-cycle-specific (Fig. 5-2). With the use of synchronized cells, the effects of radiation at different stages of cell cycle may be studied. These effects vary from cell line to cell line, although some general observation may be made: (1) cells are more sensitive at or near mitosis; (2) if the G-1 (pre-DNA synthetic gap) is appreciable in length, a resistant period may be seen early

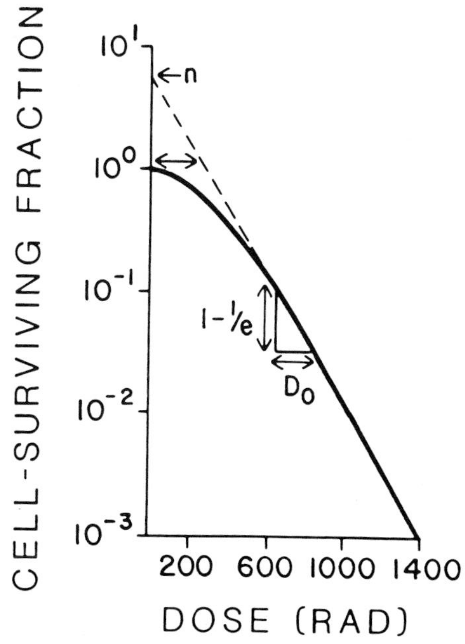

Fig. 5-1. Radiation survival curve, the proportion of surviving cells as a function of radiation dose, is shown. The shoulder depicted by the arrow is the ability of cells to repair sublethal radiation injury (see text). (From Hall EJ: Radiobiology for the Radiologist (ed 2). New York: Harper and Row, 1978. With permission.)

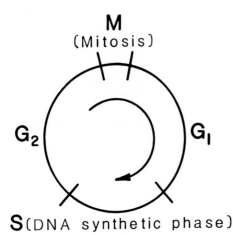

Fig. 5-2. Schematic of cell cycle. M = mitosis; G-1 = pre-DNA synthetic phase; S = DNA synthesis phase; G-2 = H premitotic phase. (From Hall EJ: Radiobiology for the Radiologist (ed 2). New York: Harper and Row, 1978. With permission.)

followed by a decline in survival toward S (period of DNA synthesis); (3) the end of G-1 may be as sensitive as M (mitosis) (in many cell lines, resistance increases during S and reaches a maximum and during the latter part of S; which usually is the most resistant part of the cycle); and (4) in most cell lines, G-2 (premitotic gap) is as sensitive as M (Fig. 5-3). The cell cycle distribution in a tumor may affect radiocurability.[7]

Repair

The threshold of response implies that damage must be accumulated in a cell before it loses reproductive integrity. A cell may have received an ionizing lesion in some, but not all, of its critical sites and may have suffered sublethal damage; that is, it may have been damaged but not killed. The cell may repair the effects of sublethal damage and recover completely. Repair of sublethal damage SLDR has been extensively studied by Elkind and his colleagues,[1] who introduced a technique by which the effect of exposure to a single dose of radiation was compared to the effect of exposure to the total dose provided at equal fractions. Figure 5-4 shows an increase in survival between fractions. This is a complex function with an enhancement, decrement, and second enhancement in survival. This is because radiation lethality and repair are cell-

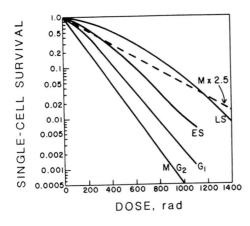

Fig. 5-3. Single cell survival as a function of cycle cell and radiation dose. (From Hall EJ: Radiobiology for the Radiologist (ed 2). New York: Harper and Row, 1978. With permission.)

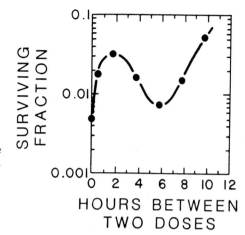

Fig. 5-4. Surviving fraction of Chinese hampster ovarian cells over time after exposure to two doses of radiotherapy (see text). (From Hall EJ: Radiobiology for the Radiologist (ed 2). New York: Harper and Row, 1978. With permission.)

cycle-specific. For example, in the case of Chinese hampster ovarian (CHO) cells shown in Fig. 5-4, the majority of survivors are located in the S phase of the cycle. If a period of time is allowed to elapse before a second dose is given, this group of initially exposed cells may progress around the period of the cell cycle. If the increase in radiosensitivity moving from S to late G-2 exceeds the repair of sublethal damage, the surviving fraction falls. The pattern shown in Figure 5-4 thus is a combination of two processes: (1) the repair of sublethal damage and (2) progression through the cell cycle. The enhancement in surviving fraction after 200 rads daily treatment due to sublethal damage repair over 30 treatment fractions may be very large since the survival after each dose is magnified to an exponent equal to the number of fractions (Table 5-1).[11]

Potentially lethal damage is operationally defined as damage that becomes lethal if it is not repaired. Environmental conditions after exposure to x-rays can influence cell survival. The fraction of cells surviving after a dose of radiation may be increased or decreased, therefore, depending on the nature of the postradiation condition. If survival after a dose of radiation is increased, it can be interpreted to mean that potentially lethal damage has been repaired. If survival is decreased, this can be interpreted that potentially lethal damage has been expressed. Repair of potentially

Table 5-1

Calculated Cumulative Survival Fraction

Survival Fraction*	x^{32} $x =$	x^{20} $x =$
10^{-11}	0.45	0.28
10^{-10}	0.49	0.32
10^{-9}	0.52	0.35
10^{-8}	0.56	0.40
10^{-7}	0.60	0.45
10^{-6}	0.65	0.50

*Calculated cumulative survival fraction for either 32 or 20 equal fractions when the fractional survival is varied.

lethal damage (PLDR) is shown in Figure 5-5. Repair of potentially lethal x-ray damage has been shown to occur both in vitro and in vivo and predominantly in noncycling cells. The effects of PLDR may be greatest in larger tumors with a small growth fraction and a large component of noncycling cells.[4]

A variety of investigators have studied in vitro radiosensitivity and ability to repair sublethal and potentially lethal x-ray damage in human tumors. For some histologic types, a large n (ability to accumulate and repair sublethal x-ray injury) has been found, whereas other histologic subtypes have been found to vary in inherent radioresistance and/or potentially lethal damage repair.

Most models for investigation for the repair of x-ray damage include the repair of DNA strandbreaks. This is studied by alkaline sucrose gradient centrifugation as well as the alkaline elution technique. There is general agreement that under physiologic conditions, most single-strand breaks are repaired; therefore, many investigators postulate that double-stranded breaks are the critical lesion that leads to the loss of reproductive activity in the cell. Another type of DNA lesion produced by ionizing radiation is base damage. The role of base damage in cell killing is unknown and may be more important for radiation induced mutagenesis and perhaps carcinogenesis rather than actual cell kill.

Hypoxic Cells in Radiation Oncology

Thomlinson and Gray studied thin sections of human lung tumors and showed necrotic areas surrounded by intact tumor cells.[9] No tumor cord that had a radius of more than 200 μm was without a necrotic center. Also, as the necrotic area increased, width of tumor cells remained relatively constant at 100–150 μm. Tumor cells could grow only if they were in close proximity to oxygen. Thomlinson and Gray concluded that oxygen concentration falls off with increasing distance from the capillary and thus that a group of radioresistant hypoxic cells might exist (Fig. 5-6). These hypoxic cells might render a tumor radioincurable since it has been shown that hypoxia may render cells resistant to ionizing radiation because molecular oxygen is important for free radical formation (Fig. 5-7).[9]

The use of electron affinic agents specific for hypoxic cells is an important area of research in clinical radiation oncology. These studies have progressed from develop-

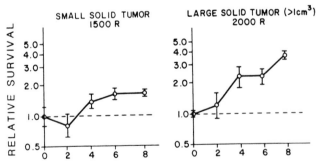

Fig. 5-5. Proportion of surviving cells over time after exposure to radiation therapy (dose shown). The repair of potentially lethal damage (PLDR) is greatest in large tumors. (From Hall EJ: Radiobiology for the Radiologist (ed 2). New York: Harper and Row, 1978. With permission.)

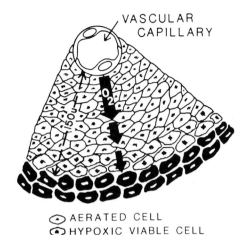

VASCULAR
CAPILLARY

Fig. 5-6. Schematic representation of a tumor in close proximity to a vascular capillary. The hypoxic and anoxic cells are depicted as shown. (From Hall EJ: Radiobiology for the Radiologist (ed 2). New York: Harper and Row, 1978. With permission.)

⊙ AERATED CELL
◉ HYPOXIC VIABLE CELL
● ANOXIC NECROTIC CELL

ments in radiation chemistry to clinical experimentation. The nitroimidazoles are efficient in sensitizing hypoxic tumor cells to the effects of radiation in experimental animals and currently are under clinical investigation. Use of high-LET radiation, which is not as dependent on molecular oxygen for production of free radical as is sparsely ionizing radiation, is also under clinical investigation to circumvent the problem of hypoxic tumor cells. Examples of high-LET radiation under clinical investigation are neutrons and stripped nuclei.

Reoxygenation of tumors may also be important in radiotherapy. In animal tumor systems, it has been determined that the proportion of hypoxic cells following various fractionated radiation treatments are the same at the end of fractionated radiotherapy as in the untreated tumor. This has been interpreted as evidence that during the course of radiation treatment, cells move from the hypoxic to the well-oxygenated component of the tumor since the proportion of hypoxic cells would increase during the course of fractionated radiation if this did not occur. This is because radiation would depopulate the more radiosensitive aerated compartment more than the hypoxic compartment. Therefore, many investigators have postulated that reoxygenation (or lack of reoxygenation) is important in human tumor radiotherapy.[10]

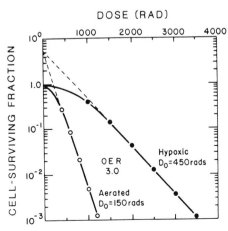

Fig. 5-7. The radiation survival curves for areated versus hypoxic tumors. The hypoxic tumors have a greater shoulder on the radiation curve (see text). (From Hall EJ: Radiobiology for the Radiologist (ed 2). New York: Harper and Row, 1978. With permission.)

Normal tissue Effects

Normal tissue reactions to radiation are related to the volume of tissue irradiated, the overall time of administration of treatment, the daily amount of radiation administered at each session (fraction size), and the total dose of radiation. Acute reactions develop as a consequence of radiation damage to proliferating cell renewal systems and, therefore, are most noticeable in tissues with rapidly proliferating cell renewal systems. These include the mucosal lining of the oral cavity and the lining of the gastrointestinal tract. A specific example of acute reactions is mucositis in the pharynx, which occurs because the destruction of cells in the basal layer exceeds their production.

In the treatment of lung cancer with ionizing radiation, acute reactions may develop in the skin, the mucosal lining of the tracheobronchial tree, the esophagus, the pericardium, and, of course, the lung parenchyma itself. With the use of supervoltage radiation equipment and multiple treatment fields, acute reactions of the skin are not dose-limiting. Esophagitis develops at approximately 3000 rads, causing dysphagia. Although esophagitis rarely is dose-limiting, most patients can maintain adequate nutrition with a change in dietary habits such as consuming softer food and even liquid diets. Acute pericarditis can develop secondary to irradiation if the whole heart or significant portions of the heart are in the treatment field. With good treatment planning, however, much of the heart can be shielded from high-dose irradiation.

The lung parenchyma itself can be a dose-limiting factor in the treatment of lung cancer with irradiation. The effects of irradiation on lung parenchyma are evident in the first 24 hours after exposure to radiation with resultant congestion and intra-alveolar edema. There is exudation of proteinacious material into the alveoli, leading to impairment of gas exchange. In a few weeks the interstitial edema organizes into collagen fibriles, which eventually lead to thickening of the alveolar septa. These changes may resolve over the source of a few weeks to a few months. However, depending on the volume of lung parenchyma irradiated, the total dose delivered to the lung parenchyma and the dose per fraction used, these pathological changes can result in a syndrome known as *acute radiation pneumonitis*. Usually this is manifested 6–24 weeks after the initiation of radiation therapy but can occur earlier or at a later time interval. The signs and symptoms of the acute radiation pneumonitis syndrome are dyspnea, low-grade fever, chest pain that usually is pleuritic, and a dry cough. If greater than 75 percent of the total lung parenchyma is irradiated in excess of 4500 rads, the acute radiation pneumonitis can be very severe and produce acute respiratory distress with the patient experiencing spiking temperatures and acute cor pulmonale that can lead to death. The radiation injury can be manifest on radiographic examination with a diffuse infiltrate appearing on chest x-ray that corresponds to the radiation field. These radiographic changes can occur even in an asymptomatic patient. In most cases, the pneumonitis will resolve clinically and radiographically, leading to no residual pulmonary problems.[6]

The higher the total radiation dose, the greater the lung parenchymal volume treated; and the higher the dose per fraction, the greater the incidence of penumonitis will be. The experience with whole lung irradiation, especially in bone marrow transplant patients from the Seattle group, has led to some understanding of lung tolerance. Of 27 patients who received a single fraction of 1000 rads to both lungs, 26 percent developed clinical pneumonitis. It should be noted that the dose rate employed in the bone marrow transplant studies is considerably lower than those employed in the treatment of lung cancer. In 26 patients who received 1200 rads to both lungs in six fractions of 200 rads each, the incidence of pneumonitis was 15 percent.[2] A 5 percent pneumonitis risk exists in patients given whole lung irradiation at 180 rads per fraction to a total dose of 1800 rads. Of course, in the treatment of lung cancer, radiation is not given to both lungs and high-dose radiation is given to considerably less volume than whole lung irradiation. Doses used can vary from 5000 to 6500 rads to the tumor. However, there are no reliable clinical data to predict what total dose can be given to what percentage of lung parenchyma and not produce clinical radiation pneumonitis. Radiation treatment planning should be meticulous to ensure that as little volume of normal lung is irradiated in a protracted radiation schedule over 5-7 weeks.

In contrast to the acute reaction, the chronic effects of radiation are observed from months to years following treatment. The mechanism of chronic complications is thought to be related to the effects of radiation on the vascular and endothelial cells or the effects on somatic cells of the organ at risk. Each organ has a unique radiation tolerance, and thus a combination of vascular damage and somatic cell damage may be important in the development of late radiation injury.

The chronic phase of lung injury can occur without a prior history of an acute radiation pneumonitis. The late lung injury is characterized by progressive fibrosis of alveolar septa with the septa being thickened by bundles of elastic fibers. The alveoli collapse and are obliterated by connective tissue. These changes can lead to the radiographic appearance of lung scarring on chest radiography, which corresponds to the shape of the radiation portal. Eventually, the previously irradiated lung can develop dense fibrotic nodules, especially in the area of previous tumor.[5]

The clinical symptomatology of such changes is proportional to the extent of the lung parenchyma involved. There is very minimal symptomatology when the late radiation fibrosis is limited to less than 50 percent of one lung. If the volume involved increases above this limit, however, dyspnea may manifest clinically and progressive chronic cor pulmonale leading to right heart failure may occur. In most cases, however, the lung parenchyma injury is not very great and patients usually become asymptomatic, with the fibrotic changes stabilizing about 1 year after completion of irradiation.

Late lung fibrosis occurs after radiation injury to the type II pneumocyte. The lack of type II pneumocytes results in the loss of surfactant, which is necessary for the integrity of the alveolus. The alveolus eventually collapses and the former alveolar spaces are replaced by fibrotic tissue. In addition, the endothelial damage of the fine vessels in the alveolus results in fibrotic changes in the blood vessels.[8]

Although tolerance doses may be exceeded, not all patients will develop complications since the likelihood of complications is a probability event. This probability is balanced against the probability of tumor control, allowing the radiation oncologist to decide on the dose that will be likely to control the tumor or having an estimate of the risk of normal tissue damage produced by the dose employed. Successful therapy requires an adequate dose of radiation, but the dose that can be employed is limited by the complications (acute and long-term) of the time/dose relationship selected. A graphic example of this shows the probability of tumor control and the probability of major complications against radiation dose (Fig. 5-8). The curves are sigmoid, indicating steep dose-response relationships for both tumor control and complications, and

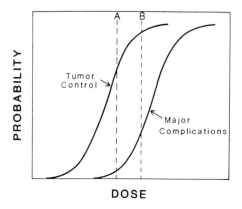

Fig. 5-8. Graphic representation of radiation benefit/toxicity curves as a function of dose. The points between A and B represent the narrow therapeutic window at which radiation therapy dose will lead to a high degree of tumor control and a relatively low complication rate. Beyond B, the control rate increases slightly but at the expense of major complications.

the separation between the tumor control curve and the complication curve usually is small. Increasing radiation dose will increase the probability of tumor control, therefore, but it will also increase the likelihood of significant radiation damage to the tissues.

REFERENCES

1. Elkind MM, Sutton GH, Moses WB, et al: Radiation response of mammalian cells in culture V. Temperature dependence of the repair of x-ray damage in surviving cells. Rad Res 25:359-376, 1965
2. Fajardo L-G: Respiratory system, in Pathology of Radiation Injury, New York, Masson, 1982, chapter 4
3. Hall EJ: Radiobiology for the Radiobiologist, 2d ed. Hagerstown, MD, Harper and Row, 1978
4. Little JB, Hahn GM, Frindell E, et al: Repair of potentially lethal radiation damage in vivo and in vitro. Radiology 106:689-694, 1973
5. Rubin P: The Franz Busche Lecture: Late effects of chemotherapy and radiation therapy: A new hypothesis. Internatl J Radiat Oncol Biol Phys 10:5-34, 1984
6. Rubin P, Casarett GW: Respiratory system, in Clinical Radiation Pathology, vol ii. Philadelphia, Saunders, 1968, chapter 12
7. Sinclair WK: Cyclic x-ray responses in mammalian cells in vitro. Rad Res 33:620-643, 1968
8. Thomas ED, Clift RA, Hersman J, et al: Marrow transplantation for acute nonlymphoblastic leukemia in first remission using fractionated or single dose irradiation. Internatl J Radiat Oncol Biol Phys 8:817-821, 1982
9. Thomlinson H, Gray L: The histological structure of some human lung cancers and the possible implications for radiotherapy. Br J Cancer 9:539-549, 1955
10. van Putten LM: Tumor reoxygenation during fractionated radiotherapy. Studies with a transplantable osteosarcoma. Eur J Cancer 4:173-182, 1968
11. Weichselbaum RR: The role of DNA repair processes in the response of human tumors to fractionated radiotherapy. Internatl J Radiat Biol Oncol Phys 110:112-124, 1984

Jacob D. Bitran
Harvey M. Golomb

6

Principles of Medical Oncology

The subspecialty of medical oncology integrates the medical care of the cancer patient with the knowledge of antineoplastic chemotherapeutic agents. Thus the medical oncologist must be a knowledgeable clinician, chemotherapist, and an expert in supportive care.

The use of chemicals to treat disease dates back to the early part of this century, when Dr. Paul Erlich found that arsenicals could be used to treat syphilis.[38] In fact, it was Dr. Erlich who coined the term "chemotherapy." Research in chemotherapy was limited to antimicrobials with the discovery of sulfanilamide, penicillin, and streptomycin in the 1930s. With the introduction of streptomycin for the treatment of tuberculosis, resistant strains developed to this antimicrobial. One could delay the emergence of resistant strains by using two or three effective antituberculosis drugs.[26]

The foundation of medical oncology as a subspecialty began with the pioneering work of Goodman and Gilman, who investigated nitrogen mustard, a derivative of mustard gas, and Saul Farber and his coworkers, who initiated clinical trials in acute leukemias with the antifol, aminopterin.[21] Since the 1960s, the number of currently available antineoplastic chemotherapeutics has rapidly grown. There are currently 50-60 drugs in clinical use and 2-3 times that amount in either preclinical screening or undergoing clinical investigation.

It is beyond the scope of this chapter to review all the aspects of medical care for the cancer patient. Complications of cancer therapy and supportive care are reviewed at great length in Chapter 27. Rather, the intent of this section is to review the biology of tumor growth, the principles involving the use of chemotherapeutic agents, and the pharmacology of some of the frequently used chemotherapeutic drugs.

BIOLOGIC PRINCIPLES OF CANCER

While the exact etiology of cancer is not clearly defined, several mechanisms can cause malignant transformation. Presumed etiologic agents that can initiate malignant transformation include genetic instability, viruses, chemicals, ultraviolet irradiation, ionizing radiation, immune deficiency, chronic inflammation, and parasites.[42]

It is well established that viruses can cause malignant tumors in animals; examples include murine leukemia virus, the feline leukemia virus, and avian leukosis virus. All of these viruses belong to the *Oncorna* group of viruses and are RNA viruses. Human viruses that have been linked to human neoplasia include herpes virus type II (cervical carcinoma), cytomegalovirus (Kaposi's sarcoma), Epstein-Barr virus (Burkett's lymphoma and nasopharyngeal carcinoma),[41] and human T-cell lymphotrophic retrovirus (HTLV-I, T-cell malignant lymphoma).[25]

The retroviruses and, in particular, HTLV-I induces neoplasia by the incorporation of the viral genome directly into the DNA of the infected cell. This is done by reverse transcriptase, an enzyme present in retroviruses that can make a DNA copy of the viral RNA genome. The severely transformed cells lose the regulatory mechanisms that govern cellular growth and differentiation.[25]

Since 1775, when Sir Percival Pott described scrotal cancer in chimney sweeps, chemical exposure has been a known cause of cancer. Known carcinogens in humans include aromatic hydrocarbons and amines, alkylating agents, tobacco and wood products, nickel, asbestos, chromates, thorium dioxide, seneco alkaloids, aflatoxin, diethylstilbestrol, and oxymetholone.[52] The presumed mechanism of action of carcinogens such as aromatic hydrocarbons, aromatic amines, and alkylating agents is the generation of the highly reactive "carbonium ion" and other oxidants.[52] These oxidants subsequently cause DNA damage that, if sublethal, will cause cellular transformation.

Factors that influence chemical carcinogenesis include age, sex, endocrine status, and immunologic status. In central Africa, aflatoxin is linked to hepatocellular carcinoma; however, while both men and women are exposed to aflatoxin, the incidence of hepatocellular carcinoma is 4–5 times greater in men.

Radiation exposure, both ionizing and ultraviolet, plays an unequivocal role in the etiology of cancer.[1] Incidence studies show an increase in basal cell carcinoma, squamous cell carcinoma, and melanoma in the southern half of the United States. Similar incidence studies performed on atomic bomb survivors in Hiroshima and Nagasaki show an increased risk of acute and chronic leukemia.[7] Similarly, when ionizing radiation was used to treat benign diseases such as facial acne or ankylosing spondylitis, the incidence of cancer is increased in the treated population. The malignancies induced by radiation therapy include acute and chronic leukemias,[7,35] malignant lymphoma (Hodgkin's and non-Hodgkin's), multiple myeloma, myelofibrosis, thyroid cancer,[43] and salivary gland cancer. Uranium mine workers have a higher incidence of lung cancer after 15–20 years of chronic exposure.

Chronic skin trauma can lead to chronic dermatitis and ultimately to squamous cell carcinoma of the skin. Parasites such as *Schistosoma haematobuim* and *Clonorchiasis sinensis* have been linked to bladder cancer and carcinoma of the pancreas and bile ducts, respectively.

THE BIOLOGY OF CANCER

The properties that are characteristic of cancer cells include unregulated cellular growth and the ability to cause local tissue invasion and metastases. These unique properties are found in all malignant cells. The complex molecular biology that leads to malignant transformation is not well understood; yet as a result of increasing research in molecular biology, some insights into the molecular events causing malignant transformation are emerging.

A cancer always arises from a single clone of transformed cells.[56] The injection of a *single* malignant clonogenic cell can ultimately lead to the death of the host animal; the larger the number of clonogenic cells injected, the shorter the survival of the host animal. While there is often phenotypic heterogeneity in any malignant neoplasm, genotypically a cancer is a clonal growth. This theory is supported by the nonrandom chromosomal abnormalities found in patients with cancers.[56] Patients with chronic myelogenous leukemia (CML) have been found to have a unique chromosomal abnormality, the Philadelphia chromosome, which represents a translocation of the long arm of chromosome 22 to chromosome 9. This unique and consistent chromosomal abnormality is found in approximately 80 percent of patients with CML. Patients with CML and a Philadelphia chromosome have a better overall prognosis than do patients with CML and an absent Philadelphia chromosome. The observation of only a *single* glucose-6-phosphate dehydrogenase (G-6-PD) isoenzyme present in red blood cells and white blood cells of patients with CML further supports the clonal origin of this cancer. Fibroblasts from these patients contain both G-6-PD isoenzymes. There is tumor cell heterogeneity in cancer despite their clonal origin. In mice with B-16 melanoma, certain tumor cells have the capacity to metastasize selectively to the lung while others do not.[22] Cell suspensions prepared from a single human cancer nodule characteristically have populations of cells sensitive to chemotherapeutic agents as well as resistant cell populations.[50]

Chromosomal analysis of cancer cells can provide prognostic and at times therapeutic information. Patients with acute myelogenous leukemia and a normal karotypic analysis have a better overall prognosis than do those with abnormal karotypes.[28] Patients with a 15/17 chromosome translocation always have acute promyelocytic leukemia; identification of a patient with acute promyelocytic leukemia is important as typically these patients have a bleeding diathesis (disseminated intravascular coagulation) that requires heparin therapy.[28,29] Patients with promyelocytic leukemia require aggressive chemotherapy and supportive care as they are potentially curable.

Cellular Kinetics

All human cells capable of replication such as the bone marrow and gastrointestinal tract enter the cell cycle (Fig. 6-1).[55] Many of the currently available chemotherapeutic drugs require cells to be in cycle (cycle-specific) or work only during a specific phase of the cell cycle (phase-specific). The cell cycle is characterized by a resting phase, G_0. Cells can then enter into cycle G_1, which is a variable pre-DNA synthetic phase. The G_1 phase may be as short as 12 hours and as long as a few days. The next phase is a phase of DNA synthesis, S phase, which usually lasts 4-6 hours. The G_2 phase, a short post-DNA synthetic phase, follows the S phase. A tetraploid quantity of DNA is found within cells during the G_2 phase which lasts for 2-4 hours. Mitosis (M phase), follows G_2 and usually lasts for 1-2 hours. The daughter cells then either enter a variable resting phase (G_0) or reenter the cellular cycle. The cell cycle may be as brief as 24 hours or may last for many days.[48] Cancer cells usually have a cell cycle of many

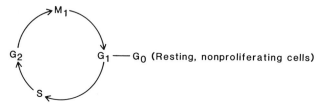

Fig. 6-1. The cell cycle. G_1 = Pre-DNA synthetic phase; S = DNA synthesis; G_2 = Post-DNA synthetic phase; M = Mitosis.

days. The generation time is the time it takes for malignant cells to enter the cycle and give rise to two daughter cells.[48]

A tumor may be thought of as having compartments of cells (Fig. 6-2). At any point in tumor growth, cells may be in cell cycle or resting and as shown in Figure 6-2.[18] Cells may move from a resting state into cell cycle and vice versa.[18] There are compartments of cells that may be resting—in a nonproliferative phase—and are incapable of ever entering into cell cycle. These cells constitute a nonproliferating compartment that accounts for tumor bulk. It is known from cell culture and animal data that small tumors have a greater percentage of cells in cycle and a greater proliferative capability. Alternatively, large tumors have fewer cells in cycle and a much lower proliferative activity.[47] Tumor growth occurs in a Gompertzian fashion; in other words, initially tumor growth is exponential, but this is followed by a plateau phase where cell death equals the rate of new daughter cells being formed (Fig. 6-3).[47]

Metastases

Cancer cells have the unique property of the ability to cause local tissue invasion and metastases. Local tissue invasion can result from tumor pressure on normal tissues that can, in turn, lead to inflammation, or the tumor may elaborate substances, such as collagenase, that lead to enzymatic destruction of normal tissues. Metastases can arise almost at the inception of a tumor.[22] Tumor cells are constantly shed into the circulation. By use of animal tumor models, it has been estimated that a 1-cm tumor will shed more than 1 million cells in the efferent venous circulation over 24 hours.[30] Circulating tumor cells have been identified in patients with early-stage breast cancer and colon cancer; however, the presence of circulating tumor cells in human malignancies does not correlate with early recurrence or limited survival. In fact, the statistical probability of a single circulating tumor cell becoming a metastatic nodule has been estimated to be a million to one.[30] Circulating tumor cells in animals usually die as a result of trauma sustained within the circulation. The longer the tumor cell spends in the circulation, the greater the chance of its death.

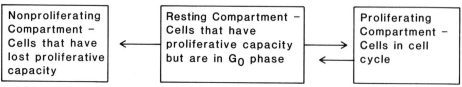

Fig. 6-2. Schematic representation of the "compartments" of cells within a malignant tumor mass.

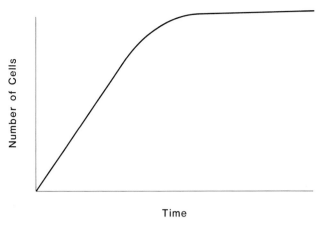

Fig. 6-3. A schematic of tumor growth as a function of time. The Gompertzian kinetics are exponential growth followed by a plateau phase.

Metastasis develops as a result of a single tumor cell or cells adhering to the vascular endothelium. As these cells grow, nutrients are provided by direct diffusion from the circulation. As tumor growth increases, local pressure and the elaboration of collagenase lead to the destruction of normal tissues; subsequently, the synthesis of tumor angiogenesis factor causes the formation of an independent vascular supply to the tumor nodule.

As a tumor continues to grow, cells are shed within the efferent circulation. Despite the fact that a majority of these cells die as a result of the circulatory trauma, a small quantity of tumor cells are capable of surviving the circulatory forces and trauma. These cells are then capable of starting an independent tumor nodule, a metastasis. The sequence of tumor growth is then resumed many times over. Thus both the primary tumor and metastases can lead to metastasis.[22]

Within an individual tumor, certain groups of cells will "home into" specific meta-static sites and not others; this homing quality has been shown in animal experiments using B-16 melanoma cells.[22] With proper cloning techniques, a line of B-16 mela-noma cells can be obtained that will preferentially metastasize only to the lung. As the number of metastases increases, metastatic nodules can themselves give rise to other metastases. Animal tumor experiments such as those with the B-16 melanoma cell line demonstrate that metastasis is not a random event. Studies with the same B-16 melanoma cell line also indicate that the primary tumor exerts an inhibitory effect on the growth of metastatic nodules. Clinicians have long observed that removal of the primary tumor will result in an explosion of metastases within a short period of time. In human hypernephroma, experimental evidence indicates a similar growth rate of the primary tumor and metastatic nodules as measured by the thymidine labeling index.

PRINCIPLES OF CANCER CHEMOTHERAPY

The ideal neoplastic chemotherapeutic agent is one that selectively destroys can-cer cells and has no toxic effects on the host's normal cells. Unfortunately, no such agent exists. Although many antineoplastic chemotherapeutics have a narrow therapeutic index, it is possible to use existing chemotherapeutic agents in the treatment of patients with cancer and to cure certain patients. In this section, the principles and pharmacology of antineoplastic chemotherapy is reviewed.

PRINCIPLES OF CHEMOTHERAPY

Cancer cells are more sensitive to chemotherapeutic agents than are normal cells.[18] Combinations of chemotherapeutic agents when used to treat a patient with cancer are more effective than a single agent or the sequential use of single agents.[18] Drugs employed in a combination chemotherapy regimen should be used at maximal dose and at a dose rate that is just long enough for the host to recover from toxic side effects but shorter than the doubling time of an individual tumor.[24] The importance of dose schedules is exemplified by the fact that in animal tumor models a twofold increase in dose can lead to a tenfold increase in cancer cell kill.[24] The dose-response curve to chemotherapeutic agents is steep and similar to the time for radiotherapy. The dose rate should be longer than the 8-10 days that is required for the host to recover from myelotoxicity yet shorter than the doubling time. Knowledge of these principles and their application has resulted in the formulation of combination regimens that have curative potential. The regimen adriamycin, bleomycin, vinblastine, and DTIC (ABVD) was formulated from four agents that are each individually effective in Hodgkin's disease and have no overlapping toxicities.[10] The ABVD regimen when used in full dose can lead to a 75 percent complete response rate in Hodgkin's Disease. The drugs in the ABVD combination have different mechanisms of action. Bleomycin, vinblastine, and DTIC are all phase- and cycle-specific, while adriamycin is neither. Finally, the toxicities of all four drugs in the ABVD regimen are all different.

The importance of employing drugs at maximal dose and at a constant interval *cannot* be overemphasized.[24] Most antineoplastic chemotherapeutic agents cause myelosuppression; however, bone marrow recovery usually occurs in 8-10 days. The treatment interval should be long enough for the host to recover from any toxicities yet shorter than the doubling time of the tumor. Each course of chemotherapy will cause a constant fractional cell kill. If a chemotherapeutic regimen causes a 90 percent cell kill with each course of administration, therefore, after 6 courses such a regimen will cause a 99.9999 percent cell kill of a malignant tumor.

Genetic Instability and Drug Resistance

It has been long appreciated that cancer cells are genetically unstable. This instability is frequently manifest by the appearance of karyotypic changes over time such as new marker chromosomes or chromosomal fragments (double minutes) and/or the appearance of novel proteins.[16,17,33] Because of this inherent genetic instability, cancer cells can quickly develop resistance to either ionizing radiation or chemotherapeutic agents. Mechanisms of antineoplastic drug resistance are as follows:

1. Pseudoresistance due to decreased plasma levels
    a. Decreased conversion of a prodrug into the active compound (6-mercaptopurine, liver disease)

    b. Increased degradation of an active drug (cytosine arabinoside–cytosine deaminase)

2. True cellular resistance

    a. Increased intracellular concentration of a target enzyme (methotrexate–dihydrofolate reductase)

    b. Decreased cellular requirements of a specific metabolic inhibitor (L-asparaginase–asparaginine)

    c. Increased energy-dependent drug efficiency due to altered cellular membrane (anthracyclines, vinca alkaloids, dactinomycin, epipodophyllotoxin derivatives–P-glycoprotein)

    d. Rapid DNA repair (ionizing radiation, alkylating agents)

The Coldman-Goldie hypothesis calculates the probability of spontaneous drug resistance as a function of time;[12,27] whereas initially 99.99 percent of the cancer cells may be entirely sensitive to a chemotherapeutic drug or regimen, after repeated exposure the percent of sensitive cells declines as resistant populations emerge.[12,27] According to the Coldman-Goldie hypothesis, brief exposure to a variety of chemotherapeutic agents or the use of non-cross-resistant regimens will lead to the delay of resistant clones of cancer cells and ultimately will cure the host. Clinical trials conducted in both Hodgkin's disease and multiple myeloma have proven the validity of this concept.[3,45]

PHARMACOLOGY OF ANTINEOPLASTIC CHEMOTHERAPEUTICS

Alkylating Agents[13]

Alkylating agents were the first compounds recognized to have therapeutic value in the treatment of human neoplasia. Many of the alkylating agents are chemically similar to mustard gas and have a chemical structure shown below and in Table 6-1.

$$R\text{———}N\diagdown\begin{matrix} CH_2CH_2Cl \\ \\ CH_2CH_2Cl \end{matrix}$$

Currently used alkylating agents include nitrogen mustard, cyclophosphamide, L-phenylalanine mustard, and chlorambucil. Alkylating agents are either electrophiles or generate electrophiles in vivo. Thus these agents attack electron-rich regions of molecules adding alkyl groups to oxygen, nitrogen, and sulfur. Proteins and nucleic acids within the cell are alkylated when exposed to such compounds. If DNA is alkylated, the single DNA strands that constitute the double helix are unable to uncoil and replicate themselves. This disruption of cellular metabolism ultimately leads to cellular death.

Nitrogen mustard is an active compound when administered intravenously; in contrast, cyclophosphamide is inert and must undergo metabolic conversion within the liver to its active forms, which are aldophosphamide and phosphamide mustard.

Table 6-1
Chemotherapeutic Agents

Mustards

$$R\text{-}N \begin{matrix} CH_2CH_2Cl \\ CH_2CH_2Cl \end{matrix}$$

Typical chemical structure of mustard compounds

R = substitution group

R = CH_3	Nitrogen mustard

R = O CH_2CH_2COOH	Chlorambucil

$$R = \text{O-}CH_2\text{-}CH_2 \begin{matrix} NH_2 \\ | \\ | \\ COOH \end{matrix}$$ L-Phenylalanine mustard

$$R = \begin{matrix} O & H \\ \| & | \\ P\text{——}N\text{-}CH_2 \\ \diagdown \qquad \diagup CH_2 \\ O\text{——}CH_2 \end{matrix}$$ Cyclophosphamide

Antimetabolites
Purine antagonists
  6-Mercaptopurine
  6-Thioguanine
Pyrimidine antagonists
  Cytosine arabinoside
  5-Fluouracil, 5-fluorodeoxyuridine
Folate antagonists
  Methotrexate
Plant alkaloids
  Vincas
    Vincristine
    Vinblastine
  Podophyllotoxins
    Etoposide
    Tenoposide
Antitumor antibiotics
  Intercalators of DNA
    Actinomycin-D
    Daunomycin and adriamycin
  Scission of DNA
    Bleomycin
  Covalent binding of DNA
    Mitomycin-C
Other agents
  Inorganic ions—*cis*-diamminedichloroplatinum II
Biologic-response modifiers
  Interferons
Enzymes
  L-Asparaginase
Endocrine therapy

The half-time of both nitrogen mustard and cyclophosphamide is approximately 15–20 minutes. These compounds are dependent on renal excretion for elimination.

Alkylating agents play an integral role in cancer chemotherapy and have activity in the treatment of Hodgkin's disease, the non-Hodgkin's lymphomas, multiple myeloma, chronic myelogenous leukemia, chronic lymphocytic leukemia, acute lymphoblastic leukemia, breast cancer, small cell cancer of the lung (SCLC), non-small cell lung cancer (NSCLC), and prostate cancer.

Toxicities of alkylating agents include nausea, vomiting, alopecia, hemorrhagic cystitis, leucopenia, thrombocytopenia, anemia, the syndrome of inappropriate ADH, and pulmonary fibrosis.

Antimetabolites

This broad category of antineoplastic chemotherapeutic drugs consists of purine antagonists, pyrimidine antagonists, and folate antagonists (Table 6-1). Antimetabolites are cycle- and phase-specific agents. They require cells to be in cell cycle and in the DNA synthetic phase (S phase) for these agents to promote their antitumor effects.

The purine antagonists 6-mercaptopurine and 6-thioguanine both inhibit de novo purine synthesis and the interconversion of purines.[20] Both drugs are administered orally and are dependent on renal excretion. Oral absorption is incomplete and variable. The major metabolites of 6-thioguanine is thiouric acid. 6-Mercaptopurine may undergo metabolic conversion to 6-thioguanine. These two purine antagonists play a role in the therapy of acute lymphocytic leukemia and acute nonlymphocytic leukemia. Toxicities include alopecia and myelosuppression.

The pyrimidine antagonists are cytosine arabinoside, 5-fluorouracil, and 5-fluorodeoxyuridine. All three drugs are administered parenterally. Cytosine arabinoside has been well studied. Its mechanism of action in inhibition of DNA synthesis is by inhibition of deoxycytidylate kinase and DNA polymerase.[32] Cytosine deaminase, an enzyme that resides in endothelial cells and liver, converts cytosine arabinoside into an inactive compound, arabinosyluridine.[46] Cytosine arabinoside has a very short plasma half-life. Cytosine arabinoside penetrates into the central nervous system with levels that are about 30–50 percent of plasma levels. Toxicities include nausea, vomiting, alopecia, myelosuppression, skin rash, and diarrhea. When cytosine arabinoside is administered in high dose, conjunctivitis and cerebellar ataxia are known adverse effects. Cytosine arabinoside plays an integral role in the therapy of acute nonlymphocytic leukemia and diffuse histiocytic lymphoma.[19]

5-Fluorouracil (5-FU) and 5-fluorodeoxyuridine (5-FUdR) are substituted pyrimidine analogues that inhibit DNA by the inhibition of thymidylate synthetase.[31,37] The therapeutic effect of 5-FU and 5-FUdR can be inhibited when reduced folate stores are depleted (see below). Both 5-FU and 5-FUdR are rapidly converted to CO_2. The plasma half-life is about 10–15 minutes following parenteral administration. Antitumor activity for 5-FU has been reported in breast cancer, colon cancer,[49] gastric cancer, and adenocarcinoma of the lung, and, when used in combination with other drugs, in squamous cell carcinoma of the head and neck. 5-FUdR, when administered as an intrahepatic arterial infusion, has been reported to have activity in colon cancer with hepatic metastases. The toxicities of 5-FU and 5-FUdR include nausea, vomiting, alopecia, mucositis (oropharyngeal and enteral), myelosuppression, and cerebellar dysfunction at high dose.[37,49]

Methotrexate is a folate antagonist.[8] Methotrexate binds tightly with the intracellular enzyme dihydrofolate reductase. It inhibits the formation of tetrahydrofolic acid, the reduced and active form of folic acid. After exposure to methotrexate, cell death results from the inability to synthesize pyrimidines.[8] By administering tetrahydrofolinic acid (leucovorin), one can bypass the enzymatic blockage caused by methotrexate. Rescue with leucovorin allows high doses of methotrexate to be administered without lethal toxicity. Resistance to methotrexate may be a result of decreased intracellular transport or elevated dihydrofolate reductase levels. Recently, amplification of the dihydrofolate reductase gene has been demonstrated in a small cell carcinoma cell line resistant to methotrexate.[16] Drugs that decrease cellular uptake of methotrexate include hydrocortisone, methylprednisone, cephalothin, and L-asparaginase; in contrast, vincristine and vinblastine increase cellular uptake of methotrexate.[51] When 5-FU is given after methotrexate, there is sequential enzymatic blockade and a synergistic antitumor effect.[11] Methotrexate is rapidly adsorbed from the gastrointestinal tract, and 50-60 percent of the drug present within the blood is protein bound. Methotrexate is eliminated unchanged in the urine. Its clearance is dependent on glomerular filtration and active tubular secretion. Methotrexate is widely distributed within the body, including the cerebrospinal fluid and effusions. Toxicities of methotrexate include myelosuppression, anemia, leucopenia, thrombocytopenia, nausea, vomiting, anorexia, stomatitis, pharyngitis, hepatocellular injury, erythematous rashes, folliculitis, hyperpigmentation, alopecia, renal failure (especially in high doses), chills, fever, and pulmonary fibrosis. Methotrexate has a wide spectrum of antitumor activity, including squamous cell carcinoma of the head and neck, breast cancer, non-Hodgkin's lymphomas, acute lymphoblastic leukemia, small cell lung cancer, ovarian carcinoma, transitional carcinoma of the bladder, and osteogenic sarcoma.

Plant Alkaloids

The use of plant derivatives in the treatment of cancer dates to antiquity. The early Egyptians (1550 B.C.) used the external application of garlic to treat skin cancer. Galen, in the second century A.D., listed woody nightshade (*Solanum dulcamara*) as a remedy for cancer, warts, and tumors. It is not surprising that a large number of traditional plant remedies do contain active antitumor agents, most often of an alkaloid nature (Table 6-2). The mechanism of action of the vinca alkaloids, podophyllotoxins, and colchicine is mitotic arrest. The vinca alkaloids (vincristine, vinblastine) and colchicine inhibit mitosis by crystallization of microtubular proteins.[5] Etoposide and tenoposide do not crystallize spindle tubular protein, and their exact mechanisms of action are unknown. The podophyllotoxins also inhibit DNA synthesis, as well as RNA and RNA-dependent protein synthesis.[54] At low doses the effect on mitosis is reversible. At high concentrations the inhibition is irreversible.[4]

Vincristine and vinblastine are administered by intravenous bolus injection and are rapidly cleared from the circulation.[5] The plasma half-life is 15 minutes for vincristine and 35 minutes for vinblastine. Vinblastine is partially metabolized by the liver, and both drugs are excreted in the bile. The antitumor activity of vincristine and vinblastine includes acute lymphoblastic leukemia, breast cancer, Ewing's sarcoma (vincristine), Wilm's tumor (vincristine), Hodgkin's and non-Hodgkin's lymphomas, testicular carcinoma (vinblastine), and renal cell carcinoma (vinblastine).

Toxicities of vinblastine and vincristine include nausea, vomiting, alopecia, myelosuppression (vinblastine), peripheral neuropathy (vincristine), ileus, myopathy (vincristine), and syndrome of inappropriate antidiuretic hormone secretion (SIADH).[53]

The podophyllotoxin derivatives, etoposide and tenoposide, are administered by slow IV infusion. When given by rapid IV bolus, these drugs precipitate severe hypotension. Etoposide and tenoposide are protein-bound. Only minimal amounts of both agents cross the blood–brain barrier. The half-life of etoposide is 11.5 hours; the half-life of tenoposide is 45 minutes. Etoposide is eliminated via the biliary tract with half of the dose being a fecally excreted metabolite.[4] In contrast, tenoposide is dependent on urinary excretion. In patients with renal insufficiency, tenoposide has a longer half-life. Accordingly, patients with renal insufficiency tend to experience greater hematologic toxicity with tenoposide. Etoposide is an active agent in the treatment of Hodgkin's disease and the non-Hodgkin's lymphomas, SCLC, and testicular cancer. Tenoposide has activity in Hodgkin's disease, the non-Hodgkin's lymphomas, and primary brain tumors. Toxicities of etoposide and tenoposide include nausea, vomiting, alopecia, myelosuppression, and peripheral neuropathy.

ANTITUMOR ANTIBIOTICS

Antitumor antibiotics are chromatogenic compounds obtained from the fermentation of *Streptomyces* species (actinomycin-D, adriamycin, and daunomycin) (Table 6-2). These compounds react with DNA and prevent cell replication by positioning themselves between planar base pairs of DNA, thus preventing the unwinding of the DNA double helix.[40] Actinomycin-D also inhibits DNA-dependent RNA synthesis. Adriamycin and daunomycin inhibit DNA polymerase and thus ultimately interfere with nucleic acid synthesis.[15] Adriamycin and daunomycin are tetracyclic molecules (anthracyclines) that differ only by a single hydroxyl at carbon position 14 in the alkyl side chain. The anthracycline moiety is linked at the B ring to the amino sugar daunosamine.

Actinomycin-D, adriamycin, and daunomycin are all administered by IV bolus, and all cause tissue necrosis if extravasation occurs. When adriamycin and daunomycin are given by IV bolus, there is rapid dispersement throughout tissues and plasma. The alpha half-time is 30 minutes, with detectable plasma levels of adriamycin for as long as 15 hours. Both adriamycin and daunomycin are extensively metabolized by the liver; these metabolites include adriamycinol and daunomycinol (active), adriamycinone (inactive), and other inactive aglycones.[6]

Actinomycin-D and daunomycin have limited antitumor activity. Actinomycin-D is an effective agent in testicular carcinoma and sarcomas.[23,24] Daunomycin is an effective agent in the therapy of acute leukemia. In contrast, adriamycin has a wide spectrum of antitumor activity. In fact, adriamycin is one of the most active antineoplastic chemotherapeutic agents ever identified. Adriamycin is an active agent in the treatment of acute leukemia, Hodgkin's disease, and the non-Hodgkin's lymphomas, breast cancer, SCLC and NSCLC, ovarian cancer, gastric cancer, thyroid cancer, bladder cancer, osteogenic sarcoma, soft-tissue sarcomas, and malignant melanoma. Toxicities of adriamycin and daunomycin include nausea, vomiting, alopecia, myelosuppression, and dose-dependent cardiotoxicity (over 550 mg/m^2).

Bleomycin is an antibiotic produced by fermentation of *Streptomyces verticillus*. Bleomycin causes scission of both single- and double-stranded DNA and is cycle- and phase-specific, with its major effect in G_2 and M phase. Bleomycin can be administered directly into a body cavity or can be given intramuscularly (IM), intravenously (IV), or subcutaneously (SC).[2,9] The peak blood level of bleomycin (IM or SC) injection is obtained about 30 minutes after the dose is administered. The IV half-life of bleomycin is 20 minutes, with detectable levels as long as 2.5 hours. Bleomycin is excreted by the kidney; hence bleomycin should be administered cautiously in patients with renal failure.[9] Bleomycin is active in the treatment of squamous cell cancer of the head and neck; cancer of the cervix, skin, penis, and rectum; Hodgkin's disease, the non-Hodgkin's lymphomas; testicular cancer; and lung cancer. Toxicities of bleomycin include anaphylactoid reactions, fever, chills, anorexia, skin changes, and a dose-dependent pulmonary fibrosis (over 200 mg/m^2).[2]

Mitomycin-C

Mitomycin-C is an antineoplastic antibiotic that inhibits DNA synthesis by acting as a bifunctional alkylating agent. This action is not cell-cycle-specific or phase-specific; however, the kinetic effects are maximized if cells are treated in late G_1 and early S phase.[14,44] Mitomycin-C is administered by slow infusion through a well-running IV line. Local tissue necrosis will occur on extravasation of the drug. On IV infusion, mitomycin-C is cleared from the vascular compartment, with only about 10-30 percent of the dose excreted in the urine.[14,44] The primary means of elimination is by hepatic metabolism. Mitomycin-C has activity in gastric adenocarcinoma, colon, breast, and lung cancer and transitional cell carcinoma of the bladder. Toxicities include myelosuppression (with leucopenia and thrombocytopenia occurring 4-6 weeks following administration of mitomycin-C), alopecia, lethargy, fever, and renal toxicity as manifested by a hemolytic-uremic syndrome.[14]

Other Agents

Other antineoplastic agents include inorganic salts such as *cis*-diamminedichloroplatinum II (Platinol; cisplatin, Bristol, Syracuse, NY). Platinol® is a bifunctional alkylating agent as well as an intercalator and thus inhibits DNA synthesis. Platinol® is neither cycle- nor phase-specific.[57] When Platinol® is administered as a slow IV infusion, it is cleared from the plasma in 25-79 minutes (alpha half-life), followed by a slower secondary phase (beta half-life) of 58-73 hours.[39] Platinol® is protein-bound and is dependent on renal clearance. Platinol® has activity in germ cell neoplasms, lymphomas, ovarian carcinoma, and squamous cell carcinoma of the head and neck. A dose-related nephrotoxicity is the major dose-limiting toxicity.[36] The renal toxicity can be overcome with the use of vigorous hydration, hypertonic saline, mannitol, or Lasix (Furosemide; Hoechst-Roussel, Somerville, NJ). Other toxicities include peripheral neuropathy, ototoxicity, anemia, and mild myelosuppression.

REFERENCES

1. Albert RE, Omran AR: Follow up study of patients treated by x-ray epilation for tinea capitis. Arch Environ Health 17:899, 1968

2. Alberts DS, Chen HSG, Liu R, et al: Bleomycin pharmacokinetics in man: I. Intravenous administration. Cancer Chemother Pharmacol 1:177-181, 1978

3. Alexanian R, Dretcher R: Chemotherapy for multiple myeloma. Cancer 53:585-588, 1984

4. Allen LM, Creaven PJ: Comparison of the human pharmacokinetics of VM-26 and VP-16, two antineoplastic epipodophyllotoxin glucopyranoside derivatives. Eur J Cancer 11:697-707, 1975

5. Bender RA, Castle MC, Margileth DA, et al: The pharmacokinetics of ^{3}H-vincristine in man. Clin Pharmacol Ther 22:430-438, 1977

6. Benjamin RS: Pharmacokinetics of adriamycin in patients with sarcomas. Cancer Chemother Rep 58:271-273, 1974

7. Bizzozero OJ Jr, Johnson KG, Cicocco A: Radiation-related leukemia in Hiroshima and Nagasaki, 1946-1964. New Engl J Med 274:1095, 1966

8. Bleyer WA: The clinical pharmacology of methotrexate. Cancer 41:36-51, 1978

9. Blum RH, Carter SK, Agre K: A clinical review of bleomycin—a new antineoplastic agent. Cancer 31:903-914, 1973

10. Bonadonna G, Zucali R, Monfardini S, et al: Combination chemotherapy of Hodgkin's disease with adriamycin, bleomycin, vinblastine, and imidazole carboxamide versus MOPP. Cancer 35:252-259, 1975

11. Cadman EC, Heimer R, Davis L: Enhanced 5-fluorouracil nucleotide formation following methotrexate: Biochemical explanation for drug synergism. Science 205:1135-1137, 1979

12. Coldman AJ, Goldie JH: A model for the resistance of tumor cells to cancer chemotherapeutic agents. Math Biosci 65:291-307, 1983

13. Colvin M: A review of the pharmacology and clinical use of cyclophosphamide, in Pinedo HM (ed): Clinical Pharmacology of Antineoplastic Drugs. Amsterdam, North Holland, 1978, pp 245-261

14. Crooke ST, Bradner WT: Mitomycin C: A review. Cancer Treat Rev 3:121-139, 1976

15. Crooke ST, DuVernay VH, Galvan L, et al: Structure-activity relationships of anthracyclines relative to effects on macromolecular synthesis. Molec Pharmacol 14:290-298, 1978

16. Curt GA, Carney DN, Dowan KH, et al: Unstable methotrexate resistance in human small cell carcinoma associated with double-minute chromosomes. New Engl J Med 308:199-202, 1983

17. Curt GA, Clendenin NJ, Chabner BA: Drug resistance in cancer. Cancer Treat Rep 68:767-769, 1984

18. DeVita VT Jr: Principals of chemotherapy, in DeVita VT Jr, Hellman S, Rosenberg SA (eds): Principles and Practice of Oncology, 2d ed. Philadelphia, Lippincott, 1985, pp 257-287

19. Early AP, Preisler HD, Slocum H, et al: A pilot study of high-dose 1-beta-D-arabino-furanosylcytosine for acute leukemia and refractory lymphoma: Clinical response and pharmacology. Cancer Res 42:1587, 1982

20. Elion GB: Biochemistry and pharmacology of purine analogs. Fed Proc 26:898-904, 1967

21. Faber S, Diamond LK, Mercer RD, et al: Temporary remissions in acute leukemia in children produced by folic acid and antagonist, 4-aminopteroyl-glutamicacid (Aminopterin). New Engl J Med 238:787, 1948

22. Fidler IJ, Posler G: The cellular heterogeneity of malignant neoplasms: Implications for adjuvant chemotherapy. Semin Oncol 12:207-221, 1985

23. Frei E: The clinical use of actinomycin. Cancer Chemother Rep 58:49-54, 1974

24. Frei E III, Canellos GP: Dose: A critical factor in cancer chemotherapy. Am J Med 69:585-594, 1980

25. Gallo RC, Sarin PS, Blattner WA, et al: T cell malignancies and human T cell leukemia virus. Semin Oncol 9:12-17, 1984

26. Glassroth J, Robbins AG, Snider DE Jr: Tuberculosis in the 1980's. New Engl J Med 302:1441-1450, 1980

27. Goldie JH, Coldman AJ: Quantitative model for multiple levels of drug resistance in clinical tumors. Cancer Treat Rep 67:923-931, 1983

28. Golomb HM, Rowley JD, Vardiman JW, et al: "Microgranular" acute promyelocytic leukemia: A distinct clinical-ultrastructural and cytogenetic entity. Blood 55:253-259, 1980

29. Golomb HM, Vardiman JW, Rowley JD, et al: Correlation of clinical findings with Q-banded chromosomes in 90 adults with acute nonlymphocytic leukemia: An eight year study (1970-1977). New Engl J Med 229:613-619, 1978

30. Gullino P: Experimental systems and invasion, in Weiss L, Gilbert H (eds): Bone Metastases. Boston, GK Hall Medical Publishers, 1981, pp. 24-38

31. Heidelberger C, Chandhari NH, Dannenberg P, et al: Fluorinated pyrimidines: A new class of tumor inhibitory compounds. Nature 179:663-666, 1957

32. Ho DHW, Frei E III: Clinical pharmacology of 1-B-D-arabinofuranosylcytosine. Clin Pharmacol Ther 12:944-954, 1971

33. Kartner N, Shales M, Riordan JR, et al: Daunorubicin-resistant Chinese hamster ovary cells expressing multidrug resistance and a cell surface P-glycoprotein. Cancer Res 43:4413-4419, 1983

34. Kennedy BJ: Mithramycin in testicular cancer. J Urol 107:429-433, 1972

35. LeBeau MM, Albain RS, Larson RA, et al: Clinical and cytogenetic correlations in 63 patients with therapy-related myelodysplastic syndrome and acute nonlymphocytic leukemia. Further evidence for characteristic abnormalities of chromosomes no. 5 and 7. J Clin Oncol 4:325-345, 1986

36. Madia NE, Harrington JT: Platinum nephrotoxicity. Am J Med 65:307-314, 1978

37. Mandel HG: Incorporation of 5-fluorouracil into RNA and its molecular consequences. Progr Molec Subcell Biol 1:82-135, 1969

38. Marshall EK Jr: Historical perspectives in chemotherapy, in Goldin A, Hawking IF (eds): Advances in Chemotherapy, vol 1. New York, Academic Press, 1964, pp 1-8

39. Patton TF, Himmelstein KJ, Belt R: Plasma levels and urinary excretion of filterable platinum species following bolus injection and i.v. infusion of cis-dichlorodiammineplatinum (II) in man. Cancer Treat Rep 63:1359-1361, 1979

40. Pigram WJ, Fuller W, Amilton LDH: Stereochemistry of intercalation: Interaction of daunomycin with DNA. Nature 235:17-19, 1972

41. Rapp F, Westmoreland D: Cell transformation by DNA containing viruses. Biochem Biophys Acta 458:167, 1976

42. Rauscher FJ Jr, Flamm: Etiology of cancer, in Holland JF, Frie III E (eds): Cancer Medicine, 2d ed. Philadelphia, (Lea & Febiger) 1982, pp 1-4

43. Rebeloff S, Harrison J, Karatilski, et al: Continuing occurrence of thyroid carcinoma after irradiation to the neck in infancy and childhood. New Engl J Med 292:171, 1975

44. Reich SD: Clinical pharmacology of mitomycin C, in Carter SK, Crooke ST (eds): Mitomycin C: Current Status and New Developments. New York, Academic Press, 1979, p 243

45. Santoro A, Bonadonna G, Bonfante V, et al: Alternating drug combinations in the treatment of advanced Hodgkin's disease. New Engl J Med 306:770-775, 1982

46. Steuart CD, Burke PJ: Cytidine deaminase and the development of resistance to arabino-syl cytosine. Nature 233:109-110, 1971

47. Tannock IF: Biology of tumor growth. Hosp Pract 81-93, 1983

48. Tannock I: Cell kinetics and chemotherapy: A critical review. Cancer Treat Rep 62:1117-1133, 1978

49. Vogel SJ, Presant CA, Ratkin GA, et al: Phase I study of thymidine plus 5-fluorouracil infusions in advanced colorectal carcinoma. Cancer Treat Rep 63:1-5, 1979

50. Von Hoff DD, Weisenthal L: In vitro methods to predict patient response to chemotherapy. Adv Pharmacol Chemother 7:133-156, 1980

51. Warren RD, Nichols AP, Bender RA: Membrane transport of methotrexate in human lymphoblastoid cells. Cancer Res 38:668-671, 1978

52. Weisburger JH, Williams GM: Chemical carcinogens, in Holland JF, Frie E III (eds): Cancer Medicine, 2d ed. Philadelphia, Lea & Febiger, 1982, pp 42-895

53. Weiss HD, Walker MD, Wiernik PH: Neurotoxicity of commonly used antineoplastic agents. New Engl J Med 291:127-133, 1974

54. Wozniak AJ, Ross WE: DNA damage as a basis for 4'-demethyl-epipodophyllotoxin-9-(4,6-0-ethylidene-beta-D-glucopyranoside (etoposide) cytoxicity. Cancer Res 43:120, 1983

55. Young RC, DeVita VT: Cell cycle characteristics of human solid tumors in vivo. Cell Tissue Kinet 3:285-295, 1970

56. Yunis J: The chromosomal basis of human neoplasia. Science 221:227-236, 1983

57. Zwelling LA, Kohn KW: Mechanism of action of cis-dichlorodiammine platinum (II). Cancer Treat Rep 63:1439-1444, 1979

Heber MacMahon
Stephen R. Ell
Mark K. Ferguson

7

Diagnostic Methods in Lung Cancer

The diagnosis of lung cancer usually occurs as a sequence of events and decisions that can be divided into three principal phases: (1) detection of a suspicious abnormality, (2) noninvasive workup, and (3) tissue diagnosis. Clinical staging follows tissue diagnosis; however, in practice, staging is often partially completed during the diagnostic workup. We shall discuss diagnostic methods in the context of these somewhat arbitrary phases in order to clarify the purpose of each procedure and to demonstrate a rational approach to the diagnostic process.

As in any area of medicine, it is important that the physician understand the specific merits and limitations of each diagnostic procedure. Sensitivity, specificity, risk factors, and monetary cost must all be considered. Finally, prompt and accurate communication between the various specialists involved in the case is essential in order to optimize the choice and sequence of diagnostic tests.[12,32]

DETECTION

The chest radiograph is still the keystone of lung cancer detection and is likely to remain so in the foreseeable future. It has the virtues of high sensitivity, low cost, and negligible risk. It has the additional merit of providing information regarding the patient's cardiopulmonary status, which may be relevant to that patient's future management.

Chest radiography for lung cancer detection should consist of frontal and lateral views performed at full inspiration. High-kilovoltage technique and the use of wide-latitude film are required to achieve good visualization of all parts of the lungs, including the retrocardiac and retrodiaphragmatic areas. Although these basic principles are widely recognized, chest radiography is often poorly performed in practice. Systematic quality control is essential to maintain optimal radiographic image quality. Errors in exposure or film processing inevitably result in impaired diagnostic capability. Such technical problems are particularly common when operation of the x-ray equipment is not supervised by a radiologist.

LUNG CANCER: A COMPREHENSIVE TREATISE
ISBN 0-8089-1876-1

Because early lung cancer is potentially curable, several studies have been performed to determine the worth of screening asymptomatic cigarette smokers by means of periodic chest radiography and sputum cytologic examination.[20,49,52] The results have been mixed. While a higher percentage of cases with early disease has been successfully detected and apparently cured as a result of screening examination, it has not yet been demonstrated that the screened population as a whole has a significantly lower death rate from lung cancer than comparable unscreened groups. Several important facts have emerged from these studies: (1) chest radiography has a higher yield for detection of asymptomatic lung cancer than does sputum cytology; (2) oat cell carcinoma and centrally located non-oat cell varieties tend to grow rapidly and hence usually have metastasized before they are detected, even with intensive periodic screening; (3)peripheral non-oat cell tumors, especially adenocarcinomas, tend to grow slowly and frequently are detected at an early stage by periodic radiography. The majority of these are AJC Stage I when detected[52] (Fig. 7-1).

Because screening of asymptomatic smokers has not been proven to be beneficial, the American Cancer Society no longer recommends annual chest radiography as a routine for smokers. It must be emphasized, however, that although the benefits of systematic screening have not been demonstrated, neither has it been proven that screening is of no value. This unsatisfactory state of affairs is related to the difficulty in monitoring a valid "control" population for such studies. Improvements in imaging

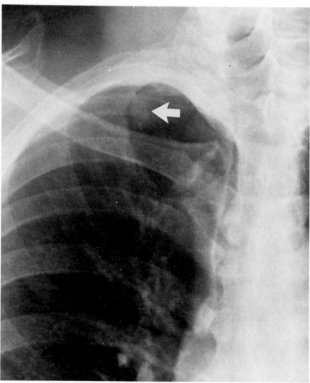

Fig. 7-1.   Early lung cancer (arrow). A 1-cm noncalcified lesion in the right apex detected on routine radiography. Surgery revealed bronchoalveolar carcinoma arising in a scar.

technology also tend to render the conclusions of earlier studies obsolete. Interestingly, the interim results of an ongoing lung cancer screening program at Memorial Sloan Kettering Cancer Center in New York are among the most optimistic to date.[49] At present, it is reasonable to obtain a baseline chest radiograph on smokers and to offer annual chest radiographs to high-risk patients (smokers over the age of 50 years) on an individual basis. For the future, digital chest radiography holds some promise, with potential for computer-assisted lesion detection, improved discrimination of benign and malignant lesions,[79] and reduced cost.

The radiographic findings of lung cancer are extremely varied and as a whole are beyond the scope of this discussion. The following points deserve emphasis, however: (1) carcinoma must be considered in the differential diagnosis of any noncalcified pulmonary nodule, especially in smokers over 40 years old; (2) lung cancer presenting as a solitary pulmonary nodule presents the best opportunity for potential cure; and (3) the only radiologic signs that have been shown to exclude malignancy reliably are "benign" patterns of calcification, or lack of growth over a period of 2 years or more.[26,27,54,74] Although a large majority of lung cancers will show visible growth over a 12-month period, lesions that grow very slowly are the best candidates for curative surgery. Therefore, it is appropriate to set conservative limits for excluding malignancy on the basis of growth rate. The presence of calcification in a nodule also strongly suggests a benign etiology. Although specific patterns of calcification more reliably indicate benignancy (i.e., central, diffuse, laminated, and "popcorn" patterns), the presence of any calcification detectable by conventional radiography or tomography in a lung nodule suggests benignancy with a high degree of reliability.[16,26,27,76] Most such calcified lesions will represent healed granulomas. The popcorn pattern can be seen in hamartomas. Most execptions to this general rule are caused by carcinomas that engulf preexisting granulomatous calcifications. This is particularly apt to occur in the hilar areas where calcified nodes may be engulfed by a malignant mass or in the lung apices when a carcinoma arises in an area of fibrocalcific scarring. Dystrophic calcification can occur within lung cancers, although it is rarely detectable by conventional radiography.[76]

In screening programs, approximately two-thirds of all lung cancers present as a pulmonary nodule; the next most common finding is a hilar mass (Fig. 7-2). In clinical practice, many cases of lung cancer will present as an apparent pneumonia due to bronchial obstruction, and a recurrent or persistent pneumonic infiltrate in a smoker should raise the question of underlying lung cancer. Significant volume loss in a consolidated lobe is also suggestive of bronchial obstruction and should be regarded with suspicion (Fig. 7-3).

NONINVASIVE PROCEDURES

When a possible lung cancer is detected by chest x-ray, a number of options are available for further investigation. While each case should be considered individually, some general rules apply. The objective should be to obtain the necessary information for diagnosis and staging with as little risk, discomfort, and expense to the patient as possible. To achieve this goal, it is useful to outline a plan and timetable at the outset.

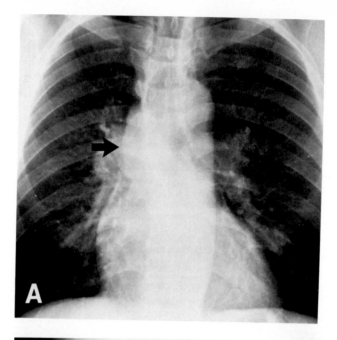

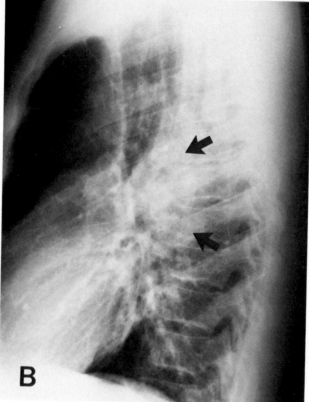

Fig. 7-2. (*A*) Right hilar carcinoma (arrow) producing increased density, obscuration of bronchus intermedius, and slight volume loss in the right lung. (*B*) Posterior mass effect (arrows) with compression of bronchus, visible on the lateral view.

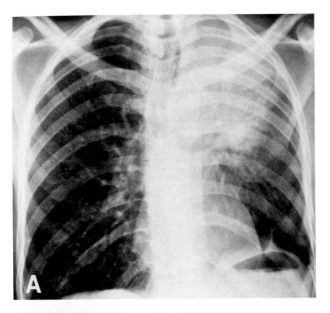

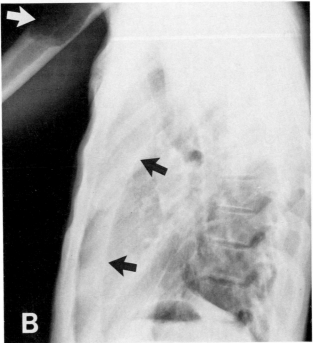

Fig. 7-3. (A) Central tumor with left upper lobe atelectasis. Note marked volume loss in left hemithorax. (B) Lateral view demonstrates collapsed left upper lobe outlined by major fissure (black arrow), which is displaced forward. Note large lytic lesion in humerus (white arrow) indicating metastatic involvement.

Chest Radiography

Almost without exception, the chest radiograph is the key that determines the specific direction of the workup. Therefore, it is fundamentally important that current, good-quality frontal and lateral chest radiographs are obtained initially. Although a radiograph may have been obtained recently, major decisions should be based on completely current information. Strict adherence to this policy may render further investigation unnecessary for resolving inflammatory lesions, previously misdiagnosed artifacts, or even cancers that have markedly progressed since the original diagnosis. By the time a patient has been referred for investigation of an abnormal chest radiograph, several weeks may have passed and the findings will often have changed.

Assuming that one is dealing with a questionable or merely suspicious finding, comparison with any previous chest radiographs that may be available is vitally important. If the lesion has been demonstrably stable for 2 years or more, further workup is unnecessary. If it has not visibly changed for 12 months, it is probably benign and should be followed.[54] In such cases, failure to obtain previous radiographs for comparison is a serious error.

Special Views of the Chest

In addition to the standard posteroanterior (PA) and lateral projections, lordotic, decubitus, and oblique views of the chest are available. However, they have been used infrequently since the advent of high-kilovoltage chest radiography and widespread availability of computed tomography (CT) scanning.

A lordotic view of the chest allows a clear view of the lung apices unobstructed by overlying clavicles and costal cartilages. This can be adequate for establishing the presence or absence of a nodule. If an intrapulmonary abnormality is clearly present on the standard examination, however, a lordotic view will not necessarily help. A more definitive procedure, such as a CT scan, may be more appropriate. Oblique views, with or without fluoroscopic guidance, can demonstrate rib or pleural lesions more clearly than the standard chest x-ray. Indeed, low-kilovoltage radiography with oblique views is the preferred technique for confirming rib invasion or metastases, and can be superior to a CT scan in this application.

The main purpose of a decubitus view of the chest is to demonstrate the presence of a free pleural effusion. When the effusion is substantial, there is inevitably some degree of consolidation in the underlying lung due to compression atelectasis. Therefore, the mere presence of "infiltrate" in the lower lobe is not helpful in determining the etiology of the effusion. However, aspiration and analysis of the fluid are simple and potentially diagnostic.[34,44]

Conventional (Film-Screen) Tomography

In the past, lung tomography was employed almost routinely in cases of suspected lung cancer. Now, since the advent of CT, its role has become quite limited. In its favor, conventional tomography is less expensive and usually more readily available than CT. However, continued improvements in image quality and, more importantly, increased experience with interpretation of cross-sectional images have rendered CT the investigation of choice in most cases of suspected or proven lung cancer. The subject remains controversial and personal preferences reflect individual experience.[42,56] In the authors' opinion, it seldom is necessary to perform conventional tomography in lung cancer assuming that a CT scanner is available. There are some situations, though, in which conventional tomography can play an important role; these are listed below:

1. When an ill-defined density is detected in the lung on a chest radiograph, conventional tomography can serve to confirm the presence or absence of a solid nodule. If a solid nodule is confirmed, however, a CT scan will probably be performed for further workup. Therefore, the preferred role of conventional tomography is to "rule out" rather than "rule in" cancer.

2. In the case of a small peripheral lung nodule ("coin" lesion) the major differential diagnosis is usually between primary carcinoma and granuloma. A high proportion of granulomata contain calcium and the large majority of lung cancers do not.[76] In many cases conventional tomography will serve to confirm the presence of calcification. Although CT is theoretically, the technique of choice for demonstrating subtle calcifications, it has some practical limitations in this respect; these limitations are addressed in further detail below. Most importantly, unless a specific meticulous technique is used, small foci of calcification may not be detected in lung nodules by CT. Conventional tomography, although slightly less sensitive, will reliably confirm any calcification that is sufficiently substantial to be even faintly visible on chest x-ray.[1] If a nodule is suspected to be calcified on the basis of the chest radiograph, therefore, the yield of conventional tomography is high. Calcium is demonstrated well on tomograms for two reasons. (a) the tomographic mechanism blurs overlying structures, thereby effectively removing superimposed detail; and (b) more importantly tomography is performed with a low-energy beam that maximizes visibility of calcium (Fig. 7-4).

3. When chest radiographs indicate possible compromise of the trachea or major bronchi by intraluminal or extrinsic tumor, conventional tomography can be helpful. In this situation, the ability of tomography to display the anatomy in coronal and sagittal planes can be an advantage, although the cross-sectional perspective of CT may provide complementary information.

4. Until recently, many radiologists preferred conventional tomography to CT for evaluating the pulmonary hila. Now, increased experience with CT interpretation aided by several excellent CT-anatomic correlation studies, have reversed this trend.[23] The authors share this prevalent opinion and consider that a well-performed CT scan with contrast enhancement of hilar blood vessels is the examination of choice for evaluating a suspicious hilum.

Therefore, while lung tomography has a role in lung cancer diagnosis, it is quite limited. Because the tomographic examination must be tailored to each particular situation, it is important that the nature of the specific clinical question be defined in advance and that the tomograms be supervised directly by a radiologist. It should be remembered that the diagnostic accuracy of any imaging examination is determined largely by the skill and experience of the individual who interprets it. Therefore, the individual radiologist's prejudices and preferences should not be ignored. If the radiologist can evaluate the lesion more confidently on conventional tomograms than a CT scan, tomograms become the procedure of choice.

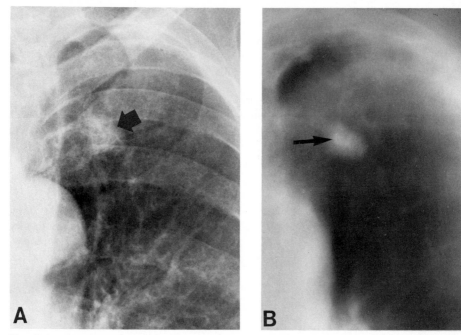

Fig. 7-4. (*A*) An abnormal density (arrow) is shown in the left upper lobe on a routine chest radiograph. Possible causes include calcified costal cartilage, granuloma, and tumor. (*B*) A representative section from a conventional tomogram confirms that the abnormality is in the lung. In addition, a small focus of central calcification is demonstrated (arrow) indicative of a healed granuloma.

Computed Tomography

CT has added greatly to our ability to diagnose and stage lung cancer.[50,79] Although precise indications for its use are widely debated, there is no doubt that it provides detailed anatomic information unavailable by other modalities. In the context of suspected or proven lung cancer, a CT scan can provide important data, as it can (1) confirm the presence and extent of a lung mass that was merely suspected from chest x-ray (Fig. 7-5, 7-6), (2) confirm or exclude the presence of additional lung lesions as it is the most sensitive imaging technique for lung nodule detection,[53,66] and (3) demonstrate the location of enlarged mediastinal and hilar lymph nodes that are likely to contain metastatic disease.[3,43,57] Extrathoracic metastases can also be identified, particularly in the liver and adrenal glands.[38,65]

When the chest radiograph shows only a small peripheral nodule, the additional yield from a CT scan is relatively low,[30] although not insignificant. In the case of central or more advanced tumors, the frequency of unexpected findings is high and clearly justifies its use, in the authors' opinion. Obviously, much of the data obtained by CT scan pertains more to staging than diagnosis, and its utility in that role is discussed elsewhere in this volume.

A major role has been advocated for CT scanning in distinguishing cancerous lung nodules from benign granulomata. This was first proposed in 1980 when Seigleman and co-workers published the results of an extensive study.[69] Their observations indicated that CT could be used to distinguish grossly noncalcified granulomas from tumors, based on their measured densities. The hypothesis was that CT, with its extreme sensitivity to small density differences in tissue, could identify small quantities of calcium in many granulomas that were apparently noncalcified on conventional tomography. Enthusiasm for this technique faded when others failed to reproduce these initial results.[24] This failure of reproducibility led to some important realizations regarding the use of CT as a quantitative technique. The Seigleman study was performed on a particular CT device of which only a few units were built. This scanner used a specific reconstruction algorithm (the formula by which the density of each pixel is computed) that differed from other CT scanners on the market. Subsequently, extensive work has been performed in this area, particularly by Zherhouni and coworkers, to determine exactly how multiple factors may influence CT density numbers in the chest.[85] Changes in the character of the x-ray beam as it passes through various structures ("beam hardening") play a major role. To correct for this, a phantom device has been developed to allow comparison of a standard artificial nodule, scanned within the phantom, with a real nodule in a patient's chest.[86] This has minimized the calibration problems that formerly beset CT density measurements in the chest. A recent multicenter cooperative study has endorsed this technique, finding thin-section CT to be useful mainly for evaluating small (<3 cm) smoothly marginated nodules. However, some calcifications were detected in 7 percent of the malignant lesions studied, and the authors of that paper conclude that there can be no completely reliable criterion for benignancy on the basis of numbers alone.[87] Although we have not employed CT density measurements in lung nodules as a criterion for surgery in the past, resection of granulomatous lesions due to suspicion of cancer has been very unusual in our experience. In areas where granulomatous disease is common, CT density measurements may have a greater role.

Dual-energy CT scanning[8] and digital radiography [19] both hold promise for accurate quantitation of calcium in pulmonary nodules, but the role of these new methods has not been established.

Mediastinal and Hilar Lymph Nodes

One of the more widely debated applications of CT scanning in the chest is the evaluation of mediastinal nodal involvement in lung cancer. This question relates to staging rather than diagnosis per se and is addressed elsewhere in this volume. Briefly, the CT scan provides accurate information regarding size and location of abnormal mediastinal nodes. Unfortunately, although markedly enlarged nodes are likely to contain metastases and normal-size nodes usually are uninvolved, exceptions to this rule do occur with sufficient frequency that biopsy is usually required, Using 1 and 2 cm as the upper limit for negative nodes and lower limit for positive nodes respectively, one can obtain a high degree of predictive accuracy. This is achieved at the cost of relegating a proportion of cases to an "indeterminate" category (nodes in the 1-2-cm range).[3]

Before the diagnosis of lung cancer has been established, identification of enlarged mediastinal lymph nodes by CT scan can have implications for tissue diagnosis. When the suspected primary lesion is very small, and if a percutaneous approach is contraindicated because of severe emphysema, or if involved mediastinal nodes would preclude resection, mediastinoscopy with nodal biopsy may be desirable. In

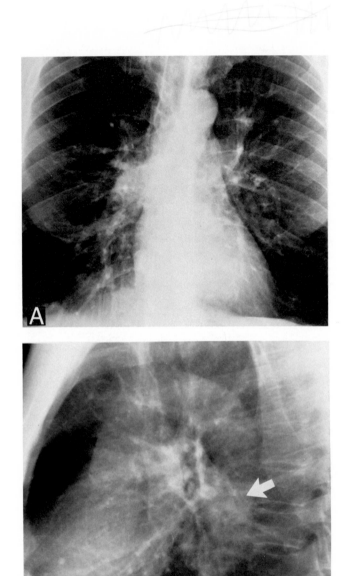

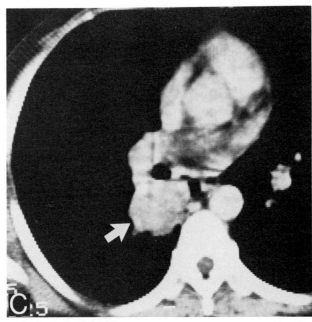

Fig. 7-5. (A) Chest radiograph of a 58-year-old man with hemoptysis. The right hilum is denser than the left, a clue to the presence of a mass. (B) The lateral view shows subtle retrohilar density (arrow). (C) A CT scan demonstrates a large mass (arrow) posterior to the right hilum. Bronchoscopic biopsy revealed squamous cell carcinoma.

such cases, identification of large pretracheal nodes by CT scan may be useful in planning the biopsy approach.

When a CT scan is performed for evaluation of suspected lung cancer, the patient should be studied from the lung apices through the level of the adrenal glands. The adrenals are located within a few centimeters of the most caudal portion of the lungs, and including these glands adds only slightly to the time and expense of the examination. The additional information is valuable for staging purposes, in the event that lung cancer is confirmed.[65] When the diagnosis is uncertain, discovery of hepatic or adrenal masses can help to confirm the nature of the lung lesion. The adrenal glands are a common site for metastases in bronchogenic carcinoma (Fig. 7-7). With increasing use of CT, however, it has become apparent that nonfunctioning adrenal adenomas are also common,[51] and unfortunately they are often indistinguishable from metastases. Therefore, when an enlarged adrenal gland is the only evidence of metastatic disease, percutaneous biopsy usually is required for confirmation.

The authors' recommendations regarding use of CT in suspected lung cancer can be summarized as follows: (1) when the chest x-ray indicates probable lung cancer, a CT scan is the most useful noninvasive procedure for diagnosis and staging; (2) the

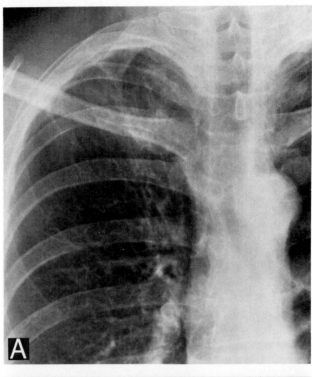

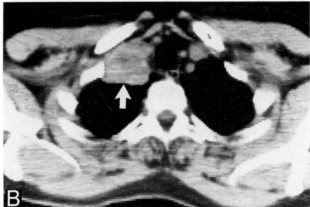

Fig. 7-6. (A) Chest radiograph of a 47-year-old man with a history of cough and chest pain for 6 months showing ill-defined density in the right apex medially but no definite mass. (B) A CT scan at the level of the upper thorax shows a large mass (arrow) invading the mediastinum and encasing the subclavian vessels. Needle biopsy revealed adenocarcinoma.

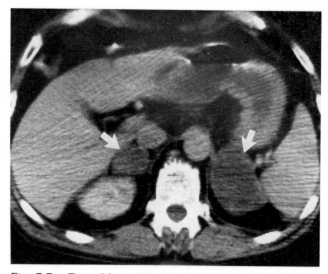

Fig. 7-7. Typical large bilateral adrenal metastases (arrows) shown on a CT scan of the upper abdomen. The adrenal glands are involved frequently by metastatic lung cancer; thus it is important to extend chest CT scans through the upper abdomen in such cases.

CT scan is the technique of choice to demonstrate hilar and mediastinal anatomy, particularly with regard to lymph node size; (3) a CT scan can detect small amounts of calcification in a nodule, but a specific, meticulous technique must be used, and the resulting density measurements should not be the only criterion used to determine management; and (4) when enlarged lymph nodes or adrenal masses are detected by CT, a biopsy usually is necessary to confirm metastatic disease.

Magnetic Resonance Imaging

In its present stage of development, magnetic resonance imaging (MRI) has little to offer in comparison to CT for diagnosis and staging of lung cancer. The equipment is expensive, and MRI studies are time-consuming to perform. In the lungs, spatial reslution is poor, mainly because of a relatively long acquisition time and resulting image degradation by patient motion. Consequently, the sensitivity of MRI for detection of small nodules is considerably less than that of CT. Neither is MRI useful for detecting calcification in benign nodules.

The principal advantages of MRI in this area at present relate to its ability to distinguish vascular from solid structures in the mediastinum and hila without use of contrast materials[21] (Fig. 7-8). The capacity of MRI to display mediastinal anatomy in sagittal, coronal, or oblique planes is also impressive, although of unproven clinical value[80] (Fig. 7-9). The lack of ionizing radiation, a much touted advantage of MRI in general, is of doubtful consequence in a patient who is evaluated for suspected or proven lung cancer. Studies that have systematically compared CT and MRI as staging techniques have indicated no clear advantage for MRI while emphasizing some limitations of the method.[31,81] The weight of opinion at present favors CT as the optimal method for initial evaluation of lung cancer. Nonetheless, MRI is still in its infancy. Although it seems unlikely to surpass CT in terms of anatomic detail, it is possible that tissue characterization by spectroscopy will become an important clinical tool in the near future. Meanwhile, the role of MRI in the chest is mainly confined to resolving specific questions in those patients in whom use of iodinated contrast material is contraindicated.[41]

Sputum Cytology

When correct techniques are used for sputum collection and analysis, cytologic examination can have a high diagnostic yield.[14,29,77] Early-morning sputum collection on several consecutive days is recommended for best results. Between 60 and 75 percent of all cases of lung cancer can be diagnosed in this way at the time that they present.[14,29,64,77,78]

Sputum examination is most commonly positive in patients with central tumors. However, the yield is less in cases where bronchial obstruction and atelectasis have occurred.[64] The cell type most frequently associated with positive sputum cytology is squamous carcinoma, in keeping with its tendency to occur in a central endobronchial location. The yield is also high for oat cell tumors. Adenocarcinomas, which are typically small and peripherally located, provide the lowest yield.

Cytopathology has developed into a major subspecialty, and an expert in this field can confidently determine the tumor cell type from a positive sputum sample in approximately 80 percent of cases.[45,59,64] The greatest difficulty arises in cytologic diagnosis of large cell and poorly differentiated cell types. However, distinction between small cell and non-small cell tumors can be made with a high level of confidence in most cases. In several large series, the false-positive rate has been extremely low (in the region of ≤ 1 percent) although such high accuracy reflects the expertise of the experienced cytopathologists involved.[10,29] Such skills may not be available in every hospital where lung cancer is diagnosed. Sputum cytology has been used for screening high-risk individuals. As noted above, the yield has been low in this application, and it seems unlikely that this method of screening will ever be economically viable.

Fig. 7-8. (A) A noninfused CT scan at the level of the hila showing an anterior left lung mass (m) and an enlarged left hilum. (B) With intravenous contrast infusion, metastatic disease in the hilum (arrow) is better defined and more clearly separable from the pulmonary artery. (C) An MRI scan clearly distinguishes vascular structures (which appear black) from tumor (arrow). (Case courtesy of Dr. Harvey Glazer, Mallinckrodt Institute of Radiology.)

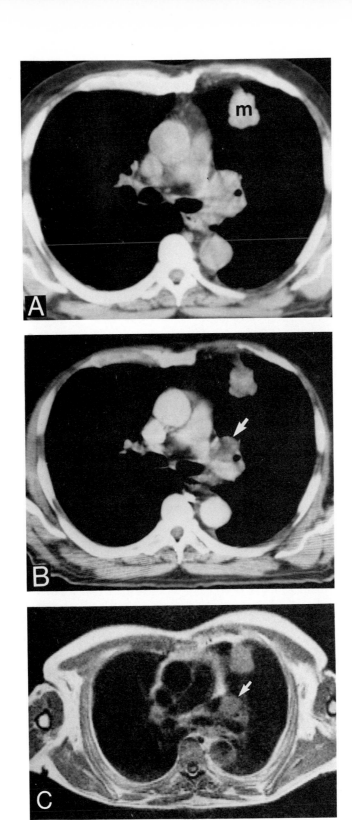

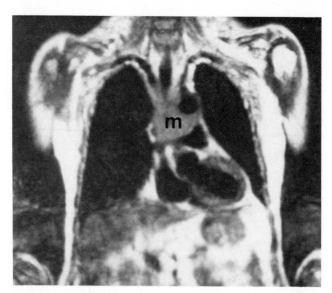

Fig. 7-9. A coronal section from an MRI scan of a patient with a large infiltrating tumor mass anterior to the carina (m). Note that the extent of the tumor and its relationship to vascular structures are clearly shown. (Case courtesy of Dr. Harvey Glazer, Mallinckrodt Institute of Radiology.)

Recent results have reemphasized the superiority of chest radiography for early detection of lung cancer.[20,49,52]

TISSUE DIAGNOSIS

Bronchoscopy

Fiberoptic bronchoscopy is an accurate and safe technique for definitive diagnosis of lung cancer. It has the unique advantage of providing direct visualization of the trachea and bronchial tree to the level of most segmental and some subsegmental divisions. Central tumors can be inspected, brushed, and biopsied for cytologic and histologic diagnosis. For staging purposes, the carina can be inspected and biopsied.[63] In cases where the lesion is located beyond the subsegmental bronchial divisions, brush or biopsy instruments can be directed into the abnormal area under fluoroscopic control. Thus, direct visualization of a tumor is not essential for diagnosis.

Fiberoptic bronchoscopy usually is performed under local anesthesia and mild sedation. Although the technique is not difficult to master, training and experience are important for optimal results. The fiberoptic instrument is currently used in approximately 95 percent of all bronchoscopic examinations in large hospitals, although the rigid instrument still has a role in some situations.[46] The main advantage of the rigid bronchoscope is its larger lumen and, consequently, improved size of biopsy and control of potential hemmorhage. However, the areas that can be reached are more limited, and the procedure sometimes requires general anesthesia.

Accuracy

Not surprisingly, diagnostic accuracy for bronchoscopic biopsy is extremely high for large central tumors and correspondingly low for small peripheral lesions.[61,75] Therefore, overall accuracy, which is in the 55–80 percent range, has little relevance in prediction of the yield in a particular case.[13,39,83] Radke and co-workers determined that the size of the primary lesion was the most important single fact in predicting diagnostic success, while location was critical for small lesions.[61] In their series, 87 percent of tumors that were greater than 2 cm in diameter and located in the inner third of either lung were accurately diagnosed by bronchoscopy. However, when the tumor was less than 2 cm in size and was in the outer third of either lung, diagnostic accuracy fell to 23 percent. This is in keeping with our own experience. Indeed, in cases where the only x-ray finding is a small peripheral nodule, it is logical to proceed directly to needle biopsy, since a negative result from bronchoscopy is virtually assured.

Two specific anatomic areas are difficult to access via the fiberoptic broncho-scope: the superior segments of the lower lobes and the most medial portions of the apical segments of the upper lobes. In such instances, it may prove impossible to achieve sufficiently acute angulation with the bronchoscope to biopsy the lesion.[39] Metastatic lung lesions are less susceptible to bronchoscopic diagnosis than primary tumors because of their usual extrabronchial origin. For the same reason, hilar or mediastinal masses without an endobronchial component cannot be diagnosed by conventional bronchoscopic technique.

A recent development, transbronchial needle aspiration, has extended the role of the bronchoscope.[68] With this technique a fine aspirating needle is inserted via the bronchoscope through the bronchial wall to obtain material for cytologic diagnosis. This method is particularly useful for identifying subcarinal nodal disease and can be employed to aspirate peripheral nodules under fluoroscopic guidance.

Complications

Fiberoptic bronchoscopy is a safe procedure when correctly performed and when patients are appropriately screened. Complications can occur as a result of premedications, anesthetics, the physical effect of the bronchoscope in the airway, or they can arise secondary to the biopsy itself.[9,60] Laryngospasm is a relatively common problem, but it usually is transient. Hypoxia can occur as a result of partial obstruction of the airway, especially in patients whose respiratory function is already compromised. Cardiac arrythmias and myocardial infarction have been reported. When transbronchial forceps biopsy is performed, pneumothorax and hemorrhage are potential complications. Although postbiopsy bleeding usually is minor, significant hemorrhage can occur, especially in those patients with abnormal hemostasis due to chemotherapy or uremia.[83] Forceps biopsy is not recommended in the presence of a platelet count of less than 50,000 mm^{-3}, and a platelet transfusion is advisable immediately prior to bronchoscopy, even at higher counts if platelet function is abnormal. Fortunately, these factors seldom are present in patients being investigated for lung cancer. The more likely hazard in this situation is bleeding due to biopsy of a highly vascular tumor such as carcinoid.

Percutaneous Needle Biopsy

Since the technique of aspiration needle biopsy became widely accepted in the 1960s, considerable experience has been accumulated and significant improvements have been made in biopsy needle design.

Formerly, two principal types of biopsy needles were used: (1) the aspirating needle, which achieved an impressive record for safety while yielding sufficient material for cytologic diagnosis in most cases;[70] and (2) the cutting needle, typified by the Tru-Cut* (Travenol, Inc., Deerfield, IL) type (Fig. 7-10), which was larger and yielded adequate tissue for histologic examination but had a high complication rate due to hemorrhage.[17,47,48]

More recently, several manufacturers have produced needles that combine many of the advantages of the old aspirating and cutting instruments.[2,33] This has been achieved by the use of fine-gauge (21-23-gauge) thin-walled needles with tips modified to obtain a small core of tissue (Fig.7-11). Development of two-tiered systems has been another significant advance. With this arrangement, a larger (19-gauge) needle is inserted into the lung as a guide. When its tip is adjacent to the target, the stylet is removed and a biopsy needle is inserted through the lumen of the larger needle. Thus the biopsy needle can be removed and reinserted for multiple tissue samples without repuncturing the pleura and without the need for time-consuming repositioning of the needle. Most of these newer aspiration cutting needles require a combination of suction and vigorous rotation during biopsy for optimal results. The tissue specimen is inevitably extremely small and requires special handling in the laboratory.[88]

Regardless of which type of needle is used, accurate placement is critical. Failure to position the needle correctly is the most common reason for nondiagnostic results. Fluoroscopy and CT are the most widely used guidance systems for percutaneous

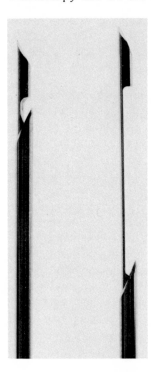

Fig. 7-10. Close-up view of the tip of a 14-gauge Trucut cutting biopsy instrument. Use of such needles is rarely indicated in the chest in view of a high risk of serious hemmorhage.

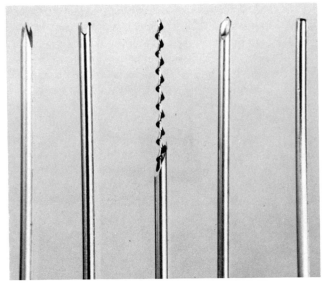

Fig. 7-11. Close-up view of five 22-gauge aspiration-cutting biopsy instruments. From the left: Franseen, EZM, Rotex, Chiba, and Greene needles.

biopsy, and ultrasound occasionally is useful for pleural-based masses. Fluoroscopy has the advantage that it is a "real-time" system, which can show the position of the needle and the target lesion while the needle is advanced and manipulated. For this reason, we favor fluoroscopic guidance for the majority of cases. Biplane fluoroscopy is helpful, especially for small nodules, although it is not essential. For an experienced operator, monoplane fluoroscopy is adequate for needle placement in most instances.

Biopsies are performed under CT guidance when the lesion is not adequately defined by fluoroscopy or in situations where particularly accurate placement is required, especially in terms of depth. Pleural or mediastinal masses usually are best defined by CT and are most easily biopsied using CT guidance. The greatest limitations of CT as a biopsy guidance system are its limited field of display and the fact that it is not a real time system. These limitations become significant when the biopsy target is an intrapulmonary nodule subject to respiratory motion. Even cooperative patients are unable to reproduce a given degree of lung inflation precisely on successive scans. Therefore, a small lesion may move out of the scan plane during the localization procedure. With a real-time system such as fluoroscopy, such respiratory variations can be monitored and corrected for more easily.

Accuracy

Needle biopsy can be highly accurate in expert hands. In several large series in which the biopsies were performed by experienced radiologists, the reported accuracy ranged from 74 to 96 percent for malignant lesions.[5,22,40,82] In practice, the success rate will depend on several factors. In addition to the skill of the individual performing the biopsy, the pathologist also plays a crucial role. The diagnostic yield will also reflect patient selection. Highest accuracy rates are achieved in hospitals where cases that yield indeterminate results are rebiopsied on a routine basis.

A significant limitation of fine-needle biopsy has been its inability to diagnose benign lesions reliably. This reflects a heavy reliance on cytologic techniques in the past that allowed confident diagnosis of malignant tumors in many cases but negative or indeterminate results for most benign inflammatory lesions. This shortcoming of the technique has been mitigated by the newer "aspirating-cutting" needles that can obtain tissue for histology.[28] The tissue sample is still small, however, and will not be adequate for confident diagnosis of benign disease in every case. Therefore, diagnostic accuracy for benign lesions such as granulomas is still considerably less than that for malignant disease. This has practical implications for the patient with an indeterminate coin lesion. Assuming that there is no evidence of metastatic disease, neither a positive nor an indeterminate biopsy result will preclude the need for a thoracotomy. Only a definitive diagnosis of benign disease will alter therapy. Therefore, when the probability of lung cancer is extremely high, on the basis of noninvasive testing, it sometimes is appropriate to proceed to thoracotomy without a tissue diagnosis. Needle biopsy is most useful for confirming metastic disease in either the lungs or elsewhere. In this application a cytologic diagnosis is usually adequate.

Complications

The most common complication of needle biopsy is pneumothorax, with a reported incidence in the range of 20 to 35 percent, although only 5 to 10 percent require treatment.[22,40] In patients with chronic obstructive pulmonary disease, the risk is markedly increased.[71] If a lesion is located in an area surrounded by bullae, a pneumothorax is virtually assured. The likelihood of pneumothorax is also greater when multiple pleural punctures are performed or when pulmonary fissures are transgressed by the biopsy needle.

Significant hemorrhage is very uncommon when small-gauge needles are used. In a collected series of 2726 cases no deaths occurred, but 2 deaths due to hemorrhage were reported among 430 cases in another series.[5,71] The two reported fatalities occurred in patients with central cavitary lesions containing air fluid levels that were biopsied with 18-gauge needles. Such cases should be approached with caution. Mild hemoptysis is very common, and some degree of localized pulmonary hemorrhage in the immediate vicinity of the biopsied lesion is almost inevitable. Air embolism is a rare complication but has been documented. It is liable to occur when a patient generates negative intrathoracic pressure when the needle tip is inserted in a pulmonary vein and the stylet has been removed. For this reason, needle biopsy should be performed only when the patient is in the recumbent position, and the stylet should be in place during manipulation.[71] The possibility of implanting tumor cells along the needle track has been a cause of concern in the past. Extensive experience has now been accumulated, and such events have proven to be very rare.[22,40] Sinner found one such example among 5300 biopsies.[71]

Contraindications

There are few absolute contraindications to fine-needle biopsy although factors that increase the likelihood of pneumothorax or reduce the patient's ability to tolerate a pneumothorax increase the risk. Inability of a patient to cooperate by maintaining a fixed position, uncontrollable cough, or inability to suspend respiration on demand are also contraindications.

Central location of the lesion is not in itself a contraindication to needle biopsy provided a fine-caliber needle (i.e., ≤ 21-gauge) is used. Accidental puncture of major vascular structures rarely results in serious hemorrhage; however, we recommend advancing the biopsy needle cautiously through hilar or mediastinal lesions with suction, prior to utilizing more vigorous biopsy techniques.[84] Abnormal hemostasis or the presence of pulmonary hypertension greatly increase the risk of hemorrhage.

Large-caliber cutting needles should be used with extreme caution in the lung. Although these instruments can obtain excellent tissue specimens, they do so at the cost of a serious risk of uncontrollable bleeding.[47,48] Reported mortality rates have been as high as 4 percent in some series.[17] We recommend using these large cutting needles only for pleural based masses, and only when fine-needle biopsy has failed to provide adequate tissue. Trephine needle biopsy, which involves the use of a compressed-gas powered cutting needle, has a diagnostic yield and complication rate similar to those for conventional large cutting needles.[37]

Mediastinoscopy

Mediastinoscopy is a surgical procedure that usually is performed under general anesthesia. The mediastinoscope, a hollow, rigid instrument, is introduced through a small incision at the supersternal notch and advanced along the pretracheal plane to the level of the carina. Lymph nodes can be visualized and biopsied. On the right side, the upper margin of the hilum can be reached; on the left, access to the hilum is limited by the aortic arch.

Mediastinoscopy is mainly a staging procedure in lung cancer, although it can be used for diagnosis when the primary lesion is not easily accessible and when enlarged nodes are identified on CT scan in the pretracheal plane.

The diagnostic yield will depend heavily on patient selection. Predictably, in cases where there is x-ray evidence of mediastinal involvement, the yield of mediastinoscopy is very high. Stanford and co-workers reported positive results in 24 out of 27 patients who had chest x-ray evidence of mediastinal adenopathy, while only 1 out of 16 with a radiographically normal mediastinum was positive.[73]

Superior venacaval obstruction, previous mediastinal surgery, or previous radiation therapy are relative contraindications to mediastinoscopy. The procedure is safe in experienced hands, with an average mortality of less than 1 percent.[18] The principal risk from the procedure itself is hemorrhage secondary to laceration or inadvertent biopsy of a blood vessel. Recurrent laryngeal nerve paralysis, pneumothorax, and mediastinal emphysema can also occur.[25] Infection and tumor spread have been reported although they are rare.[11,62] Several mediastinal nodal groups are not accessible via mediastinoscopy, particularly posterior subcarinal, left hilar and paraesophageal, and 5 to 36 percent of patients with negative mediastinoscopy will be found to have involved mediastinal nodes at surgery.[36]

Parasternal Exploration

A limited parasternal mediastinotomy can be performed for diagnostic purposes. This provides access to areas of the mediastinum that are beyond the reach of the mediastinoscope, particularly the hilum and aortopulmonary window regions on the left and the hilum on the right. Portions of the lung may also be palpated by entering the pleura.

The procedure is more invasive than mediastinoscopy and has a slightly higher complication rate. Wound infection, pneumonia, pleural effusion, and hematoma have been reported.[15,35] In general, however, it is a well-tolerated procedure with lower risks than a conventional thoracotomy. The diagnostic yield will largely reflect patient selection.

Thoracentesis and Thoracoscopy

When the presence of pleural effusion is uncertain, a lateral decubitus view is usually diagnostic. CT is also highly accurate for identifying pleural fluid, although simpler techniques usually suffice. In a patient with suspected lung cancer, a pleural effusion may be secondary to direct pleural invasion by the primary lesion, metastatic involvement of the pleura, reactive effusion secondary to postobstructive pneumonia, or lymphatic obstruction. Other etiologies such as cardiac failure, pulmonary embolism, or infection may also play a role. These causes may be impossible to distinguish on radiological grounds alone, but thoracentesis and cytologic analysis of the fluid provide more specific information.[34,44] In all cases of lung cancer with pleural effusion, a positive cytologic diagnosis can be made from the fluid in 40 to 75 percent, with the highest yield in adenocarcinomas.[34,35] Other characteristics of the effusion can be helpful. For instance, more than 100,000 RBCs mm^{-3} is strongly suggestive of malignancy if infarct and trauma can be excluded.[44] A predominance of polymorphs suggests inflammation, while a predominance of lymphocytes favors tumor or tuberculosis.[44]

When a pleural effusion is the sole abnormality and both thoracentesis and pleural biopsy are nondiagnostic, thoracoscopy should be considered.[4,6,67] Either a modified bronchoscope or a rigid thoracoscope can be used. The instrument is inserted through a small incision in an intercostal space under general anesthesia to allow direct inspection and biopsy of the pleural surfaces. Significant complications are rare although hemorrhage, infection, and tumor seeding have been reported.

Scalene and Supraclavicular Node Biopsy

Routine biopsy of nonpalpable scalene or supraclavicular nodes produces a very low diagnostic yield in patients with lung cancer and thus is not recommended. However, in selected cases with palpable supraclavicular nodes, the yield for detection of metastases is in the region of 90 percent.[7,58] Major complications are uncommon although injuries to adjacent structures can occur, resulting in neurologic damage, lymphatic leaks, and pneumothorax.[72] We reserve this procedure for patients with palpable supraclavicular nodes. The information gained can be valuable for both diagnosis and staging.

CONCLUSION

The optimal diagnostic approach to the patient with suspected lung cancer is one that leads to a conclusive diagnosis while minimizing monetary cost and patient morbidity. To achieve this requires some flexibility and careful planning.[52] A diagnostic study should be selected with specific questions and likely answers in mind. The results of one test may render the next test unnecessary.

Regardless of the particular circumstances of a case, a thorough history, physical examination, and chest radiography should be the starting point of the investigation. As the workup proceeds, direct communication between the various specialists involved becomes vital in order to achieve a coherent approach and to ensure that available resources are used efficiently.

REFERENCES

1. Austin JHM, Sagel SS: Tomography, Sagel SS (ed): Special procedures in Chest Radiology. Philadelphia, Saunders, 1976, pp 1-22
2. Ballard GL, Boyd WR: A specially designed cutting aspiration needle for lung biopsy. Am J Roentgenol 130:889-903, 1978
3. Baron RL, Levitt RG, Sagel SS, et al: computed tomography in the preoperative evaluation of bronchogenic carcinoma. Radiology 145:727-732, 1982
4. Ben-Isaac FE, Simmons DH: Flexible fiberoptic pleuroscopy: Pleural and lung biopsy. Chest 67:573-576, 1975
5. Berquist TH, Bailey PB, Cortese DA, et al: Transthoracic needle biopsy. Accuracy and complications in relation to location and type of lesion. Mayo Clin Proc 55:475-481, 1980
6. Boutin C, Viallat JR, Cargnino P, et al: thoracoscopy in malignant pleural effusions. Am Rev Respir Dis 24:588-592, 1981
7. Brantigan JW, Brantigan CO, Brantigan OC: Biopsy of nonpalpable scalene lymph nodes in carcinoma of the lung. Am Rev Respir Dis 107:962-974, 1974
8. Cann CE, Gamusu G, Birnberg FA, et al: Quantification of calcium in solitary pulmonary nodules using single-and dual-energy CT. Radiology 145:493-496
9. Credle WF, Smiddy JF, Elliott RC: Complications of fiberoptic bronchoscopy. Am Rev Resp Dis 109:67-72, 1974
10. Dahlgren SE, Lind B: Comparison between diagnostic results obtained by transthoracic needle biopsy and by sputum cytology. Acta Cytolog 16:53-58, 1972
11. Doctor AH: Mediastinoscopy: A critical evaluation of 220 cases. Ann Surg 174:965-968, 1971
12. Elkin M: Issues in radiology related to the new technologies. Radiology 143:1-6, 1982
13. Ellis JH Jr: Transbronchial lung biopsy via the fiberoptic bronchoscope: Experience with 107 consecutive cases and comparison with bronchial brushing. Chest 68:524-532, 1975
14. Erozan YS, Frost JK: Cytopathologic diagnosis of lung cancer. Semin Oncol 1:191-198, 1974
15. Evans DS, Hall JH, Harrison GK: Anterior mediastinotomy. Thorax 28:444-447, 1973
16. Felson B: Thoracic calcifications. Dis Chest 56:330-343, 1969
17. Forrest JV, Sagel SS: Comment on lung biopsy techniques. Chest 67:737-738, 1975
18. Foster DE, Munro DD, Dobell ARC: Mediastinoscopy: A review of anatomical relationships and complications. Ann Thorac Surg 13:273-386, 1972
19. Fraser RG, Barnes GT, Hickey N, et al: Potential value of digital radiography. Preliminary observations on the use of dual-energy substraction in the evaluation of pulmonary nodules. Chest 89:249-252, 1986
20. Frost JK, Ball WC Jr, Levin ML, et al: Early lung cancer detection: Results of the initial (prevalence) radiologic and cytologic screening in the Johns Hopkins study. Am rev Resp Dis 130:549-554, 1984

21. Gamsu G, Webb WR, Sheldon P, et al: Nuclear magnetic resonance imaging of the thorax. Radiology 147:473-480, 1983

22. Gibney RTN, Man GCW, King EG, et al: Aspiration biopsy in the diagnosis of pulmonary disease. Chest 80:300-303, 1981

23. Glazer GM, Francis IR, Shirazi KK, Evaluation of the pulmonary hilum: comparison of conventional radiography, 55° posterior oblique tomography, and dynamic computed tomography. J Comput Assist Tomogr 983-989, 1983

24. Godwin JD, Speckman JM, Fram EK, et al: distinguishing benign from malignant pulmonary nodules by computed tomography. Radiology 144:349-351, 1982

25. Goldberg EM, Shapiro CM, Glicksman AS: Mediastinoscopy for assessing mediastinal spread in clinical staging of lung carcinoma. Semin Oncol 3:205-214, 1974

26. Good CA, Wilson TW: The solitary circumscribed pulmonary nodule: Study of seven hundred five cases encountered roentgenologically in a period of three and one-half years. JAMA 166:210-215, 1958

27. Good CA, Hood RT Jr, McDonald JR: Significance of a solitary mass in the lung. Am J Roentgenol 70:543-554, 1953

28. Greene R, Szyfelbein WM, Isler RJ, et al: Supplementary tissue-core histology from fine-needle transthoracic aspiration biopsy. Am J Roentgenol 144:787-792, 1985

29. Grunze H: A critical review and evaluation of cytodiagnosis in chest diseases. Acta Cytol 4:175-198, 1960

30. Heavey LR, Glazer GM, Gross BH, et al: The role of CT in staging radiographic $T_1N_0M_0$ lung cancer. Am J Radiology 146:285-290, 1986

31. Heelan RT, Martini N, Westcott JW, et al: Carcinomatous involvement of the hilum and mediastinum: Computed tomographic and magnetic resonance evaluation. Radiology 156:111-115, 1985

32. Heilman RS: What's wrong with radiology. New Engl J Med 306:477-479, 1982

33. House AJS, Thomson KR: Evaluation of a new transthoracic needle for biopsy of benign and malignant lung lesions. Am J Roentgenol 129:215-220, 1977

34. Jarvi OIl, Kunnas RJ, Laitio MT, et al: The accuracy and significance of cytologic cancer diagnosis of pleural effusions (A followup study of 338 patients). Acta Cytol 16:152-158, 1972

35. Jolly PC, Hill LD, Lawless PA, et al: Parasternal mediastinotomy and mediastinoscopy: Adjuncts in the diagnosis of chest disease. J Thorac Cardivasc Surg 66:549-556, 1973

36. Kagan AR, Steckel RJ, Bein ME, et al: Diagnostic oncology case study. Pulmonary mass in a smoker: Preoperative imaging for staging of lung cancer. Am J Roentgenol 136:739-745, 1981

37. King EG, Bachynski JE, Mielke B: Percutaneous trephine lung biopsy: Evolving role. Chest 70:212-216, 1976

38. Knopf DR, Torres WE, Fajman WJ, et al: Liver lesions: Comparative accuracy of scintigraphy and computed tomography. Am J Radiology 138:623-627, 1982

39. Kvale PA, Bode FR, Kini S: Diagnostic accuracy in lung cancer. Comparison of techniques used in association with flexible fiberoptic bronchoscopy. Chest 69:752-757, 1976

40. Lalli AF, McCormack LJ, Zelch M, et al: Aspiration biopsies of chest lesions. Radiology 127:35-40, 1978

41. Levitt RG, Glazer HS, Roper CL, et al: Magnetic resonance imaging of mediastinal and hilar masses: Comparison with CT. Am J Radiology 145:9-14, 1985

42. Lewis JW Jr, Madrazo BL, Gross SC, et al: The value of radiographic and computed tomography in the staging of lung carcinoma. Ann Thorac Surg 34:553-557, 1982

43. Libshitz HI, McKenna RJ, Haynie TP, et al: Mediastinal evaluation in lung cancer. Radiology 151:295-299, 1984

44. Light RW, Erozan YS, Ball WC: Cells in pleural fluid: Their value in differential diagnosis. Arch Intern Med 132:854-860, 1973

45. Lukeman JM: Reliability of cytologic diagnosis in cancer of the lung. Cancer Chemother Rep, Part 3, Vol 4:79-93, 1973

46. Marsh BR, Wang KP: Bronchoscopy in the diagnosis of pulmonary disease, in Siegelman SS, Stitik FP, Summer WR (eds): Pulmonary System: Practical Approaches to Pulmonary Diagnosis. Orlando Fl; Grune & Stratton, 1979, pp 161-181

47. McCartney RL: Hemorrhage following percutaneous lung biopsy. Radiology 112:305-307, 1974

48. Rehnert JH, Brown MJ: Percutaneous needle core biopsy of peripheral pulmonary masses. Am J Surg 136:131-156, 1978

49. Melamed MR, Flehinger BJ, Zaman MB, et al: Screening for early lung cancer. Results of the Memorial Sloan-Kettering study in New York. Chest 86:44-51, 1984

50. Mintzer RA, Malave SR, Neiman III, et al: Computed vs. conventional tomography in evaluation of primary and secondary pulmonary neoplasms. Radiology 132:653-659, 1979

51. Mitnick JS, Bosniak MA, Megibow AJ, et al: Non-functioning adrenal adenomas discovered incidentally on computed tomography. Radiology 148:495-499, 1983

52. Muhm JR, Miller WE, Fontana RS, et al: Lung cancer detected during a screening program using four-month chest radiographs. Radiology 148:609-615, 1983

53. Muhm JR, Brown LR, Crowe JK, et al: Comparison of whole lung tomography and computed tomography for detecting pulmonary nodules. Am J Roentgenol 131:981-984, 1978

54. Nathan MH, Collins VP, Adams RA: Differentiation of benign and malignant pulmonary nodules by growth rate. Radiology 79:221-232, 1962

55. Naylor B, Schmidt RW: The case for exfoliative cytology of serous effusions. Lancet 1:711-712, 1964

56. Osborne DR, Korobkin M, Ravin CE, et al: Comparison of plain tomography, conventional tomography, and computed tomography in detecting intrathoracic lymph node metastasis from congestive heart failure, lymph node enlargement, and neoplastic infiltration. Radiology 179:551-559, 1981

57. Osborne DR, Korobkin M, Ravin CE, et al: Comparison of plain radiography, conventional tomography, and computed tomography in detecting intrathoracic lymph node metastases from lung carcinoma. Radiology 142:157-161, 1982

58. Palumbo LT, Sharpe WS: Scalene node biopsy: Correlation with other diagnostic procedures in 550 cases. Arch Surg 98:90-93, 1969

59. Payne CR, Hadfield JW, Stovin PG, et al: Diagnostic accuracy of cytology and biopsy in primary bronchial carcinoma. J Clin Pathol 34:773-778, 1978

60. Percira W, Kovnat DM, Khan MA, et al: Fever and pneumonia after flexible fiberoptic bronchoscopy. Am Rev Resp Dis 112:59-64, 1975

61. Radke JR, Conway WA, Eyler WR, et al: Diagnostic accuracy in peripheral lung lesions. Factors predicting success with flexible fiberoptic bronchoscopy. Chest 76:176-179, 1979

62. Reynders H. Mediastinoscopy in bronchogenic cancer. Dis Chest 45:606-611, 1964

63. Robbins HM, Sweet ME, Jefferson SE, et al: The determination of resectability of lung cancer by fiberoptic bronchoscopy. Arch Intern Med 141:649-650, 1981

64. Rosa UW, Prolla JC, Gastal ES: Cytology in diagnosis of cancer affecting the lung: Results in 1,000 consecutive patients. Chest 63:203-207, 1973

65. Sandler MA, Pearlberg JP, Madrazo BL, et al: Computed tomographic evaluation of the adrenal gland in the preoperative assessment of bronchogenic carcinoma. Radiology 145:733-736, 1982

66. Schaner EG, Chang AE, Doppman JL, et al: Comparison of computed and conventional whole lung tomography in detecting pulmonary nodules: A prospective radiologic-pathologic study. Am J Roentgenol 131:51-54, 1978

67. Senno A, Moallem S, Quijano ER, et al: Thoracoscopy with the fiberoptic bronchoscope:

A simple method in diagnosing pleuropulmonary diseases. J Thorac Cardiovasc Surg 67:606-611, 1974

68. Shure D, Fedullo PF: The role of transcarinal needle aspiration in staging of bronchogenic carcinoma. Chest 86:693-696, 1984

69. Siegelman SS, Zerhouni EA, Leo FP, et al: CT of the solitary pulmonary nodule. Am J Roentgenol 135:1-13, 1980

70. Sinner WN: Transthoracic needle biopsy of small peripheral malignant lung lesions. Invest Radiol 8:305-314, 1973

71. Sinner WN: Complications of percutaneous transthoracic needle aspiration biopsy. Acta Radiol Diagn 17:813-827, 1976

72. Skinner DB: Scalene Lymph Node Biopsy. Reappraisal of risks and indications. New Engl J Med 268:1324-1329, 1963

73. Stanford W, Steele S, Armstrong RG, et al: Mediastinoscopy: Its applicaiton in central versus peripheral thoracic lesions. Ann Thorac Surg 19:121-126, 1975

74. Steele JD: The solitary pulmonary nodule: Report of a cooperative study of resected asymptomatic solitary pulmonary nodules in males. J Thorac Cardiovasc Surg 46:21-39, 1963

75. Stringfield JT, Markowitz DJ, Bentz RR, et al: The effect of tumor size and location on diagnosis by fiberoptic bronchoscopy. Chest 72: 474-476, 1977

76. Theros EG: Varying manifestations of peripheral pulmonary neoplasms: A radiologic-pathologic correlative study. Am J Roentgenol 128:893-914, 1977

77. Umiker WO: Diagnosis of bronchogenic carcinoma: An evaluation of pulmonary cytology, bronchoscopy and scalene lymph node biopsy. Dis Chest 37:82-90, 1960

78. Umiker WO: The current role of exfoliative cytopathology in the routine diagnosis of bronchogenic carcinoma. Dis Chest 40:154-159, 1961

79. Webb WR: Computed tomography in the diagnosis of bronchogenic carcinoma, in Margolis AR, Gooding CA (eds): Diagnostic Radiology. San Francisco, University of California Department of Radiology, 1982, pp 239-249

80. Webb WR, Gamsu G, Crooks LE: Multisection sagittal and coronal magnetic resonance imaging of the madiastinum and hila. Radiology 150:475-478, 1984

81. Webb WR, Jensen BG, Sollitto R, et al: Bronchogenic carcinoma: Staging with MR compared with staging with CT and surgery. Radiology 156:117-124, 1985

82. Westcott JL: Percutaneous needle aspiration of hilar and mediastinal masses. Radiology 141:323-329, 1981

83. Zavala DC: Pulmonary hemorrhage in fiberoptic transbronchial biopsy. Chest 70:584-588, 1976

84. Zelch JV, Lalli AF: Diagnostic percutaneous opacification of benign pulmonary lesions. Radiology 108:559-561, 1973

85. Zerhouni EA, Spivey JF, Morgan RH, et al: Factors influencing quantitative CT measurements of solitary pulmonary nodules. J Comput Assist Tomogr 6:1075-1087, 1982

86. Zerhouni EA, Bukadoum M, Siddiky MA, et al: Standard phantom for quantitative CT analysis of solitary pulmonary nodules. Radiology 149:767-773, 1983

87. Zerhouni EA, Stitik FP, Siegelman SS, et al: CT of the pulmonary nodule: A cooperative study. Radiology 160:319-327, 1986

88. Zerhouni EA, Frederick PS, Siegelman SS, et al: CT of the pulmonary nodule: A cooperative study. Radiology 160:319-327, 1986

Mark K. Ferguson, Heber MacMahon
Carlos Bekerman, James W. Ryan

_____ **8** _____

Noninvasive and Invasive Staging
of Lung Cancer

The staging of cancer is a process in which the extent of disease is assessed and patients are accordingly assigned to groups with similar prognoses for which similar treatments are recommended. Staging of lung cancer is particularly relevant because of the significant differences in survival among the various stages and the multiple therapeutic modalities available for this disease. The use of a formal staging system in the management of lung cancer provides many benefits. Staging assists in planning treatment by assigning patients to groups that require local (surgery or radiation therapy) versus systemic (chemotherapy) treatment. Because the staging systems are based on retrospective studies comparing the anatomic extent of cancer to survival rates, staging also provides the patient with an estimate of prognosis. Communication between one physician and another regarding treatment of an individual patient is immeasurably aided by reference to a standardized staging system for lung cancer. Finally, clinical research depends on accurate pretreatment staging to provide comparable groups for randomization between treatment options. Staging thus assists in comparing results between treatment programs within an institution and is indispensable in comparing results from one institution to those of another.

DEFINITIONS

The American Joint Committee for Cancer Staging and End Results Reporting (AJC)[51] provides a staging method based on the TNM system adopted by the International Union Against Cancer.[54] The AJC staging system is used throughout this text and is the most widely used system for staging of lung cancer in the Western hemisphere.

LUNG CANCER: A COMPREHENSIVE TREATISE
ISBN 0-8089-1876-1

Primary Tumor (T)

WHen the TNM system is used to describe the anatomic extent of disease, the letter "T" refers to the primary tumor, with appropriate suffixes to describe the size and extent of primary tumor involvement. "T_X" designates a tumor proven cytologically by the presence of cancer cells in sputum or bronchial washings but not evident broncho- scopically or radiographically. Such primary tumors are commonly detected in high- risk screening programs. "T_0" and "T_{IS}" are other uncommonly used headings that indicate no evidence of primary tumor or carcinoma in situ, respectively.

"T_1" designates a tumor that is completely surrounded by lung or visceral pleura, does not invade proximal to a lobar bronchus at bronchoscopy, and measure 3.0 cm or less in greatest diameter. Primary tumors of this size, because of their lack of involvement of pleura or proximal airways, frequently are asymptomatic and often are diagnosed as a result of a routine chest radiograph.

A tumor indicated by "T_2" measures more than 3 cm in maximum diameter. The category also includes tumors of any size associated with atelectasis or obstructive pneumonitis involving less than an entire lung, or tumors of any size that invade the visceral pleura (Fig. 8-1). Bronchoscopically, these tumors must be at least 2 cm distal to the carina. Such tumors cannot have an associated pleural effusion. Because of the involvement of visceral pleura, associated atelectasis, or invasion of major airways, T_2 tumors are more likely than T_1 tumors to be symptomatic.

"T_3" refers to a tumor of any size with one or more of the following characteristics: (1) direct extension into an adjacent structure, including the mediastinal pleura or its contents, diaphragm, parietal pleura, or chest wall; (2) a tumor that bronchoscopically extends to within 2 cm of the carina; (3) a tumor associated with atelectasis or obstructive pneumonitis of an entire lung; or (4) any tumor associated with a pleural effusion (benign or malignant) (Fig. 8-2). T_3 tumors usually are symptomatic because of pain from chest wall involvement, respiratory symptoms from obstruction and/or pleural effusion, or hoarseness from involvement of a recurrent laryngeal nerve.

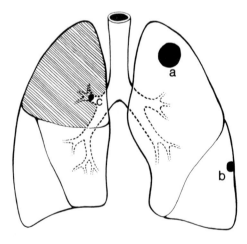

Fig. 8-1. In the T_2 classification, the pri- mary tumor is greater than 3 cm in diameter (a) or invades visceral pleura (b) or is associ- ated with atelectasis extending to the hilum (c).

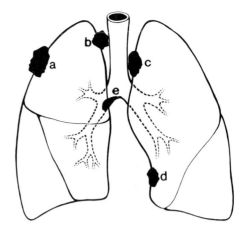

Fig. 8-2. T_3 tumors have extension into the chest wall (*a*) or mediastinum (*b*), directly invade the great vessels or recurrent or phrenic nerves (*c*), involve pericardium or diaphragm (*d*), or are demonstrable bronchoscopically to extend to within 2 cm of the carina (*e*).

Nodal Involvement (N)

The status of regional lymph nodes with regard to involvement by tumor metastases is designated by the letter "N" with appropriate subscripts. "N_0" refers to the absence of demonstrable metastases to regional lymph nodes, including hilar and mediastinal nodes. "N_1" designates metastases to nodes in the intrapulmonary, peribronchial, or ipsilateral hilar region, all of which are normally encompassed by visceral pleura (Fig. 8-3). "N_2" refers to the presence of metastases in mediastinal lymph nodes, including paratracheal, subcarinal, tracheobronchial, para-aortic, paraesophageal, inferior pulmonary ligament, aortopulmonary, and anterior mediastinal lymph nodes (Fig. 8-4). Scalene and supraclavicular lymph node metastases are specifically excluded from the N_2 designation as they represent metastatic diseases.

Distant Metastases (M)

The presence or absence of distant metastases is designated by the letter "M" with modifying subscripts. "M_X" refers to instances in which the presence of distant metas-

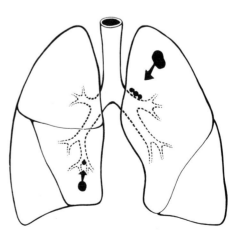

Fig. 8-3. N_1 lymph nodes are those in the ipsilateral hilar region or the peribronchial region or are intrapulmonary.

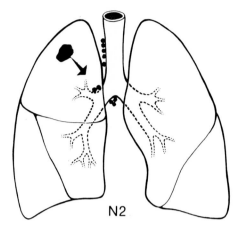

N2

Fig. 8-4. N_2 lymph nodes include those in the subcarinal region and ipsilateral or contra-lateral paratracheal, paraaortic, aorto-pulmonary, paraesophageal or pulmonary lig-ament nodes.

tases is not adequately assessed. "M_0" indicates no known distant metastases. "M_1" signifies the presence of distant metastases, with additional subscripts employed to identify the specific site of metastatic spread when possible (PUL—contralateral pulmonary; OSS—osseous; HEP—hepatic; BRA—brain; LYM—lymph nodes; MAR—bone marrow; PLE—pleura; SKI—skin; EYE—eye; OTH—other).

Stages

On the basis of the TNM classification the AJC has defined three stages for lung cancer (Table 8-1). Any tumor that is classified as T_1 without metastases or T_1 with metastases to peribronchial and/or ipsilateral hilar regional lymph nodes, or any tumor that is classified as T_2 in the absence of metastases is included in stage I disease. (Fig. 8-5). Stage II is a single subset consisting of patients with a T_2 primary tumor with metastases to lymph nodes in the ipsilateral hilum (Fig. 8-6).

Stage III disease encompasses all other patients, including those with T_3 tumors, N_2 nodal metastases, or metastatic disease (M_1). Because of the wide variability of

Table 8-1

AJC Lung Cancer Stages

Stage I	$T_XN_0M_0$
	$T_{IS}N_0M_0$
	$T_1N_0M_0$
	$T_1N_1M_0$
	$T_2N_0M_0$
Stage II	$T_2N_1M_0$
Stage III	
III_{M_0}	T_3 with any N; M_0
	N_2 with any T; M_0
III_{M_1}	M_1 with any T; any N

After Staging of Lung Cancer 1979. American Joint Committee for Cancer Staging and End Results Reporting: Task Force on Lung Cancer. Chicago, Il, 1979.

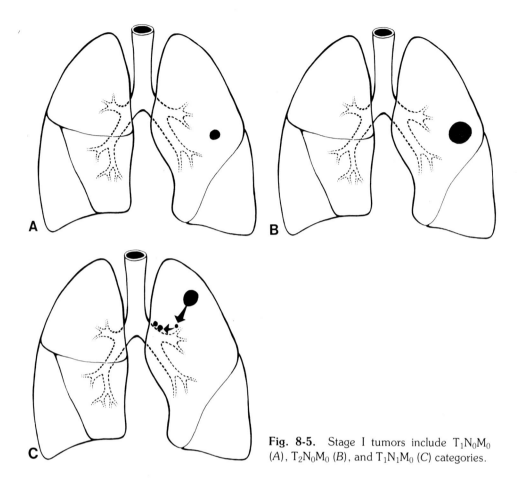

Fig. 8-5. Stage I tumors include $T_1N_0M_0$ (*A*), $T_2N_0M_0$ (*B*), and $T_1N_1M_0$ (*C*) categories.

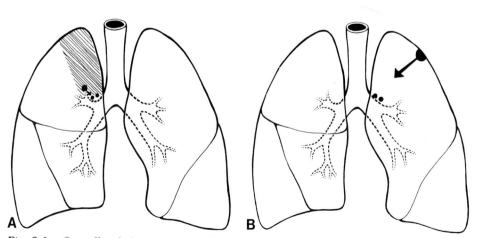

Fig. 8-6. Stage II includes tumors classified as $T_2N_1M_0$, with T_2 tumors classified on the basis of obstructive pneumonitis (*A*), involvement of visceral pleura (*B*), or size larger than 3 cm.

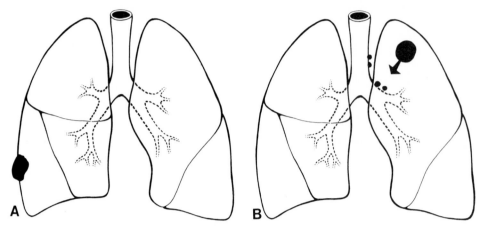

Fig. 8-7. Stage III tumors may be categorized as such on the basis of a locally advanced primary tumor, $T_3N_0M_0$ (A), on the basis of spread to mediastinal (N_2) lymph nodes (B), or because of distant metastases.

disease spread in stage III, ranging from a small peripheral tumor involving the parietal pleura without nodal or distant metastases ($T_3N_0M_0$) (Fig. 8-7) to a large central tumor invading the mediastinum with mediastinal nodal and distant metastases ($T_3N_2M_1$), it is useful to refer to specific TNM categories when discussing patients with stage III disease. Clinically it is our practice to subdivide this group into patients with and without distant metastases, as prognosis is strongly related to the presence or absence of M_1 disease. Thus, stage III is subdivided into stage III_{M0} and stage III_{M1} disease.

Staging Classification

Staging of lung cancer is an ongoing process that parallels the initial evaluation, treatment, and natural course of the disease. Pretreatment staging is based on the anatomic extent of disease that is detected prior to thoracotomy or initiation of therapy. This Clinical-Diagnostic stage (cTNM) is based on information obtained during history and physical examination, bronchoscopy, radiographic and scintigraphic examination, mediastinoscopy, thoracentesis, or thoracoscopy. In some patients, particularly those with metastatic disease or those who are unable to undergo thoracotomy, the Clinical-Diagnostic stage is the final stage available prior to institution of therapy.

Other patients will go on to have Surgical-Evaluative staging and Postsurgical Treatment–Pathologic staging. Surgical-Evaluative staging (sTNM) is based on data obtained during Clinical-Diagnostic staging and on information available during exploratory thoracotomy but does not include information obtained from examination of a resected specimen. Those patients who undergo palliative or therapeutic resection are entered into the Postsurgical Treatment–Pathological stage group (pTNM).

During therapy or in the course of follow-up examinations, recurrence or progression of disease can indicate treatment failure. At this point in time, the anatomic extent of tumor is reassessed, including radiographic and scintigraphic examinations and biopsy techniques when indicated, and the patient is assigned a Retreatment Stage (rTNM). Ultimately, the most accurate method of assessing cancer stage is at autopsy following death of a cancer patient. All information obtained in this manner is used in assigning a final Autopsy stage (aTNM).

Other Staging Systems

A variety of other systems exist for staging lung cancer. These include the system adopted by the International Union Against Cancer,[54] which is nearly identical to the AJC system used throughout this text, as well as another more disparate system promulgated by the American Thoracic Society.[8] At a recent meeting of the IV World Conference on Lung Cancer, a new international staging system for lung cancer was proposed that has had input from a variety of organizations, including the American Cancer Society, the National Cancer Institute, the American College of Surgeons, the American College of Physicians, and the American College of Radiology. The present text is organized according to the AJC staging system. However, the newly proposed system, as outlined in Table 8-2, is likely to be extensively used in the future as it is based on more thorough evaluation and followup of a larger number of lung cancer patients than has previously been available.[41,50]

Table 8-2
Proposed International Staging
for Lung Cancer

Occult carcinoma	$T_X N_0 M_0$
Stage 0	$T_{1S} N_0 M_0$
Stage I	$T_1 N_0 M_0$
	$T_2 N_0 M_0$
Stage II	$T_1 N_1 M_0$
	$T_2 N_1 M_0$
Stage IIIa	$T_3{}^* N_0 M_0$
	$T_3{}^* N_1 M_0$
	$T_{1-3} N_2{}^\dagger M_0$
Stage IIIb	Any T with N_3; M_0
	T_4 with any N; M_0
Stage IV	Any T; Any N; M_1

After Mountain CF: A new international staging system for lung cancer. Chest 89:225S–233S, 1986 and Staging of lung cancer. American Joint Committee on Cancer, in press.
*T_3 differs from current AJC definition only in that involvement of chest wall and mediastinum is limited to regions amenable to surgical resection. All other primaries, including those involving aorta, main pulmonary artery, myocardium, trachea, esophagus, or vertebral body, or those associated with a malignant pleural effusion, are classified as T_4.
†N_2 disease, in contradistinction to the current AJC classification, refers to metastases to ipsilateral mediastinal and subcarinal lymph nodes. Involvement of contralateral hilar, contralateral mediastinal, or any supraclavicular or scalene lymph nodes is considered N_3 disease.

STAGING PROCESS

The staging process is a sequentially performed series of examinations or tests designed to elucidate the anatomic extent of disease in a manner that is time-efficient, is cost-effective, and has both low morbidity and high patient acceptance. Only objective data are used to define a cancer stage, but subjective information is invaluable in selecting tests.

Noninvasive Staging Techniques

Patient Evaluation

A carefully performed history and physical examination constitute the most important first step in evaluation of any patient with suspected lung cancer. Information is obtained relating to performance status as judged by the Karnofsky or the AJC/Zubrod scale (Table 8-3).[9,51] This initial assignation is important in identifying patients who are capable of meeting future rigorous demands provided by invasive tests or by treatment options such as surgery, radiation therapy, or chemotherapy. In addition, clues may be uncovered that direct the investigation to specific organ systems and thus maximize staging efficiency. Common clinical findings that suggest metastatic disease include weight loss, bone pain, neurologic symptoms, hepatomegaly, and elevation of serum alkaline phosphatase or calcium levels.

Radiography

The first test acquired in the staging process is that customarily used for diagnosis: posteroanterior and lateral chest radiography. Accurate interpretation of the chest film gives many clues as to the stage of a lung cancer. In peripheral tumors, estimation of the size, location, and relationship to the chest wall yields an estimate of T classification. Although it is difficult to recognize specific nodal groups with metastases, the impression of an enlarged hilum or enlarged mediastinal lymph nodes frequently provides a clue to N status. Other important findings may include a pleural effusion, elevation of a hemidiaphragm suggesting involvement of the ipsilateral phrenic nerve, lobar collapse indicating a T_2 tumor, or collapse of an entire lung identifying a T_3

Table 8-3
AJC/Zubrod Performance Scale (PS)

Grade	Description
0	Fully active, able to carry on all predisease activities without restriction
1	Restricted in physically strenuous activity but ambulatory and able to carry out work of a light or sedentary nature
2	Ambulatory and capable of all self-care but unable to carry out any work activities; up and about $>50\%$ of waking hours
3	Capable of only limited self-care, confined to bed or chair $\geq 50\%$ or more of waking hours
4	Completely disabled; cannot carry out any self-care; totally confined to bed or chair

After Staging of lung cancer 1979. American Joint Committee for Cancer Staging and End Results Reporting: Task Force on Lung Cancer. Chicago, Il, 1979.

tumor. In addition to findings in the bronchopulmonary tree and lung parenchyma, careful examination of the bony thorax may yield evidence for pathologic rib fractures or metastases to other areas in the spine or shoulder girdle.

Special plain radiographic techniques, including tomography and oblique hilar tomography, have been used extensively in the past and continue to be used at some centers to further elucidate the identity of peripheral lung nodules and the anatomy of the pulmonary hila. For evaluation of the mediastinum and hilum, oblique hilar tomography has reasonable accuracy but, in general, is less useful than computed tomography for estimation of the size of hilar lymph nodes.[30,42,53]

Computed tomography (CT) currently is the most accurate of our noninvasive staging techniques. Its popularity has increased over the past 10 years, and currently the combination of rapid scanners and radiologists experienced in CT interpretation makes this examination highly useful. We employ CT scanning on all patients diagnosed as having possible lung cancer and rely on its accuracy to direct other noninvasive or invasive staging procedures. Correct application of scanning techniques is important in providing accurate information. Scans should be performed from the apices of the hemithoraces through the liver and adrenal glands. Scans are performed by using contiguous slices 8–10 mm thick and interpreted by employing separate window settings for both lung parenchyma and mediastinal soft tissues. Intravenous contrast agents are infused continuously, and a bolus infusion is used for selected cases with hilar or aortopulmonary window region abnormalities.

Interpretation of the CT scan includes assessment of the primary lung mass with respect to its margins, dimensions, and location relative to the mediastinum or chest wall and the presence or absence of calcifications. If there is a suggestion of chest wall involvement, bone window settings are of value in resolving this question (Fig. 8-8). Frequently it is difficult to determine with accuracy whether soft tissues of the chest wall are infiltrated by tumor. Many tumors abut the chest wall or mediastinum, and some may cause sufficient distal confluent atelectasis to result in an indeterminate reading. Only surgical exploration can resolve this question.

In addition to evaluation of the primary tumor, CT is valuable in assessing possible enlargement—and by inference, tumor involvement—of hilar and mediastinal lymph nodes. There is continued disagreement regarding size criteria for lymph node enlargement in these regions. Nodes in patients without lung cancer typically measure less than 10 mm,[20,22] but the size in patients with cancer may be greater as a result of atelectasis or obstructive pneumonitis causing reactive enlargement.[19]

Evaluation of hilar lymph nodes for enlargement is the least accurate aspect of CT staging. Because of the confluence of nerves, vessels, and bronchi in these regions, the presence of lymph nodes, much less their size, is often difficult to determine. Frequently only a reading of hilar enlargement can be given for what appears to be an abnormal region. Nevertheless, CT of the hilum still retains an overall accuracy in the range of 70 percent.[17]

More benefit from CT is gained in the assessment of mediastinal lymph nodes (Fig. 8-9). Sensitivity, specificity, and predictive indices may vary considerably depending on limits chosen for normal lymph node size. When an upper limit of 9–10 mm is selected, sensitivity is good, approaching 80 percent, but specificity and overall accuracy are relatively poor at 75 and 77 percent, respectively (Table 8-4). When nodes larger than 15 mm are considered positive, specificity and accuracy rise to 93 and 86 percent, making this criterion much more useful. Despite the large numbers of

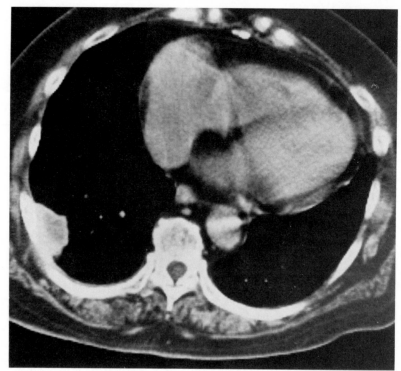

Fig. 8-8. The CT scan frequently is helpful in evaluating involvement of chest wall or mediastinum by the primary tumor, as in this patient, who had a right lower lobe squamous cell cancer involving the seventh rib.

Table 8-4
Accuracy of CT in Mediastinal Staging

Patients (No.)	Abnormal Size (mm)	Sensitivity (%)	Specificity (%)	Accuracy (%)	PPI* (%)	NPI† (%)	Reference
35	>10	29	46	43	12	72	14
94	>9	92	80	85	77	94	2
73	>10	91	94	93	88	95	30
41	>10	76	67	71	62	80	39
42	>10	72	83	79	76	80	42
49	>10	95	64	78	67	95	21
48	>9	95	68	79	68	95	48
102	>10	60	60	61	32	84	36
484		78.0	71.8	75.1	61.2	88.2	
51	>15	88	94	92	88	94	15
94	>15	74	98	88	97	84	2
41	>15	50	97	83	86	82	40
41	>15	57	85	76	67	79	23
97	>15	75	89	86	69	92	11
324		71.3	92.9	85.9	82.0	87.1	

*Positive Predictive Index.
†Negative Predictive Index.

122

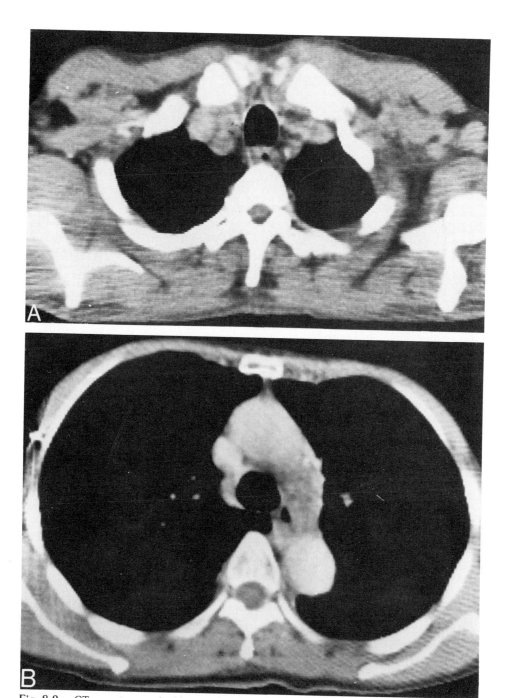

Fig. 8-9. CT scanning is valuable in assessment of mediastinal lymph node size. Most mediastinal regions are adequately assessed, frequently showing discrete enlarged lymph nodes as in the paratracheal region (A), while an estimation of discrete adenopathy in the aortopulmonary region usually is less reliable (B).

Table 8-5

CT of the Mediastinum. Accuracy According to Tumor Histology

Histology	Patients	Sensitivity (%)	Specificity (%)	Accuracy (%)	PPI* (%)	NPI† (%)
Adenocarcinoma	22	87.5	100	100	91.7	94.7
Squamous cell	24	100	58.3	50	100	70.6
All cell types	61	95	83.3	79.2	96.1	88.0

After reference 17 with permission.
*Positive Predictive Index.
†Negative Predictive Index.

data already collected, the optimal size criteria for staging mediastinal lymph nodes remain undefined. We have chosen to classify all lymph nodes measuring less than 10 mm in size as "uninvolved," those measuring greater than 20 mm as "involved," and those between 1.0 and 2.0 cm "indeterminate" (less than 10 percent of all mediastinal nodes in our experience). This provides optimal sensitivity, positive predictive index, and negative predictive index with an acceptable overall accuracy (Table 8-5). The accuracy of mediastinal lymph nodes assessment by CT scan is worse for squamous cell carcinoma than for adenocarcinomas. In addition, the aorto-pulmonary window region is less accurately assessed than most mediastinal regions, again illustrating the need for bolus contrast infusion when scanning through tumors likely to involve this region.

Scanning through the upper abdomen provides evaluation of the liver and adrenal glands for metastases. Because of the high frequency of liver and adrenal metastases in lung cancer, the CT scan can provide evidence for distant spread that may otherwise go unsuspected.

Scintigraphy

Scintigraphic examinations are also useful in the noninvasive staging of lung cancer. At our institution we use a tomographic ^{67}Ga scan in all patients with suspected lung cancer as part of the initial staging evaluation.[12] The technique used in performing the ^{67}Ga scan is of utmost importance in obtaining accurate and dependable results. Following an injection of 10 mCi (millicuries) of ^{67}Ga citrate,* tomographic images over the entire body are obtained 72 hours following injection. In interpreting the scan results, only abnormalities 2 cm or greater in diameter will be reliably detected. The use of the ^{67}Ga scan as a screening test for lung cancer is not recommended, as its specificity is considerably reduced in the presence of other malignant or inflammatory diseases.

For purposes of interpretation, scan results may be divided into three categories: primary tumor, mediastinal uptake, and evidence for distant metastases. Proven lung cancers are positive in 85–96 percent of ^{67}Ga scans.[18,32,43,47]. A positive scan in the presence of a suspected primary lung cancer carries a sensitivity of 96 percent, a specificity of 59 percent, a positive predictive index of 91 percent and an overall accuracy of 89 percent. In evaluations of the mediastinum and whole body for nodal

---

*Injection of 10 mCi ^{67}Ga citrate is usually permitted only for investigational purposes. The more standard dose is 5 mCi.[3]

metastases or distant metastases respectively, only those patients with ^{67}Ga uptake in the primary tumor should be included in analysis. The overall accuracy for positive mediastinal scan in patients with peripherally located primary tumors is 80 percent, with a specificity of 89 percent and a sensitivity of 69 percent (Table 8-6). Patients with primary tumors near the mediastinum have an overall accuracy of mediastinal evaluation of 61 percent because of the difficulty in separating the uptake of the primary from the uptake of mediastinal lymph nodes. In patients with ^{67}Ga uptake in the primary tumor and distant organ metastases, the accuracy is 92 percent with a sensitivity of 88 percent and a specificity of 100 percent, considering only discrete areas of uptake.[12] A ^{67}Ga scan can correctly identify otherwise occult metastatic lesions in 11 percent of patients with known lung cancer (Fig. 8-10). Although we rely heavily on findings in positive ^{67}Ga scans to make the diagnosis of M_1 disease, we do not rely on normal ^{67}Ga scans to serve as evidence for the absence of metastatic disease.

A number of other scintigraphic examinations are used routinely at other institutions in the noninvasive staging of lung cancer, including bone, brain, and liver scans. When used as screening tests for patients known to have cancer, the scans reveal a low overall incidence of metastatic disease.[24,25,45,46] The liver and bone scans are rarely abnormal in patients without symptoms or signs on history and physical examination of metastases (Table 8-7). When clinical signs of metastatic disease are present, the liver scan has an appreciable incidence of false-negative results, while it is generally agreed that the sensitivity of the nuclide brain scan is too poor to be of benefit in confirming suspected brain metastases (Table 8-8).[33] Computed tomography of the brain is more accurate than nuclide brain scan and should be obtained when a clinical suspicion of central nervous system (CNS) metastases exists.[5,26,37] The incidence of abnormal findings for bone scans is higher than that for the other scintigraphic studies in asymptomatic patients and is caused in part by a significant number of false-positive results, which necessitate further investigation. The bone scan is able to detect clinically unsuspected metastases in 8 percent of patients, however, and confirms metastatic disease in a large percentage of patients with clinical symptoms.[13,25,45]

We normally require two positive tests to diagnose a metastasis and confidently assign a clinical stage of M_1. In other cases, particularly those in which only a single

Table 8-6
Accuracy of ^{67}Ga Scan in Mediastinal Staging

Patients (No.)	Sensitivity (%)	Specificity (%)	Accuracy (%)	PPI* (%)	NPI† (%)	Reference
25	100	71	84	73	100	1
34	89	67	79	77	83	29
66	56	94	74	90	67	12
70	88	86	87	93	76	18
50	55	97	82	91	79	47
75	92	70	85	87	80	32
51	56	100	80	100	74	56
51	23	82	67	30	76	35
422	68.9	88.7	79.9	82.0	77.4	

*Positive Predictive Index.
†Negative Predictive Index.

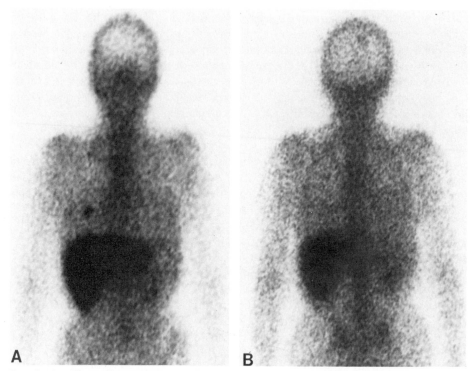

Fig. 8-10. The gallium scan normally is positive in primary tumors greater than 2 cm in diameter, as in this patient with a right middle lobe cancer (*A*). Sometimes it is valuable in detecting asymptomatic metastases, such as this left parietal cerebral metastasis in the same patient (*B*).

study suggests metastatic disease, histologic documentation is necessary. This normally requires invasive staging procedures as described below.

Invasive Staging Techniques

All patients with lung cancer should undergo bronchoscopy. While this normally serves a diagnostic role for the purpose of obtaining histologic confirmation of suspected lung cancer by biopsy or cytology, bronchoscopy can also provide valuable and necessary staging information. It is important to ascertain the location of central tumors relative to the carina, as this measurement is an important criterion for T

Table 8-7
Incidence* of Abnormal Organ Scans

Clinical Findings Suggesting M_1 Disease	Scan		
	Liver	Brain	Bone
Absent	3/145	0/155	10/124
Present	21/153	16/147	43/126

Data from references 25, 45, and 46.
*Expressed as number positive/number performed.

Table 8-8

Results of Organ Scans in Patients with Lung Cancer

Scan	Patients	Sensitivity (%)	Specificity (%)	Accuracy (%)	PPI* (%)	NPI† (%)
Liver	151	28	88	78	32	86
Brain	131	71	97	95	77	97
Bone	113	96	70	76	49	98

Data from references 24, 45, and 46.

*Positive Predictive Index.

†Negative Predictive Index.

classification. The presence of endobronchial lesions other than the primary tumor should also be sought as evidence for a concurrent synchronous lung cancer[16] or submucosal lymphatic spread suggesting M_1 disease. The carina should be examined bronchoscopically for evidence of widening. Newer techniques of transcarinal bronchoscopic needle biopsy may provide a cytologic diagnosis of N_2 disease in subcarinal lymph nodes, obviating the necessity for mediastinoscopy or exploratory thoracotomy in some patients.[4,49,55]

In patients with suspected N_2 disease, mediastinoscopy may be used to histologically document disease status in paratracheal and subcarinal lymph nodes.[10,44] Reports illustrate the anatomic advantage in using a selective approach for mediastinal lymph node biopsy.[27,28] When indicated, we use cervical mediastinoscopy for right-sided primary tumors and generally reserve left parasternal mediastinotomy for left-sided tumors unless obvious subcarinal or paratracheal lymph node enlargement is present.

Many situations occur in which a suspicion of metastatic disease is raised and histologic documentation is necessary prior to final staging. Patients with large or persistent pleural effusions are stage III solely on the basis of the usual T_3 classification. In the absence of other metastatic disease, however, it is important to determine whether the effusion is the result of obstruction of lymphatics, permitting surgical treatment in some cases, or is due to pleural seeding by tumor. Thoracentesis frequently can provide cytologic documentation of malignancy in pleural fluid, making a diagnosis of M_1 disease. When thoracentesis is negative, blind pleural biopsy sometimes is performed. The accuracy of this technique is only moderately good because pleural seeding generally occurs in sites that are poorly amenable to blind pleural biopsy.[7] When differentiation between benign and malignant pleural effusions is mandatory, we generally employ diagnostic pleuroscopy (thoracoscopy), which allows a thorough inspection of both the visceral and parietal pleural surfaces, complete evacuation of effusion for cytology, and biopsy of suspected sites under direct vision.[6]

Occasional patients will present at the time of diagnosis with enlarged lymph nodes, particularly in the supraclavicular region. By definition, these nodes, if positive, satisfy the criterion for metastatic spread of disease. Biopsy in this case, usually under local anesthesia, will provide both histologic diagnosis and staging. However, routine blind biopsy of scalene nodes in the absence of abnormalities on physical examination or positive findings on ^{67}Ga scan yields evidence for metastatic disease in less than 10 percent of patients and is not recommended.

Occasionally, localized bone pain in a patient leads to a bone scan that reveals isolated positive uptake in ribs in the absence of rib abnormalities on plain radiographs. If there is no suspicion of direct chest wall involvement by the primary tumor in such patients, and no other evidence for metastatic disease is present, a rib biopsy sometimes is necessary to complete the staging process. A recent technique using a bone scintiscan and a local methylene blue injection to identify the rib abnormalities is of value in directing open biopsy and obtaining accurate results in these patients.[31]

The ultimate and perhaps most important invasive staging technique is exploration and biopsy at the time of thoracotomy. Valuable clinical information is available regarding the site and extent of primary tumor. In addition, biopsy of mediastinal lymph nodes from multiple sites, including subcarinal, paraaortic, paraesophageal, and paratracheal regions, should be performed to complete the staging process. Clinical stage I and stage II patients have mediastinal lymph node metastases in many cases, and failure to document this will lead to improper staging and "unexpected" recurrences in many cases.[34,52]

OPTIMAL STAGING PLAN

An idealized algorithm for staging lung cancer is illustrated in Fig. 8-11. In our institution we typically use a sequential staging process[38] because not all investigations are required for all patients. At the end of the initial evaluation, encompassed by history and physical examination, chest x-ray, bronchoscopy, and blood chemistries, almost half of all patients have evidence for metastatic disease. This group of patients can go on to specific tests to document metastases and then to appropriate treatment without further delay. In those in whom staging is incomplete following initial evaluation, additional examinations are performed, which typically include chest CT and

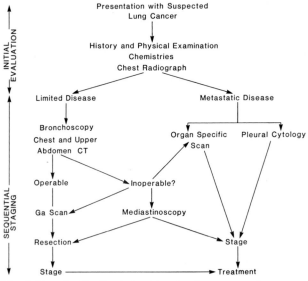

Fig. 8-11. An idealized algorithm for the sequential staging of lung cancer.

⁶⁷Ga scans. The necessity for histologic examination of suspected mediastinal lymph nodes remains controversial. It is our practice to be very aggressive from a surgical standpoint, exploring and resecting patients in whom enlarged mediastinal lymph nodes are confined to the ipsilateral hemithorax or subcarinal region. In other circumstances, we require documentation of tumor involvement of matted ipsilateral nodes or of contralateral nodes by mediastinoscopy. Following the algorithm, it is our belief that the accuracy of preoperative clinical staging is maximized and unnecessary testing is eliminated.

REFERENCES

1. Alazraki NP, Ramsdell JW, Taylor A, et al: Reliability of gallium scan chest radiography compared to mediastinoscopy for evaluating mediastinal spread in lung cancer. Am Rev Resp Dis 117:415-420, 1978

2. Baron RL, Levitt RG, Sagel SS, et al: Computed tomography in the preoperative evaluation of bronchogenic carcinoma. Radiology 145:727-732, 1982

3. Bekerman C, DeMeester TR, Skinner DB: The value of "high-count" ⁶⁷gallium citrate scans in the staging of lung carcinoma, in Medical Radionuclide Imaging, vol 2. Vienna, Internatl Atomic Energy Agency, 1976, p 351

4. Brynitz S, Struve-Christensen E, Borgeskov S, et al: Transcarinal mediastinal needle biopsy compared with mediastinoscopy. J Thorac Cardiovasc Surg 90:21-24, 1985

5. Butler AR, Leo JS, Lin JP, et al: The value of routine cranial computed tomography in neurologically intact patients with primary carcinoma of the lung. Radiology 131:399-401, 1979

6. Canto A, Rivas J, Saumench J, et al: Points to consider when choosing a biopsy method in cases of pleurisy of unknown origin. Chest 84:176-179, 1983

7. Canto A, Ferrer G, Romagosa V, et al: Lung cancer and pleural effusion. Clinical significance and study of pleural metastatic locations. Chest 87:649-652, 1985

8. Clinical staging of primary lung cancer. American Thoracic Society. Am Rev Resp Dis 127:659-664, 1983

9. Coscarelli-Schag C, Heinrich RL, Ganz PA: Karnofsky performance status revisited: Reliability, validity and guidelines. J Clin Oncol 2:187-193, 1984

10. Coughlin M, DesLauriers J, Beaulieu M, et al: Role of mediastinoscopy in pretreatment staging of patients with primary lung cancer. Ann Thorac Surg 40:556-560, 1985

11. Daly BDT Jr, Faling LJ, Pugatch RD, et al: Computed tomography: An effective technique for mediastinal staging in lung cancer. J Thorac Cardiovasc Surg 88:486-494, 1984

12. DeMeester TR, Golomb HM, Kirchner P, et al: The role of gallium-67 scanning in the clinical staging and preoperative evaluation of patients with carcinoma of the lung. Ann Thorac Surg 28:451-464, 1979

13. Donato AT, Ammerman EG, Sullesta O: Bone scanning in the evaluation of patients with lung cancer. Ann Thorac Surg 27:300-304, 1979

14. Ekholm S, Albrechtsson U, Kugelberg J, et al: Computed tomography in preoperative staging of bronchogenic carcinoma. J Comput Assist Tomogr 4:763-765, 1980

15. Faling LJ, Pugatch RD, Jung-Legg Y, et al: Computed tomographic scanning of the mediastinum in the staging of bronchogenic carcinoma. Am Rev Resp Dis 124:690-695, 1981

16. Ferguson MK, DeMeester TR, DesLauriers, J, et al: Diagnosis and management of synchronous lung cancers. J Thorac Cardiovasc Surg 89:378-385, 1985

17. Ferguson MK, MacMahon H, Little AG, et al: The regional accuracy of computed tomog-

raphy of the mediastinum in staging of lung cancer. J Thorac Cardiovasc Surg 91:498–504, 1986

18. Fosburg RG, Hopkins GB, Kan MK: Evaluation of the mediastinum by gallium-67 scintigraphy in lung cancer. J Thorac Cardiovasc Surg 77:76–82, 1979

19. Friedman PJ, Feigin DS, Liston SE, et al: Sensitivity of chest radiography, computed tomography, and gallium scanning to metastasis of lung carcinoma. Cancer 54:1300–1306, 1984

20. Genereux GP, Howie JL: Normal mediastinal lumph node size and number: CT and anatomic study. Am J Radiol 142:1095–1100, 1984

21. Glazer GM, Orringer MB, Gross BH, et al: The mediastinum in non-small cell lung cancer: CT—surgical correlation. Am J Radiol 142:1101–1105, 1984

22. Glazer GM, Gross BH, Quint LE, et al: Normal mediastinal lymph nodes: Number and size according to American Thoracic Society mapping. Am J Radiol 144:261–265, 1985

23. Goldstraw P, Kurzer M, Edwards D: Preoperative staging of lung cancer: Accuracy of computed tomography versus mediastinoscopy. Thorax 38:10–15, 1983

24. Gutierrez AZ, Vincent RG, Bakshi S, et al: Radioisotope scans in the evaluation of metastatic bronchogenic carcinoma. J Thorac Cardiovasc Surg 69:934–941, 1975

25. Hooper RG, Beechler CR, Johnson MC: Radioisotope scanning in the initial staging of bronchogenic carcinoma. Am Rev Resp Dis 118:279–286, 1978

26. Jacobs L, Kinkel WR, Vincent RG: "Silent" brain metastasis from lung carcinoma determined by computerized tomography. Arch Neurol 34:690–693, 1977

27. Jolly PC, Hill LD, Lawless PA, et al: Parasternal mediastinotomy and mediastinoscopy. J Thorac Cardiovasc Surg 66:549–556, 1973

28. Jolly PC, Li W, Anderson RP: Anterior and cervical mediastinoscopy for determining operability and predicting resectability in lung cancer. J Thorac Cardiovasc Surg 79:366–371, 1980

29. Lesk DM, Wood TE, Carroll SE, et al: The application of ^{67}Ga scanning in determining the operability of bronchogenic carcinoma. Radiology 128:707–709, 1978

30. Lewis JW Jr, Madrazo BL, Gross SC, et al: The value of radiographic and computed tomography in the staging of lung carcinoma. Ann Thorac Surg 34:553–558, 1982

31. Little AG, DeMeester TR, Kirchner PT, et al: Guided biopsies of abnormalities on nuclear bone scans. J Thorac Cardiovasc Surg 85:396–403, 1983

32. Lunia SL, Ruckdeschel JC, McKneally MF, et al: Noninvasive evaluation of mediastinal metastases in bronchogenic carcinoma: A prospective comparison of chest radiography and gallium-67 scanning. Cancer 47:672–679, 1981

33. Lusins JO, Chayes Z, Nakagawa H: Computed tomography and radionuclide brain scanning. Comparison in evaluating metastatic lesions to brain. NY State J Med 80:185–189, 1980

34. Matthews MJ, Kanhouwa S, Pickren J, et al: Frequency of residual and metastatic tumor in patients undergoing curative surgical resection for lung cancer. Cancer Chemother Rep 4:63–67, 1973

35. McKenna RJ Jr, Haynie TP, Libshitz HI, et al: Critical evaluation of the gallium-67 scan for surgical patients with lung cancer. Chest 87:428–431, 1985

36. McKenna RJ Jr, Libshitz HI, Mountain CE, et al: Roentgenographic evaluation of mediastinal nodes for preoperative assessment in lung cancer. Chest 88:206–210, 1985

37. Mintz BJ, Tuhrim S, Alexander S, et al: Intracranial metastases in the initial staging of bronchogenic carcinoma. Chest 86:850–853, 1984

38. Mintz U, DeMeester TR, Golomb HM, et al: Sequential staging in bronchogenic carcinoma. Chest 76:653–657, 1979

39. Moak GD, Cockerill EM, Farber MO, et al: Computed tomography vs standard radiology in the evaluation of mediastinal adenopathy. Chest 82:69–75, 1982

40. Modini C, Passariello R, Iascone C, et al: TNM staging in lung cancer: role of computed tomography. J Thorac Cardiovasc Surg 84:569-574, 1982

41. Mountain CF: A new international staging system for lung cancer. Chest 89: 225S-233S, 1986

42. Osborne DR, Korobkin M, Ravin CE, et al: Comparison of plain radiography, conventional tomography, and computed tomography in detecting intrathoracic lymph node metastases from lung carcinoma. Radiology 142:157-161, 1982

43. Pannier R, Verlinde I, Puspowidjono I, et al: Role of gallium 67 thoracic scintigraphy in the diagnosis and staging of patients suspected of bronchial carcinoma. Thorax 37:264-269, 1982

44. Pearson FG: An evaluation of mediastinoscopy in the management of presumably operable bronchial carcinoma. J Thorac Cardiovasc Surg 55:617-625, 1968

45. Quinn DL, Ostrow LB, Porter DK, et al: Staging of non-small cell bronchogenic carcinoma: Relationship of the clinical evaluation to organ scans. Chest 89:270-275, 1986

46. Ramsdell JW, Peters RM, Taylor AT Jr, et al: Multiorgan scans for staging lung cancer. Correlation with clinical evaluation. J Thorac Cardiovasc Surg 73:653-658, 1977

47. Richardson JV, Zenk BA, Rossi NP: Preoperative noninvasive mediastinal staging in bronchogenic carcinoma. Surgery 88:382-385, 1980

48. Richey HM, Matthews JI, Helsel RA, et al: Thoracic CT scanning in the staging of bronchogenic carcinoma. Chest 85:218-221, 1984

49. Shure D, Fedullo PF: The role of transcarinal needle aspiration in the staging of bronchogenic carcinoma. Chest 86:693-696, 1984

50. Staging of lung cancer. American Joint Committee on Cancer, in press

51. Staging of lung cancer 1979. American Joint Committee for Cancer Staging and End Results Reporting: Task Force on Lung Cancer. Chicago, Ill, 1979

52. Suemasu K, Ogata T, Yoneyama T, et al: Evaluation of the clinical TNM in comparison with the surgico-pathological TNM in peripheral type lung cancer. Jap J Clin Oncol 7:9-14, 1977

53. Thermann M, Poster H, Muller-Hermelink KH, et al: Evaluation of tomography and mediastinoscopy for the detection of mediastinal lymph node metastases. Ann Thorac Surg 37:443-447, 1984

54. TNM classification of malignant tumors. Geneva, International Union Against Cancer, 1974

55. Wang KP, Brower R, Haponik EE, Siegelman S: Flexible transbronchial needle aspiration for staging of bronchogenic carcinoma. Chest 84:571-576, 1983

56. Waxman AD, Julien PJ, Brachman MB, et al: Gallium scintigraphy in bronchogenic carcinoma. The effect of tumor location on sensitivity and specificity. Chest 86: 178-183, 1984

Stage I Non-Small Cell Lung Cancer

Tom R. DeMeester
Mario Albertucci

9

Surgical Therapy

CLINICAL CHARACTERISTICS OF STAGE I DISEASE

Clinically, stage I lung cancer presents in two ways. If the lesion arises in the central portion of the bronchial tree, it can cause three symptoms associated with early carcinoma: (1) the lesion may bleed, causing hemoptysis; (2) the lesion may irritate the mucosa, causing a persistent cough that differs from the ordinary smoker's cough; and (3) the lesion may obstruct the bronchus, causing a distal infection. Of the three signs, hemoptysis is most worrisome to both the patient and the physician. Cough receives the least attention, and persistent pneumonitis is the most overlooked symptom. These early signs and symptoms of lung cancer indicate the need for chest x-ray; if that is normal, bronchoscopy is appropriate. If done, a substantial number of patients will be diagnosed at an early stage of the disease. If the symptoms are not attended to, or if the patient fails to experience them, the lesion will most likely be diagnosed at an advanced stage when it metastasizes or invades adjacent structures.

A coin lesion is the second way a stage I lung cancer can present on a chest roentgenogram. A coin lesion, or lung nodule, is a roughly spherical density on the chest roentgenogram of 1-6 cm in its greatest diameter.[12] It seldom is associated with the atelectasis or pneumonitis that occurs with more central endobronchial lesions. There are a number of facts or aphorisms about solitary lung nodules that most experienced surgeons agree upon.[12] The aphorisms listed below are helpful in managing a patient with a lung nodule and can be categorized according to those that are encouraging or discouraging.
The encouraging aphorisms are:

1. Solitary lung nodules are benign in 50-85 percent of cases.
2. The probability of a lung nodule being benign in a patient under 30 is 99 percent.
3. Virtually all lung nodules in which deposits of calcium can be demonstrated are benign.

LUNG CANCER: A COMPREHENSIVE TREATISE
ISBN 0-8089-1876-1

4. Lung nodules that remain unchanged in size for 4 years can be considered benign.
5. Operative mortality for resection of a benign lung nodule is less than 1 percent.

The discouraging aphorisms are:

1. Asymptomatic solitary lung nodules are malignant in 15–50 of cases.
2. The probability of a lung nodule being malignant in patients over the age of 40 is directly related to the patient's age, that is, 40 percent for 40 years old, 50 percent for 50 years old, and so on.
3. The 5-year survival of a resected, asymptomatic lung nodule is 50 percent, whereas once the symptoms occur, it is 20 percent.
4. As the size of malignant lung nodules increases, the 5-year survival decreases.
5. The location of a malignant lung nodule affects the patient's survival; a midlung nodule has a 50 percent 5-year survival, whereas a subpleural nodule has an 8 percent 5 year survival.
6. The operative mortality for the resection of a malignant lung nodule ranges from 3 to 10 percent.

The goal in the management of a lung nodule is twofold: (1) to limit the number of thoracotomies performed for benign nodules or malignant nodules that have metastasized and (2) to avoid prolonged delays prior to the resection of a malignant nodule with a high probability for cure. Fig. 9-1 shows that survival from a malignant lung nodule decreases as the size of the nodule increases.[3] Delaying therapy in order to observe whether a lung nodule enlarges before removing it is not in the patient's best interest. A common cause of inadvertent delay in the treatment of lung nodules is poor communication between the radiologist and the primary physician. Primary physicians frequently rely on the reports they receive from the radiologist. As a consequence, the primary physician can miss information about the chest roentgenogram if the report is not read carefully. To avoid this problem, the reports should be stamped with a large red-letter statement, "Carcinoma until proven otherwise." The

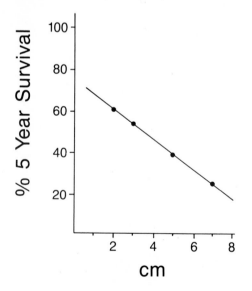

Fig. 9-1. Five-year survival of patients with a resected lung nodule according to the size of the nodule based on 887 patients reported by Brewer.[3] (Used by permission of the author.)

same stamp should be placed on the chest roentgenogram as a reminder to those reviewing the film to determine whether the lesion has been investigated and treated.

Every solitary lung nodule should be resected unless the patient's general condition contraindicates surgery, there is evidence the lesion is benign, or there is evidence that metastatic spread has already occurred. Because of the high resectability rate of a solitary lung nodule, the prognosis is excellent, and patients should be encouraged to undergo surgery.

CLINICAL EVALUATION OF LUNG NODULES

Special studies have been designed to help the physician differentiate a malignant from a benign lung nodule. The most common is tomography, which defines the borders of the nodule and whether it contains calcium.[23] Benign nodules tend to have sharp borders and satellite lesions, whereas the borders of malignant nodules are irregular and radiating or smooth and dimpled. The presence of calcification is a strong indication that the lesion is benign. If calcium is present, its location in the nodule is important. Central or laminated calcifications strongly suggest a benign nodule, whereas marginally located or tiny diffused flecks of calcium suggest malignancy. The latter results from a malignant growth within or adjacent to a benign lesion, the so-called scar carcinoma. Theros, on reviewing 1269 roentgenograms of lung nodules that contained calcium, found only 7 that were malignant.[25] An air fluid level or air density within a nodule indicates cavitation. If the walls of the cavity are irregular and thick, this is a sign of malignancy. Thin wall cavities are more apt to be benign. The most common tumors that produce cavitary lesions in the lung are primary squamous cell carcinomas and metastatic lung nodules from a rectal or colon primary.[25] Computed tomographic scans can detect additional lung nodules in 48 percent of patients with a single nodule on conventional tomography.[23] However, 60 percent of the additional nodules observed are benign granulomas or pleural based nodes. Actually, computerized tomography adds very little in the evaluation of lung nodules except to better define the contours of the lesion and its location.

Another way to differentiate benign from malignant lung nodules is to estimate the doubling time of the nodule by comparing prior and recent chest roentgenograms.[28] If the doubling time is less than 1 month or greater than 16 months, it is more likely to be benign; if it is between these periods, it is more likely to be malignant.[19] The calculation of growth rate is based on the assumption that growth remains constant during the time lapse between the two chest roentgenogram.[4]

Percutaneous needle biopsy or endoscopic brushing under fluoroscopic guidance is useful for determining the histology of a lung nodule. A radiologist who has experience with percutaneous needle biopsy can obtain a cytologic diagnosis of a malignancy in 90 percent of malignant nodules biopsied.[20] Repeating the procedure increases the yield to 95 percent. The method is applicable to nodules as small as 1 cm in diameter. A pneumothorax occurs in 5–30 percent of patients biopsied. A positive preoperative needle aspirate obviates the need for an interoperative biopsy of the nodule prior to resection and reduces the likelihood of tumor cell dissemination during operation. Poe and Tobin observed that of 1826 needle biopsies performed on patients with lung nodules suspected to be carcinoma, 1569 were confirmed as malignant and 256 benign.[20] On the basis of this experience, the sensitivity of the technique—its ability to detect disease when it is present—is 83 percent. The specificity—the ability to exclude disease when it is absent—is 98 percent. The problem with the technique is that 48 percent of benign needle aspirates come from patients with known cancer. Therefore, a benign aspirate is not dependable information for clinical management.

The intensity of clinical investigations expended to differentiate a primary malignant lung nodule from a pulmonary metastasis is controversial.[24] Some authors believe that in the absence of gastrointestinal complaints or blood in the stools, no search for a hidden primary is necessary and the lung lesion should be treated as though it were a primary malignancy. Others have suggested that an upper and lower gastrointestinal series, intravenous pyelograms, and pancreatic ultrasounds should be performed on all patients. The latter is rather expensive in view of the low probability of finding an extrapulmonary asymptomatic primary lesion. A current compromise is to obtain a CT scan from the brain to the midabdomen. This excludes primary or metastatic lesions in the major organs while at the same time evaluates the location and contour of the lung lesion and the presence of metastatic lymph nodes in the mediastinum.[17] Resection of a metastatic pulmonary nodule after such an evaluation is unlikely to harm the patient and may prolong survival.[10,15]

THE PROBLEM OF SYNCHRONOUS LUNG NODULES

Carcinoma of the lung can be a multifocal disease, and it is possible for patients to present with synchronous lung nodules, each representing separate primary tumors. Synchronous tumors are defined as primary lung tumors with different cell types or with similar cell types but arising in different lobes or lungs.[6] The evaluation of two pulmonary nodules presenting simultaneously is complex because the nodules may represent metastatic disease from an extrapulmonary cancer, lung cancer with a pulmonary metastasis, lung cancer with an associated benign tumor, two synchronous lung cancers, or two benign lesions. The incidence of synchronous lung tumors is low but so important in regard to therapy that the possibility must be considered prior to any therapeutic plan. In the absence of hilar or mediastinal node involvement, synchronous tumors have a mean survival of 26 months after resection. However, synchronous tumors in patients with stage II or III disease have a median survival of 11 months after resection.[6] Pneumonectomy is the operation of choice for synchronous unilateral tumors. Sequential resection, starting with the most advanced lesion, is indicated in bilateral tumors. A careful preoperative evaluation of pulmonary function is critical in these patients in order to plan a curative resection while preserving as much functional lung as possible.[29]

PREOPERATIVE EVALUATION OF PATIENTS WITH STAGE I DISEASE

With the decision to resect a primary malignant lung nodule or a more central endobronchial lung cancer comes the necessity to evaluate the patient's physiological status. The patient's cardiac and pulmonary functions must be sufficient to allow for recovery and an active life after resection. Preoperative pulmonary function tests should be obtained with specific attention given to the FEV_1.[29] The postresection FEV_1

should be at least 800–1000 cm.[3] If the planned resection is apt to reduce function below this critical value, the patient should have quantitative pulmonary ventilation and perfusion scans to assess the contribution of that portion of the lung to be removed to the overall lung function. In marginal patients, one week of intense respiratory therapy can make a dramatic difference as pulmonary function can be improved considerably in patients who are chronic smokers and have chronic obstructive lung disease.[26] Prior to excluding a curative resection in a patient with marginal pulmonary function, the ability to function on one lung can be tested by catheter occlusion of the pulmonary artery on the side to be resected.[11]

If the patient has a history of cardiac disease, a suggestion of cardiac failure on physical examination, or is over the age of 75, cardiac ejection fraction should be measured with either radioisotopes or an echocardiogram. A resting ejection fraction below 0.4, or the failure of the ejection fraction to increase with exercise, indicates a lack of cardiac reserve and increases the risk of resection.[21] In such patients, a thorough cardiac evaluation should be performed prior to resection. If poor ventricular wall motion is observed, a coronary arteriogram should be performed to exclude coronary artery disease. If coronary artery disease is present and a bypass is possible, most surgeons would perform the bypass prior to the lung resection. Others have advocated performing both the lung resection and a coronary bypass procedure at the same time. It is our opinion that the lung resection, if at all possible, should be done with careful cardiac monitoring prior to the coronary artery bypass because of the deleterious effect extracorporeal heart–lung bypass has on host immune mechanisms.[22]

MEDIASTINOSCOPY IN PATIENTS WITH STAGE I DISEASE

Mediastinoscopy should be performed prior to resection on all patients in whom CT scans identify mediastinal hymph nodes greater than 1 cm in diameter. When mediastinal nodes are smaller than 1 cm, the possibility of detecting involved nodes by mediastinoscopy is less than 5 percent.[1] Cervical mediastinoscopy is used to biopsy lymph nodes in the peritracheal region as far inferiorly as the azygos vein on the right and the aortic arch on the left. In some patients the subcarinal nodes can also be biopsied. Left parasternal mediastinoscopy is used to biopsy[16] para-aortic nodes in patients with lesions located in the left upper lobe. The survival rate of patients with mediastinal lymph node disease biopsied by mediastinoscopy is so poor that resection is not justified.[1] An algorithm outlining the preoperative evaluation of patients with lung cancer is shown in Fig. 9-2. On the basis of this algorithm, patients with T_1 or T_2 tumors who undergo surgical resection are likely to have stage I or II disease depending on whether the hilar lymph nodes are involved. A few patients will have stage III disease because of the unsuspected involvement of mediastinal lymph nodes.

SURGICAL CONSIDERATION IN STAGE I DISEASE

A posterior lateral thoracotomy is the most common exposure used to resect a lung lesion. The entrance into the pleural cavity is through the fourth intercostal space over the superior border of the fifth rib. This gives excellent exposure of the hilum, where 90 percent of the dissection will occur, regardless of whether the lesion is

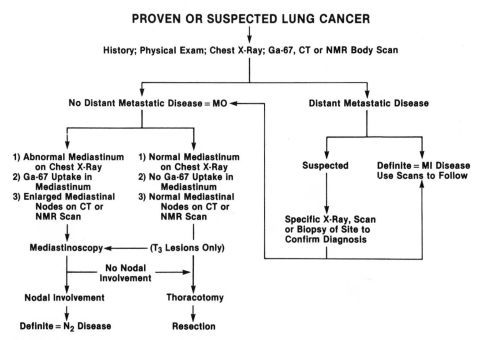

Fig. 9-2. Approach for staging patients with known or suspected carcinoma of the lung. (Used by permission of the author.)

located in the upper or lower lobe. On entering the chest, the surgeon identifies the lesion by palpating the lung. If a preoperative cytological diagnosis has not been made, the surgeon must decide on the basis of the gross pathology whether to biopsy the lesion or to proceed directly with a lobectomy. It is difficult, even with considerable experience, to properly identify a carcinoma by palpation when it is embedded within the substance of a lobe. Such tumors are also impossible to remove by an excisional biopsy without considerable operative damage to the lobe. The use of a Tru-Cut® (Tranvenol, Inc., Deerfield, IL) needle biopsy in this situation results in less pleural cavity contamination with tumor cells than that following incision of the lung and obtaining a biopsy directly from the nodule. Lesions located just under the surface are easier to identify by gross appearance and are suitable for an excision biopsy with little chance for tumor spillage.

Once malignancy has been confirmed, a decision must be made as to the extent of the resection. To make this decision, the size of the lesion, its location within the lung, the presence of involved hilar lymph nodes, and the patient's pulmonary function must be considered. The algorithm shown in Fig. 9-3 is based on our experience regarding the initial site of tumor recurrence in patients following surgical resection.[8] In those who had a lobectomy for T_1N_0 and T_2N_0 disease, the overall recurrence rate was 27.8 percent. Eight out of ten recurrences were local. Seventy-five percent of the local recurrences were in the hilar lymph nodes and 25 percent in the bronchial stump. This indicates that involvement of the hilar nodes is difficult to ascertain at operation when the nodes are deep within the hilum and that the disease can be present in the bronchial stump despite the reported absence of microscopic tumor in the resected margin. Patients with a primary tumor greater than 4 cm in diameter were particularly

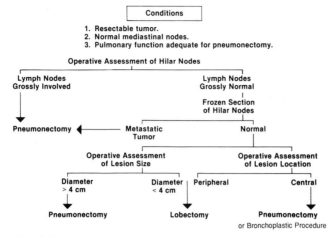

Fig. 9-3. Algorithm of operating room action based on the size of the primary tumor and its location and the involvement of the hilar nodes. (Used by permission of the author.)

prone to develop local recurrences, and a more extensive resection would have provided better local control. On the basis of this experience, we would recommend that an intrapericardial pneumonectomy be performed in patients with a primary tumor 4 cm or greater in diameter, regardless of location. In patients with a peripheral primary tumor less than 4 cm in diameter, it is safe to proceed with a lobectomy. A pneumonectomy or bronchoplastic procedure should be done for central lesions less than 4 cm in diameter.

When a resection is performed for stage I carcinoma of the lung, the peritracheal, tracheobronchial, subcarinal, and paraesophageal nodes should be removed for staging purposes. The subcarinal nodes are removed by dissecting along the inferior border of the right or left main-stem bronchus up to the carina and then down the opposite main-stem bronchus. The tracheobronchial nodes, which traverse the pleural reflection at the hilum, should be properly identified, since they can lead to inaccurate staging by the pathologist, who, on the basis of their location on the surgical specimen, assumes they are hilar nodes.[13]

A sleeve lobectomy should be performed in patients where resection of the tumor would ordinarily require a pneumonectomy but the predicted pulmonary function following resection is insufficient to sustain an active life.[9] Fig. 9-4 shows examples of (A) a central tumor at the opening of a lobar bronchus, (B) a tumor that invades the main-stem bronchus from outside, and (C) a peripheral tumor with metastatic lymph nodes around the lobar bronchus. In each situation, the patient should be free of mediastinal lymph node involvement. The surgeon should have considerable experience with the operation since it can lead to life-threatening complications such as bronchopleural fistula, bronchovascular fistula, and an anastomotic stenosis.

The second indication for a sleeve lobectomy is a central tumor less than 4 cm in diameter located in the right upper lobe bronchial orifice with uninvolved hilar lymph nodes.[27] In such patients, a pneumonectomy would cause the needless loss of functional lung tissue. If the hilar lymph nodes are involved, however, the patient is better treated with an intrapericardial pneumonectomy provided the loss of one lung will not jeopardize the pulmonary function in the remaining lung.

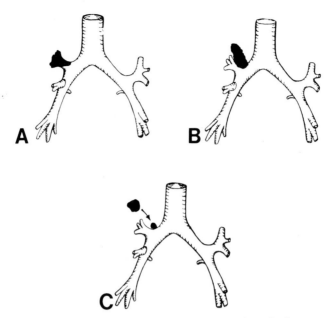

Fig. 9-4. Indications for sleeve lobectomy in bronchial-carcinoma: (*A*) central tumor in any lobe bronchus; (*B*) tumor with invasion of the main bronchus from outside; (*C*) peripheral tumor with metastatic lymph nodes around the lobar bronchus. (Used by permission of the author.)

When the extent of the tumor necessitates sleeve resection of the pulmonary artery, alone or in combination with the bronchus, a pneumonectomy should be done if possible, since infiltration of the main trunk of the pulmonary artery indicates that embolization of the tumor into the distal pulmonary arterial bed probably has occurred. If a pneumonectomy will result in insufficient pulmonary function to sustain an active life, however, a sleeve resection of both the bronchus and artery may be done. Situations appropriate for this procedure are a central tumor that has directly infiltrated the main pulmonary artery trunk and can be removed by taking a segment of the pulmonary artery, or peripheral tumors with a hilar lymph node metastasis that have infiltrated the main pulmonary artery. A rare indication for a sleeve resection of either the bronchus or pulmonary artery is the presence of a contralateral synchronous lung tumor that will need subsequent resection.

When performing a sleeve resection of either the bronchus or pulmonary artery, it is important to cover the anastomosis with a pedicel flap of pleura, pericardium, or azygos vein to provide protection against anastomotic breakdown and fistula formation.

RESULTS OF OPERATIVE THERAPY

According to the American Joint Committee for Cancer Staging, stage I patients are those classified with $T_1N_0M_0$, $T_2N_0M_0$, or $T_1N_1M_0$ disease.[2] Experience has shown that patients with T_1 tumors and hilar lymph node involvement (N_1) have a similar recurrence pattern and survival rate as stage II patients (i.e., $T_2N_1M_0$), and both differ considerably from patients without nodal involvement. For this reason, it is useful to modify stage I to include only patients with $T_1N_0M_0$ and $T_2N_0M_0$ classification and stage II to those with $T_1N_1M_0$ and $T_2N_1M_0$ classification.[5,7,14]

The results of surgical therapy for modified stage I disease are based on our experience with 96 patients who have been followed for a mean of $6\frac{1}{2}$ years after the removal of T_1 or T_2 primary tumors with no evidence of lymph node involvement.[14] Five patients were lost to follow-up between 20 and 70 months. Both were without evidence of recurrence at the time they were last seen. The actuarial overall survival of the 91 operative survivors and survival by classification of the primary tumor is shown in Fig. 9-5. The 5-year survival rate for the whole group was 70 percent, with a median survival of 71.4 months. The 5-year survival rate was 72.1 percent for T_1N_0 patients and 68.3 percent in T_2N_0 patients. There was no significant difference between these two classifications. Survival was not affected by the tumor cell type or by the age, sex, or race of the patient. Five patients died within 30 days of the operation; three from pulmonary sepsis caused by aspiration, one from a cerebral vascular

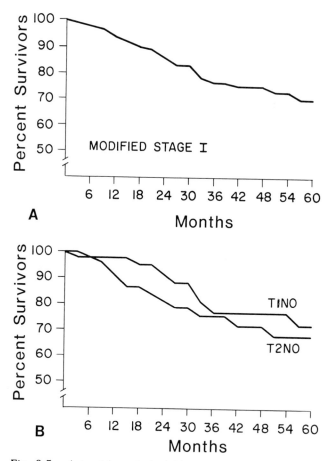

Fig. 9-5. Actuarial survival of 91 patients: (A) all modified stage I patients; (B) survival according to the classification of the primary tumor.

occlusion, and another from a myocardial infarction; thus the operative mortality rate was 5.2 percent. The operative mortality was not affected by the extensiveness of the procedure.

Recurrent cancer occurred in 16.5 percent of patients who did not have lymph node involvement, 9.1 percent of the patients with T_1N_0 disease, and 23.4 percent of the patients with T_2N_0 disease. This was a statistical difference and suggested that T_2 disease (i.e., tumors >3 cm in diameter) are associated with a higher incidence of recurrence. This can be partially explained by insufficient use of a more extensive procedure in these patients, since 27 percent of the recurrences were local and 73 percent were distant. For this reason, we have developed the algorithm for surgical resection shown in Fig. 9-3. The observation that most of the recurrences in patients with T_1 or T_2N_0 disease were distant suggests the presence of undetectable micrometastasis at the time of resection.

Six patients without lymph node involvement developed a new primary lung cancer at a mean interval of $65^1/2$ months (range 30-192) after the initial resection. Four of the six patients were able to undergo a second resection, and all had stage I disease without hilar lymph node involvement. All four are alive with no evidence of disease at 3, 4, 4, and 5 years after the second operation. Two patients could not undergo a resection because of insufficient pulmonary reserve, and both were treated with radiation therapy and died from progressive disease.

THE ROLE OF ADJUVANT INTRAPLEURAL THERAPY IN STAGE I DISEASE

The use of intrapleural bacillus Calmette-Guerin (BCG) immunotherapy as adjuvant therapy in patients with carcinoma of the lung has been shown to be ineffective.[8] It was hoped that immunotherapy with BCG would destroy existing micrometastatic disease following operative resection and improve the hosts immunity against the developement of a subsequent, second primary tumor. We have applied immunotherapy utilizing BCG in patients with very early disease, that is, with T_1 or T_2 tumors without lymph node involvement.[14] The organism was applied by scarification over a 5 × 5 cm skin grid. Treatments were started 6 weeks after surgery and given weekly for 13 weeks, monthly for 3 months, and then every 3 months for 5 years. A total of 29 patients were randomized over a period of 8 years; 15 patients received BCG, and 14 served as control subjects. The original lung cancer recurred in 6 patients, 2 treated with BCG and 4 controls. A second primary occurred in three patients, two treated with BCG and one control. Fig. 9-6 shows the overall results of this randomized trial with BCG scarification. The 5-year survival for patients receiving BCG was 85.9 percent compared to a 63.9 percent for the control patients and 69.6 percent for patients who had the same stage of disease but did not enter the study. The survival differences closely approached statistical significance (BCG patients vs control patients $p = .075$ and BCG vs nonstudy patients, $p = .077$). The results obtained with repetitive adjuvant immunostimulation with BCG skin scarification are surprising in light of the previous lack of success with intrapleural BCG. The difference between the two studies was the site of the administration, skin versus pleura; and the duration of treatment, 5 years versus 1 month. An earlier unpublished analysis of our study

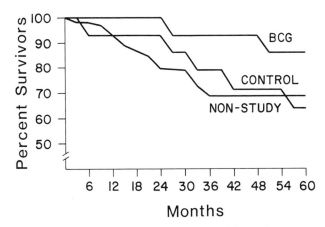

Fig. 9-6. Actuarial survival is shown (BCG, study patients randomized to receive BCG; CONTROL, study patients randomized not to receive BCG; NON-STUDY, patients not enrolled in the study).

suggested no improvement in survival, and we closed the study. After an additional 3-year follow-up, the results have shown a real and nearly statistical trend toward increased survival. Consequently, an evaluation of BCG adjuvant immunotherapy for patients with early disease should be continued. If the results hold, BCG scarification immunotherapy would then appear to have an effective adjuvant role in patients with early disease. Overall, the recurrence rate in patients undergoing resection with N_0 disease is not high enough to warrant the routine use of postoperative chemotherapy. This opinion is based on the absence of a chemotherapy regiment that is highly active against non-oat cell lung cancer and the toxicity of current regiments. If a nontoxic, effective regiment were available, its use as an adjuvant in patients with T_1 or $T_2N_0M_0$ disease would be more attractive.

EDITORIAL COMMENT FOR SURGICAL THERAPY FOR STAGE I NON-SMALL CELL LUNG CANCER

No patient with a potentially curable lung cancer should be denied that opportunity. The editors thus strongly support the contention made in this chapter that patients with solitary pulmonary nodules should be approached as though they have lung cancer until proven otherwise, either by definitive histologic evidence or by extremely convincing circumstantial clinical evidence. This means thoracotomy should be performed—assuming that the patient is physiologically able—if cancer cannot be definitely excluded. When regarding surgery for patients without involvement of any lymph nodes, however, it is our feeling that lobectomy is the procedure to be considered as the standard one. We agree, as pointed out in this chapter, that when there is a large central tumor or when hilar lymph nodes are involved, a pneumonectomy must be carefully considered, but these patients do not fall into the modified stage I category, which is the focus of this chapter.

REFERENCES

1. Albertucci M, DeMeester TR, Iascone C, et al: Use and prognostic value of staging mediastinoscopy in non oat cell lung cancer. Surgery, in press
2. American Joint Committee for Cancer Staging and End Result Reporting: Clinical staging system for carcinoma of the lung. Chicago, 1973
3. Brewer LA: Patterns of survival in lung cancer. Chest 71:644, 1977
4. Collins VP, Loeffler RK, Rivey H: Observation on growth rate of human tumors. Am J Roentgenol Radium Ther Nucl Med 76:988, 1956
5. DeMeester TR: The staging issue: Unification of criteria—discussion, in Delarue NC, Eschapasse H (eds): International Trends in General Thoracic Surgery, vol. I: Lung Cancer. Philadelphia, Saunders, 1985, p 37
6. Ferguson MK, DeMeester TR, Deslauries J, et al: Diagnosis and management of synchronous lung cancer. J Thorac Cardiovasc Surg 89:378, 1985
7. Ferguson MK, Little AG, Golomb HM: The role of adjvant therapy following resection of $T_1N_1M_0$ and $T_2N_1M_0$ non small cell lung cancer. J Thorac Cardiovasc Surg 91:344, 1986
8. Mountain CF, Gail MH: Surgical adjuvant intrapleural BCG treatment for stage I non-small cell lung cancer. J Thorac Cardiovasc Surg 82:649, 1981
9. Jensik RJ, Faber LP, Kittle CF: Sleeve lobectomy for bronchogenic carcinoma: The Rush-Presbyterian-St. Luke's Medical Center experience. Internatl Surg 71:207, 1986
10. Joseph WL, Morton DL, Adkins PC: Prognostic significance of tumor doubling time in evaluating operability in pulmonary metastatic disease. J Thorac Cardiovasc Surg 61:23, 1971
11. Laros CD, Swierenga J: Temporary unilateral pulmonary artery occlusion in the preoperative evaluation of patients with bronchial carcinoma. Med Thorac 24:269, 1967
12. Lillington GA: The solitary pulmonary nodule. Am Rev Respir Dis 110:699, 1974
13. Little AG, DeMeester TR, MacMahon H: The staging of lung cancer. Semin Oncol 10:56, 1983
14. Little AG, DeMeester TR, Ferguson MK, et al: Modified stage I (T1N0M0, T2N0M0), nonsmall cell lung cancer: Treatment results, recurrence patterns, and adjuvant immunotherapy. Surgery 100:621, 1986
15. McCormack PM, Bains MS, Beattie EJ, et al: Pulmonary resection in metastatic carcinoma. Chest 73:163, 1978
16. McNeill TM, Chamberlain JM: Diagnostic anterior mediastinoscopy. Am Thorac Surg 2:532, 1966
17. Modini C, Passariello R, Iascone C: TNM staging in lung cancer: role of computed tomography. J Thorac Cardiovasc Surg 84:569, 1982
19. Nathan MH, Colling VP, Adams RQ: Differentiation of benign and malignant pulmonary nodules by growth rate. Radiology 79:221, 1962
20. Poe RH, Tobin RE: Sensitivity and specificity of needle biopsy in lung malignancy. Am Rev Resp Dis 112:725, 1980
21. Port S, Cobb FR, Coleman E, et al: Effect of age on the response of the left ventricular response to exercise. New Engl J Med 303:1133, 1980
22. Ryhanen P, Herva E, Hollmen A, et al: Changes in peripheral blood leucocyte counts, lymphocytes subpopulations, and in vitro transformation after heart valve replacement. J Thorac Cardiovasc Surg 77:259-266, 1979
23. Schaner EG, Chang AE, Doppman SL, et al: Comparison of computed and conventional whole lung tomography in detecting pulmonary nodules. A prospective radiologic-pathologic study. Am J Roentgenol 131:51, 1978
24. Stewart JF, Tattersall MHN, Woods RL, et al: Unknown primary adenocarcinoma: Incidence of over-investigation and natural history. Br Med J 1:1530, 1979

25. Theros EG: Varying manifestation of peripheral pulmonary neoplasm: A radiologic-pathological correlative study. Am J Roentgenol 128:893, 1977
26. Tisi GM: Preoperative preparation of pulmonary function. Am Rev Resp Dis 119:293, 1979
27. Toomes H, Vogt-Moyropf I: Conservative resection for lung cancer, in Delarue NC, Eschapasse H (eds): International Trends in General Thoracic Surgery, vol. I: Lung Cancer. Philadelphia, Saunders, 1985, p 88
28. Weiss W: Tumor doubling time and survival of men with bronchogenic carcinoma. Chest 65:3, 1974
29. Wernly JA, DeMeester TR, Kirchner PT: Clinical value of quantitative ventilation-perfusion lung scans in the surgical management of bronchogenic carcinoma. J Thorac Cardiovasc Surg 80:535, 1980

Azhar M. Awan
Ralph R. Weichselbaum
George T. Y. Chen

10

Radiation Therapy

The principal therapy for stage I non-small cell carcinomas of the lung is surgery. The majority of the patients presenting with lung cancer usually are diagnosed with disease that is not amenable to surgery, however, and a significant number of patients thought to be clinically resectable will be found at thoracotomy to have unresectable lung cancer. In the American Joint Committee for Cancer Staging and End Results Reporting (AJC) staging system[1], stage I lung cancers are those with disease that is classified as $T_1N_0M_0$ and $T_2N_0M_0$ (see Chapter 8).

DOSE-TUMOR VOLUME RELATIONSHIPS IN CLINICAL RADIATION ONCOLOGY

The basic physical and radiobiological principles of radiation oncology have been outlined in Chapter 5. Since radiation kills a fixed proportion of tumor cells, the greater the tumor cell burden, the greater is the dose needed for local control. Most of the clinical data regarding dose-tumor control relationships is derived from epithelial tumors of the aerodigestive tract and breast carcinoma since most of these tumors are accessible to measurement during and after a course of radiotherapy. There is a direct relationship between the dose delivered and the probability of tumor control. For example, to achieve a greater than 90 percent probability of controlling subclinical disease, a dose of approximately 5000 rads is required. At 3000–4000 rads, the probability of control of subclinical disease drops to between 60 and 70 percent. Fletcher has shown that 6000 rads is needed to control gross disease less than 2 cm in size.[8,9] Gross disease between 2 and 4 cm in size requires 7000 rads to achieve a 90 percent probability of control.[8,9] A large analysis of dose and tumor volume as it relates to operable lung cancer has not been performed. Sherman et al, however, analyzed time-dose relationships in unresectable lung cancer in patients who survived at least 18 months and found that there was a survival advantage in patients treated

Table 10-1

Local Failure as a Function of Dose in Inoperable Lung Cancer

Dose (Rad)	Total Patients	Number of Local Failure	Percent Local Failure
≥4000-<5000	8	4	50
≥5000-<5500	27	6	22
≥5500-<5900	11	2	18
≥5900	20	1	5

Modified from Sherman DM, Weichselbaum RR, Hellman S: The Characteristics of long term survivors of lung cancer treated with radiation. Cancer 47:2575, 1981. With permission.

with high doses (> 5500 rads).[17] The local control was also higher in patients receiving aggressive, well-planned radiation therapy. Table 10-1 shows the local failure rate as a function of dose.

It is important to keep dose-tumor volume relationships in mind when analyzing the efficacy of radiation therapy in controlling any neoplasm. Radiation therapy cannot be dismissed as being ineffective if doses effective in controlling only microscopic disease are applied to gross disease. Currently in the treatment of non-small cell carcinoma of the lung (NSCLC), we employ 5000 rads in the treatment of microscopic disease whereas gross disease is treated with doses ranging between 6000 and 6500 rads.

RADIOTHERAPY EXPERIENCE IN OPERABLE NON-SMALL CELL CARCINOMA OF THE LUNG

Reports of radiation for operable lung cancer are not numerous since most patients with early disease are treated surgically. The comparison of the efficacy of surgery and radiation in the treatment of early-stage lung cancer is influenced by the inherent inadequacies of clinical staging. The surgical series contain true stage I patients since these patients have undergone resection with node sampling or dissection. Those patients who are presumed to be stage I clinically and who undergo radiation may be understaged since a significant portion of clinical stage I patients who undergo thoracotomy for possible resection are upstaged on the basis of involvement of hilar and/or mediastinal lymph nodes. Differences in the results of surgical resection based on clinical staging and postsurgical pathologic staging are highlighted in the AJC study on cancer staging and end results. The 5-year survival for patients with clinical stage I carcinoma of the lung is lower than the percent 5-year survival for those who are true stage I patients based on postsurgical pathologic staging.[19]

Most experience on radiation for surgically resectable lung cancer is derived from patients who were too ill to undergo surgical treatment. Some reports, however, address the use of radiotherapy in operable lung cancer in medically fit patients. One of the earliest reports on the use of radiation for operable lung cancer was that from Hilton in London.[6] The report does not indicate the clinical stage of the patients but states that all the patients treated were candidates for resection. Thirty-eight patients were treated with radiation alone. Eighteen patients lived for at least 2 years, and 8 patients were alive at least 5 years posttreatment. This results in a crude 5-year survival of 21 percent. This paper does not detail the dose of radiation or the volume of lung irradiated. In addition, Hilton compared some of these patients to a group of surgically treated patients and noted that at 5 years the survival rates for both groups were very similar. The 1-year survival was superior in the radiotherapy treated patients, 96 percent compared to 62 percent for surgery, due to the immediate operative mortality as well as delayed mortality from surgical complications.

Smart updated Hilton's series and analyzed 40 patients who received radiation alone for operable lung cancer.[18] These patients were all men ranging in age from 34 to 81 years and who had either histologic proof of bronchogenic carcinoma by bronchoscopic biopsy or had evidence of lung cancer by sputum cytology. Eight patients were classified as undifferentiated carcinoma (oat cell or anaplastic), 27 were classified as squamous cell carcinoma, and 5 patients had only cytological diagnosis of malignant cells without a specific tissue type. The doses delivered were 5000 to 5500 rads for squamous cell carcinomas and 4000 to 4500 rads for undifferentiated carcinomas. Specific details of the volume treated are not given, but it appears that undifferentiated lesions were treated with an extended portal covering the mediastinum. Squamous cell lesions were treated with local radiation only. The total course of the treatment lasted between 7 and 8 weeks. This protraction of treatment was a result of varying daily doses dependent on the patient's tolerance to the treatment. The 5-year survival for these patients was 22.5 percent. Smart does not outline the sites of relapse for the various histologies, but the 5-year survival might have been better if the oat cell carcinomas were omitted from the analysis. Also, on the basis of current knowledge regarding time–dose relationships and tumor control, a higher local dose may have resulted in even better survival rates.

There is one randomized trial comparing surgery to radiotherapy in the treatment of bronchogenic carcinoma. The results of this trial were reported by Morrison et al. from the Hammersmith Hospital in London.[14] The patients who participated in this trial were all under 70 years of age and were in sufficiently good physical condition to undergo a pneumonectomy. All patients showed histologic proof of malignancy. The treatment was randomly assigned. The radiation was delivered by means of an 8-MV (megavolts) linear accelerator with a mean tumor dose of 4500 rads delivered in 4 weeks. The volume treated included the primary tumor with a 2-cm margin of normal tissue and included the ipsilateral hilum and the mediastinum. The surgically treated patients had a radical resection of the tumor with associated hilar and mediastinal node dissection. Patients randomized were not all clinical stage I or II. There were 9 patients in the surgical group who had N2 disease and 10 patients in the radiotherapy group who had N2 disease. The 1-year survival for patients who received radiation therapy was 64 percent and for surgically treated patients, 43 percent. However, the surgically treated patients had a 23 percent 4-year survival, compared to a 7 percent 4-year survival for the radiotherapy patients. These differences were significant at the $p = .05$ level. The authors concluded that surgery was a better treatment than radiation for operable lung cancer. However, the patients who were treated with radiotherapy had inadequate doses (4500 rads) for control of gross disease. In bronchogenic carcinoma, doses of 6000 to 6500 rads are employed for gross disease. It is possible that if higher doses were employed, the outcome in the radiotherapy treated patients would have been better than the results achieved.

A more recent report by Cooper et al. analyzed a group of 72 patients who were treated with radiation therapy alone for operable lung cancer.[6] Operability was confirmed by bronchoscopic examination, and all patients had mediastenoscopic evidence of negative mediastinal lymph nodes. The results of radiotherapy in this group of patients were compared to a group of 123 patients undergoing thoracotomy for lung cancer and meeting the same criteria of technical operability on the basis of bronchoscopic examination and having negative mediastinal lymph nodes. The cumulative 5-year survival using the life table method for the patients receiving radiotherapy was 6 percent, compared to a 46 percent 5-year cumulative survival for patients undergoing thoracotomy. Individuals who received radiotherapy alone constituted a cohort who were at a high risk for postoperative morbidity and mortality because of poor cardiac or pulmonary status. The radiation dose administered was stated for 66 out of the 72 patients. Of significance is the fact that about half the patients received doses of less than 4000 rads. Fourteen (21 percent) of the patients received doses of 3000–4000 rads. Seventeen (27 percent) of the patients received doses of less than 3000 rads. Of the 35 patients (53 percent) who received doses of 4000 rads or more, details are not provided regarding the range of doses. Those patients who underwent thoracotomy were not comparable to the radiotherapy patients in that the surgically treated patients were able to undergo thoracotomy. Patients who were treated with radiotherapy (because of their medical condition) were destined to do poorly no matter what form of therapy was chosen. Therefore, a favorable bias for the thoracotomy patients existed. All but one of the 123 patients taken to surgery were resected and completed the planned therapy prescribed. Most of the patients assigned to radiotherapy received less than curative doses of radiation and, therefore, did not undergo the planned therapy. The only conclusion from this report is that patients who are technically resectable but medically inoperable can be expected to do poorly with radiotherapy alone, especially if less than curative doses of radiation are delivered. Conversely, it can be concluded that patients who are technically resectable and who are medically fit to undergo a thoracotomy can expect a successful outcome if the planned resection is carried out.

SIDE EFFECTS AND COMPLICATIONS OF RADIATION THERAPY IN THE TREATMENT OF OPERABLE LUNG CANCER

The sequelae of radiation therapy can be divided into acute side effects and delayed complications. The biological and clinical aspects of the acute and delayed effects of radiation in regard to lung parenchyma are outlined in Chapter 5. The acute morbidity experienced by patients undergoing radiation therapy for lung cancer is dependent on the anatomic structures included in the treatment portal. The acute side effects are also dependent on the dose per fraction used in treating the patient. In general, lung cancer is treated using daily fractions of 180–300 rads.

With the use of supervoltage radiotherapy equipment, acute skin effects are minimal and usually well tolerated by the patient. Most patients will experience only a first- or second-degree epithelial reaction—specifically, erythema and dry desquamative epidermitis, respectively. When the mediastinal structures are irradiated, there is injury to the epithelial lining of the esophagus, and this results in an esophagitis at approximately 3000 rads. The esophagitis is manifest clinically by dysphagia and odynophagia. The esophagitis is usually limited and subsides 2–3 weeks after completion of radiation therapy. In some instances, the esophagitis might be sufficiently severe to necessitate a break in treatments or result in the patient being admitted for nutritional support. A similar epithelial reaction can occur in the tracheobronchial tree, and this can result in thickening of the respiratory secretions. The patient can develop a dry, nonproductive cough during and after radiation; again, this usually is self-limited. In rare instances, symptoms can persist for several months and years after the completion of radiation therapy. If significant portions of the heart are irradiated, an asymptomatic pericardial effusion may develop in some patients 3–7 months after completion of radiation.[11] Radiation pneumonitis may occur 6–24 weeks after radiation. The acute effects on lung parenchyma have been described in Chapter 5.

With the use of modern supervoltage equipment, delayed complications of the skin are rarely of concern. Esophageal stenosis as a delayed complication of radiation is rare. Late cardiac effects are dependent on the volume of heart irradiated and the total dose delivered. In some cases, an acute pericarditis can eventually lead to a constrictive pericardial syndrome. A delayed complication of mediastinal irradiation can be radiation myelitis. Radiation induced transverse myelitis usually appears within 6–24 months after exposure of the spinal cord to high doses of radiation. The tolerance of the spinal cord is usually said to be approximately 5000 rads in 5 1/2 weeks when doses of 180 rads per fraction are employed. Most radiation oncologists, however, do not exceed a spinal cord dose of 4500 rads because of the devastating nature of this complication. It should be pointed out that the risk of transverse myelitis increases with increasing length of spinal cord irradiated and also with higher doses per fraction. With good treatment planning and attention to the spinal cord dose, the risk of radiation-induced transverse myelitis as a consequence of radiation therapy for lung cancer can be virtually eliminated.

For the most part, the above-outlined acute and delayed complications of radiation are not dose-limiting factors in the treatment of early-stage lung cancer. The lung, however, is a major dose-limiting structure, since the majority of patients referred for radiotherapy have very poor pulmonary reserve. The patients with chronic pulmonary disease must be assessed carefully prior to radiotherapy planning so that as little nontumor containing lung parenchyma is irradiated as possible. Large extended field irradiation in patients with severe pulmonary disease can be very morbid and lead to treatment related deaths. Green and Weinstein reviewed 20 patients with lung cancer and chronic pulmonary disease who were treated with local involved field irradiation.[11] They compared this group to 41 patients with lung cancer and chronic pulmonary disease who were treated using an extended field technique. The incidence of radiation pneumonitis was 7 percent for patients receiving involved field irradiation, compared to a pneumonitis rate of 17 percent for those receiving extended field irradiation. The 1-year disease-free survival for those patients undergoing involved field irradiation was 41 percent, compared to a 19 percent 1-year disease-free survival for those undergoing extended field radiation.

NEW DIRECTIONS IN LUNG TREATMENT PLANNING

Ideally, a uniform dose to the tumor/target volume is delivered while minimizing the dose to the uninvolved lung, heart, and spinal cord. This must be achieved under the following complicating considerations: (1) there are substantial variations in external patient contour and dimensions, (2) lung density is significantly less than soft-tissue density and will affect the attenuation of radiation beams, and (3) radiation-sensitive structures are in close proximity to the target region. In conventional treatment planning for this site, fields are arranged and weighted to cover the target volume with the 100 percent isodose in the central plane. Frequently, one level above and one level below the central plane are also calculated. In this way, variations in target shape and anatomy are assessed. The three-level approach has been in use for over a decade, and several good reviews of current treatment planning considerations are described elsewhere.[16]

In this section we describe an experimental approach to three-dimensional dosimetry for treatment planning lung lesions. With advanced treatment planning systems, it is now feasible to calculate three-dimensional dose matrices. Combined with the anatomic information provided by volumetric computed tomography (CT) studies, the dose to specific organs may be calculated. By assessing the dose delivered in three dimensions, a more quantitative interpretation of the treatment plan is possible. The three-dimensional dose matrix is analyzed by examining isodose distributions and dose–volume histograms. Dose–volume histograms have been found to be useful in (1) evaluating the relative merit of treatment plans employing different field configurations or different types of ionizing radiation, and (2) estimating the partial organ tolerance of critical structures. The technique is summarized here and described in more detail elsewhere.[2-4,5,10]

First, CT scans in the treatment position are obtained, typically specifying 1-cm contiguous slices. The region scanned includes the entire target volume and lungs. Radiation portals may be delineated in the usual manner on simulator films, in which case the dimensions (widths) of the fields are transferred to the corresponding CT level by registering the two data sets through bony landmarks and other structures. Alternatively, interactive computer programs are used to delineate the target on axial CT images and used to deduce the port shapes and position. In either case, target, lungs and heart are contoured on the axial image data.

Tissue density is determined from the CT study and may be used in the dose calculation.[7,15] A dose matrix is calculated for each CT level. Dose–volume histograms are generated by tabulating those dose matrix points within a specific organ contour. The integral dose—volume histogram displays the fractional organ volume receiving a dose in excess of D. To illustrate the use of dose–volume histograms in planning for lung lesions, a case study of a patient who underwent radiation therapy for a carcinoma of the right lung is presented in the following paragraph.

Several multiple-field treatment plans usually are calculated and evaluated in the course of treatment planning. In determining the optimal treatment plan, the dose–volume histograms are examined to analyze which plan irradiates the least volume of normal tissue to the least dose, while simultaneously irradiating the target uniformly. In some situations, there may not be important clinical differences between field arrangements for a treatment plan. Figure 10-1 shows the dose–volume histogram for a patient with a tumor in the right lung. This patient had previously had her left lung removed because of disease. It was, therefore, important to devise a treatment plan for her remaining lung that would spare the most lung tissue in her remaining lung. Multiple treatment plans were generated on the central slice, with subsequent discussion of their relative plan merits. Plan variations included a heavily weighted lateral and anterior right-angle pair of fields, a combination arc and right posterior field, and a simple oblique parallel opposed pair. When the dose-volume histograms for the right

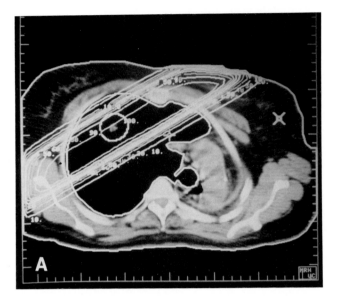

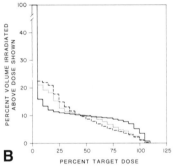

Fig. 10-1. (A) Isodose distribution for a right lung lesion. In this plan, opposed oblique radiation fields are used. (B) Integral dose volume histograms for three plan variations: dotted line—right angled wedged pair; dashed line—arc with posterior oblique; solid line—opposed oblique fields.

lung were calculated, the differences observed between these plans were quite small. Taking 20 Gy* as a threshold for lung damage, all of the plan variations irradiated 11-14 percent of the right lung to a dose in excess of this. In this case, the various field arrangements resulted in differences of only 3 percent in lung irradiated in excess of 20 Gy. Generally, this is not the case, and field arrangements can result in substantially different dose-volume histograms.

It is envisioned that CT scans of patients who may have radiation-induced pneumonitis in the course of therapy may be collected and analyzed to correlate the region of pneumonitis with the dose and volume of irradiation. A similar analysis has been performed with liver irradiated with heavy charged particles,[7] resulting in an estimate of liver radiation tolerance.

---

*Unit of absorbed dose, equal to the energy imparted by ionizing radiation to a mass of matter corresponding to 1 joule per kilogram; termed *gray*, symbolized *Gy*.

ANALYSIS OF RISK IN THERAPY FOR LUNG CANCER

McNeil and colleagues investigated the importance of evaluating therapeutic results with an index that includes consideration of patient attitudes toward risk.[13] They proposed to demonstrate the limitation of a 5-year survival rate for this type of decision. They examined attitudes of a small group of patients being treated with surgery or radiotherapy for carcinoma of the lung. The investigators specifically chose lung cancer since the alternative treatments for this disease, surgery versus radiotherapy, differ in survival rates rather than quality of life. By studying carcinoma of the lung, therefore, the investigators needed to make only one utility assessment; life now versus life later (because surgery carries an immediate mortality risk, and, presumably, superior 5-year survival and radiotherapy carries very little or no immediate mortality and presumably an inferior 5-year survival). Unexpectedly, a group of patients preferred radiotherapy to surgery, even with a stated inferior 5-year survival. These individuals were older patients who were risk-averse (who wanted guaranteed life now vs superior survival later) and preferred radiotherapy. The authors caution that their results do not necessarily indicate that radiation is superior to surgery for patients with operable lung cancer, since their population was too small and selected. Their investigation, however, is considered a prototype concerned with the choice between two therapies offering an increased chance for prolonged survival versus another offering a smaller chance for prolonged survival, but with no early death risk. The authors stress that all clinicians should consider patient attitudes toward risk and differing timeframes of survival.

SUMMARY

In this chapter we have presented the radiation therapy experience in operable lung cancer. The limited data available suggests that high-dose, well-planned radiotherapy may be an alternative to surgical resection for stage I lung cancer. Surgery remains the standard treatment for stage I non-small cell lung cancer (NSCLC). There is a subset of patients, however, for whom surgery is not optimal and for whom radiation therapy may be the better form of treatment. If cases for radiotherapy are selected carefully, the patients with stage I lung cancer who are treated with radiotherapy may expect a good outcome.

REFERENCES

1. American Joint Committee on Cancer: Manual for Staging of Cancer, 2d ed. Philadelphia, Lippincott, 1983
2. Austin-Seymour M, Chen GTY, Castro JR, et al: Dose volume histograms in the analysis of liver radiation tolerance. Internatl J Rad Onc Biol Phys 12:31-36, 1986
3. Chen GTY: Dose volume histograms in treatment planning evaluation of carcinoma of the Pancreas, in Proceedings of 8th International Conference on Computers in Radiology, Toronto 1984, Silver Springs, MD, IEEE Computer Press, ISBN 81860551-6, pp 264-268
4. Chen GTY, Pelizzari C, Spelbring D, et al: Evaluation of treatment plans with dose volume

histograms, in Vaeth J(ed): Treatment Planning of Radiation Therapy. Krager-Basel, 1987, pp 44-55

5. Chin LM, Kijewski PK, Svensson GK, et al: A computer controlled radiation therapy machine for pelvic and para-aortic nodal areas. Internatl J Rad Oncol Biol Phys 7:61-70, 1981

6. Cooper JD, Pearson G, Todd TR, et al: Radiotherapy alone for patients with operable carcinoma of the lung. Chest 87:289, 1985

7. Cunningham JR: Tissue heterogeneity characterization and correction, in Advances in Radiation Therapy Treatment Planning, AAPM Monograph 9, New York, American Institute of Physics, (1983)

8. Fletcher GH: Local results of irradiation in primary management of localized breast cancer. Cancer 29:545, 1972

9. Fletcher GH: Textbook of Radiotherapy, 3d ed. Philadelphia, Lea & Febiger, 1980

10. Goitein M, Miller T: Planning proton therapy of the eye. Med Phys 10:275-283, 1983

11. Green N, Weinstein H: Reassessment of radiation therapy for management of lung cancer in patients with chronic pulmonary disease. Internatl J Rad Oncol Biol Phys 9:1891-1896, 1983

12. Hilton G: Present position relating to cancer of the lung: Results with radiotherapy alone. Thorax 15:17, 1960

13. McNeil BJ, Weichselbaum RR, Paulker SG: Fallacy of the five year survival in lung cancer. New Eng J Med 299:1397, 1978

14. Morrison R, Deeley, TJ, Cleland, WP: The treatment of carcinoma of the bronchus: Clinical trial to compare surgery and supervoltage radiotherapy. Lancet 1:683, 1963

15. Orton CG, Mondalek PM, Spicka JT, et al: Lung corrections in photon beam treatment planning: Are we ready? Internatl J Rad Oncol Biol Phys 10:2191-2199, 1984

16. Purdy J, Perez C: Treatment strategies: Thorax, in Advances in Radiation Therapy Treatment Planning. New York, American Association of Physicists in Medicine/American Institute of Physics, (1983), pp 373-402

17. Sherman DM, Weichselbaum RR, Hellman S: The characteristics of long term survivors of lung cancer treated with radiation. Cancer 47:2575, 1981

18. Smart J: Can cancer of the lung be cured by radiation alone? JAMA 195:1034, 1966

19. Staging of Lung Cancer/1979 American Joint Committee for Cancer Staging and End-Results Reporting. Chicago, Task Force on Lung, 1978

PART III

Stage II Non-Small Cell Lung Cancer

Alex G. Little
Mark K. Ferguson
David B. Skinner

11

Surgical Therapy of Patients with Modified Stage II ($T_1N_1M_0$ and $T_2N_1M_0$) Non-Small Cell Lung Cancer

Standard AJC staging criteria define stage I patients as those with $T_1N_0M_0$, $T_2N_0M_0$ and $T_1N_1M_0$ disease, whereas stage II contains only patients with $T_2N_1M_0$ disease.[1] Several groups of investigators have observed that patients with $T_1N_1M_0$ and $T_2N_1M_0$ non-small cell lung cancer (NSCLC) have prognoses and responses to treatment that are similar within that group but are significantly different from those in patients with $T_1N_0M_0$ and $T_2N_0M_0$ lung cancers.[6,12] As patients with similar prognoses should receive the same treatment for their lung cancers, patients with T_1 or T_2 primary tumors and involvement of N_1 nodes should be grouped as a modified stage II; stage I should include only patients without involvement of any lymph nodes.

We are, then, reviewing in this chapter surgical considerations for patients with T_1 or T_2 primary tumors and metastases to N_1 nodes. This includes lymph nodes from three anatomic levels: intraparenchymal, intersegmental, and hilar. Patients with T_3 primary tumors, or involvement of N_2 nodes, are not included in this discussion as they are in stage III, and their prognosis and surgical considerations are quite different.

SURGICAL CONSIDERATIONS

Principles of thoracic surgery and preoperative diagnostic and staging techniques and considerations are reviewed in Chapters 4 and 8. Following the appropriate clinical staging, the most important function of which is to identify stage III patients whose surgical considerations are more complicated, all patients in clinical stage I or II are candidates for potentially curative resections. In fact, most patients eventually proved by pathologic staging to be in modified stage II are in clinical stage I at the time of thoracotomy. When the patients' physiologic status is sufficient, as reviewed in Chapter 4, standard treatment for these patients is surgical resection, with the extent of resection being determined by intraoperative assessment of the ability to remove all identifiable pathologic tissue with a lobectomy. When this is not possible, even with a bronchial sleeve resection, a pneumonectomy is necessary. The two surgical considerations are the resectability of the primary tumor and the ability to remove all the involved N_1 nodes.

With regard to the first consideration, there are no conclusive data showing that an extensive margin or distance between the tumor and the end of the resected bronchus is necessary.[11] One study shows a difference in local recurrence favoring pneumonectomy over lobectomy in patients with modified stage II disease[3] and, therefore, suggests that overly conservative resections for these patients may increase the risk of local recurrence. Most reports differ however, revealing that the majority of postresection recurrences are distant rather than local and that the extent of resection (lobectomy vs pneumonectomy) does not affect recurrence or survival. Obviously, there must not be tumor in the bronchial margin.[11] Fortunately, skip lesions do not seem to occur, in contrast to the gastrointestinal tract, where, for example, 10-cm margins are necessary for esophageal cancers because of skip involvement of both the mucosa and the submucosal lymphotics. Our experience, that survival is not related to the distance between the tumor and the bronchial stump, thus is not surprising.[2] Apparently, there is no definite benefit to pneumonectomy over lobectomy with regard to the primary tumor when the smaller operation encompasses all tumor. Obviously, a pneumonectomy is more likely to be required for a T_2 than a T_1 primary tumor, particularly if it is T_2 because of a central location.

Intraoperative assessment of lymph node groups prior to the resection, the second consideration, is based on a combination of their gross appearance and frozen-section histologic analysis. When the N_1 nodes are not enlarged or abnormal in any way, and a lobectomy will suffice to remove the primary tumor, this operation is an appropriate procedure. In its technical performance, all accessible N_1 nodes should be taken with the specimen regardless of appearance. This is important for staging and perhaps for therapy by removal of unsuspected micrometastases within N_1 nodes. When enlarged or abnormal-appearing N_1 nodes are encountered, a frozen-section analysis should be obtained and, the patient's physiologic status permitting, a pneumonectomy performed if the biopsy is positive in order to extirpate all involved regional lymphatics. This is based on the intuitive, but unproved, assumption that when a N_1 nodal metastasis is of sufficient size to be recognizable, this implies a greater likelihood of occult involvement of other N_1 nodes than when all nodes appear normal.

Although results have varied, 5-year postresection survival rates for $T_1N_1M_0$ and $T_2N_1M_0$ patients are 14 percent to 39 percent[2,4,5,7,9,10] (Table 11-1). It appears that it is the N_1 nodal involvement per se that is the primary determinant of survival. Although none of these series has documented a definite relationship between the number of involved nodes or level of N_1 nodal involvement (intraparenchymal, intersegmental or hilar) and prognosis, the best survival for modified stage II patients was obtained in a group of patients with a relatively low (37.3 percent) incidence of hilar nodal involvement.[7] In comparison, our patients had a 70.6 percent incidence of involvement of nodes at this level.[2] In contrast to the importance of the nodal involvement for prognosis, neither the histologic cell type, the classification of the primary tumor (T_1 vs. T_2), the presence or absence of visceral pleural involvement, nor the type of resection performed have any definite relationship to survival in our experience.[2] Kirsh found that patients with squamous cell carcinoma had a better prognosis than

Table 11-1
Reported Survival in Patients with Modified Stage II NSCLC

Number of Patients	TNM Status	5-Year Survival (%)	Reference
80	T_1 and $T_2N_1M_0$	22	9*
54	T_1 and $T_2N_1M_0$	30	9†
?	T_1 and $T_2N_1M_0$	31.1	5
35	$T_1N_1M_0$	6.9	10
147	$T_2N_1M_0$	25.5	10
22	T_1 and $T_2N_1M_0$	14	4
17	$T_1N_1M_0$	56	7
58	$T_2N_1M_0$	48	7
75	T_1 and $T_2N_1M_0$	49	7
8	$T_1N_1M_0$	30.2	2
26	$T_2N_1M_0$	30.2	2
34	T_1 and $T_2N_1M_0$	30.2	2

*Study conducted during 1950-1959.
†Study conducted during 1960-1969.

those with adenocarcinoma,[5] but others[7] agree with our conclusion that although adenocarcinoma is more likely to be advanced at the time of diagnosis than is squamous cell carcinoma, when the stage is the same, the prognosis is similar.

The recurrence rates and patterns following resection in these patients are shown in Table 11-2. Except for the one conflicting report,[4] there is a consistent observation that most patients with involvement of N_1 nodes recur at sites outside the operative hemithorax, that is, with distant or metastatic disease. In addition, over half of these distant recurrences are in the brain, primarily in patients with adenocarcinoma. This suggests that failure is most often due to undetected micrometastases at time of surgery, that is, that there is a failure of staging. This strengthens the conclusion that a lobectomy usually is the most appropriate resection as most failures are due to distant rather than local recurrences.

The roles of adjuvant therapies, radiation therapy, or chemotherapy are addressed in detail in Chapter 12. Our experience[2] strongly suggests the need for postoperative adjuvant therapy of some type.

Table 11-2
Postresection Recurrence Rates and Patterns in Patients with Modified Stage II NSCLC

Number of Patients	TNM Status	Recurrence*			Reference
		Local	Distant	Total	
22	T_1 and $T_2N_1M_0$	9 (41)	5 (23)	14 (64)	4
17	$T_1N_1M_0$	0 (0)	8 (47)	8 (47)	7
58	$T_2N_1M_0$	8 (13.8)	21 (36.2)	29 (50)	7
75	T_1 and $T_2N_1M_0$	8 (10.7)	29 (38.7)	37 (49)	7
18	$T_1N_1M_0$	5 (41.7)	7 (58.3)	12 (66.7)	8
8	$T_1N_1M_0$	0 (0)	3 (37.5)	3 (37.5)	2
26	$T_2N_1M_0$	3 (11.5)	10 (38.5)	13 (50)	2
34	T_1 and $T_2N_1M_0$	3 (8.8)	13 (38.2)	16 (47.1)	2

*n (% of patients).

EDITORIAL COMMENT

The new staging system defines stage II tumors to be exactly those we had grouped in our modified approach to the previous staging system, that is $T_1N_1M_0$ and $T_2N_1M_0$ lung cancers. Accordingly, there is in this chapter no difference between the present and the new proposed system.

REFERENCES

1. American Joint Committee for Cancer Staging and End-Results Reporting. Staging of lung cancer, 1979
2. Ferguson MK, Little AG, Golomb HM, et al: The role of adjuvant therapy after resection of T1N1M0 and T2N1M0 non-small cell lung cancer. J Thorac Cardiovasc Surg 91:344-349, 1986
3. Iascone C, DeMeester TR, Albertucci M, et al: Local recurrence of resectable non-oat cell carcinoma of the lung: A warning against conservative treatment for N_0 and N_1 disease. Cancer 57:471-476, 1986
4. Immerman SC, Vanecko RM, Fry WA, et al: Site of recurrence in patients with stages I and II carcinoma of the lung resected for cure. Ann Thorac Surg 32:23-27, 1981
5. Kirsh MM, Rotman H, Argenta L, et al: Carcinoma of the lung: Results of treatment over 10 years. Ann Thorac Surg 21:371-377, 1976
6. Little AG, DeMeester TR, Ferguson MK, et al: Modified stage I (T1N0M0, T2N0M0) non-small cell lung cancer: Treatment results, recurrence patterns and adjuvant immunotherapy. Surgery, in press
7. Martini N, Flehinger BJ, Nagasaki F, et al: Prognostic significance of N_1 disease in carcinoma of the lung. J Thorac Cardiovasc Surg 86:646-653, 1983
8. Pairolero PC, Williams DE, Bergstralh EJ, et al: Postsurgical stage I bronchogenic carcinoma: Morbid implications of recurrent disease. Ann Thorac Surg 38:331-338, 1984
9. Paulson DL, Reisch JS: Long-term survival after resection for bronchogenic carcinoma. Ann Surg 184:324-332, 1976
10. Shields TW, Keehn RJ: Postresection stage grouping in carcinoma of the lung. Surg Gynecol Obstet 145:725-728, 1977
11. Soorae AS, Stevenson HM: Survival with residual tumor on the bronchial margin after resection for bronchogenic carcinoma. J Thorac Cardiovasc Surg 76:175-180, 1979
12. Williams DE, Pairolero PC, Davis CS, et al: Survival of patients surgically treated for stage I lung cancer. J Thorac Cardiovasc Surg 82:70-76, 1981

Thomas J. Fitzgerald
Joel S. Greenberger

_____ **12** _____

Adjuvant Radiotherapy and Its Role in the Treatment of Stage II Lung Cancer

Lung carcinoma remains an enormous clinical challenge for all health care personnel involved in the care of these patients. In the most favorable anatomic and histologic presentations (which represent no more than 20 percent of the total lung cancer population), 5-year survivals of 70–80 percent can be achieved by surgical resection of the disease.[4] However, the percentage of patients coming to surgical exploration decreases as diagnostic and presurgical imaging techniques become more sophisticated.[5] Those patients with unresected primary lung carcinoma are ultimately referred for radiation therapy in order to control local regional disease. It is important to recognize that great gains in longevity have not materialized with the addition of adjuvant therapy. However, a very real benefit in the quality of life for most patients with carcinoma of the lung can be achieved with the judicious and thoughtful application of sophisticated radiation therapy, for a small but significant portion of the population, a cure will result from this treatment. This chapter will review the role of radiation therapy as an adjuvant to definitive surgical treatment.

STAGING AND PROGNOSTIC FACTORS

The clinical staging system proposed by the American Joint Committee for Cancer Staging is reviewed in Chapter 8. The anatomic extent of disease prior to treatment may be established by history, physical examination, x-ray studies, endoscopy (including mediastinoscopy), and radioisotopic scans for distant metastases. At our institution the patients undergo computerized tomography (CT) scanning of the chest for anatomic definition of the primary target volume as well as scans of the brain and abdomen for evaluation of potential sites of metastatic disease. These studies are not presently required for staging purposes.

In addition to the anatomic extent of the disease and histology, other manifestations of lung cancer have been shown to have a strong correlation with reduced survival.[18] These are, specifically, weight loss and performance status. Patients requir-

LUNG CANCER: A COMPREHENSIVE TREATISE
ISBN 0-8089-1876-1

ing more than 25-50 percent of normal active time in bed and those who have lost 10-15 percent of body weight have a much more limited prognosis than do patients without these findings. For the surgeon who deals primarily with limited disease, the proposed system is reasonably predictive of the overall prognosis of the patient. For the radiotherapist, who deals almost exclusively with stage III disease, it will be necessary to identify the subsets of patients within this stage with respect to the location and size of the primary lesion and extent of mediastinal metastasis in order to assess the prognosis for each individual patient. It is equally demanding on the radiotherapist to be able to identify patients whose normal tissue reserves could not withstand the rigors of aggressive radiation treatment. The normal tissue restraints of each individual patient will greatly influence the radiotherapist in choosing each individual patient's treatment volume, daily fraction size, and total treatment dose.

OPERATIVE IRRADIATION TREATMENT

With the overall unsatisfactory results of the surgical therapy of lung cancer, many investigators began to use radiation therapy on a preoperative basis in an attempt to increase cure rates. The rationale for preoperative irradiation is as follows: the ability of radiation therapy to convert unresectable lesions to resectable lesions, the efficacy of subtherapeutic radiation treatment in eliminating potential microscopic disease, and the possible reduction of the number of cells capable of implantation at the time of thoracotomy in local and/or distant sites. Bloedorn[1] and Hellman et al.[7] carefully demonstrated in the preoperative setting that irradiation doses from 48 to 60 Gy eliminated biopsy-proven tumor in at least 30 percent of patients when the radiation was delivered on a preoperative basis. Studies on the effectiveness of radiation therapy to control local tumor also include those of Rissanen, who found persistent tumor in all patients treated with 20-30 Gy and no carcinoma in 18 out of 60 patients (30 percent) of patients treated with 45-62 Gy.[13] This initial sense of optimism has been tempered by studies by Shields[16] and Warren,[21] who both failed to demonstrate a survival advantage in patients treated with radiation therapy on a preoperative basis. In 1978 Sherman et al. published a series of 53 patients treated at the Harvard Joint Center for Radiation Therapy.[15] The majority of patients had stage III disease at presentation. Because the tumor volume was judged to be of borderline resectability, the patients were treated with 30-40 Gy of radiation on a preoperative basis. Of the 53 original patients, 38 ultimately went to surgical resection, and of these remaining 38, there were 12 patients (32 percent) alive with a median followup of 48 months. In 1984 a series was published from the University of Nijmegem that demonstrated the results of a randomized study in patients with resectable carcinoma of the bronchus.[8] In this group, 14 patients underwent 20-Gy preoperative irradiation and 14 patients had surgery as their only mode of therapy. At a follow-up time of 10 years, 59 percent of patients who received radiation treatment and surgery were alive, compared to 43 percent of the patients treated with surgery alone.

In favorable series, the survival advantage to preoperative radiation therapy has been modest; therefore, few institutions practice this form of treatment. The advantage to postoperative treatment is that it does not interfere with the surgical procedure and allows for a better definition of staging. Most institutions now favor postoperative treatment on this basis.

POSTOPERATIVE IRRADIATION TREATMENT

The 5-year survival rate for patients treated with lobectomy and pneumonectomy varies from 20 to 50 percent, depending on the indications for the surgical procedure and the careful pathologic staging of the disease. In patients with a completely resected primary lesion and no lymph node metastasis, the survival rates are good.[4] For those patients with metastatic hilar lymph nodes, however, the survival rate decreases to 20 to 30 percent, and among those with mediastinal lymph nodes, long-term survivors are, unfortunately, rare. As in other anatomic locations, patients with metastatic regional lymph nodes do have a higher risk of developing distant metastasis. When there are positive lymph nodes identified in the pathology specimen, there is a significant probability of tumor remaining in unresected tissue. Because of this potential for residual disease, it is thought that irradiation treatment to the tumor bed site and draining lymph nodes would sterilize any remaining disease and potentially offer the patient increased local control and possible increased benefit in survival.

In a randomized study reported by Patterson and Russell, there was no significant difference in survival when pneumonectomy alone was compared to pneumonectomy followed by mediastinal irradiation.[11] The 3-year survival rate for the pneumonectomy-alone group was 36 percent, and that for the postoperative radiotherapy group was 33 percent. It is important to acknowledge that there was no stratification of patients with respect to size of the primary lesion, pathologic stage, performance status, or histology. The portals used for irradiation were small by today's standards (10×15 cm), and the tumor dose was limited to 4500 cGy. There is no information available regarding the pattern of failure in these patients. Therefore, in spite of the negative results, there are several missing variables within the study that may partially explain the data. Another important feature is that performance status was not noted in these patients, and this is reflected in the fact that 24 of the 103 patients in the study did not complete their course of postoperative irradiation because of declining constitutional status during the course of treatment. Van Houtte et al. reported on 224 patients receiving postoperative radiation therapy. In this group, 175 were randomized to receive either surgery alone (pneumonectomy or lobectomy) or combined with thoracic irradiation (6000 cGy in 6 weeks delivered with ^{60}Co).[20] There was no significant difference in survival between the two groups; however, it should be noted that many patients in this study were without hilar lymph node metastasis and had complete resection of the primary lesion. Since there is minimal evidence that patients such as these benefit from postoperative irradiation, the negative results are not surprising in this series.

More favorable reports have indicated increased survival when patients with hilar or mediastinal lymph nodes are treated with postoperative irradiation. Chung et al. reported the 40 percent 3-year survival in a group of 38 patients with positive lymph nodes receiving postoperative irradiation treatment, as compared to 10 percent of 29 patients treated with surgery alone.[3] Kirsch et al. described improved survival in a nonrandomized series of 69 patients with metastatic mediastinal lymph nodes treated with doses of 5000–5500 cGy after surgical resection.[9] Of those patients receiving postoperative radiotherapy, 23 percent survived for 5 years, whereas no survivors were reported at 5 years in a group of 20 patients treated by surgery alone.

Pavlov et al. reported on 616 patients treated either with surgery alone or surgery combined with postoperative radiotherapy (4000–5000 cGy).[12] The 5-year survival rate was 24 percent in the patients treated with surgery and 38 percent in those treated with combined therapy. The authors noted in this study that there was surprisingly higher incidence in survival in irradiated patients with no evidence of regional lymph node metastasis (48 percent), as opposed to those with negative lymph node metastasis treated with operation alone (30 percent). Green et al. described 35 percent 5-year survival in 66 patients with non-small-cell carcinoma of the lung (NSCLC) and positive hilar or mediastinal nodes receiving postoperative radiotherapy (5000 cGy), as opposed to 3 percent (1 out of 30) in patients treated with surgery alone.[6] The 5-year survival was 22 percent in a group of 64 patients with negative lymph nodes treated with surgery alone, which is similar to the survival in this series in patients receiving combined therapy (27 percent).

Choi et al. reported on 55 patients treated by surgery alone and 93 patients treated with surgery and postoperative radiotherapy.[2] A group of patients with adenocarcinoma receiving postoperative radiotherapy demonstrated a 43 percent 5-year survival, in contrast to 8 percent of 21 patients who had surgery alone. In patients with squamous cell carcinoma, there was no difference in survival, 42 percent versus 33 percent in patients treated with combined therapy or surgery alone. Intrathoracic recurrences, however, were significantly decreased in the patients with squamous cell carcinoma who received postoperative irradiation.

In summary, recent literature seems to indicate that there is a survival advantage for patients treated with postoperative irradiation therapy. With respect to the available data, the authors presently recommend surgical resection as the current treatment for patients with operable, non-small cell bronchogenic carcinoma, and then suggest selecting a group of patients with metastatic regional lymph nodes in the thorax and treat them with postoperative irradiation. However, several significant variables are not currently addressed and need to be explored with well-controlled studies. The issue of histology needs to be clarified because some series demonstrate improved survival in patients with adenocarcinoma only, and other series demonstrate an increased survival in patients with squamous cell carcinoma. The optimal postoperative treatment dose and discrete target volume are likewise not fully studied. The optimal doses of treatment, fractionation schedule, and planning techniques are crucial factors in obtaining optimal tumor control and low treatment morbidity, and these issues need to be appropriately investigated.

TECHNIQUES OF IRRADIATION; VOLUMES, IRRADIATION PORTALS, AND X-RAY BEAM ARRANGEMENT

The volume of tissue to be irradiated and the configuration of the portals should be determined by the size and location of the primary tumor, the lymphatic drainage of the area in which the primary tumor arose, and the equipment and beam energy available for each individual patient.[7] It is common radiation practice to design treatment portals with a 2-cm margin around the areas of gross tumor defined on CT scans and a minimum of 1.5 cm around electively treated regional lymph node areas that were thought to contain microscopic residual disease. In order to include the appropriate lymph node draining areas, careful attention must be considered to the given lymphatic pathways of each lobe of both right and left lungs. Field sizes within an irregular shape are preferred, and these fields require special secondary blocking to spare as much normal tissue as possible. In patients with potentially curable lesions to be treated with high doses of irradiation, complicated portal arrangements are necessary. Oblique or lateral portals are quite useful in combination with anteroposterior-posteroanterior (AP-PA) portals in order to boost the dose to the particular target volume in the lung and mediastinum without excessive irradiation to normal tissues. Spinal cord shielding blocks must be used judiciously, and it is important to recognize that 1-cm variance in the daily setup of the patient on the oblique block could result in either overirradiation of the spinal cord or underirradiation of the mediastinal structures.

The choice of appropriate beam energies in addition to the volume to be treated is crucial to the delivery of adequate doses of irradiation to the tumor without producing toxicity to adjacent normal tissues. Because of the large diameter of the chest, there is much improved target volume dosimetry when one uses high-energy photons.

The most significant problems encountered in treatment planning for bronchogenic carcinoma include the sloping surface of the chest with decreased diameter at the level of the thoracic inlet; the presence of nonunidensity tissues such as the lung; the proximity to the target volume of sensitive structures such as the spinal cord, heart, esophagus, and uninvolved lung; and the frequent need for irregular isodose computations necessary in order to treat target volumes in the lower and upper lung fields.[5,13]

The sloping surface of the chest results in a varied source to tumor distance over the treatment field, and the cause of the differences and separation produces a nonuniform dose distribution. If one chooses to calculate the radiation at the level of the isocenter, this could potentially lead to underdosing of inferior structures where the chest wall diameter is larger. If one chooses to calculate the specific radiation dose at the level of greatest separation, this would lead to excessive high irradiation of tissues located within the area of the chest with a smaller separation. One method of addressing this problem is to correct for the source to to surface discrepancy by use of compensating filters. At our institution, the separation of the patient is taken along the central axis in many different points and is compared to the CT distribution of the target volume and the slope of the patient. This allows for the appropriate compensator to be fitted to each patient and for administration of homogenous dose to the target volume without excessive radiation to normal tissue structures. The compensating filter can be designed to accommodate for changes in the slope in both the cephalocaudad and lateral axis.

The lung air cavity within the irradiation treatment volume is not of tissue unit density; therefore, the primary radiation beam is not attenuated in a uniform fashion; likewise, the scatter function generated from the primary beam is also nonuniform. To correct fully for these inhomogeneities, it is necessary to know the size, shape, and position of the target volume relative to the amount of lung volume within the irradiation treatment portal. The problems of air cavity inhomogeneity has led to a new era in the field of radiation treatment planning. Many investigators have begun to look at target volume inhomogeneities within the radiation field because of this change in unit density material. Some investigators have noted relative inhomogeneities of 25 percent at the central and peripheral portions of the target volume.[10] The central portion of the target volume has received excessively high irradiation doses because of decreased attentuation of the primary radiation beam; however, the periphery of the target volume is thought to receive a decreased irradiation dose because of the lack of scatter located at the boundary of the target volume and lung tissue. The recent advent of CT will create new perspectives in order to assess the effect of target volume inhomogeneities in radiation dose distribution within the thorax.[10] This is becoming of increasing importance because radiation therapists need to reassess target volume inhomogeneities with respect to reporting data concerning local control of thoracic malignancies.

At the University of Massachusetts all patients who are being planned for irradiation treatment to the lung are treated with CT directed planning. The initial target volume is chosen by the radiation therapist. The patient then undergoes CT scanning in the radiation treatment position. This allows for appropriate delineation of the therapy target volume with respect to the patient's contour and proximity to adjacent normal structures. The isocenter of treatment is then chosen with respect to the position of the target volume and the patient's contour, and the patient is then brought back to the radiation simulator where the appropriate imaging films are taken. Most patients are treated with a two- to four-field plan that will allow for a maximal irradiation within the target volume and minimal irradiation as possible to normal tissue structures. The amount of lung within the irradiation field is calculated as a percentage volume, and individual patient blocks are templated in order to protect normal tissue structures.

FUTURE DIRECTIONS IN RADIATION THERAPY IN TREATING PATIENTS WITH PRIMARY LUNG CARCINOMA

Because of the continued problem in local tumor control, current Radiation Therapy Oncology Group studies are being directed towards ways to improve the results of primary radiation treatment. Changes in time dose fractionation schedules include increasing the total x-ray dose with one fraction per day by combining large field treatment to the primary tumor and likely area of nodal involvement with a smaller boost field to grossly involved areas of the primary tumor and lymph nodes. The total x-ray dose to the target volume is 7500 cGy in trials that are presently being conducted. In addition, the Radiation Therapy Oncology Group is completing a pilot study in which two fractions per day of 120 cGy were given 4–6 hours apart to a total dose of 5040 cGy to a large field, with subsequent small field boost to 6960 cGy.[14]

The boost volume includes only that area where gross tumor is involved as demonstrated on CT scan. Other attempts are being made to improve the therapeutic ratio with the use of neutrons, in which the Radiation Therapy Oncology Group study is now randomizing patients to treatment with photons alone, neutrons alone, and mixed photon and neutron beam therapy. The data from these studies will be utilized in developing future therapy treatment protocols.

Attempts have been made to enhance the radiation effect with radiation sensitizers such as the simultaneous administration of misonidazole. Other groups have examined the use of iridium afterloading technique in conjunction with Neodymium Yag laser in the treatment of malignant airway obstruction. Hopefully, the results of these ongoing studies may eventually directly influence the primary management in patients with lung carcinoma.

REFERENCES

1. Bloedorn F, Cawley R, Cuccia C: Preoperative irradiation in bronchogenic carcinoma. Am J Roentgenol 92:77, 1964
2. Choi N, Grillo A, Gardiello M, et al: Basis for new strategies in postoperative radiotherapy of bronchogenic carcinoma. Internatl J Radiat Oncol Biol Phys 6:31, 1980
3. Chung C, Stryker J, O'Neill M: Evaluation of adjuvant postoperative radiotherapy for lung cancer. Internatl J Radiat Oncol Biol Phys 8:900, 1982
4. Gail M, Eagan R, Feld R, et al: Prognostic factors in patients with resected Stage 1 non small cell lung cancer. Cancer 54:1802, 1984
5. Glatstein E, Lichter A, Frass B, et al: The imaging revolution and radiation oncology: Use of CT, ultrasound, and NMR for localization, treatment planning and treatment delivery. Internatl J Radiat Oncol Biol Phys 11:299, 1985
6. Green N, Kuromara S, George F, et al: Postresection irradiation for primary lung cancer. Radiology 116:405, 1975
7. Hellman S, Kligerman M, Von Essen C, et al: Sequelae of radical radiotherapy of carcinoma of the lung. Radiology 82:1055, 1964
8. Kazem I, Jongerius C, Languet L: Evaluation of short course preoperative irradiation in the treatment of resectable bronchus carcinoma: Long term analysis of a randomized pilot study. Internatl J Radiat Oncol Biol Phys 10:981, 1984
9. Kirsh M, Dickerman R, Fayos J, et al: The value of chest wall resection in the treatment of superior sulcus tumors of the lung. Ann Thorac Surg 15:339, 1973
10. Mira J, Potter J, Fullerton G, et al: Advantages and limitations of computed tomography scans for treatment planning of lung cancer. Internatl J Radiat Oncol Biol Phys 8:1617, 1982
11. Patterson R, Russell M: Clinical trials in malignant disease. Part IV-Lung cancer. Value of postoperative radiotherapy. Clin Radiol 13:141, 1962
12. Pavlov A, Pirosov A, Trachtenberg A: Results of combination treatment in lung cancer patients: Surgery plus radiotherapy and surgery plus chemotherapy. Cancer Chemother Rep 4:133, 1973
13. Rissanem P, Tikka U, Holsti L: Autopsy findings in lung cancer treated with megavoltage radiotherapy. Acta Radiol (Ther) (Stockh) 7:433, 1968
14. Seydel GH: External beam treatment of unresectable lung cancer. Internatl J Radiat Oncol Biol Phys 10:573, 1984
15. Sherman D, Neptune W, Weichselbaum R, et al: An aggressive approach to marginally resectable lung cancer. Cancer 41:2040, 1978
16. Shields T, Higgins G, Lawton R, et al: Preoperative x-ray therapy as an adjuvant in the treatment of bronchogenic carcinoma. J Thorac Cardiovasc Surg 59:49, 1970
17. Smart J: Can lung cancer by cured by irradiation alone? JAMA 159:1034, 1966
18. Stanley K: Prognostic factors for survival in patients with inoperable lung cancer. J Natl Cancer Inst 65:299, 1980
19. Thomlinson R, Gray L: The histological structure of some human lung cancers and the possible implications for radiotherapy. Br J Cancer 9:539, 1955
20. Van Houtte P, Rocimans P, Zmets P: Postoperative radiation therapy in lung cancer: A controlled trial after resection of curative design. Internatl J Radiat Oncol Biol Phys 6:983, 1980
21. Warren J: Preoperative irradiation of cancer of the lung. Final report of a therapeutic trial. Cancer 36:914, 1975
22. Weichselbaum R, Nove J and Little J. X-ray sensitivity of human tumor cells in vitro. Internatl J Radiat Oncol Biol Phys 6:437, 1980

Thomas Lad

13

Adjuvant Therapy of Stage II Non-Small Cell Lung Cancer

The current staging recommendations by the American Joint Committee on Cancer define stage II lung cancer as $T_2N_1M_0$, using the TNM nomenclature.[1] A T_2 primary tumor is greater than 3 cm in maximum diameter and must be surrounded by lung tissue, except that visceral pleural involvement is allowed. In addition, a tumor causing lobar atalectasis or obstructive pneumonitis is a T_2 lesion regardless of size. N_1 nodal status consists of metastasis to ipsilateral intrapulmonary and/or hilar lymph nodes. This staging classification is based on a detailed analysis of 2155 lung cancer cases collected by the Task Force on Lung Cancer of the American Joint Committee, which was published in 1974.[19] This analysis resulted in a grouping of various TNM subsets according to survival. Survival of the $T_2N_1M_0$ group was intermediate between that for smaller tumors and that for the T_3, N_2, and/or M_1 groups; hence its designation as stage II. Of the 2155 patients included in the analysis, 6 percent were stage II, making this stage the least common.

STAGING DEFINITIONS

A new international staging system for lung cancer has been proposed.[17] This new system was constructed mainly to separate the many subgroups within AJCC stage III. For example, the prognosis for $T_3 N_0 M_0$ patients is quite different from that for patients with M_1 status despite the fact that both of these TNM subsets fall within the AJCC definition of stage III. The new staging proposal does change the definition of stage II to include both $T_1 N_1 M_0$ and $T_2 N_1 M_0$ subsets. However, since the available literature pertinent to adjuvant therapy of lung cancer has been reported prior to the new staging proposal, this chapter will use the "old" AJCC staging system as defined by the AJCC Task Force.

LUNG CANCER: A COMPREHENSIVE TREATISE
ISBN 0-8089-1876-1

Table 13-1

AJCC Task Force on Lung Cancer: 2-Year
Survival (Percent) by Clinical Stage and Histology

	Stage		
Histology	I	II	III
Squamous cell	46	40	11
Adenocarcinoma	46	14	8
Undifferentiated large cell	43	12	13
Undifferentiated small cell	6	5	4

Modified from Mountain CF, Carr DT, Anderson WAD: A system for the
clinical staging of lung cancer. Am J Roentgenol Radiat Ther Nucl Med
120:130–138, 1974. With permission.

PROGNOSIS FOR STAGE II LUNG CANCER

Table 13-1 shows the 2-year survival figures from the AJCC Task Force analysis
according to stage and histology. Two important biologic aspects of lung cancer are
illustrated by this table: (1) small cell carcinoma separates itself from the other histologies in that the TNM stage does not correlate with survival; and (2) squamous cell
carcinoma is different from adenocarcinoma and large cell carcinoma in that N_1 status
is associated with a better prognosis in squamous cell patients.

It is important to point out that the assignment of T, N, and M status for the 1974
Task Force analysis was based on clinical, not surgical, staging methods.[19] The patients were collected during the 1960s, at which time clinical staging methods were not
nearly as sensitive as they are today. It remained to be shown that the proposed
staging system would hold true for surgically staged patients. An identical analysis was
undertaken using 835 of the 2155 patients, for whom pulmonary resection was
completed and surgical and pathologic staging data were available.[18] The results of the
surgical staging analysis justified the proposed staging system in that the survival for
stages I, II, and III were distinctly different. Table 13-2 shows 5-year survival figures for
the surgically staged patients. In this group, 13 percent (103 out of 794) of the
resected non-small cell lung cancer (NSCLC) patients were stage II, and their 5-year
survival rate was 29 percent.

At this point it will be useful to examine the published large series of resected lung
cancer patients staged according to the TNM system in order to corroborate the

Table 13-2

Resected Non-Small Cell Lung Cancer: 5-Year
Survival (Percent) by Surgical Stage and Histology

	Stage		
Histology	I	II	III
Squamous	54	35	20
Nonsquamous	51	18	10
Both	53	29	16

From Mountain CF: A new international staging system for lung cancer.
Chest 89:225s–235s, 1986. With permission.

prognosis established by the AJCC Task Force. For patients with stage II lung cancer, the largest group of patients was provided by the Veterans Administration Surgical Adjuvant Group (VASAG).[25] Between the years 1957 and 1973, 2341 patients underwent pulmonary resection and were subsequently enrolled in prospective randomized control adjuvant chemotherapy trials. These trials failed to show either beneficial or adverse effects of chemotherapy, and so all patients were considered together for survival analysis. Single institution retrospective analyses have been reported from the University of Michigan,[10] Roswell Park,[28] and Memorial–Sloan Kettering.[9] The Michigan series was comprised of 371 patients collected between 1959 and 1969, Roswell Park reported 295 patients resected between 1963 and 1974, and the Memorial series contained 175 patients treated between 1968 and 1972. Table 13-3 lists the 5-year survival rates from all four of these series according to nodal status. Table 13-4 shows the prognostic implication of cell type in two of these series in which sufficient numbers of patients were available for such an analysis. One can see the wide range of survival figures for each nodal category, which illustrates the problem of retrospective analysis. The major criterion for inclusion in these analyses was "complete" or "potentially curative" resection, except for the Roswell series, which included 67 (23 percent) incomplete resections. This can explain the relatively poor survival in the Roswell group. The VASAG patients were collected prospectively, but there was no uniform staging protocol or central pathologic review mechanism for this large multicenter effort.[6] The retrospective studies[9,10,28] did not make use of a prospective staging protocol, although two of these series[9,10] show remarkably similar results. The discrepancy between these results and those of the VASAG reflects the multicenter composition of the latter group and perhaps its exclusively male population.[6]

The VASAG and Michigan series did not analyze their cases according to AJCC stage grouping, but rather according to TNM node status. Stage I includes $T_1N_1M_0$, and the portion of N_1 patients represented in Tables 13-3 and 13-4 who were stage I was not reported. The Roswell Park group found such a poor survival rate in their N_1 patients that their data did not support the inclusion of $T_1N_1M_0$ into stage I. This issue has been discussed for years, and although the current AJCC system considers T_1N_1 to be stage I,[1] a new international proposal[17] classifies this combination as stage II. The AJCC Task Force 5-year survival of 29 percent for stage II patients[18] is essentially the same as the observations for N_1 disease in the Michigan[10] and MSK[9] series. Consequently, the prognosis for stage II lung cancer patients treated by curative-intent pulmonary resection has been reasonably well defined for retrospectively staged patients.

Table 13-3
5-Year Survival (Percent) According to Node Status

Series	Samples (Pts)	N_0	N_1	N_2	Reference
VASAG	2341	34	19	9	25
Michigan	371	49	31	23	10
Roswell	295	25	0	4	28
MSK	175	45*	27†	18	9

*Stage I: includes $T_1N_1M_0$.
†Stage II: $T_2N_1M_0$ only.

Table 13-4
5-Year Survival (Percent) by Histology and Node Status

Node Status	Series	Squamous	Adenocarcinoma	Reference
N_0	VASAG	34	35	25
	Michigan	53	44	10
N_1	VASAG	20	15	25
	Michigan	47	0	10
N_2	VASAG	11	3	25
	Michigan	34	13	10

RATIONALE FOR ADJUVANT THERAPY

The 5-year survival rate for stage I lung cancer treated by "curative" pulmonary resection is only about 50 percent, and the prognosis for the more advanced stages is worse. Furthermore, the lung cancer survival curves do not plateau at 5 years, but continue a downward slope, and at 10 years the survival rates are only about half those of the 5-year figures. It has long been recognized that occult metastatic disease is quite common in surgically treated lung cancer patients and is the major cause of subsequent mortality, although 10–20 percent of resected lung cancer patients die of causes other than lung cancer.[9,10,28,25]

It stands to reason that adjunctive antineoplastic treatment would be appropriate for resected lung cancer patients, provided that effective treatment could be identified. The choice of an adjuvant treatment modality for a given clinical situation depends on the location of occult residual disease. An autopsy study conducted on patients dying within 30 days of apparent curative pulmonary resection has shown a surprisingly high incidence of both persistant local disease and extrathoracic metastases identifiable grossly so soon after surgery.[14] Squamous carcinoma patients had a 33 percent incidence of local persistence and a 17 percent incidence of distant metastasis, and adenocarcinoma patients had a 40 percent incidence of disease in both categories. Half of the squamous patients with residual disease had local persistance as the only identifiable site, whereas this was almost never valid for the other histologies. A survey of metastatic sites in 681 autopsy patients dying with lung cancer has produced similar findings in that distant metastatic involvement was less frequent in squamous than in nonsquamous cancers.[12] These data, together with the better prognosis for squamous patients with hilar and mediastinal node metastases at the time of surgical treatment, suggest that postoperative radiation therapy would more likely be useful in squamous cell patients than for those with nonsquamous disease where presence of lymph node metastasis is a stronger indication of systemic metastasis. Systemic adjuvant treatment would be more appropriate for nonsquamous patients.

ADJUVANT RADIATION THERAPY

Since only 10–15 percent of surgical lung cancer patients are in stage II, it would be difficult to collect a sufficient number of patients to support a clinical trial testing the efficacy of adjuvant therapy in this stage of disease. The literature pertinent to adjuvant radiation therapy does not address stage II disease specifically. The University of Michigan series discussed earlier[10] employed postoperative radiation therapy for patients with N_2 disease only. Adjuvant radiation therapy was an established policy for N_2 patients in that series. None of the 10 patients who for various reasons did not receive radiation therapy survived 5 years, compared to 23 percent survival for those who were irradiated. The survival rate was 34 percent for squamous patients and 12 percent for non-squamous patients (Table 13-4). The study concluded that adjuvant irradiation appeared to be beneficial in squamous cell carcinoma and justified surgical treatment of N_2 squamous cell carcinoma.

A retrospective trial from San Diego Naval Hospital[5] analyzed survival rates for 219 patients resected between 1954 and 1966; of these, 125 received postoperative radiation therapy. The average dose was 4400 rads in 22 fractions, and the target induced the mediastinum and both hila and supraclavicular regions. In this study, 59 out of 123 patients with negative lymph nodes were irradiated and no advantage was found for this N_0 group. The 5-year survival for N_0 patients was 24 percent, and 64 patients were N_1 stage and 32 were N_2. These patients were combined into a single group to augment the size of the group for more meaningful analysis. The 5-year survival was 35 percent for 66 irradiated patients and 3 percent for those not irradiated. A beneficial effect of radiotherapy was seen for all histologic types. Considering all stages together, the adjuvant irradiation group had double the 5-year survival (31 percent vs 16 percent) of the surgery-alone group. No comment is made regarding patient selection in this trial. Another retrospective trial, from Massachusetts General Hospital, analyzed 148 patients who were surgically staged to be N_1, N_2, or T_3 between 1971 and 1977.[3] In this group, 93 patients received adjuvant irradiation averaging 5000 rads in 25 fractions, and 55 patients were not irradiated. Assignment to adjuvant treatment was made on an individual basis; there was no policy of routine adjuvant radiotherapy at the time. Fifty-seven percent of the patients had N_1 stage (either T_1 or T_2), and 19 out of 35 N_1 adenocarcinoma patients and 22 out of 43 N_1 squamous patients were irradiated. Results were reported for the entire group but not for the N_1 group separately. An advantage was seen in adenocarcinoma, with the 5-year survival for the irradiated group at 43 percent, compared to 5 percent for the surgery-alone group. In contrast, no advantage was found for squamous cell carcinoma, with the 5-year survival at 40 percent for both groups.

In summary, the three retrospective series cited above show three different results of adjuvant radiotherapy: a benefit for squamous cell carcinoma only,[10] a benefit for adenocarcinoma only,[3] and a benefit for all histologies.[5] It is therefore difficult to appeal to this literature for guidance. Obviously, patient selection, lack of a prospective staging protocol, and lack of uniform inclusion criteria in these studies can either alone or together account for the discordant results. A prospective randomized control trial would avoid these problems. Unfortunately, there are none that deal specifically with stage II disease; however, two prospective randomized control trials involving post-surgical adjuvant radiation therapy in lung cancer have been reported. The first was a European trial.[26] Eligibility criteria for this trial included a complete "curative" resection and negative regional lymph nodes (N_0). The adjuvant radiation dose was 6000 rads in 6 weeks to the mediastinum beginning 1 week after surgery. In total, 175 patients were enrolled, 92 in the control arm and 83 in the irradiated arm. The 5-year survival rates were 43 percent for the control arm and 24 percent for the irradiated arm. A local effect of radiation therapy was observed in that there were only four local relapses in the treated arm as opposed to 19 in the control. Extrathoracic failure occurred 75 percent of the time, but again a local effect of radiotherapy was appreciated because extrathoracic failure occurred in 92 percent of the treated group and in 67 percent of the controls. The reasons for a deleterious effect of radiotherapy in this trial are not readily apparent. Balanced randomization was achieved for histology and type of operation. There was no prospective staging protocol, however, and it is conceivable that an imbalance in microscopic node involvement occurred as the result of lack of standardized node sampling rules.

In an attempt to provide some definitive data regarding the efficacy of modern adjuvant treatment for lung cancer, the Lung Cancer Study Group (LCSG) was formed in 1977.[22] A great deal of care was taken to ensure the collection of accurate, detailed, and high-quality clinical data in a small cooperative group setting. Eligibility requirements for all LCSG studies include mandatory sampling of intrapulmonary, hilar, subcarinal, and paratracheal nodes. The sampling must be documented to the Pathology Reference Center at M. D. Anderson Hospital in Houston, Texas, where histologic type and pathologic stage are referreed. A mean of 11 lymph nodes per patient has been sampled in these studies.[15] Complete resection is defined by the LCSG to include histologically negative resection margins and histologically negative highest resected paratracheal node (a "negative margin" of lymph node resection, in a certain sense). LCSG study No. 773 was begun in 1978 to evaluate adjuvant irradiation, 5000 rads in 5 weeks to the mediastinum and ipsilateral hilum, of completely resected stage II and III squamous cell carcinoma.[13] The rationale for limiting eligibility for this study to squamous cell carcinoma patients was the interpretation of the Michigan study previously cited[10] as well as autopsy data[12,14] regarding incidence of distant metastatic sites of squamous and nonsquamous cancers, and finally the differences in prognostic significance of lymph node metastasis in squamous versus nonsquamous cancer. Between 1978 and early 1985, 190 patients fulfilled eligibility requirements and were randomly assigned treatment with radiotherapy or no adjuvant treatment. Stratification for weight loss, stage (II or III), and participating institution ensured balanced randomization for these factors. Two-thirds of the patients had stage II disease. At a mean of 3.5 years after randomization, no difference in survival could be found between the irradiated group of 102 patients and the control group of 108 patients. The biologic effect of radiation therapy was appreciated, however. Only 1 out of the 24 patients in whom the first site of recurrence was purely local was in the irradiated group. Systemic recurrence rates were 97 percent in the treatment arm and 59 percent in the control arm. Twenty-two percent of the deaths have been due to causes other than cancer. The 5-year survival projection for the entire group is about 40 percent.

As we can see, the literature concerning adjuvant irradiation runs the gamut between beneficial effects for squamous cell carcinoma,[10] adenocarcinoma,[3] and both histologies,[5] a detrimental effect,[26] and no survival difference.[13] The LCSG trial is the most carefully done randomized prospective trial and has made the definitive statement so far.[13] It has been pointed out that since lung cancer is most often a systemic disease, the efficacy of radiation therapy should be measured by other means than survival.[23] Both prospective trials have shown the local benefit of adjuvant radiotherapy. Of the first recurrences in the LCSG trials, 75 percent were systemic, 97 percent in the treatment arm and 60 percent in the control arm, which are nearly identical to the findings of the European randomized trial.[26]

ADJUVANT CHEMOTHERAPY

Since systemic metastasis is the major problem in lung cancer, at least in terms of limiting the effectiveness of local treatments, systemic treatment is a logical choice for adjuvant therapy. Adjuvant chemotherapy after pulmonary resection for lung cancer is by no means a novel idea. The Veterans Administration Surgical Adjuvant Group began a series of prospective randomized control adjuvant chemotherapy trials almost 30 years ago.[27] A summary report of the VA adjuvant experience in over 3700 lung cancer patients shows no benefit of adjuvant chemotherapy.[7] Four trials were conducted over a 20-year period, testing the single agents nitrogen mustard and cyclophosphamide, and then the combinations of cyclophosphamide–methotrexate and CCNU-hydroxyurea. The survival of these patients according to stage and histology has been listed in Tables 13-3 and 13-4. A Swiss study using cyclophosphamide adjuvant to "radical resection" of lung cancer showed a detrimental effect of chemotherapy in the 95 treated patients compared to 95 controls.[2] Forty percent of each group had negative lymph nodes. The AJCC staging system was not used in this study, and it is not known how many patients had stage II disease. The Working Party on Lung Cancer adjuvant trial tested CCNU in a prospective randomized trial of 72 surgically staged stage I and II patients between 1973 and 1976.[21] No advantage was observed for CCNU treatment. Twenty-six percent of the patients had stage II disease.

It is not surprising that adjuvant therapy with the chemotherapy regimens utilized in the studies mentioned above was not effective, since the drugs involved are not very active against NSCLC.[11] Combinations, especially those containing adriamycin, platinum, or both, were found to cause a response rate of 30-40 percent in a large number of series throughout the 1970s,[11] and the chance of observing a benefit in the adjuvant situation would be higher employing one of these combination regimens.

The literature contains only one stage II adjuvant chemotherapy series.[4] This series consists of 34 patients, 5 of whom have $T_1N_1M_0$ disease. The patients were treated with various combinations of surgery, radiation therapy, and the cytoxan, adriamycin, methotrexate, and procarbazine (CAMP) chemotherapy regimen in uncontrolled fashion. It is difficult to interpret the significance of this study, although the study concludes that chemotherapy is advantageous. The Lung Cancer Study Group has conducted a trial of adjuvant cytoxan, adriamycin, and platinum (CAP) for stages II and III completely resected nonsquamous lung cancer.[8] This trial (LCSG No. 772) began in 1978 in parallel to the LCSG adjuvant irradiation trial for squamous carcinoma described above. Adjuvant chemotherapy was felt to be more appropriate for nonsquamous histology because of its worse prognosis but its higher response rate to combination chemotherapy in comparison to squamous cancer. Stages II and III were combined in this trial because of their similar survival rates (Tables 13-3 and 13-4) and because the relative infrequency of pathologic stage II lung cancer would prohibit prospective randomized trial for this stage alone. The CAP regimen was chosen as a representative combination regimen using the most modern chemotherapeutic agents available at the time. The equivalence of CAP to other active combination regimens has subsequently been demonstrated by large prospective randomized trial in advanced disease.[24] Eligibility requirements, staging protocol, and stratifications were the same for the CAP study as for the radiotherapy study, except for histology. Between 1978 and 1984, 130 eligible patients were randomized to receive either 6 monthly cycles of CAP chemotherapy or immediate postoperative intrapleural BCG.[8] At the time when the study was designed, it was felt that adjuvant BCG had shown some evidence of benefit in lung cancer,[15,16] and most members of the LCSG were hesitant to allow a no-treatment control arm for patients with such a poor prognosis. An additional LCSG study (No. 771) has shown subsequently that intrapleural BCG does not confer survival benefit in stage I resected lung cancer,[20] and thus the CAP versus BCG trial can be viewed as a chemotherapy versus no treatment trial. At a mean of 4 years after randomization, an advantage in median survival of about 8 months has been observed for the chemotherapy arm. A similar difference in relapse-free survival has occurred. These differences are significant, log rank $p = 0.013$ for survival and 0.018 for recurrence when the respective life table curves are compared. The 2-year survival of the BCG arm is 30 percent and the projected 5-year survival is 15 percent, which is consistent with survival figures for untreated historical controls (Tables 13-2 and 13-4). Eighty-three percent of initial recurrences have been extrathoracic in both CAP and BCG arms.

SUMMARY

As the review presented in this chapter has indicated, there are no controlled studies concerning adjuvant treatment of stage II lung cancer alone. This is due to the relative infrequency of this stage. However, the Lung Cancer Study Group has completed two trials that include stages II and III disease together. Although this has been done because of expediency, the survival curves for resected lung cancer patients support this behavior. This review of the data concerning adjuvant radiation therapy for squamous cell lung cancer concludes that there is no indication for routine postoperative irradiation for squamous cell lung cancer patients after complete resection of the disease regardless of stage (II vs III). If no benefit can be established for squamous disease, a benefit for nonsquamous disease would be extremely unlikely, given the pattern of first recurrence for these histologies.[8,13] Adjuvant chemotherapy with a regimen containing platinum and adriamycin has delayed relapse and prolonged survival for nonsquamous patients,[8] but the magnitude of benefit is marginal from a clinical standpoint. It remains to be determined whether the same benefit can be realized for squamous cell carcinoma with adjuvant chemotherapy. An LCSG study is in progress to answer this question. Clearly, the efficacy of adjuvant chemotherapy depends on the antitumor activity of the drug or drugs chosen. The major problem in lung cancer treatment has been the lack of effective systemic treatment,[11] and until this problem is solved, adjuvant treatment of lung cancer will have limited success.

The proposed new international staging system for lung cancer is an international agreement endorsed by the American Joint Committee.[17] The new system expands to four stages, defines subsets within the current stage III, and alters the definitions of stages I and II to include $T_1N_1M_0$ in stage II rather than I. If this system is accepted by the oncologic community, the existing literature will have to be interpreted accordingly and care will have to be taken in designing future clinical trials to build on the experiences already achieved within the framework of the new staging system.

REFERENCES

1. American Joint Committee on Cancer: Manual for Staging of Cancer, 2d ed. Philadelphia, Lippincott, 1983, pp 99-105

2. Brunner KW, Marthaler T, Muller W: Adjuvant chemotherapy with cyclophosphamide (NSC-26271) for radically resected bronghogenic carcinoma: 9-year follow-up. Progr Cancer Res Ther 11:411-420, 1979

3. Choi NCH, Grillo HC, Cardiello M, et al: Basis for new strategies in postoperative radiotherapy of bronchogenic carcinoma. Internatl J Radiat Oncol Biol Phys 6:31-35, 1980

4. Ferguston MK, Little AG, Golomb HM, et al: The role of adjuvant therapy after resection of $T_1N_1M_0$ and $T_2N_1M_0$ non-small cell lung cancer. J Thorac Cardiovasc Surg 91:344-349, 1986

5. Green N, Kurohara SS, George FW, et al: Postresection irradiation for primary lung cancer. Radiology 116:405-407, 1975

6. Higgins GA, Beebe GW: Bronchogenic carcinoma: Factors in survival. Arch Surg 94:539-549, 1967

7. Higgins GA, Shields TW: Experience of the Veterans Administration Surgical Adjuvant Group. Progr Cancer Res Ther 11:433-442, 1979

8. Holmes EC, Gail M, The Lung Cancer Study Group: Surgical adjuvant therapy for stage II and stage III adenocarcinoma and large-cell undifferentiated carcinoma. J Clin Oncol 4:710-715, 1986

9. Kemeny MM, Block LR, Brain DW, et al: Results of surgical treatment of carcinoma of the lung by stage and cell type. Surg Gynecol Obstet 147:865-871, 1978

10. Kirsh MM, Rotman H, Argentaly, et al: Carcinoma of the lung: results of treatment over 10 years. Ann Thorac Surg 21:371-377, 1976

11. Lad TE, McGuire WP: Chemotherapy for non-small cell lung cancer, in Aisner J (ed): Lung Cancer. New York, Churchill-Livingstone, 1985, pp 155-182

12. Line DH, Deeley TJ: The necropsy findings in carcinoma of the bronchus. Br J Dis Chest 65:238-242, 1971

13. The Lung Cancer Study Group: Effects of postoperative mediastinal radiation on completely resected stage II and stage III epidermoid cancer of the lung. N Engl J Med 315:1377-1381, 1986

14. Matthews MJ, Kanhouwass, Pickren J, et al: Frequency of residual and metastatic tumor in patients undergoing curative surgical resection for lung cancer. Cancer Chemother Rep 4:63-67, 1973

15. McGuire WP, for the Lung Cancer Study Group: Clinical trials of the Lung Cancer Study Group, in Jones SE, Salmon S (eds): Adjuvant Therapy of Cancer II. Orlando, FL, Grune & Stratton, 1979, pp 561-569

16. McKneally M, Mauer C, Lininger L, et al: Four year follow-up of the Albany experience with intrapleural BCG in lung cancer. J Thorac Cardiovasc Surg 81:485-492, 1981

17. Mountain CF: A new international staging system for lung cancer. Chest 89:225S-233S, 1986

18. Mountain CF: Assessment of the role of surgery for control of lung cancer. Ann Thorac Surg 24:365-373, 1977

19. Mountain CF, Carr DT, Anderson WAD: A system for the clinical staging of lung cancer. Am J Roentgenol Radiat Ther Nucl Med 120:130-138, 1974

20. Mountain CF, Gail MN, for the Lung Cancer Study Group: Surgical adjuvant BCG treatment for stage I non-small cell lung cancer. J Thorac Cardiovasc Surg 82:649–657, 1981

21. Mountain CF, Vincent RG, Sealy R, et al: A clinical trial of CCNU as surgical adjuvant treatment for patients with surgical stage I and stage II non-small cell lung cancer: Preliminary findings. Progr Cancer Res Ther 11:421–431, 1979

22. Muggia FM, McGuire WP: Adjuvant systemic therapy of lung cancer. Cancer Clin Trials 1:235–241, 1978

23. Perez CA: Radiation therapy in the management of carcinoma of the lung. Cancer 39:901–916, 1977

24. Ruckdeschel JC, Finkelstein DM, Mason BA, et al: Chemotherapy for metastatic non-small cell bronchogenic carcinoma: EST 2575, generation V—a randomized comparison of four cis-platin-containing regimens. J Clin Oncol 3:72–79, 1985

25. Shields TW, Yee J, Conn JH, et al: Relationship of cell type and lymph node metastasis to survival after resection of bronchial carcinoma. Ann Thorac Surg 20:501–510, 1975

26. Van Houtte PR, Rocmans P, Smets P, et al: Postoperative radiation therapy in lung cancer: A controlled trial after resection of curative design. Internatl J Radiat Oncol Biol Phys 6:983–906, 1980

27. Veterans Administration Surgical Adjuvant Cancer Chemotherapy Group: Evaluation of chemotherapeutic agents as adjuvant to surgery in 22 Veterans Administration hospitals: Experimental design. Cancer Chemother Rep 20:81–87, 1962

28. Vincent RG, Takita H, Lane WW, et al: Surgical therapy of lung cancer. J Thorac Cardiovasc Surg 71:581–591, 1976

PART IV

Stage III$_{M_0}$ Non-Small Cell Lung Cancer

Douglas J. Mathisen
Hermes C. Grillo

14

Management of T_3N_0–T_3N_1 Non-Small Cell Carcinoma of the Lung

The American Joint Committee for cancer staging[2] defines a T_3 tumor as "a tumor of any size with direct extension into an adjacent structure such as the parietal pleura or chest wall, the diaphragm, or the mediastinum and its contents; or a tumor demonstrable bronchoscopically to involve a main bronchus less than 2.0 centimeters distal to the carina; or any tumor associated with atelectasis or obstructive pneumonitis of an entire lung or pleural effusion."* Under the current staging system, T_3 lesions are considered to be stage III. It is clear from many reports that certain T_3 tumors have a more favorable prognosis than others.[6,8,11,17,21,24,40,43,47] It is imperative, therefore, that everyone dealing with lung cancer understand this and not condemn patients with T_3 tumors as being surgically incurable.

Patients with T_3 lesions must be carefully evaluated for metastatic disease and from a functional standpoint. Surgery remains the optimal treatment for appropriate patients but may carry greater risk because of the more extensive resection required to extirpate these tumors.[11,14,20,27,44] Because of these increased risks, one must be certain that there is no evidence of metastatic disease (stage III M_1). It is unwise to subject these patients to the risks of surgery only to find at a later date that the patient was harboring occult metastatic disease. It is justified in this group of patients to examine the brain, bones, liver, adrenals, and mediastinal nodes for the presence of metastases. We have used postinfusion brain computerized axial tomography (CAT) to detect brain metastases and bone scans to detect bone metastases. Chest and upper abdominal CAT scanning is used to evaluate the mediastinal nodes, adrenals, and liver and to search for visceral invasion. We routinely perform mediastinoscopy even in the presence of a negative CT scan because of the false-negative rate[9,16] and the implications of N_2 disease in this group of patients.[21,41,42,44] Mediastinoscopy should be carried out prior to any adjuvant therapy in order not to obscure the presence of N_2

---

*Reprinted from Anderson WAD, Carr DT: Clinical staging system for carcinoma of the lung. American Joint Committee for Cancer Staging and End-Results Reporting, Chicago, 1979. With permission.

disease by preoperative radiation or chemotherapy. Open biopsy or needle biopsy should be performed to rule out the possibility of metastatic disease when abnormalities are discovered on scans. The goal of surgery in the management of lung cancer should be primarily curative rather than palliative, especially in advanced stages, where operative risks are greater.

Surgery for T_3 tumors may be extensive and lengthy. The functional status of each patient should be precisely assessed to determine tolerance for the planned surgical procedure. In addition to assessment of the overall medical condition, pulmonary function tests (PFT) and quantitative ventilation/perfusion (V/Q) lung scan are extremely helpful to determine the patient's ability to tolerate the proposed pulmonary resection. The use of PFTs and V/Q scans to estimate the postoperative FEV_1 is invaluable.[58] We rarely have found it necessary to do more extensive testing.

Bronchoscopy by the operating surgeon is mandatory for assessment of endobronchial disease, even if done previously; endoscopic evaluation allows the surgeon to determine whether a bronchoplastic procedure will be required. It also permits the surgeon to put the results of preoperative functional testing into better perspective. Bronchoscopy with biopsies to determine extent of tumor should be done prior to preoperative treatment.

The surgeon and anesthesiologist should be well versed in airway management and techniques of bronchoplastic repair for tumors involving the proximal mainstem bronchi or carina. One should not deny or compromise a patient's chance of cure by performing lesser procedures. Bronchoplastic procedures can be performed safely with an excellent chance for cure in many cases.[4,11,20,27,43,54]

CHEST WALL INVASION

Direct invasion of the chest wall by lung cancer is amenable to surgical therapy. Approximately 8 percent of patients undergoing resection for carcinoma of the lung at the Massachusetts General Hospital have involvement of the chest wall.[21] Suspicion of chest wall involvement is based on the location of a peripheral lesion on x-ray, complaints of pain localized to the area of suspected involvement, a bone scan positive in the suspected area, or a CT scan suggestive of chest wall involvement. Patients' complaints probably are the most reliable indication of chest wall involvement since invasion between the ribs may lead to a negative bone scan or CT scan may fail to demonstrate frank invasion.

Extensive resection of a portion of the chest wall allows paradoxic motion unless prosthetic replacement is utilized. Patients undergoing chest wall resection experience increased pain and may require measures beyond the standard use of narcotics. Epidural narcotics have been helpful in the management of severe postoperative pain. Chest wall resection may render PFTs and V/Q scans less predictable in determining which patients can tolerate pulmonary resections. Marginal patients should be carefully scrutinized. Chest wall stabilization for these few patients is mandatory.

The histologic type of carcinoma that involves the chest wall has been predominantly squamous cell in most series. The combined cases from the Massachusetts General Hospital, Mayo Clinic, Toronto General Hospital, and Memorial Hospital for Cancer and Allied Diseases show the following distribution: squamous cell, 63 percent; adenocarcinoma, 20 percent; and large cell, 17 percent.[21] Rare cases with alveolar cell or small cell carcinoma are reported.

Survival is related to the presence or absence of positive mediastinal lymph nodes and not the presence of chest wall invasion. Mediastinoscopy is thus invaluable in assessing operability. The presence of positive nodes precludes surgical intervention in most patients. Grillo[21] and Patterson[40] reported no 5-year survivors with positive N_2 nodes. Piehler et al. found only 7 percent 5-year survival in patients with N_1-N_2 disease as compared to 54 percent of patients with N_0 disease.[44] Mishina et al. noted only 1 out of 10 patients with positive nodes as a 5-year survivor.[37]

There is controversy regarding the role of preoperative radiation therapy in patients with suspected chest wall invasion.[40,44] Proponents argue that it may limit the extent of resection required and lessen the incidence of local recurrence. Opponents argue that the amount of chest wall spared is small, damage to unresected lung complicates the postoperative course, and local recurrence can be controlled by postoperative radiation therapy. We have often used preoperative radiation therapy when chest wall invasion is suspected. This is especially true with large, posterior tumors where resection margins may be close. We have given 3500 rads over a 3-4 week-period and then waited about 3 weeks before surgery.

Knowledge of chest wall involvement preoperatively is important in planning the incision and where to enter the chest, especially when prosthetic replacement of the chest wall is anticipated. The cutaneous incision should be remote from the area of involvement so that the prosthetic material does not lie directly beneath the incision. Entering the chest at a site remote from the chest wall involvement will lessen the risk of tumor spillage and allow the surgeon to assess the extent of involvement.

Invasion of the parietal pleura necessitates removal of chest wall in most cases. Extrapleural dissection alone has been associated with a high incidence of local recurrence.[44] We feel that segments of ribs above and below actual invasion should be taken with approximately 3-4 cm margins away from the gross limits of the tumor. It is often easier to do the chest wall resection initially and then proceed with the pulmonary resection.

The majority of chest wall resections can be done without need for prosthetic replacements. Functional and cosmetic consideration should be given to each patient. The risk of infection should be balanced against the potential benefits of prosthetic replacement. Resection of a portion of three or fewer ribs posteriorly rarely requires prosthetic replacement as the scapula lessens the cosmetic and functional impact of the chest wall resection. Resection of larger portions of chest wall, especially anteriorly or laterally, may require a prosthetic substitute for the chest wall to provide stability and improve cosmetics.

We have utilized methylmethacrylate between two layers of Marlex as described by Eschapasse[15] and McCormack.[34] A tracing of the defect is made on paper and then drawn on the Marlex. The methylmethacrylate is spread onto the Marlex to cover an area slightly smaller than what has been drawn to prevent overriding or bulging of the prosthesis. A second piece of Marlex is placed on top of the methacrylate. The exact contour desired can be obtained by molding a sheet of malleable lead and adding the methacrylate to the Marlex placed over the lead. Approximately 2 cm of excess Marlex should be left as a sewing ring to secure the prosthesis to the chest wall. Absolute sterility is required when using a chest wall substitute. Both pre- and postoperative antibiotics should be used. Air leaks should be kept to a minimum by covering the raw surface of lung with a pleural tent if necessary. The results of chest wall reconstruction using this technique have been very good.

The survival of patients undergoing chest wall resection has ranged from 15 to 38 percent (Table 14-1). The presence of positive nodes has been the most important determinant of long-term survival.[6-8,17,18,21,23,37,40,44,45,47] Gronquist et al.[23] and Mishina et al.[37] both expressed the belief that depth of invasion of the chest wall by carcinoma was an indication of prognosis. Invasion of the pleura only was more favorable than invasion into the intercostal muscles, while invasion into the ribs gave the worst prognosis. These observations must be corrected for the histologic character of the tumor and for the extent of nodal spread. At present, there do not seem to be enough cases recorded in detail to provide unequivocal information. Most authors agree that if the parietal pleura is involved, full thickness chest wall resection provides the best chance for cure. Patterson and colleagues made the interesting observation that resection can be done in discontinuous fashion with good results.[40] Three of their six patients who underwent discontinuous resection of the chest wall were alive in follow-up. Trastek et al. compared 14 patients who had $T_3N_0M_0$ lung cancers that invaded parietal pleura and who underwent extrapleural resection similar to eight patients from a previous study who had chest wall resection for parietal pleural invasion.[55] Survival at 5 years was greater in patients who underwent chest wall resection (75 percent vs. 27.9 percent), although the difference was of only borderline significance ($p = .057$). This suggests that chest wall resection may be a more adequate method of treatment than extrapleural dissection when parietal pleura is invaded.

The value of radiation therapy remains controversial. All reports of results of chest wall resection have been retrospective; therefore, it is difficult to discern the benefit of radiation therapy. Patterson reported on five patients with preoperative radiation therapy and 8 with postoperative irradiation.[40] The radiation doses ranged from 2000 to 5000 rads. Another 22 patients in this series had no irradiation. The 5-

Table 14-1
Long-Term Survival After Resection of
Carcinoma of Lung with Chest Wall
Involvement (Survival 3-5 Years)

Year	Number of Cases	Long-Term Survival (%)	Reference
1947	5	—	7
1957	12	0	18
1957	16	25	23
1959	38	20	47
1966	19	16	22
1967	41	35	17
1968	27	10	45
1974	30	23	6
1978	43	19	37
1979	43	10	26
1979	19	21	8
1982	35	38	40
1982	66	33	44

year survival of unirradiated patients was 30 percent, while that of the 13 irradiated patients was 56 percent. Piehler et al. reported that 16 out of 66 patients underwent postoperative irradiation.[44] These patients had a 53 percent 5-year survival, in comparison with 54 percent for those without irradiation. These two studies express the lack of uniformity of opinion regarding the value of radiotherapy either pre- or postoperatively. Clarification awaits the results of a randomized prospective study. We add postoperative irradiation for positive mediastinal nodes or if the surgical margins are positive.

SUPERIOR SULCUS TUMORS

A high index of suspicion is necessary in order to detect these lesions in an early state. The typical complaints of arm and shoulder pain with a lack of pulmonary symptoms often direct these patients to an orthopedist or neurosurgeon. Pain is initially localized to the shoulder and the vertebral border of the scapula. As the tumor involves the brachial plexus, symptoms develop in the distribution of the T_1 nerve root (ulnar distribution of the arm to the elbow) and the C_8 nerve root (ulnar surface of the forearm and small and ring fingers). Involvement of the stellate ganglion and sympathetic chain leads to Horner's syndrome.

Diagnosis is made by history and the presence of a shadow at the extreme apex of the chest x-ray. Histologic confirmation is mandatory. Sputum cytology and bronchoscopy are positive less frequently than in more centrally placed tumors.[42] Open biopsy as described by McGoon[35] rarely should be necessary now with needle biopsy techniques, which have proved to be very reliable. In our series of superior sulcus tumors, needle biopsy has been positive in 19 out of 20 cases. The need to establish a diagnosis preoperatively is important since preoperative radiation therapy may make histologic interpretation difficult.

Since these tumors may involve the upper ribs and vertebral bodies, bone scans are extremely helpful. Valuable information can be obtained from CT scans as to extent of vertebral body involvement or the likelihood of vascular invasion when contrast material is given. Caution should be exercised in diagnosing vertebral body involvement. Unless invasion through the cortex of the vertebral body is seen, patients should not be deemed inoperable on the basis of minor deformity of the vertebral body. The tumor may abut the vertebral body without invading it. Nuclear magnetic resonance offers additional capabilities in defining the extent of tumor invasion. It is especially helpful in defining invasion of the neural foramen; spinal cord, or subclavian artery.

Positive mediastinal nodes may be found in as many as 25 percent of patients. In Paulson's series, no patients survived beyond 1 to 2 years when hilar or mediastinal nodes were involved.[42] This underscores the need for mediastinoscopy following initial diagnosis prior to preoperative radiation therapy. Presence of positive nodes remains the worst prognostic factor, followed by vascular invasion and extensive vertebral body invasion. Rib involvement and involvement of the lowest limb of the brachial plexus are not contraindications to surgery. Shahian and co-workers suggest that even positive nodes may be associated with prolonged survival in highly selected cases when completion radiotherapy is given postoperatively.[46]

Superior sulcus tumors were initially considered inoperable and were treated by radiation therapy. Results were often disappointing from a palliative or curative stand-point. Chardack and MacCallum reported the first 5-year survival following complete en bloc resection of a superior sulcus tumor followed by radiation therapy.[42] It remained for Shaw and Paulson to demonstrate prolonged survival using preoperative radiation therapy followed by en bloc resection.[47] Their results have been confirmed by others.[3,36,42] When such an approach is employed, a 30–35 percent 5-year survival can be anticipated. Additional radiation therapy postoperatively may allow survival even in the presence of positive nodes or incomplete resection of all gross disease in highly selected patients.[46]

We stage these patients carefully at initial presentation. Precise functional assessment is made to determine their ability to withstand the planned resection. Presence of positive mediastinal nodes at mediastinoscopy or extensive invasion of a vertebral body generally precludes surgery. In such patients, we rely on primary irradiation (see Chapter 16). Recent reports suggest improved results with primary irradiation for palliation and even cure in some cases.[1,12,29,56] Van Houtte et al. report symptomatic relief in 21 out of 23 patients although median duration of palliation was only 11 months.[56] They reported four long-term survivors. These were in patients without rib involvement, which raises the question as to whether these were true superior sulcus tumors.

If evaluation indicates potential curability, 3500 rads are given over 3 to 4 weeks. Patients are allowed to recover for approximately 3 weeks and are then restaged. If no signs of metastatic disease is found, we proceed with surgery. Our surgical approach is essentially that described by Paulson.[42] An extended posterolateral thoractomy is used, carrying the incision cephalad toward the base of the neck halfway between the scapula and spine. This allows for mobilization of the shoulder to gain access to the first rib and structures at the thoracic inlet. The ribs are detached posteriorly by exposing the transverse process and dividing it. This allows access to the first rib, where it articulates with the vertebral body. Great care is needed in dividing the neurovascular bundles at this level. If they are not adequately secured, the vessels may retract. Bleeding should be controlled by ligation and not packing since this may lead to hemorrhage into the spinal canal, causing cord compression and possible serious neurologic sequelae. Involvement of the vertebral bodies often is the last thing to be determined. Portions of the vertebral body may be removed, but prudence is advisable. There are few documented cases of 5-year survivors following partial excision of vertebral bodies for direct tumor invasion.[42] Lobectomy, segmentectomy, or even wedge resection of the lung may be used. Procedures lesser than lobectomy require careful intraoperative sampling of hilar and mediastinal nodes that may not have been studied preoperatively.

These patients require diligent postoperative care. Because of previous smoking history, preoperative radiation, extent of surgery, some chest wall instability, and pain, many patients have a problem with sputum retention. Pain control, chest physiotherapy, and bedside fiberoptic bronchoscopy are invaluable in management.

For residual disease, we have not utilized afterloading catheters or radioactive seeds as described by others.[24,46] We have given additional external beam radiotherapy. Our general policy has been to employ additional radiotherapy if nodes or margins were positive. Routine postoperative radiotherapy has not been employed because of the potential for long-term brachial plexus injury from high-dose radiotherapy.

INVOLVEMENT OF THE MAIN-STEM BRONCHUS WITHIN 2 CM OF THE CARINA

Until recently, cancers that involved the main-stem bronchi within 2 cm of the carina were considered inoperable and were treated primarily by radiation. As techniques of sleeve resection of the airway have become better understood and more widespread, surgeons have reconsidered this challenging group of patients. Although no one institution has accumulated a large experience[11,14,20,27,43,60] operative mortality has generally been high, ranging from 8.3 to 30 percent (see Table 14-2).

Because of the high operative mortality, one must carefully evaluate each patient. Each should be screened for any sign of metastatic disease. Radiologic evaluation to determine the extent of the lesion is mandatory. We have utilized CT scanning, tomograms of the carina, and barium swallows to determine the extent of disease and involvement with adjacent structures. Complete functional assessment is essential. Mediastinoscopy should be done to document the status of mediastinal nodes. Mediastinoscopy is best performed at the time of resection. The fibrosis and inflammation that follow mediastinoscopy will make assessment of the degree of tumor involvement and the technical aspects of reconstruction more difficult if this is separated in time from the resection and reconstruction. Involvement of mediastinal nodes in most cases makes resection unwise.

In patients who are deemed inoperable or in patients who will undergo resection, it may be necessary to re-establish a patent airway. The use of a rigid bronchoscope to "core out" the tumor has been very effective in our hands. The combination of biopsy forceps and use of the tip of the bronchoscope to morcellate the tumor has been successful in opening up the airway with minimal bleeding in most cases. More recently, there have been many enthusiasts for the use of the laser to achieve this goal. The laser is believed to lessen the risk of bleeding. The use of the laser, however, is often tedious and time-consuming and requires multiple procedures in order to open up obstructed airways. We feel that the added expense, the risk of multiple anesthesias, and the inability to achieve a patent airway in some cases at the first examination makes the use of a laser less desirable than the more conventional endoscopic means of removing obstructing tumor. In our hands there have been few complications and no deaths, and bleeding has been at a minimum. Providing a satisfactory airway at the beginning of an operative procedure facilitates the anesthetic management.

Problems of carinal resections have been classified into three categories: (1) technical considerations, (2) intraoperative anesthetic management of the airway, and (3) postoperative care. Each of these can present formidable challenges. The surgeon

Table 14-2
Mortality and Survival for Carcinal Resections

Mortality (%)	Patients (No.)	Survival (%)	Reference
27	26	23	11
17	18	—*	14
8.3	12	—*	20
29	34	15	27
31	29	—*	43
10.4	29	3.9	60

*Survival figures unavailable

and anesthesiologist duo must be well versed in the techniques of reconstruction and the methods of airway management necessary to successfully complete the surgery undertaken. Lack of experience of either part of the duo may lead to catastrophic complications and death of the patient.

At the time of surgery, bronchoscopic measurements are made to determine the extent of airway involvement. Three specific anatomic locations of tumor can be considered for surgical resection: (1) tumor originating in the right upper lobe and extending proximally to the level of the carina, sparing the bronchus intermedius; (2) tumor involving the entire right lung and carina; and (3) tumor of the left upper lobe involving the left main-stem bronchus extending to the carina. All are potentially resectable. The right side is more commonly involved.

Anesthetic management in these lesions is complicated. Double lumen tubes are not preferable in these circumstances. High-frequency ventilation catheters passed from the oral endotracheal tube into a main-stem bronchus provides one method of ventilation during this type of surgery. We usually have elected to use an extra long endotracheal tube with a flexible tip to start the operative procedure and then intubate across the operative field into the opposite main-stem bronchus once the carina has been divided. This allows for complete collapse of the lung to be resected and ventilation of the other lung. The endotracheal tube can then be removed periodically to place sutures as necessary. At the end of the procedure, the extra-long oral endotracheal tube is advanced into the main-stem bronchus as the sutures are tied. Other publications describe specific details of these techniques of airway management.[59]

The surgical reconstructive possibilities of right-sided cancers depend on the extent of involvement of the bronchus intermedius in these lesions. A right posterolateral thoracotomy is the best approach. When the tumor also involves the bronchus intermedius, a "sleeve right pneumonectomy" usually is all that is feasible. The airway is reconstructed by approximating the distal trachea to the left main-stem bronchus. When the bronchus intermedius has been spared, reconstruction can be accomplished by approximating the distal trachea to the proximal left main-stem bronchus and then reimplanting the bronchus intermedius into the side of the proximal trachea. This requires division of the inferior pulmonary ligament and pericardial attachments of the hilar structures to allow enough mobility of the bronchus intermedius to reach the side of the trachea. On occasion the lower lobe bronchus may be implanted into the side of the left main bronchus. The anastomosis is accomplished by using an elliptical incision in the cartilaginous portion of the trachea approximately 1 cm proximal to tracheal suture line. This will help to stabilize the anastomosis and keep it patent. We have utilized an interrupted technique with 4-0 Vicryl sutures for anastomosis. At the completion of the anastomosis, a pleural flap is designed to wrap around each suture line. This lessens the risk of air leak, separation, and separates the bronchial anastomosis from the pulmonary artery, thus lessening the likelihood of bronchopulmonary artery fistula.

Tumors extending from the left upper lobe to involve the left main-stem bronchus and carina are very rare but may present a most challenging situation. These lesions can be approached through a left posterolateral thoracotomy if there is minimal involvement of the carina. The distal trachea can be reapproximated to the proximal right main-stem bronchus after mobilization of the aortic arch. Others have described transection of the proximal left main-stem bronchus, presumably through tumor, and then at a later date, through a right thoracotomy excising the carina.[19] We have not employed this approach because of concern about cutting through tumor. When it does not seem feasible to approach tumors through a left thoracotomy because of extensive involvement of the carina, we have employed a right thoracotomy approach. The carina is resected, and the trachea is then reattached to the right mainstem bronchus as previously described. The thoracotomy is then carried across the sternum and a left pneumonectomy carried out. Others have described a similar approach dividing the bronchus and removing the left lung at a later date.[43] We have employed this technique in only one patient for benign disease and were forced to remove the left lung because of excessive shunting through the atelectatic lung. We do not advise this for malignant neoplasms. The transternal bilateral thoracotomy approach is very demanding of the patient. This should be reserved for only the fittest of patients. Postoperative ventilation usually is required.

Close attention is needed postoperatively. Mechanical ventilation should be avoided when possible. Whenever mechanical ventilation is required, the endotracheal tube should be positioned above the anastomosis, checked bronchoscopically, and the ventilatory pressures kept as low as feasible. The flexible bronchoscope is invaluable in clearing secretions. Perioperative fluid management is critical in these patients. Peters had identified postpneumonectomy pulmonary edema secondary to fluid overload.[62] Peters attributes this, among other things, to excessive fluid administration and an inability of the single lung to clear it. He argues for restriction of fluids during the operation and in the postoperative period. Patients undergoing carinal resection with division of additional lymphatics may be even more susceptible to this problem. Two patients in our series died from such problems. Consequently we monitor the amount of fluid given intraoperatively and postoperatively.

The greatest challenge facing the surgeon in dealing with lung cancer involving the carina has been the operative mortality. As familiarity with the procedure and its many complexities increases, the operative mortality should decrease. Jensik et al.[27] Deslauriers,[11] Eschapasse,[14] and Wu[60] have reported operative mortality of 29, 27, 17, and 10.4 percent, respectively. Deslauriers's operative mortality has fallen to 12.5 percent in his last 16 patients over the past 5 years. We have had one operative death in 12 patients undergoing carinal resection for lung cancer and a 12 percent operative mortality in 50 carinal resections for all indications.

We are concerned that preoperative radiation therapy may interfere with healing in these patients and rarely use it. We reserve its use postoperatively for patients with positive nodes or margins. Prior to initiation of radiotherapy, we advise bronchoscopy to ensure adequate healing. Jensik et al. express less concern about preoperative radiotherapy and in fact utilized between 3200 and 5000 rads in 28 out of 34 patients undergoing sleeve pneumonectomy.[27]

Long-term survival is possible in these patients. Jensik[27] and Deslauriers[11] respectively report 15 and 23 percent 5-year survival in their series. Careful patient selection, attention to technical detail, and precise postoperative care should allow this aggressive approach to be utilized with the expectation of prolonged survival in many patients.

INVASION OF EXTRAPULMONARY INTRATHORACIC STRUCTURES

Results of surgery for invasion of structures other than the chest wall are difficult to find. Reports in many cases are anecdotal, and therefore treatment must be individualized. The reports suggest that good results are achievable when lung cancer invades structures other than the chest wall in highly selected patients. We feel that invasion of the recurrent laryngeal nerve especially on the right side is a contraindication to surgery. There have been very few expectations of this reported in the literature.

Pulmonary Artery

Invasion of the pulmonary artery may dictate intrapericardial pneumonectomy if the tumor extends to the main pulmonary artery. Involvement more distally in the pulmonary artery may lend itself to sleeve resection of the pulmonary artery. Centrally placed lesions should be suspected of involving the pulmonary artery. Ventilation perfusion studies may show diminished perfusion to the involved lung. Pulmonary arteriograms define the extent of involvement and therefore may detect unresectability.[31,33] Presence of at least 1.5 cm of uninvolved proximal main pulmonary artery should allow resection in most cases. When pulmonary artery involvement is found at surgery, the pericardium is opened to determine the extent of proximal involvement. Structures are not divided until one has determined that the artery, veins, and bronchus can all be safely divided.

Involvement of the pulmonary artery more peripherally by either direct extension of tumor or cancerous lymph nodes may be found at surgery. Toomes and Vogt Moykopf combined sleeve resections of the bronchus with sleeve resections of the pulmonary artery.[54] They have demonstrated that this can be safely performed with results that justify the procedure. The two suture lines should be separated by a pleural flap wrapping the bronchus. This will diminish the likelihood of delayed bronchopulmonary artery fistula.

Diaphragm

Local invasion occurs less commonly in the diaphragm than in other structures. Resection of the tumor with a portion of the diaphragm is justified if the patient's pulmonary function can tolerate this. In many cases, it is possible to preserve some function of the diaphragm by sparing the phrenic nerve. Reconstruction of the diaphragmatic defect often can be accomplished by suture repair. If the defect is too large, prosthetic materials, such as Dacron, Marlex, or Gortex patches, can be used. Anecdotal reports in the literature make it difficult to determine long-term survival results, but one would expect results to be similar to those of chest wall invasion.[51,55,57]

Pericardium and Phrenic Nerve

Invasion of the phrenic nerve at the level of the pericardium is a relative contraindication to surgery. Invasion of the phrenic nerve more proximally as it traverses the mediastinum seems to be an absolute contraindication to surgery. This usually implies invasion of the mediastinum. Lesions at the level of the pericardium in certain cases can be removed after intrapericardial assessment of the possibility of dividing pulmonary veins, pulmonary artery, and bronchus. It is possible to remove small cuffs of the left atrium in extended resections of this nature. Central lesions requiring this type of surgery carry a worse prognosis;[30] however, if resection is technically feasible, the results justify this aggressive approach in selected patients.[47,48]

Superior Vena Cava

Invasion of the superior vena cava may range from limited involvement to obstruction manifest as a severe superior vena cava syndrome. Presence of superior vena cava syndrome is a contraindication to pulmonary resection. Radiation therapy offers palliation and in some prolonged survival.[39] Invasion of the superior vena cava on a more limited extent, however, may lend itself to techniques of resection.[55,61] Introduction of the spiral vein graft as a method of reconstruction of the superior vena cava has provided a substitute for the superior vena cava that will remain patent.[13] In the course of resection, central venous pressure must be monitored to diminish the likelihood of cerebral edema. By-pass techniques are available to allow this to be accomplished safely.[13,60] Special heparin-bonded catheters may be used to shunt blood from the superior vena cava to the right atrium during the course of reconstruction. Experience with this type of resection is limited, and only anecdotal evidence has been reported. Therefore, it is impossible to draw conclusions about survival. If invasion of the vena cava is limited and the procedure can be accomplished safely, it would seem to be justified.

Pleural Effusion

Presence of a pleural effusion, whether positive or negative for malignant cells, qualifies a patient as having a T_3 lesion. The presence of a pleural effusion, whether positive for malignant cells or not, has not been associated with prolonged survival.[8,38] Positive malignant pleural fluid should contraindicate any type of surgical undertaking. Surgery is not necessarily contraindicated in patients with obstructive pneumonitis with an associated pleural effusion. Decker et al. reported 73 patients with cytologically negative pleural effusions.[10] In this group, 66 underwent exploration, with resection accomplished in only 4 (5.5 percent). The 4 patients with resectable tumors survived from 3 to 14 years. Lesions accompanied by bloody effusions were unresectable in 17 out of 18 patients. Despite these figures, surgical exploration in carefully selected patients is justifiable in the hope of long-term survival.

Nodal Involvement

All patients with advanced lung cancers considered for surgical resection should be evaluated for the presence of nodal metastases. In the presence of N_2 disease, only the most unusual situation should justify surgical resection as few reports show long-term survival from T_3N_2 tumors.[28,41,46,49,55,60] The goal of surgery for carcinoma of the lung should be for cure and only rarely for palliation. When N_2 disease is discovered at thoracotomy, the surgeon should proceed with a lobectomy or pneumonectomy and attempt to remove all nodal disease. Postoperative radiotherapy should be employed, as it may improve survival. It has been our practice to utilize postoperative radiotherapy when N_1 disease is discovered histologically in the resected specimen. Survival in the presence of nodal metastasis can be expected in certain patients, but they must be selected carefully.[46,55]

Future Prospects in Management

Aggressive surgical approaches to advanced carcinomas of the lung have their limitations. Careful patient selection is required in all cases. Improved surgical techniques, perioperative management, and postoperative care will continue to improve operative mortality figures in this difficult group of patients, but further success in long-term survival will require a multidisciplinary approach. Recent developments in chemotherapeutic management of lung cancer provides some hope that there may be effective agents.[5,25] Response rates of between 35 and 90 percent have been reported in recent series of non-small cell carcinoma of the lung (NSCLC). Preliminary studies of preoperative radiation and chemotherapy in advanced NSCLC have shown early encouraging results in some patients.[25,32,50,53] It will require careful integration of the best aspects of chemotherapy, radiation therapy, surgical therapy, and possibly immunotherapy[52] to improve the overall results in advanced stages of lung cancer.

EDITORIAL COMMENT

This chapter realistically portrays the appropriate role of surgery in these patients with locally advanced disease. Aggression should be used to identify patients with potentially resectable but locally invasive lung cancer, but prudence should be used to select for operation those in whom cure is truly possible and operative morbidity and mortality is not prohibitive.

In the newer AJC staging system, the lesions clearly amenable to resection are those with $T_3N_0M_0$ and $T_3N_1M_0$ cancers. Patients with T_4 primary tumors or N_3 nodal metastases clearly are not appropriate candidates for resection. A small question still remains regarding patients with T_3N_2 tumors, that is, those with metastases to ipsilateral mediastinal or subcarinal nodes. These patients may prove to have a sufficiently good prognosis to warrant multimodality treatment that includes surgery.

REFERENCES

1. Ampil FL: Radiotherapy for carcinomatous brachial plexopathy. Cancer 56:2185-2188, 1985
2. Anderson WAD, Carr DT: Clinical staging system for carcinoma of the lung. American Joint Committee for Cancer Staging and End-Results Reporting, Chicago, 1979
3. Attar S, Miller JE, Satterfield J, et al: Pancoast's tumor: Irradiation or Surgery? Ann Thorac Surg 28:578-585, 1979
4. Belli L, Meroni A, Rondinara G, et al: Bronchoplastic procedures and pulmonary artery reconstruction in the treatment of bronchogenic cancer. J Thorac Cardiovasc Surg 90:167-171, 1985
5. Bitran JD, Golomb HM, Albain K, et al: Chemotherapy of advanced lung (stage III$_{M1}$): A randomized trial comparing platinol (P) and vindesine (V) versus V. etoposide (E), P, versus cyclophosphamide, adriamycin, methotrexate, and procarbazine (CAMP). Invest New Drugs 2:13, 1984
6. Burnard RJ, Martini N, Beattie EJ Jr: The value of resection in tumor involving the chest wall. J Thorac Cardiovasc Surg 68:530-535, 1974
7. Coleman FP: Primary carcinoma of lung with invasion of ribs: Pneumonectomy and simultaneous block resection of chest wall. Ann Surg 126:156-158, 1947

8.   Cromartie RS III, Parker EF, May JE, et al: Carcinoma of the lung: A clinical review. Ann Thorac Surg 30:30–35, 1980

9.   Dale BDT, Faling LJ, Pugatch RD, et al: Computed tomography: An effective technique for mediastinal staging in lung cancer. Presented at the American Association for Thoracic Surgery, 64th Annual Meeting, May 7–9, 1984, New York

10. Decker DA, Dines DE, Payne WS, et al: The significance of a cytologically negative pleural effusion in bronchogenic carcinoma. Chest 74:640–642, 1978

11. Deslauriers J: Involvement of the main carina. Internat Trends Gen Thorac Surg 1:139–145, 1985

12. Devine JW, Mendenhall WM, Million RR, et al: Carcinoma of the superior pulmonary sulcus treated with surgery and/or radiation therapy. Cancer 57:941–943, 1986

13. Doty DB: Bypass of superior vena cava. J Thorac Cardiovasc Surg 83:326–338, 1982

14. Eschapasse H: Les tumeurs tracheales primitives: Traitement chirurgical. Rev Fr Mal Respir 2:425, 1974

15. Eschapasse H, Gaillard J, Henry F, et al: Repair of large chest wall defects. Ann Thorac Surg 31:45, 1981

16. Friedman PJ, Feigin DS, Liston SE, et al: Sensitivity of chest radiography, computed tomography, and gallium scanning to metastasis of lung carcinoma. Cancer 54:1300–1306, 1984

17. Geha AS, Bernmatz PE, Woolner LB: Bronchogenic carcinoma involving the thoracic wall: Surgical treatment and prognostic significance. J Thorac Cardiovasc Surg 54:394–402, 1967

18. Gibbon JH Jr, Templeton JY III, Nealon TF Jr: Factors which influence the long-term survival of patients with cancer of the lung. Ann Surg 145:637–641, 1957

19. Gilbert A, Deslauriers J, McClish A, et al: Tracheal sleeve pneumonectomy of carcinomas of the proximal left main bronchus. Can J Surg 27:583–585, 1984

20. Grillo HC: Carinal reconstruction. Ann Thorac Surg 34:356–373, 1982

21. Grillo HC: Pleural and chest wall involvement. Internatl Trends Gen Thorac Surg 1:134–138, 1985

22. Grillo HC, Greenberg JJ, Wilkins EW, Jr: Resection of bronchogenic carcinoma involving the thoracic wall. J Thorac Cardiovasc Surg 51:417–421, 1966

23. Gronqvist YKJ, Clagett OT, MacDonald JR: Involvement of thoracic wall in bronchogenic carcinoma: Study of 16 cases in which pneumonectomy or lobectomy and simultaneous resection of the thoracic wall were done. J Thorac Surg 33:487–495, 1957

24. Hilaris BS, Gomez J, Nori D, et al: Combined surgery, intraoperative brachytherapy, and postoperative external radiation in stage III non-small cell lung cancer. Cancer 55:1226–1231, 1985

25. Israel L, Clavier J, David PH, et al: Preoperative cisplatinum and bleomycin in 53 squamous cell carcinoma of lung. Proc Am Soc Clin Oncol 3:213, 1984

26. Jamieson, MPG, Walbaum PR, McCormack RJM: Surgical management of bronchial carcinoma invading the chest wall. Thorax 34:612–615, 1979

27. Jensik RJ, Faber LP, Kittle CF, et al: Survival in patients undergoing tracheal sleeve pneumonectomy for bronchogenic carcinoma. J Thorac Cardiovasc Surg 84:489–496, 1982

28. Kemeny MM, Block LR, Braun DW Jr, et al: Results of surgical treatment of carcinoma of the lung by stage and cell type. Surg Gynecol Obstet 147:865–871, 1978

29. Komaki R, Roh J, Cox JD, et al: Superior sulcus tumor: Results of irradiation of 36 patients. Cancer 48:1563–1568, 1981

30. Lawrence GH, Walker JH, Pinkers L: Extended resection of bronchogenic carcinoma. A reappraisal and suggested plan of management. New Engl J Med 263:615–618, 1960

31. Levett JM, Darakjian HE, DeMeester TR, et al: Bronchogenic carcinoma located in the aortic window. J Thorac Cardiovasc Surg 83:551–562, 1982

32. Madej PJ, Bitran JD, Golomb HM, et al: Combined modality therapy for stage III$_{M0}$ non small cell lung cancer (NSCLC): A five year experience. Cancer 54:5-12, 1984

33. Maruyama Y, Wilkins EW Jr, Wyman SM: An evaluation of angiocardiographic in pulmonary carcinoma with particular emphasis on prognosis. Radiology 79:617-624, 1962

34. McCormack P, Bains MS, Beattie EJ, et al: New trends in skeletal reconstruction after resection of chest wall tumors. Ann Thorac Surg 31:45, 1981

35. McGoon DC: Transcervical technic for removal of specimen from superior sulcus tumor for pathologic study. Ann Surg 159:407, 1964

36. Miller JI, Mansour KA, Hatcher CR Jr: Carcinoma of the superior pulmonary sulcus. Ann Thorac Surg 28:44-47, 1979

37. Mishina J, Suemasu K, Yoneyama T, et al: Surgical pathology and prognosis of the combined resection of chest wall and lung in lung cancer. Jpn J Clin Oncol 8:161-168, 1978

38. Mountain CF: Assessment of the role of surgery for control of lung cancer. Ann Thorac Surg 24:365-373, 1977

39. Nogeire C, Mincer F, Botstein C: Long survival in patients with bronchogenic carcinoma complicated by superior vena caval obstruction. Chest 75:325-329, 1979

40. Patterson GA, Ilves R, Ginsberg RJ, et al: The value of adjuvant radiotherapy in pulmonary and chest wall resection for bronchogenic carcinoma. Ann Thorac Surg 34:692-697, 1982

41. Paulson DL, Reisch JS: Long-term survival after resection for bronchogenic carcinoma. Ann Surg 184:324-332, 1976

42. Paulson DL: The "superior sulcus" lesion. Internat Trends Gen Thorac Surg 1:121-131, 1985

43. Perelman M, Koroleva N: Surgery of the trachea. World J Surg 4:583-593, 1980

44. Piehler JM, Pairolero PC, Weiland LH, et al: Bronchogenic carcinoma with chest wall invasion: Factors affecting survival following en bloc resection. Ann Thorac Surg 34:684-692, 1982

45. Ramsey HG, Clifton EE: Chest wall resection for primary carcinoma of lung. Ann Surg 167:342-351, 1968

46. Shahian DM, Neptune WB, Ellis FH Jr: Pancoast tumors: improved survival with pre- and postoperative radiation. Paper presented at the Twenty-second Annual Meeting of the Society of Thoracic Surgeons, 1986, Washington, DC

47. Shaw RR, Paulson DL: The Treatment of Bronchial Neoplasms. Springfield, IL, Charles C Thomas, 1959, p 95

48. Sherman DM, Neptune W, Weichselbaum R, et al: An aggressive approach to marginally resectable lung cancer. Cancer 41:2040-2045, 1978

49. Shields TW: Bronchial Carcinoma. Springfield, IL, Charles C Thomas, 1974

50. Skarin A, Veeder M, Malcolm A, et al: Chemotherapy (CAP) prior to radiotherapy (RT) and surgery in marginally resectable non small cell lung cancer (NSCLC). Proceed Am Soc Clin Oncol 1:143, 1982

51. Smith RA: The results of raising the resectability rate in operations for lung carcinoma. J Thorac Cardiovasc Surg 48:418-429, 1964

52. Takita H: Surgical adjuvant immunotherapy for lung cancer: A review. Current Surg 254-261, 1984

53. Taylor SG, Trybula M, Bomoni PD, et al: Simultaneous Cisplatin/5-FU infusion and radiation followed by surgical resection in regionally localized stage III, non-small cell lung cancer. Ann Thorac Surg 43:87-91, 1987, in press

54. Toomes H, Vogt-Moykopf I: Conservative resection for lung cancer. Internat Trends Gen Thorac Surg 1:88-99, 1985

55. Trastek VF, Pairolero PC, Piehler JM, et al: En bloc (non-chest wall) resection for bronchogenic carcinoma with parietal fixation. J Thorac Cardiovasc Surg 87:352-358, 1984

56. Van Houtte P, MacLennan I, Poulter C, et al: External radiation in the management of superior sulcus tumor. Cancer 54:223-227, 1984

57. Weissberg D: Extended resections of locally advanced stage III lung cancer. Thorac Cardiovasc Surg 29:238-241, 1981

58. Wernly JA, DeMeester TR, Kirchner PT, et al: Clinical value of quantitative ventilation-perfusion lung scans in the surgical management of bronchogenic carcinoma. J Thorac Cardiovasc Surg 80:535-543, 1980

59. Wilson RS: Tracheostomy and tracheal reconstruction, in Kaplan JA (ed): Thoracic Anesthesia. New York, Churchill-Livingstone, 1983, pp 421-445

60. Wu SF, Huang OL, Wu HS, et al: Critical evaluation of results of extension of indication for surgery for primary bronchogenic carcinoma. Semin Surg Oncol 1:23-37, 1985

61. Yoshimura H, Kazama S, Asari H, et al: Lung cancer involving the superior vena cava: Pneumonectomy with concomitant partial resection of superior vena cava. J Thorac Cardiovasc Surg 77:83-86, 1979

62. Zeldin RA, Normandin D, Landtwing D, et al: Postpneumonectomy pulmonary edema. J Thorac Cardiovasc Surg 87:359-365, 1984

F. Griffith Pearson

_____ **15** _____

Surgical Therapy of Mediastinal (N₂) Disease

N_2 disease is identified when spread occurs to mediastinal lymph nodes in any of the following locations: paratracheal and pretracheal, tracheobronchial, subcarinal, subaortic, paraesophageal, or inferior pulmonary ligament. As in other malignancies, the N status is of major prognostic importance. When lymph node metastases do occur, the prognosis is further affected by the level of nodal station involved (adjacent or distant from the primary tumor), the number of nodes and levels or stations involved, and the extent of involvement (microscopic and intranodal vs gross or extranodal spread). Multiple levels of involvement, spread to stations distant from the primary tumor, and extranodal spread all adversely affect survival.

Although some physicians contend that any case with N_2 disease is inoperable, there is persuasive published evidence that surgical treatment is the best therapy for non-oat cell N_2 tumors that can be *completely* resected. There is practically no indication for palliative resection in patients with lung cancer, and the potential for cure in N_2 tumors managed by nonsurgical means (radiotherapy, chemotherapy) is negligible. Unfortunately, a majority of N_2 tumors are inoperable at the time of presentation by virtue of either hematogenous spread or extension to mediastinal node locations, which preclude a complete and thus potentially curable resection. The challenge to surgeons is to optimize the preoperative selection of N_2 tumors that are amenable to a complete resection at thoracotomy and minimize the number of patients who are explored with tumors that are nonresectable or incompletely resectable.

PROGNOSIS IN RESECTED N₂ LUNG CANCER

Survival data are difficult or impossible to interpret from a review of most earlier publications. The reported studies were retrospective, provided no information on the extent and anatomic location of the nodal metastases, survival data were calculated without the inclusion of unresectable cases or operative mortality, and results were not analyzed on the basis of complete or incomplete resections. Predictably, such reported results were extremely variable and 5-year survival ranged from 0 to 29 percent. Five

LUNG CANCER: A COMPREHENSIVE TREATISE
ISBN 0-8089-1876-1

of these earlier publications (between 1972 and 1981) reported 5-year survival data in resected cases of N_2 disease in which the N_2 status was identified at preoperative mediastinoscopy.[3,4,8,17,19] There were no 5-year survivors in three of these five reports,[3,4,19] and the remaining two publications reported an 18 and 20 percent 5-year survival.[8,17]

Between 1969 and 1978 another five papers reported 5-year survival data with a range of 0-29 percent in patients with resected N_2 nodes in whom the N status of the disease was identified only at the time of thoracotomy.[1,2,7,13,18] It is emphasized that all of these 10 earlier publications lack basic information and uniformity in defining the location of involved mediastinal nodes and suffer the deficiencies of retrospective chart reviews.

In recent years there are several reports that document an appreciable and more consistent 5-year survival of patients with N_2 disease when a conscious attempt was made to resect all mediastinal nodal disease.[9-12,14,16] In each of these reports the location of involved mediastinal nodes was documented at the time of prethoracotomy invasive staging (mediastinoscopy or mediastinotomy) or at the time of thoracotomy. Survival data include operative mortality. A variety of adjuvants were used in the majority of patients. These papers report 5-year survival ranging between 15 and 30 percent of completely resected, non-oat cell tumors. It is apparent, however, that complete and potentially curative resection is possible in only a minority of patients presenting with N_2 disease. Two of these reports (references 12 and 10) identify that a majority of the N_2 cases operated on had incomplete, noncurative resections.

Naruke et al.[12] developed a mapping system for mediastinal lymph nodes that they have used at the time of operation since 1967. This group performed a radical lymphadenectomy in all resected cases to obtain accurate staging information. In 1986 Naruke reported a 5-year survival rate of 15.7 percent in 181 patients with non-oat cell carcinoma who had a complete and potentially curative resection with mediastinal lymph node dissection.[11] The 5-year survival for squamous tumors was 24.2 percent and for adenocarcinoma, 14.3 percent.

Martini and associates reported on 241 patients with N_2 tumors who were submitted to thoracotomy.[10] A mediastinal lymphadenectomy is performed in all resectable cases, and the resection is considered complete if all of the resected margins, including the highest mediastinal node, are negative for tumor in the final pathology. In these 241 N_2 cases, 80 (33 percent) had a complete resection and an actuarial 3-year survival of 48 percent. Martini and associates have recently updated this review[9] and document an actuarial 5-year survival of 29 percent in 151 patients with completely resected, non-small cell lung cancer (NSCLC). Survival in this series was adversely affected when multiple nodal stations were involved and when there was spread to the subcarinal compartment. There was no statistical difference in 5-year survival between cases of squamous cell carcinoma and adenocarcinoma.

In 1982 we reported on 141 patients who had undergone resection for NSCLC that had metastasized to mediastinal nodes.[16] Results of mediastinoscopy, which was performed in all, were used to divide these patients into two groups: 79 patients in whom N_2 involvement was determined at prethoracotomy mediastinoscopy, and a second group of 62 patients, all of whom had negative results at mediastinoscopy, in whom the N_2 status was established only at subsequent thoracotomy. Of the 79 "mediastinoscopy positive cases," 67 (85 percent) were resected, and 51 of these resections were complete. The 5-year survival was 9 percent for all 79 group 1 cases and 15 percent in the 51 patients undergoing complete resection. Survival was significantly better for the 62 group 2 patients, all of whom had negative mediastinoscopies and proved to have N$_2$ tumors only at subsequent thoracotomy. The actuarial 5-year survival rate for all 62 patients was 24 percent. The projected 5-year survival rate for the 25 curative resections was 41 percent. If the two groups are combined, there were 76 complete resections with an actuarial 5-year survival of 24 percent.[9]

These recent reports support a recommendation for surgical resection of non-oat cell N$_2$ lung cancer so long as a complete resection is possible. The current challenge is to improve the accuracy of the prethoracotomy selection of such cases.

STAGING FOR POTENTIALLY RESECTABLE N$_2$ LUNG CANCER

Noninvasive Staging

It is widely accepted that neither plain chest films nor conventional mediastinal tomography are accurate determinants of N$_2$ disease. Computerized axial tomography (CAT) is the procedure of choice for the imaging of mediastinal lymph nodes, although it is possible that in the future magnetic resonance imaging (MRI) will prove equal or better in this regard. In a recent review, Heitzman[6] suggests that if lymph nodes are smaller than 1 cm in diameter they should be considered normal, with the realization that such nodes may harbor microscopic foci of tumor. Lymph nodes 1 cm to 1.5 cms should be considered suspicious, and those greater than 1.5 cms should be considered abnormal, with the realization that some lymph nodes in this category may ultimately prove to be reactive, particularly if the lung harbors pneumonia in addition to tumor. The role of CAT as an alternative to mediastinoscopy is still controversial. Using 1-cm diameter as the upper limit of normal, there is general agreement that mediastinoscopy should still be done in all CAT-positive cases because of the high incidence of false-positive reports. Glazer et al. demonstrated that a negative CAT is "highly accurate in excluding mediastinal metastases and makes screening mediastinoscopy unnecessary."[5] There is increasing enthusiasm for this approach to staging, although we continue to employ mediastinoscopy in our patients since we have identified false-negative results in 15 percent of CT scans in a recent study comparing mediastinoscopy, CAT, and magnetic resonance imaging for the identifications of N$_2$ disease.[14]

Invasive Staging

Cervical mediastinoscopy is recommended as a staging procedure for most cases of presumably operable lung cancer in the author's institution. Mediastinoscopy provides a tissue diagnosis and identifies cell type. Furthermore, prethoracotomy mediastinoscopy may clearly indicate extranodal spread of tumor with fixation to structures such as the trachea or great vessels, findings that preclude a complete and potentially curative resection. Left anterior mediastinotomy and extended cervical mediastinoscopy are used in selected patients with primary tumors of the left hilum or left upper lobe.[14]

INDICATIONS FOR RESECTION OF N₂ DISEASE

If the diagnosis of N_2 involvement is established at prethoracotomy mediastinoscopy in patients with non-small cell tumors that appear otherwise operable, there will be some cases in which a complete resection appears feasible. These will be cases in which the nodal extension is ipsilateral, without extracapsular spread and fixation to unresectable mediastinal structures such as the trachea or great vessels. In our experience, these more favorable "mediastinoscopy-positive" cases comprise about 5 percent of all resections for lung cancer. Another 5 percent are added when N_2 disease is encountered at thoracotomy in locations that are inaccessible at mediastinoscopy or mediastinotomy.

When N_2 disease is encountered, a radical lymphadenectomy is recommended with the objective of extending resection beyond the highest level of nodal involvement. Intraoperative frozen-section facilities are essential for such surgery, and the pathologist should ultimately examine all the resected nodes and identify the total number removed and the number and level of those containing metastases. The nodal map described by Naruke[12] is recommended for labeling the location and is in current use by the Lung Cancer Study Group for the multicenter North American trials of adjuvant therapy in resected lung cancer.

The role of adjuvant therapy in N_2 disease remains unclear. There have been no reported results from randomized trials of adjuvant therapy in resected N_2 disease. Adjuvant radiotherapy and chemotherapy have frequently been used in combination with resection for N_2 tumors,[15] but to date no conclusion is possible regarding benefit. A clear understanding of the indications for resection and the application of adjuvant therapy awaits the type of evaluation that can only be achieved by randomized prospective trials.

EDITORIAL COMMENT

The focus in this chapter is on the problem of patient selection for surgical intervention when mediastinal lymph nodes are involved. As Dr. Pearson points out, surgery, either alone or as part of a multimodality approach, can be potentially curative in some patients, and it is crucial for them to be included in this opportunity. However, palliative and/or incomplete surgery is not useful in any way and should be avoided.

The new AJC staging system takes into account the considerations discussed in this chapter. Specifically, according to the new definitions, N_2 means that there are metastases to ipsilateral mediastinal lymph nodes or subcarinal lymph nodes. The editors would agree with Dr. Pearson that these are the patients for whom surgery is appropriate. In contrast, by the new definitions, N_3 disease means that there are metastases to contralateral mediastinal lymph nodes, contralateral hilar lymph nodes, ipsilateral or contralateral scalene nodes, or supraclavicular lymph nodes. Patients with this extent of nodal involvement are not candidates for surgical resection at the present time.

REFERENCES

1. Abbey-Smith R: The importance of mediastinal lymph node invasion by pulmonary carcinoma in selection of patients for resection. Ann Thorac Surg 25:5-11, 1978
2. Bergh NP, Schersten T: Bronchogenic carcinoma. A follow-up study of a surgically treated series with special reference to the prognostic significance of lymph node metastases. Acta Chir Scand (Suppl) 347:1-42, 1965
3. Fosberg RG, O'Sullivan MJ, Ah-Tye P, et al: Positive mediastinoscopy: An ominous finding. Ann Thorac Surg 18:346-356, 1974
4. Gibbons JRP: The value of mediastinoscopy in assessing operability in carcinoma of the lung. Br J Dis Chest 66:162-166, 1972
5. Glazer GM, Orringer MB, Gross BH, et al: The mediastinum in non-small cell lung cancer: CT surgical correlation. Am J Radiology 142:1101-1105, 1984
6. Heitzman ER: The role of computed tomography in the diagnosis and management of lung cancer: An overview. Chest (Suppl) 89:237S-241S, 1986
7. Kirsh MM, Ksahn DR, Gago O, et al: Treatment of bronchogenic carcinoma with mediastinal metastases. Ann Thorac Surg 12:11-21, 1971
8. Kirschner PA: Lung cancer—preoperative radiation therapy and surgery. NY State J Med 198:339-342, 1981
9. Martin N, Flehinger BJ, Bains MS, et al: Alternative approaches to the management of mediastinal adenopathy. Internatl Trends Gen Thorac Surg 1:108-120, 1985
10. Martini N, Flehinger BJ, Zaman MB, et al: Prospective study of 445 lung carcinomaa with mediastinal lymph node metastases. J Thorac Cardiovasc Surg 80:390-399, 1980
11. Naruke T: Staging of N$_2$ disease. Chest (Suppl) 89:3385-3395, 1986
12. Naruke T, Suemasu K, Ishikawa S: Lymph node mapping and curability at various levels of metastasis in resected lung cancer. J Thorac Cardiovasc Surg 76:832-839, 1978
13. Paulson DL, Urschel HC Jr: Selectivity in the surgical treatment of bronchogenic carcinoma. J Thorac Cardiovasc Surg 62:554-562, 1971
14. Pearson FG: Lung cancer: The past 25 years. Chest (Suppl) 89:200S-205S, 1986
15. Pearson FG: Mediastinal adenopathy—the N2 lesion. Internatl Trends Gen Thorac Surg 1:104-107, 1985
16. Pearson FG, Delarue NC, Ilves R, et al: Significance of positive superior mediastinal nodes identified at mediastinoscopy in patients with resectable cancer of the lung. J Thorac Cardiovasc Surg 83:1-11, 1982
17. Pearson FG, Nelems JM, Henderson RD, et al: The role of mediastinoscopy in the selection of treatment for bronchial carcinoma with involvement of superior mediastinal lymph nodes. J Thorac Cardiovasc Surg 64:382-390, 1972
18. Ramsey HE, Cahan WG, Beattie EJ, et al: The importance of radical lobectomy in lung cancer. J Thorac Cardiovasc Surg 58:225-230, 1969
19. Viikari SJ, Inberg MV, Puhakka H, et al: The role of mediastinoscopy in the treatment of lung carcinoma. Bull Soc Internatl Chir 2:119-126, 1974

Thomas J. Fitzgerald
Joel S. Greenberger

___ 16 ___

Radiation Treatment for Locally Advanced Stage III $_{M_0}$ Non-Small Cell Carcinoma of the Lung

Even though earliest-stage lung carcinoma can be treated with curative intent with surgical resection, the majority of patients who are diagnosed with non-small cell carcinoma of the lung (NSCLC) have disease that is, unfortunately, so locally advanced that surgical resection is not possible. Those patients with unresected primary lung carcinoma are ultimately referred for radiation therapy in order to control the local-regional disease and are also considered for systemic therapy for control of potential disseminated disease. At the outset, it is important to recognize that there is only at best a modest survival benefit with treatment for unresectable primary lung carcinoma. However, a very real benefit in the quality of life for most patients with carcinoma of the lung can be achieved with the careful application of sophisticated radiation therapy techniques, and for a small but significant portion of the population, a potential cure may result from treatment.[11]

Unresectable lung carcinoma is generally considered to be stage III disease (T_1N_2, T_2N_2, T_3N_0, T_3N_1, T_3N_2) non-small cell carcinoma of the lung (NSCLC).

Application of successful radiation therapy requires careful medical judgment with respect to the patient's constitution status. Patients with Karnofsky performance status of less than 60 and those who have lost a significant amount of weight (15 percent of overall body mass) do have significant difficulty completing a definitive course of radiation therapy.[26] Therapy-associated toxicity to pulmonary parenchyma has long been recognized as a dose–volume limiting factor in treating patients with lung cancer. Pretherapy evaluation of pulmonary function is an important part in evaluating a patient when one is considering definitive radiation therapy as a treatment option. The minimal pulmonary requirements recommended for patients suitable for definitive treatment are as follows: vital capacity of 45 percent of the predicted value; FEV, 40 percent of the predicted value; Pao_2 equal to or over 60 mm Hg; and $PaCO_2$, equal to or under 49 mm Hg.[2]

At the present time, there is no clear evidence that defines the best dose of

LUNG CANCER: A COMPREHENSIVE TREATISE
ISBN 0-8089-1876-1

radiation to treat non-small cell bronchogenic carcinoma that is surgically unresectable. From experience in the treatment of other malignancies, we know that in order to sterilize gross tumor, definitive radiation doses are necessary in order to provide optimal tumor kill.[11] There are some interesting preoperative studies that give us a sense of the amount of dose required for optimal treatment for these patients. Bromley and Szur reported that localized lung carcinoma could be eradicated in approximately 40 percent of patients given doses in excess of 4700 cGy.[4] Bloedorn et al. reported no recognizable tumor cells at the primary site in 14 out of 26 patients who received 6000 rads in 6 weeks on a preoperative basis.[3] The mediastinum in this series showed positive tumor in only 8 percent of the patients. Hellman et al. reported residual tumor at the primary site in 17 out of 24 patients with lung carcinoma treated with 5500-6000 cGy in 5-6 weeks.[12] In 15 patients who had preoperative radiographic evidence of hilar or mediastinal adenopathy, only 20 percent had pathologic specimens that demonstrated residual tumor. Rissanem et al. reported no carcinoma in the tumor volume in 18 out of 60 patients treated with doses of 4500-6250 cGy.[21] In contrast, viable tumor was found frequently in patients treated with doses below 4500 cGy; 7 patients whose therapy was interrupted after doses of 3000 cGy all showed evidence of malignancy at autopsy.[21]

These preoperative studies have helped to guide the radiation therapy community in establishing therapeutic strategies and fractionation schemes that would eradicate gross viable tumor with minimal morbidity to normal tissue structures. However, one of the most challenging problems in determining the optimal dose of irradiation for this disease is the unfortunate high incidence of distant metastasis, which results in an unrelentingly poor prognosis without regard to the status of the intrathoracic tumor volume. Roswit et al. reported a slightly increased 1-year survival rate in a group of patients treated with 5000 cGy in 5 weeks, in contrast to a group that received placebo (18 vs 14 percent).[22] In general, many definitive radiation studies have failed to demonstrate a difference in survival when patients are treated with 4000, 5000, or 6000 cGy. Deeley et al. reported a 6 percent survival rate of 2 years in 51 patients treated with 3000 cGy in 20 sessions and no survivors in 51 patients receiving 4000 cGy in 20 sessions.[6]

In 1971 the Cooperative Oxford Group published their experience in delivering radiation treatment to patients either (1) at the time of initial diagnosis of the primary lung tumor or (2) delaying treatment until distressful symptoms occurred, such as shortness of breath or superior vena caval obstruction.[9] The mean survival times for both treatment groups were equivalent. In 1977 this experience was updated by Berry et al., and again the same conclusion was established.[1] Both studies are flawed, however, in that suboptimal radiation equipment (orthovoltage) dose and fractionation schemes were used (4000 cGy/13-14 fractions/28 days). Many groups feel that this suggests that radiation therapy is ineffective for treating primary lung carcinoma; however, many other investigators feel that this suggests that suboptimal treatment is not adequate to control primary tumors.

Several investigators have begun to show improved survival rates with higher doses of radiation therapy. Eisert et al. reported local tumor control in only 14 out of 51 patients (27 percent) receiving less than 1450 RET, in contrast to 75 out of 146 patients (51 percent) treated with higher doses.[10] These authors very nicely demonstrated that an improved survival (24 percent) was correlated with control of the primary tumor of the lung. In 1981 Noah Choi published a series of 162 patients from the Massachusetts General Hospital treated with definitive radiotherapy.[5] All patients had unresectable non-small cell bronchogenic carcinoma and were treated with a curative intent by a multifield arrangement. The median survival and short-term survival up to 1.5 years were both independent of radiation doses (40-64 Gy) and specific target volumes. However, long-term survival (greater than or equal to 2 years) was dependent on radiation dose and target volume; actuarial survival rates of 36 and 28 percent were obtained, in contrast to 10 and 3 percent for the high-dose (greater than 60 Gy) versus low-dose (less than or equal to 40 Gy) treatment, respectively (p < .05). The data were reported at 2 and 3 years, respectively, with a minimal follow-up of 2 years. The actuarial survival rate was 7.5 percent with an irradiation dose of greater than or equal to 50 Gy. However, it is important to note that there were no 5-year survivors among patients who were treated with an irradiation dose of less than 50 Gy. Local control of tumor was radiation-dose-dependent; local tumor control rates at greater than or equal to 18 months were 76 versus 29 percent in patients treated above and below 5000 Gy, respectively (p < .05).

The observations of Choi were again confirmed in a paper from the Harvard Joint Center for Radiation Therapy published by Sherman et al. in 1981.[25] This particular analysis involved an initial 348 patients who had presented at the time of diagnosis with non-small cell bronchogenic carcinoma, and the target volumes were not considered to be amenable to surgery because of the advanced nature of the primary lesion. Of this entire population, only 66 patients survived a minimum of 18 months, and these patients were studied in depth with respect to irradiation dose, fractionation scheme, and target volume. This is an important publication because, since most data concerning primary lung carcinoma is contaminated by the dominance of distant disease, it often is difficult to demonstrate an effectiveness of involved field radiation treatment with respect to dose and target volume relationships. A local failure rate of 50 percent (4 out of 8) was observed for patients who received less than 50 Gy. The local failure rate of 22 percent (6 out of 27) was observed for patients receiving 50-55 Gy. A local failure rate of 10 percent was observed for patients who received 55-59 Gy, and only 1 out of 20 patients who received greater than 60 Gy failed in the local irradiation volume. The authors comment that the radiotherapy technique was also a significant variable for the presence of local failure. Forty-six percent of treatment failures identified were related to what the authors described as inadequate radiation technique. Five patients suffered recurrences under the posterior spinal cord block, which was used in treating patients with an anterior-posterior technique. The authors do suggest in the publication that oblique field irradiation may have eliminated this problem. One patient suffered a marginal recurrence in a partially treated perihilar region, and another patient had unrecognized chest wall involvement that, in retrospect, most likely could have been detailed with computerized tomography (CT), if that technique had been available at the time of treatment.

These recent studies also detailed the important observation that patient survival is dependent on local control. Eisert notes in a population of 229 patients, that a disease-free survival of 25 percent was obtained in patients in whom local control of the primary lesion was established.[10] No patient with a local failure was a survivor at 24 months. These data are important in illustrating that definitive irradiation dose, and careful attention to the irradiation treatment volume is critical when one is attempting curative treatment for these patients.

In June 1973 the Radiation Therapy Oncology Group initiated a randomized

study to determine the most effective and best tolerated irradiation dose and fractionation schedule in patients with inoperable or unresectable stage III NSCLC.[19] Randomization was carried out in the following manner: 4000 cGy split course delivering 2000
CGy in 1 week, five fractions, 2 weeks' rest, and an additional 2000-cGy dose in five
fractions, or 4000-, 5000-, or 6000-cGy tumor doses in continuous courses delivered
in five weekly fractions with daily doses of 200 cGy per day. The treatment portals
were designed to include all areas of parenchymal involvement in the hilar and
mediastinal lymph nodes, with at least a 2-cm margin around areas of gross disease. A
2-cm-wide, 5 half-value layer spinal cord block was used for a portion of the treatment
to limit the dose to the spinal cord to 4500 cGy with a continuous schedule and to
2500 cGy with a split-course schedule. Higher maximum doses frequently were delivered to the anterior portal with unequal loading in order to maximize the mediastinal
dose in both the split-course and continuous-course groups. In total, 375 cases were
analyzed. Only 8 out of 100 patients in the 4000-cGy split course group showed a
complete regression of tumor, in contrast to 18–21 percent of those treated with
continuous schedules. The overall complete and partial regression rate was 46 percent
in the patients who received 4000 cGy split course, 51 percent with the 4000-cGy
continuous course, and 65 percent in those who were treated with 5000 and 6000
cGy. The split-course group had a significantly lower complete response rate than did
groups on the other regimens ($p < .02$). When the 4000-cGy split-course patients
were compared to the patients receiving continuous course with a higher irradiation
dose, the overall response rates were significantly different (49 vs 63 percent, $p =
.005$). Because of this experience, most institutions now favor utilizing a continuous
course of irradiation treatment as opposed to a split-course regimen.

The overall survival data were updated in the 1982 publication from the Radiation Oncology Therapy Group (RTOG).[20] The survival rate at 1 year was 35–41
percent in all treatment groups. However, the 2-year survival was 10 percent for
patients treated with the split-course regimen versus 19 percent for patients treated to
a total dose of 6000 cGy. This series also demonstrated a difference in survival when
the stage on presentation was evaluated as a single variable. Patients with T_3N_0 or
T_1N_2 tumors had a 2-year survival of greater than 25 percent, in contrast to a survival
of less than 11 percent in patients with T_3N_1 tumors or those with both an advanced
primary lesion on presentation and mediastinal adenopathy. A detailed analysis of the
patterns of recurrence revealed that local control was dependent on the treatment
program. Patients treated with a split-course schedule had a 51 percent incidence of
local failure, in contrast to a 35 percent incidence of local failure in patients treated to a
total dose of 6000 cGy via a continuous regimen.

This experience was also evaluated with respect to the size of the primary lesion.
When the tumor response was correlated with the dose of irradiation and tumor size,
patients with tumor size of less than 3 cm treated to 6000 cGy had complete response
rates of 31 percent, in contrast to 16 percent of patients treated with the split-course
regimen. The complete and partial response rate was 48 percent in patients treated to
4000 cGy, in contrast to 71 percent to patients treated with 6000 cGy. The greater
tumor response was correlated with a lower incidence of local failure with no local
failures noted in patients who were treated to 6000 cGy, in contrast to a local failure
rate of 58 percent in patients treated to 4000 cGy. In patients who had primary tumors
measuring 4–6 cm, the local failure was 35 percent in those treated to 6000 cGy, in
contrast to 57 percent in those treated to 4000 cGy.

In analysis of this data, most institutions now favor a continuous course of radiation treatment, with therapy delivered to a high total x-ray dose in order to maximize local control and, hopefully, improve the overall survival in patients with locally advanced primary lung carcinoma. The issue of tissue histology in treating NSCLC patients remains controversial, with no clear-cut evidence that tissue type would influence the primary management in treating patients with definitive radiation treatment.

DIAGNOSIS AND MANAGEMENT OF CARCINOMAS OF THE SUPERIOR PULMONARY SULCUS

A clinical and x-ray syndrome due to tumor arising in the extreme apex of the lung or the thoracic inlet was described by Pancoast in 1924.[17] The clinical syndrome is characterized by pain around the shoulder, which can radiate to the axilla, toward the scapula, or down the arm, usually in an ulnar distribution. Atrophy or weakness of the hand muscles can occur, and pressure on the blood vessels may cause swelling of the affected extremity. These symptoms and signs are due to tumor involvement of the lower trunk of the brachial plexus, pleura, upper ribs, lower cervical and upper thoracic vertebrae, and the subclavian vessels. Horner's syndrome often accompanies these findings because cervical sympathetic nerves are likewise involved with tumor. On chest x-ray, the tumor presents with a small homogeneous shadow at the extreme apex of the lung, usually associated with local rib destruction and often with vertebral body infiltration. Pain is the dominant sign on clinical presentation, and it is often steady, severe, and unrelenting. Frequently the tumors in this setting are squamous carcinomas; however, large cell and adenocarcinoma can also occur in this site.

Paulson has pioneered an aggressive approach to these patients, which includes a preoperative course of irradiation followed by an extended surgical resection.[18] This strategy was prompted by the observation that these tumors usually grow slowly and present with a less frequent incidence of nodal metastasis. From the publication in 1975, 8 out of 30 patients were alive, disease-free at 10 years following the diagnosis of malignancy, and after 3 years no patient died of tumor recurrence. At the 3-year time point, 18 out of 54 patients were surviving with disease-free status. The preoperative irradiation dose was generally 3000 cGy in 10 treatments over 12 days and was delivered to the apex of the lung, upper ribs, upper mediastinum, ipsilateral hilum, and lower cervical spine. This permitted a surgical resection 3–6 weeks after completion of radiation therapy. Higher doses of irradiation were not used routinely because of the worry of increased radiotherapeutic operative morbidity associated with higher x-ray doses. An extended en bloc resection of the chest wall was then carried out. This involves an extended radical lobectomy or segmental resection. The posterior portions of the first three ribs, portions of the upper thoracic vertebrae, including the transverse processes, intercostal nerves, the lower trunk of the brachial plexus, the stellate ganglion, and the portion of the dorsal sympathetic chain are resected, along with the involved lung. Long-term complications from the procedure include permanent ulnar nerve neurologic deficits and Horner's syndrome. Immediate surgical complications are of respiratory origin and include instability of the chest wall. These patients generally require a ventilary support for 2–4 postoperative days and bronchoscopy for removal of secretions in the immediate postoperative period. Contraindications to resection include extensive invasion of a brachial plexus, subclavian artery, vertebral bodies, esophagus, mediastinum, and the presence of distant metastasis. Patients with hilar, mediastinal, or scalene node involvement have such a limited prognosis following the procedure, and these metastatic sites should probably also be considered as contraindications for a definitive procedure. Since the advent of this aggressive approach, however, many authors have been unable to reproduce such favorable results.

In a 1972 publication from the University of Michigan, Kirsch et al. published a series of 35 patients treated over a 16-year period.[14] Twelve patients underwent preoperative irradiation, followed by radical end block excision of the chest wall. None of these patients survived to 5 years. Twenty-three patients received radiation therapy, and three of those patients survived at 5 years free of disease. This was one of the first studies to question the role of radical chest wall excision in the treatment of patients with a superior sulcus tumor. In 1981 Komaki et al., in a publication from the Medical College of Wisconsin, examined a series of 36 patients treated with definitive irradiation alone with superior sulcus tumor.[15] In this group, 86 percent of patients had relief of symptoms for a median of 12 months after irradiation. Seventeen patients (47 percent) achieved local control and enjoyed a significantly longer median survival (26.5 vs 6.5 months) and a higher probability of 5-year survival (45 vs 0 percent), compared to those patients who did not achieve local control. Of 19 patients with local failure, distant metastases developed in 9. The prognosis was related to local control. The actuarial 5-year survival rate for the entire population was 23 percent. In general, patients were treated to a tumor dose of 6000 cGy, and no major complications were reported in this study.

In 1984 Van Houtte et al., in a study reported from the University of Rochester, reviewed a series of 31 patients with superior sulcus tumor.[28] The overall survival in patients treated with definitive irradiation was 18 percent; however, patients without bone erosion or scalene lymph node involvement had a 5-year survival of 40 percent. Local control was associated with the total tumor dose and tumor extent. Irradiation doses of less than 5000 cGy were associated with a higher rate of local failure; 6 out of 7 (86 percent) patients failed locally with doses of less than 5000 cGy, and 4 out of 16 (25 percent) patients failed locally with doses of greater than 5000 cGy. There were no major complications reported in this series.

In a 1986 publication from the University of Florida, Devine et al. reported a series of 50 patients with carcinoma of the superior pulmonary sulcus treated between October 1964 and October 1981.[7] Of seven patients who were treated with irradiation therapy alone, two were alive and disease-free at 5 years. The dose that these patients received ranged from 6130 rads in 33 fractions to 7070 rads in 35 fractions, with a mean dose of 6600 rads in 35 fractions. Local control was obtained in 8 out of 26 evaluable patients (31 percent) treated with preoperative radiation therapy and surgery and in 2 out of 6 patients treated with radiation therapy alone. Thirty percent of patients receiving planned preoperative radiation therapy did not undergo definitive surgery. The absolute disease-free survival rate at 5 years by treatment group for these patients was 3 out of 30 (10 percent) with preoperative radiation therapy and surgery and 2 out of 7 (18 percent) with radiation therapy alone. These series in concert argue that the aggressive approach advocated by Paulson et al.[18] is difficult to repeat in other series examining the same question. The issue of how best to approach these patients remains controversial; however, a general principle would be that if the patient has the constitutional status and tumor anatomy that is acceptable to excision, a definitive surgical procedure should be part of the patient's overall therapeutic strategy. If the lesion is thought to be unresectable by radiographic study, or if the patient does not have the constitutional status to withstand a definitive surgical procedure, that patient should be treated with definitive radiation treatment, and in a small but significant portion of these patients a cure will result.

Techniques of Irradiation: Volumes, Irradiation Portals, and X-ray Beam Arrangement

The volume of tissue to be irradiated and the configuration of the treatment portals should be determined by the following characteristics: (1) the size and the location of the primary tumor, (2) the lymphatic drainage of the area in which the primary tumor arose, (3) the equipment and beam energy available for each individual patient, and (4) special attention must be paid to the patient's overall constitutional status and preradiation pulmonary status in order to avoid significant acute or long-term normal tissue sequalae from therapy.

Of paramount importance is accurate tumor localization relative to the patient's target volume. Although it has never been proven in randomized prospective studies, CT scanning of the chest is now of great importance in the radiation treatment planning of patients with primary lung carcinoma.[2] CT scanning can now very accurately predict the size and location of the primary tumor, as well as successfully delineate gross tumor volume in the hilar region and mediastinum.[23] With accurate delineation of the target volume on CT scan, one will be able to more accurately delineate the tumor volume and, hopefully, decrease the possibility of tumor recurring at the margin of the treatment field. It is common radiation therapeutic practice to design treatment portals with a 2-cm margin around the areas of gross tumor defined on CT scanning and a minimum of 1.5 cm around electively treated regional lymph node areas that would be thought to contain microscopic residual disease. In order to include the appropriate lymph node draining areas, careful attention must be considered to the given lymphatic pathways of each lobe of the right and left lung (Fig. 16-1). The treatment field sizes within an irregular shape generally are preferred, and these fields do require special individual secondary blocking to spare as much normal tissue as possible within the target volume. In patients with potentially curable lesions to be treated with high doses of irradiation, complicated portal arrangements are necessary (Fig. 16-2). Oblique or lateral portals are quite useful in combination with AP/PA portals in order to boost the dose to the particular region of the target volume in the lung and mediastinum without excessive irradiation to normal tissue structures. Spinal cord shielding blocks must be individually cut for every patient and these must be used judiciously. It is very important to recognize that 1-cm variance in the daily setup of the patient on the oblique block could result in either overirradiation of the spinal cord or underirradiation of mediastinal structures.

The choice of appropriate beam energies in addition to the volume to be treated are crucial to the delivery of adequate doses of irradiation to the tumor without producing toxicity to adjacent normal tissue structures. Because of the large diameter of the chest, there is much improved target volume dosimetry with the use of high-energy photons for individual patient care.

Clinically, the most significant problems encountered in treatment planning for

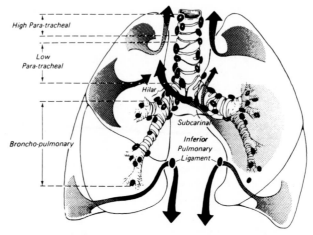

Fig. 16-1. Distribution of lymph nodes in relation to the trachea and bronchi. (Reproduced from Fletcher G: Textbook of
Radiotherapy. Philadelphia, Lea & Febiger, 1980. With permission.)

bronchogenic carcinoma include (1) the sloping surface of the chest with decreased
sagittal diameter at the lower of the thoracic inlet; (2) the presence of non-unit-density
tissues such as the lungs within the target volume; (3) the toxicity of irradiation for
sensitive structures such as the spinal cord, heart, esophagus, and uninvolved lung;
and (4) the frequent need for irregular isodose computations necessary in order to
treat target volumes.

The sloping surface of the chest results in a varied source to target distance over
the treatment field, and the cause of the differences in separation produces a nonuni-

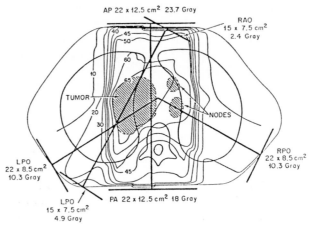

Fig. 16-2. Composite isodose distribution for a four-field radiation technique (Reproduced from Choi N, Poucette J: Improved survival of patients with unresectable non-small cell
bronchogenic carcinoma by an innovative high dose en bloc
radiotherapeutic approach. Cancer 48:101, 1981. With permission.)

form dose distribution within the patient. If one chooses to calculate the irradiation dose at the level of the isocenter, this could potentially lead to underdosing of inferior structures where the chest wall diameter is larger. If one chooses to calculate the specific radiation dose at the level of greatest separation, this could potentially lead to excessively high irradiation of tissues located in the superior aspect of the chest, which has a smaller overall separation. The favored method of addressing this problem in correcting for the source to surface discrepancy is using appropriately designed compensating filters. At our institution, the separation of the patient is taken along the central axis at many different points and is compared to the CT distribution of the target volume. This allows for the appropriate compensator to be fitted for every individual patient and subsequently allows for homogeneous dose to the target volume without excessive irradiation to normal tissue structures. The compensating filter can be designed to accommodate for changes in the slope in both the cephalocaudad and lateral axes.

The lung air cavity within the irradiation target volume is not of tissue unit density; therefore, the primary irradiation beam is not attenuated in a uniform fashion, and likewise the scatter function generated from the primary beam is also nonuniform. To correct fully for these inhomogeneities, it is necessary to know the size, shape, and position of the target volume relative to the amount of lung volume within the irradiation treatment portal. The problems of air cavity inhomogeneity have led to a new era in the field of irradiation treatment planning. Many investigators have begun to examine the target volume inhomogeneities within the irradiation field because of this change in the unit density material.[27] Some investigators have noted relative inhomogeneities as great as 25 percent at the central and peripheral portions of the target volume. The central portion of the target volume has received excessively high irradiation doses because of reduced attentuation of the primary radiation beam. However, the periphery of the target volume is thought to receive a decreased irradiation dose because of the lack of scatter located at the interface between the tumor and lung tissue. The recent advent of CT will create new perspectives in order to assess the effect of target volume inhomogeneities with respect to radiation dose distribution within the thorax, allowing accurate prediction of the amount of lung volume within the treatment field. It is the goal of many institutions to develop appropriate computer algorithms that will generate the correction factors necessary to accurately describe the irradiation target dose. The is becoming of increasing importance because radiation therapists need to reassess target volume inhomogeneities with respect to reporting data concerning local control of all thoracic malignancies.

At the University of Massachusetts, all patients who are being planned for irradiation treatment to the lung are treated with CT-direct planning. The initial target volume to be treated is chosen by the radiation therapist. The patient then undergoes CT scanning in the radiation treatment position. This allows for appropriate delineation of the therapy target volume with respect to the patient's contour and accurately delineates the proximity of the target volume with respect to the adjacent normal tissue structures. The isocenter of the treatment is then chosen in relation to the position of the tumor volume and the patient's contour, and the patient is then returned to the radiation simulator, where appropriate imaging films are subsequently taken. Most patients are treated with a two- to four-field plan that will allow for maximal irradiation within the target volume and minimal irradiation to normal tissue structures. The amount of lung within the irradiation field is then calculated as a percentage volume, and individual patient blocks are templated in order to protect as much normal tissue as possible.

Complications of Radiation Treatment

Complications of radiation treatment in patients with carcinoma of the lung carry both acute and long-term effects from therapy. Patients will tolerate daily doses of 180–200 cGy, calculated to the midplane, without major problems during the course of therapy. At approximately the 3000-cGy level, the patient will develop mild to moderate dysphagia secondary to desquamation of the esophageal mucosa. This will persist during the remaining course of radiation treatment and may precipitate an unplanned therapy break because of persistent discomfort or subsequent weight loss. Approximately 3 weeks after completion of definitive therapy, the discomfort will begin to abate and the patient will have an improved sense of well-being. Bronchial secretions will become altered during the course of therapy, and a nonproductive cough can develop.[8]

Long-term problems associated with radiation treatment are thought to involve the lung, esophagus, and spinal cord. Radiation pneumonitis rarely occurs during a patient's primary therapy course; however, it becomes clinically apparent in the first few months following completion of treatment. All patients who are treated with definitive doses of irradiation develop pulmonary fibrosis within the target volume. Severe complications from this side effect are rare, fortunately, provided one uses careful attention to the amount of lung within the primary target volume. Most patients will be clinically asymptomatic while radiographic manifestations of these changes occur and coincide with the radiation treatment portals. If the patient develops short-ness of breath or fever accompanying these radiographic changes, corticosteroids are recommended, and some patients will show a profound benefit in clinical symptoma-tology.[8]

Acute radiation esophagitis occurs during the course of x-ray treatment; however, once the mucosal surface has repopulated, the acute discomfort quickly abates. Long-term esophageal problems are rare, fortunately, and usually are seen only when a patient is treated with relatively large daily fractions (250–300 cGy/day). One has to be careful in radiation therapy planning since the esophagus is in a relatively posterior region of the chest diameter. Even though the dose at midplane may be calculated to a relatively small dose, the inhomogeneity from the treatment beam may put the esoph-ageal mucosa at a relatively higher daily fraction size.[8]

Spinal cord injuries should be avoided by careful treatment planning. Careful delineation of dose distribution within the patient at the level of the tumor and spinal cord will allow the radiation therapist to avoid this long-term problem. In 1980 the Radiation Therapy Oncology Group published a randomized series of 365 patients with histologically proven unresectable NSCLC treated with definitive radiation ther-apy. Table 16-1 is reprinted from that publication and confirms the relative infrequency of long-term morbidities secondary to radiation treatment.

FUTURE DIRECTIONS IN RADIATION THERAPY IN THE TREATMENT OF PATIENTS WITH PRIMARY LUNG CANCER

Because of the continued problem in local tumor control, current radiation ther-apy oncology group studies are being directed toward ways to improve the therapeutic

Table 16-1

Severe Complications of Radiation Treatment

	4000 Rads Split		4000 Rads Continuous		5000 Rads Continuous	6000 Rads Continuous	
Pneumonitis	—	(2)*	—		3	3	(1)
Pulmonary fibrosis	7		1		—	3	
Esophagitis	1		2	(1)	1	1	
Pneumothorax	1		—	(1)	—	—	
Bronchial obstruction	—		—		—	—	(2)
Pleural effusion	—		1		—	—	
Esophageal stricture	—		1		—	1	
Costochondritis	—		—		—	1	
Subcutaneous fibrosis	1		—		—	—	
Pulmonary embolus	—		—		1	—	
	10 +	(2)	5 +	(2)	5	9 +	(3)

From Perez C, Stanley K, Grundey G, et al: Impact of irradiation technique and tumor extent in tumor control and survival of patients with unresectable non-oat cell carcinoma of the lung. Cancer 50:1091, 1982. With permission.

*Life-threatening case indicated in parentheses.

window for patients treated with primary radiation therapy. Changes in the time/dose fractionation schedules include increasing the total x-ray dose with one fraction per day by combining wide-field treatment to the primary tumor and likely area of nodal involvement with a smaller boost field to the grossly involved areas of the primary tumor and lymph nodes. The total x-ray dose to the target volume is 7500 cGy in trials that are presently being conducted.[16] In addition, the Radiation Therapy Oncology Group is completing a pilot study in which two fractions per day of 120 cGy were given 4–6 hours apart, to a total dose of 5040 cGy to a large field with a subsequent small field boost to 6960 cGy.[24] The boost volume includes only that area where gross tumor is involved as demonstrated on CT scan. These studies will provide very good data with respect to local tumor control and normal tissue tolerance.

Alternative forms of radiation treatment have also been used in an attempt to improve local control. Nonrandomized studies with fast neutron beams have shown greater tumor sterilization rates than from photon therapy.[24] The RTOG subsequently embarked on a randomized trial, and to date preliminary data from that analysis shows no overall survival difference.[24] Trials now randomize patients to treatment with photons alone, neutrons alone, and mixed photon and neutron beam therapy. The data from these studies will be utilized in developing future therapy treatment protocols.

Attempts have been made to enhance the radiation effect with radiation sensitizers. A recent study of the Radiation Therapy Oncology Group employed once-a-day fractionation to 6000 cGy with a simultaneous administration of misonidazole. However, at this time point there has been no improvement in the local tumor control or prevention of distant disease with tumor cell sensitizers available to date.[2,24] Newer sensitizers such as RO-03-H099 or SI-2508 may permit greater and clinically useful hypoxic cell radiosensitization without dose-limiting toxicity.

There are no randomized studies that present conclusive evidence of major improvements in local control or long-term survival when chemotherapy is added to radiotherapy in the treatment of non-small cell bronchogenic carcinoma.[2,24] Nevertheless, the theoretical potential advantages are such that further phase III studies comparing such combined modality therapy with radiation alone need to be conducted. The overall feeling in the treatment community is that the present position is probably due to the inadequacy of the present chemotherapy regimens and more effective systemic therapy would hopefully change this position. Further improvements in local control could also be achieved by the application of interstitial radiation therapy during the time of primary surgery or the use of intraoperative electron beam radiation therapy.[13]

Treating patients with primary unresectable bronchogenic carcinoma continues to remain an enormous clinical challenge to all health care professionals involved in the care of these patients, and it is a challenge to the medical community to continue to explore new modes of therapy in order to improve the present survival rates. It continues to be important to recognize that there is only at best a modest survival benefit for these patients at this time. However, a very real benefit in the quality of life for most patients with carcinoma of the lung can be achieved with careful application of sophisticated radiation therapy techniques.

REFERENCES

1. Berry R, Laing A, Newman C, et al: The role of radiotherapy in treatment of inoperable lung cancer. Internatl J Radiat Oncol Biol Phys 2:433, 1977
2. Bleehan N, Cox J: Radiotherapy for lung cancer. Internatl J Radiat Oncol Biol Phys 11:1001, 1985
3. Bloedorn F, Cawley R, Cuccia C, et al: Preoperative irradiation in bronchogenic carcinoma. Am J Radiol 92:77, 1964
4. Bromley L, Szur L: Combined radiotherapy and resection for carcinoma of the bronchus: Experiences with 66 patients. Lancet 2:937, 1955
5. Choi N, Poucette J: Improved survival of patients with unresectable non-small cell bronchogenic carcinoma by an innovative high dose en bloc radiotherapeutic approach. Cancer 48:101, 1981.
6. Deeley T: A clinical trial to compare two different tumor dose levels in treatment of advanced carcinoma of the bronchus. Clin Radiol 17:299, 1966
7. Devine J, Mendenhall W, Million R, et al: Carcinoma of the superior pulmonary sulcus treated with surgery and/or radiation therapy. Cancer 47:941, 1986
8. Devita V, Hellman S, Rosenberg S: Cancer. Principles and Practice of Oncology. Philadelphia, Lippincott, 1982, Chapter 14.
9. Durrant K, Ellis F, Black J: Comparison of treatment policies in inoperable bronchial carcinoma. Lancet 1:715, 1971
10. Eisert D, Cox J, Komaki R: Irradiation for bronchial carcinoma: Reasons for failure. I. Analysis as a function of dose time fractionation. Cancer 37:2665, 1976
11. Fletcher G: Textbook of Radiotherapy. Philadelphia, Lea & Febiger, 1980
12. Hellman S, Kiligerman M, Von Essen C, et al: Sequelae of radical radiotherapy of carcinoma of the lung. Radiology 82:1055, 1964
13. Hilaris B, Gomez J, Nori D, et al: Combined surgery, intraoperative brachytherapy, and postoperative external radiation in Stage III non-small cell lung cancer. Cancer 55:1226, 1985
14. Kirsh M, Dickerman R, Fayos J, et al: The value of chest wall resection in the treatment of superior sulcus tumors of the lung. Ann Thorac Surg 15:339, 1973

15. Komaki R, Roh J, Cox J, et al: Superior sulcus tumors: Results of irradiation of 36 patients. Cancer 48:1563, 1981

16. Mohuiddin M: Extended fractionation for the treatment of non-oat cell carcinoma of the lung. Paper presented at Third World Conference on Lung Cancer, Tokyo, 1982

17. Pancoast H: Importance of careful roentgenray investigations of apical chest tumors. JAMA 83:1407, 1924

18. Paulson D. Carcinoma of the superior pulmonary sulcus. J Thorac Cardiovasc Surg 70:1095, 1975

19. Perez C, Stanley K, Rubin P, et al: A prospective randomized study of various irradiation doses and fractionation schedules in the treatment of inoperable non-oat carcinoma of the lung. Preliminary report by the Radiation Therapy Oncology Group. Cancer 45:2744, 1980

20. Perez C, Stanley K, Grundey G, et al: Impact of irradiation technique and tumor extent in tumor control and survival of patients with unresectable non-oat cell carcinoma of the lung. Cancer 50:1091, 1982

21. Rissanem P, Tikka V, Holsti L: Autopsy findings in lung cancer treated with megavoltage radiotherapy. Acta Radiol Ther (Sotckh) 7:433, 1968

22. Roswit B, Patano M, Rapp R, et al: The survival of patients with inoperable lung cancer. A large-scale randomized study of radiation versus placebo. Radiology 90:688, 1968

23. Seydel H, Kutcher G, Steiner R, et al: Computed tomography in planning radiation therapy for bronchogenic carcinoma. Internatl J Radiat Oncol Biol Phys 6:601, 1980

24. Seydel H: External beam treatment of unresectable lung cancer. Internatl J Radiat Biol Phys 10:573, 1984

25. Sherman D, Weichselbaum R, Hellman S: The characteristics of long-term survivors of lung cancer treated with radiation. Cancer 47:2575, 1981

26. Stanley K: Prognostic factors for survival in patients with inoperable lung cancer. J Natl Cancer Inst 65:25, 1980

27. Van Dyk J, Keane T, Rider W: Lung density as measured by computerized tomography: Implications for radiotherapy. Internatl J Radiat Oncol Biol Phys 8:1363, 1982

28. Van Houtte P, MacLemnan I, Poulter C, et al: External radiation in the management of superior sulcus tumor. Cancer 54:223, 1984

Renee H. Jacobs
Jacob D. Bitran

_____ **17** _____

Chemotherapy as an Adjuvant to Surgery or Radiotherapy in Stage III$_{M0}$ Non-Small Cell Lung Carcinoma

Lung cancer is a major healthcare problem in the United States, whose incidence continues to increase in both men and women. It is estimated that 149,000 new cases of lung cancer will be diagnosed in 1986.[34] Of these 149,000 cases of lung cancer, 75 percent will be non-small cell lung carcinoma (NSCLC). Approximately 30 percent of patients with NSCLC will have stage I or stage II disease that when treated with surgery are associated with 5-year survivals of 65 and 30 percent, respectively (see Chapters 9 and 11).[31] The best approach to patients with locally advanced (stage III M$_0$) NSCLC has yet to be defined and has been the subject of much clinical investigation. We intend to review the evolution of chemotherapy following surgery or radiation therapy in NSCLC and examine its role in the current management of this disease.

EARLY STUDIES IN ADVANCED NSCLC USING BIMODALITY THERAPY

It is difficult to draw firm conclusions from many of the earlier trials in bimodality therapy in radiation and chemotherapy in lung cancer.[10,13,22] Response criteria were not always defined in a uniform manner, and many trials in unresectable bronchogenic carcinoma of the lung included patients with small cell lung carcinoma (SCLC). As SCLC is sensitive to a variety of chemotherapeutic agents and radiation therapy, the inclusion of these patients can favorably bias interpretation of the data. Nonetheless, these trials established the feasibility of this approach in the therapy of lung cancer.

In a study by Carr et al. patients with unresectable carcinoma of the lung were treated with radiotherapy or radiotherapy plus 5-fluorouracil (5-FU).[10] The radiotherapy was administered in a split course or continuously at doses of 4500–5000 rads, and 5-FU was administered concurrently. The response rate for all patients with

NSCLC varied from 21 to 39 percent and 3-year survival, from 0 to 13 percent. Carr et al. concluded that the addition of 5-FU in this schedule did not improve local tumor control and did not offer a survival benefit.[3]

In 1971 Cohen et al. evaluated 62 patients with unresectable bronchogenic carcinoma and compared 2000 rads to the chest alone, 2000 rads with the concurrent administration of 5-FU, and 4000 rads.[13] Excluding patients with SCLC, the latter two programs resulted in equivalent regression in tumor, and both were superior to 2000 rads given alone. No significant differences were noted in survival among these patients.

Bergsagel et al.[2] reported a trial in which patients with inoperable lung cancer were randomized to receive 4000 rads alone or in combination with four or eight cycles of cyclophosphamide in a dose of 1.0 g/m^2. These investigators observed that cyclophosphamide delayed the time to appearance of metastatic disease outside the irradiated field; however, there was no significant prolongation of survival among patients with NSCLC.

Other early studies that attempted to combine nitrogen mustard[17] and vinblastine[15] with radiation therapy were similarly unsuccessful in improving the results of treatment over radiation therapy alone.

OPTIMAL USE OF CHEMOTHERAPY AND RADIATION THERAPY

As clinical research in bimodality therapy advances, it is imperative that each modality be used as effectively as possible. Thus any interaction between chemotherapy and radiation therapy must be well understood and used in an advantageous manner.

Chemotherapy of Advanced (Stage III M_0 and Stage III M_1) Non-Small Cell Lung Cancer

Admittedly, the role of chemotherapy in NSCLC is controversial. There is no standard single agent or combination regimen that has demonstrated convincingly a survival benefit to patients. For the best single agents, response rates in NSCLC are 11 to 29 percent.[30] Objective response rates with combination chemotherapy have been variable but have ranged from 0 to 60 percent. Investigators using cisplatin-based regimens in phase II trials have generally reported higher than 30 percent response rates in patients with advanced NSCLC (stage III M_0 and stage III M_1.[18,20,24] However, investigators conducting large randomized trials in patients with metastatic NSCLC have not shown that cisplatin-based regimens are any more effective than cyclophosphamide, adriamycin, methotrexate, and procarbazine (CAMP). In these randomized trials, cisplatin-based regimens are significantly more toxic than CAMP.[25,32]

Woods et al. reported preliminary results of a clinical trial involving 103 patients with inoperable NSCLC who were randomized to receive either cisplatin and vindesine or supportive care.[42] Although a 30 percent response rate was reported for the chemotherapy arm, this arm was associated with moderate to severe toxicity and did not result in a survival benefit (nearly identical survival times were reported for each group). Thus an optimal chemotherapeutic approach has not yet been defined for patients with NSCLC.

Radiation Therapy of Advanced and Inoperable NSCLC

Radiation therapy is reviewed in great detail in Chapter 16 and is beyond the scope of this chapter; however, an optimal treatment schedule may be 5000–6000 rads. This dose will control gross local disease in the majority of patients with NSCLC.

BIMODALITY THERAPY IN NSCLC: RECENT CLINICAL TRIALS

Bimodality therapy has been employed in an adjuvant and neoadjuvant setting with surgery and as primary therapy in patients with stage III M_0 and inoperable NSCLC. While some studies have demonstrated a benefit to the use of postoperative adjuvant radiation therapy or postoperative adjuvant bimodality therapy in patients with microscopic nodal disease and for T_3 tumors, the superiority of bimodality therapy compared to radiation therapy alone in patients with clinical (grossly apparent) stage III M_0 NSCLC is yet to be proven. The reason for this apparent discrepancy is not surprising; there is clearly a difference in the two patient populations as patients with stage III M_0 lung cancer found at the time of thoracotomy (pathologically staged) with *microscopic mediastinal nodal involvement* represent a group of patients who have a smaller total tumor burden than do those patients with clinically apparent (clinically staged) mediastinal nodal involvement. One would anticipate adjuvant therapy helping patients in the former subset and having a marginal impact in the latter subset of patients. A similar clinical observation has been made in patients with breast cancer and axillary nodal involvement who undergo adjuvant chemotherapy.[6] Among the premenopausal patients, *every adjuvant study has shown an improved disease-free survival;* yet benefit to adjuvant chemotherapy is limited to the subset of women with nine or less involved axillary nodes. In contrast, premenopausal women with greater than nine involved nodes have no demonstrable benefit to adjuvant chemotherapy.

Radiation therapy alone has a clearly defined role in NSCLC when given as an adjuvant to surgery. Studies by Green et al.,[21] Kirsch et al.,[27] and Choi et al.[11,12] have demonstrated a benefit for patients with N_1, N_2 (microscopic disease discovered at the time of surgery), and T_3 tumors when treated with 5000 rads postresection. The Lung Cancer Study Group (LCSG) recently reported results of adjuvant bimodality therapy in patients with incompletely resected NSCLC.[28] This prospective study randomized patients to receive either radiotherapy alone (4000 rads given in split fraction) or radiotherapy and cyclophosphamide, doxorubicin, and cisplatin (CAP) chemotherapy. The group receiving bimodality therapy demonstrated significant improvements in disease-free and overall survival.

Randomized trials evaluating bimodality therapy versus radiotherapy alone in patients with inoperative NSCLC are summarized in Table 17-1. Studies to date have not demonstrated a survival benefit with the use of bimodality therapy. Trovò and his colleagues reported the results of a randomized trial that compared radiotherapy alone to radiotherapy plus CAMP chemotherapy.[37] The response rates and median survivals in each arm were comparable, and there was no benefit in the addition of CAMP. Cardillo et al. asked a similar question in their trial comparing 5500 rads (split course) to radiation therapy plus CAP.[9] Again, no statistically significant benefit was demonstrated by the addition of CAP. Whereas the LCSG adjuvant studies employing bimo-

Table 17-1
Radiation Therapy Alone Versus Radiation Therapy Plus Chemotherapy in NSCLC

Treatment*	RT Dose (GY)	Number of Patients	Response Rate (%)	Median Survival (Months)	Reference
RT	45 over 6 weeks	38	50	12	37
versus					
RT + CAMP		28	43	10	
RT	55, split course	51	—†		9
versus					
RT + CAP					

*Abbreviations: RT = radiation therapy; CAMP = Cyclophosphamide, doxorubicin, methotrexate, and procarbazine; CAP = Cyclophosphamide, doxorubicin, and cisplatin.
†No difference in response rates was reported; however, the actual numbers are not given.

dality therapy in patients with stage III M_0 NSCLC and microscopic residual disease showed survival benefit to adjuvant therapy, the aforementioned studies showed no benefit to bimodality therapy in patients having grossly evident stage III M_0 NSCLC.

Several nonrandomized single arm studies have been conducted in an attempt to evaluate the feasibility of various drug combinations and radiation therapy schedules in unresectable NSCLC (see Table 17-2). Schultz et al. reported a 2-year survival of 21.5 percent in 78 patients treated with split-course radiation therapy and CAVe (CCNU, doxorubicin, vinblastine).[33] Eagan et al. evaluated four doxorubicin-containing regimens with split-course radiation therapy administered concurrently.[19] Response rates ranged from 57 to 81 percent, according to the histology. These results were superior to prior studies conducted at the Mayo Clinic and were not accompanied by an increase in treatment-related toxicity.

Booser et al. evaluated two cisplatin-based drug programs in combination with chest and prophylactic cranial irradiation.[7] Esophagitis was more severe, and the

Table 17-2
Combined Thoracic Irradiation and Chemotherapy in Unresectable NSCLC

Chemotherapy*	RT Dose (Gy)	Number of Patients	Response Rate (%)	Median Survival (Months)	Reference
CAP, VP-16-CAP, B-CAP, DAP	40, split course	107	68	13.3 (3-year survival of 17%)	19
MVP	51, split course	17	50	5.1	16
A, V, CCNU	40, split course	78	84	11 (2-year survival of 21.5%)	33
CAMP	30-42, continuous	101	64	8.8	29

*Abbreviations: C = cyclophosphamide, A = doxorubicin, P = cisplatin, B = bleomycin, V = vinblastine, D = dianhydrogalactitol, M = mitomycin C, CAMP (see Table 17-1).

median survival was shorter for patients on the doxorubicin-containing arm of their study.

Umsawasdi et al. evaluated a schedule of hyperfractionated chest irradiation with CAP therapy.[39] They report a response rate of 75 percent in a small group of patients able to receive both radiation and chemotherapy. Toxicities included a mild to moderate esophagitis. Severe esophagitis was not a significant complication of therapy, and this was attributed to the twice-daily radiation therapy schedule.

Crowley et al. reported preliminary results of a pilot study involving 17 patients with inoperative lung cancer.[16] In this study, radiation therapy was given sequentially and alternating with MVP (mitomycin C, vinblastine, cisplatin). A 50 percent response rate was observed, and the feasibility of this program was demonstrated.

At the University of Chicago, CAMP chemotherapy was initially evaluated in patients with metastatic NSCLC and achieved an objective response rate in 11 out of 23 (48 percent) patients.[3] In 1978 Bitran et al. reported preliminary results of bimodality therapy in 38 patients with unresectable NSCLC using radiation therapy (3000 rads to the chest) followed by CAMP.[4] The median survival for all patients was 9.6 months, which was statistically superior to historical control groups. A recent update of 101 patients treated with radiation therapy and CAMP demonstrated an overall response rate of 64 percent.[29] In 1977 the dose of chest radiation therapy was increased to 4200 rads; however, this did not improve disease-free survival. The higher dose of chest radiation therapy significantly improved local tumor control in patients with adenocarcinoma and large cell carcinoma; however, this benefit was not observed for patients with squamous cell carcinoma. In addition, 33 percent of the recurrences in patients with adenocarcinoma and large cell carcinoma were in the central nervous system. These data suggest a possible role for prophylactic cranial irradiation in these patients.

Although the aforementioned studies have failed to demonstrate a definite role for bimodality therapy in NSCLC, many interesting questions are raised that require investigation:

1. What is the "best" chemotherapy program in NSCLC? To date no single program has been shown to be superior to other commonly used regimens. While cisplatin-based regimens give the highest response rates, this is offset by significant toxicity and no conclusive evidence that this will improve survival. Analysis of failure patterns suggest that the majority of patients treated with bimodality therapy will relapse in both distant and local sites.[14,29]
2. What is the optimal dose and schedule of radiation therapy? The answer to this question may be determined in part by the specific chemotherapy program and the toxicities that arise from the use of both modalities.

More recently, neoadjuvant chemotherapy and radiation therapy has been the subject of clinical investigation in NSCLC (Table 17-3). The rationale for this approach in patients with stage III M_0 NSCLC is at initial diagnosis to destroy clinically occult metastases by the administration of chemotherapy, and in addition by delivering chemotherapy to the local tumor whose blood supply *has not* been altered by prior surgery or radiation therapy, exerting a tumoridal effect so that weeks later the patient may be approached surgically with curative intent. In a report by Skarin et al., patients with T_3 or "minimal N_2" disease were treated with CAP and 3000 rads of chest radiation therapy prior to surgery.[35] In this study, all patients except one were free of

Table 17-3

Neoadjuvant Chemotherapy and Radiation Therapy in NSCLC

Treatment*	Number of Patients Total/Taken to Surgery	Response Rate Prior to Surgery (%)	Survival	Reference
CAP × 2 + 30 Gy → Surgery → 20 Gy → CAP × 6	12/11	50	Median survival 9+ mo	35
VP × 2 + 30 Gy → Surgery → 25–30 Gy → VP × 2	13/8	73	Not reported	36
5-FU/P + concurrent RT × 4	59/33	61	Median time to recurrence 9.5 mo; 30% are disease-free after 16 mo	38
VEP × 2, RT given postoperatively	20/3	70	Not reported	5

*Abbreviations: CAP = cyclophosphamide, doxorubicin, cisplatin; VP = vindesine, cisplatin; 5-FU/P = 5-fluorouracil, cisplatin; VEP = Vindesine, etoposide, cisplatin.

gross disease following surgery. In a similarly designed study, Strauss et al. treated patients with vindesine and cisplatin and 3000-rad chest irradiation prior to surgery.[36] Eighty seven percent of these patients were able to have complete tumor resection. Trybula et al. reported their experience using cisplatin and 5-FU concurrently with radiation therapy.[38] The response rate was 61 percent prior to surgery. Twenty-one percent (7 out of 33 patients) were free of disease following surgery. Unlike the previous trials, all patients evaluated in the University of Chicago trial had T_3N_2 disease.[5] Of the seven patients eligible for surgery after initial treatment, only three patients consented to surgical resection. In all cases, patients were able to undergo complete resection of their disease. The impact of this intensive multimodality approach on patient survival has not been defined.

Future success with bimodality or multimodality therapy in NSCLC may rely on gaining a better understanding of the interactions between radiation therapy and chemotherapy in terms of application to future clinical trials. It has been recognized that both chemotherapy and radiation therapy can alter the blood supply in tumors and normal tissues. Enhanced blood circulation to transplanted tumors has been demonstrated in laboratory animals following radiation.[8] This phenomenon may facilitate drug delivery to the tumor and result in an improved response to therapy. In addition, transplanted tumors in animals grow more slowly in previously irradiated sites compared to unirradiated sites. This reduction in tumor growth is known as the "tumor bed effect." Several investigators have established that this phenomenon is due to the reduced ability of irradiated endothelial cells to provide vascular support to a rapidly growing tumor.[23,40] Jirtle et al. demonstrated a 50 percent reduction in blood flow to tumors in previously irradiated versus unirradiated sites.[26] This phenomenon may have an adverse effect on the ability to treat tumors that regrow in previously treated areas. Other investigators have observed an increased incidence in distant metastases in animals with irradiated primary tumors, suggesting a theoretical role for radiation therapy in the development of metastatic disease.[41] A more detailed understanding of these observations in animals may provide information that would be useful in designing combined-modality treatment programs in humans. The impact of chemotherapy and radiation therapy on host immune response may also have a role in tumor metastases.

From earlier studies it is recognized that certain independent prognostic variables have a significant impact on treatment outcome.[1] These include the patient's initial performance status, the extent of disease, and a history of significant weight loss during the time preceding diagnosis. Histology has not been recognized as an independent prognostic variable for NSCLC. However, consideration of the differences in relapse patterns among the histologic subtypes of NSCLC may be important for treatment design and outcome.

To date there is no proven role for combined modality therapy in stage III M_0 NSCLC, however, with modern radiotherapeutic approaches and new chemotherapeutic regimens, this approach may have an impact on the survival of patients with this disease.

REFERENCES

1. Aisner J, Hanson HH: Commentary: Current status of chemotherapy for non-small cell lung cancer. Cancer Treat Rep 65:979-986, 1981
2. Bergsagel DE, Jenkin RDT, Pringle JF: Lung cancer: Clinical trial of radiotherapy alone vs. radiotherapy plus cyclophosphamide. Cancer 30:621-627, 1972
3. Bitran JD, Desser RK, DeMeester TR, et al: Cyclophosphamide, adriamycin, methotrexate, and procarbazine (CAMP)—effective four-drug combination chemotherapy for metastatic non-oat cell bronchogenic carcinoma. Cancer Treat Rep 60:1225-1230, 1976
4. Bitran JD, Desser RK, DeMeester T, et al: Combined modality therapy for stage III M_0 non-oat cell bronchogenic carcinoma. Cancer Treat Rep 62:327-332, 1978
5. Bitran JD, Golomb HM, Hoffman PC, et al: Protochemotherapy in non-small cell lung carcinoma. Cancer 57:44-53, 1986
6. Bonadonna G, Valagussa P, Rossi A: A ten-year experience with CMF-based adjuvant chemotherapy in resectable breast cancer. Breast Cancer Res Treat 5:95-116, 1985
7. Booser DJ, Farha P, Umsawasdi T, et al: Combined chemoradiotherapy (CCRT) in limited inoperable adeno. and squamous cell lung cancer (ASCLC) with cyclophosphamide (C), platinum (P) and either etoposide (E or VP-16213)—CEP—or adriamycin (A)—CAP. Proc Am Soc Clin Oncol 1:148, 1982
8. Brown JM: Drug or radiation changes to the host which could affect the outcome of combined modality therapy. Internatl J Radiat Oncol Biol Phys 5:1151-1163, 1979
9. Cardillo C, Blanco Villalba J, Anac S, et al: Combined radiochemotherapy (RtCt) versus radiotherapy (Rt) in limited inoperable nonsmall cell carcinoma of the lung (NSCLC). Proc Am Soc Clin Oncol 4:177, 1985
10. Carr DT, Childs DS Jr, Lee RE: Radiotherapy plus 5-FU compared to radiotherapy alone for inoperable and unresectable bronchogenic carcinoma. Cancer 29:375-380, 1972
11. Choi NCH, Grillo HC, Gardiello M, et al: Basis for new strategies in postoperative radiotherapy of bronchogenic carcinoma. Internatl J Radiat Oncol Biol Phys 6:31-35, 1980

12. Choi NC: Reassessment of the role of postoperative radiation therapy in resected lung cancer. Internatl Radiat Oncol Biol Phys 8:2015-2018, 1982

13. Cohen JL, Krant MJ, Shnider BI, et al: Radiation plus 5-FU (NSC-19893): Clinical demonstration of an additive effect in bronchogenic carcinoma. Cancer Chemother Rep 55:253-258 1971

14. Cox JD, Yesner R, Mietlowski W, et al: Influence of cell type on failure pattern after irradiation for locally advanced carcinoma of the lung. Cancer 44:94-98, 1979

15. Coy P: A randomized study of irradiation and vinblastine in lung cancer. Cancer 26:803-807, 1970

16. Crowley T, Jensen B, Phillips T, et al: Radiation therapy (RT) sandwiched between cycles of combination chemotherapy in inoperable non-small cell carcinoma of the lung. Proc Am Soc Clin Oncol 4:182, 1985

17. Durrant RK, Ellis F, Black JM, et al: Comparison of treatment policies in inoperative bronchial carcinoma. Lancet 1:715-719, 1971

18. Eagan RT, Frytak S, Creagan ET, et al: Phase II study of cyclophosphamide, adriamycin and cis-dichlorodiammineplatinum (II) by infusion in patients with adenocarcinoma and large cell carcinoma of the lung. Cancer Treat Rep 63:1589-1591, 1979

19. Eagan RT, Lee RE, Frytak S: Thoracic radiation therapy and adriamycin/cisplatin-containing chemotherapy for locally advanced non-small-cell lung cancer. Cancer Clin Trials 2:381-388, 1981

20. Gralla RJ, Casper ES, Kelsen DP, et al: Cisplatin and vindesine combination chemotherapy for advanced carcinoma of the lung: A randomized trial investigating two dose schedules. Ann Intern Med 95:414-420, 1981

21. Green N, Kurohara SS, George FW, et al: Postresection irradiation for primary lung cancer. Radiology 116:405-407, 1975

22. Hansen HH, Muggia FM, Andrews R, et al: Intensive combined chemotherapy and radiotherapy in patients with nonresectable bronchogenic carcinoma. Cancer 30:315-324, 1972

23. Hewitt HB, Blake ER: The growth of transplanted murine tumors in pre-irradiated sites. Br J Cancer 22:808-824, 1968

24. Higby DJ, Wilbur D, Wallace HJ Jr, et al: Adriamycin, cyclophosphamide and adriamycin, cis-dichlorodiammineplatinum (II) combination chemotherapy in patients with advanced cancer. Cancer Treat Rep 61:869-873, 1977

25. Hoffman PC, Bitran JD, Golomb HM, et al: Do high-dose cisplatin regimens add to the therapy of metastatic non-small cell lung cancer (MNSCLC)? Proc Am Soc Clin Oncol 4:177, 1985

26. Jirtle R, Rankin JHG, Clifton KH: Effect of X-irradiation of tumor bed on tumor blood flow and vascular response to drugs. Br J Cancer 37:1033-1038, 1978

27. Kirsch MM, Rotman H, Argenta L, et al: Carcinoma of the lung: results of treatment over ten years. Ann Thorac Surg 21:371-377, 1976

28. Lad T, Weisenburger T: Adjuvant therapy of incompletely resected non-small cell bronchogenic carcinoma: A Lung Cancer Study Group trial. Proc Am Soc Clin Oncol 4:179, 1985

29. Madej PJ, Bitran JD, Golomb HM, et al: Combined modality therapy for stage III M_0 non-small cell lung cancer: A five-year experience. Cancer 54:5-12, 1984

30. Minna JD, Higgins GA, Glatstein EG: Cancer of the lung, in DeVita V, Hellman S, Rosenberg SA (eds): Principles and Practice of Oncology. Philadelphia, Lippincott, 1985, pp 507-597

31. Mountain CF: Therapy of stage I and stage II non-small cell lung cancer. Semin Oncol 10:71-80, 1983

32. Ruckdeschel JC, Finkelstein DM, Ettinger DS, et al: Chemotherapy of metastatic non-

small cell bronchogenic carcinoma (NSCBC): A randomized comparison of the four most active regimens. Proc Am Assoc Cancer Res 25:171, 1984

33. Schultz HP, Overgaard M, Sell A: Inoperable lung cancer treated by x-ray therapy and combination chemotherapy with CCNU, adriamycin and vinblastine (CAVe). Internatl J Radiat Oncol Biol Phys 6:1071-1074, 1980

34. Silverberg E, Lubera J: Cancer statistics, 1986. Ca—Cancer J Clin 36:9-41, 1986

35. Skarin A, Veeder M, Malcolm A, et al: Chemotherapy (CAP) prior to radiotherapy (RT) and surgery in marginally resectable non-small cell lung cancer (NSCLC). Proc Am Soc Clin Oncol. 1:143, 1982

36. Strauss G, Sherman D, Schwartz J, et al: Combined modality approach to regionally advanced stage III non-small cell carcinoma of the lung (NSCCL) employing neoadjuvant chemotherapy (CT) with vindesine and high dose platinum, radiotherapy (RT) and surgery (S)—a preliminary report. Proc Am Soc Clin Oncol 4:175, 1985

37. Trovó MG, DePaoli A, Veronesi A, et al: Combined radiotherapy (RT) and CAMP regimen vs RT alone in locally advanced epidermoid bronchogenic carcinoma (EBC): A randomized study. Proc Am Soc Clin Oncol 2:191, 1983

38. Trybula M, Taylor SG, Bonomi P, et al: Preoperative simultaneous cisplatin/5-fluorouracil and radiotherapy in clinical stage III non-small cell bronchogenic carcinoma. Proc Am Soc Clin Oncol 4:182, 1985

39. Umsawasdi T, Barkley HT, Murphy WK, et al: Chemotherapy + hyperfractionated chest irradiation (HF-CI) for limited disease inoperable adeno. squamous cell lung cancer (LI-ASCLC). Proc Am Soc Clin Oncol 2:204, 1983

40. Urano M, Suit HD: Experimental evaluation of tumor bed effect for C3H mouse mammary carcinoma and for C3H mouse fibrosarcoma. Radiat Res 45:41-49, 1971

41. Van den Brenk HAS, Sharpington C: Effect of local X-irradiation of a primary sarcoma in the rat on dissemination and growth of metastases: Dose-response characteristics. Br J Cancer 25:812-830, 1971

42. Woods RL, Levi JA, Page J, et al: Non-small cell cancer: A randomized comparison of chemotherapy with no chemotherapy. Proc Am Soc Clin Oncol 4:177, 1985

PART V

Stage III$_{M_1}$/Stage IV Non-Small Cell Lung Cancer

John C. Ruckdeschel

_____ 18 _____

Chemotherapy of Disseminated Non-Small Cell Lung Cancer

The majority of patients with non-small cell lung cancer (NSCLC) will either present with, or develop, metastatic disease, and this development will invariably lead to their death.[5] The sole treatment modality available to deal with metastatic disease remains chemotherapy. Controversy exists, however, as to whether the use of chemotherapy contributes in a positive way to either the quantity or quality of life.[1] NSCLC is notorious for the extent of primary resistance to chemotherapeutic agents, and this de novo resistance has led many investigators to advocate that patients with disseminated NSCLC are prime candidates for phase I (determining the maximum tolerated dose) and II (efficacy) trials of new agents. Other investigators and some clinicians have developed sufficient nihilism about the results of therapy to suggest that patients with metastatic NSCLC should receive only supportive care. With the advent of cisplatin-containing regimens, most practicing oncologists feel that a trial of chemotherapy is warranted for patients in reasonably good shape. These differences in approach to a nearly uniformly fatal condition are, in part, a reflection of the confusion that exists in the literature about "response" and "survival" as a function of therapy. This chapter reviews the characteristics of both patients and treatments in clinical trials that permit an appropriate evaluation of chemotherapy and then review the regimens suggested as useful.

PATIENT CHARACTERISTICS

Any discussion of therapy for NSCLC is dependent on a careful description of the patient population involved. In many ways the search for dramatic advances in chemotherapeutic efficacy will not be hindered by a mixed patient population. A truly quantum leap in therapy will be obvious regardless of how poorly the study is designed. However, the history of progress in this disorder has been related to small, incremental advances. The necessity for a uniform patient population, then, becomes increasingly paramount.

LUNG CANCER: A COMPREHENSIVE TREATISE
ISBN 0-8089-1876-1

Many of the characteristics of a uniform patient population are obvious. Uniformity in histologic classification and stratification is the first priority. Patients whose tumors reflect complete or partial expression of neuroendocrine markers, characteristic of small cell carcinoma, will invariably have a higher response rate. Recent evidence suggests that many of the patients classified previously as having large cell anaplastic carcinoma may, in fact, have a form of neuroendocrine carcinoma that is a variant population of small cell lung cancer (SCLC).[6,14,17] Consequently, inclusion of these patients in a trial of chemotherapy for NSCLC will tend to overestimate the response rate; however, there may be only a marginal impact on survival.

This author believes that it is critical to carefully select patients by stage. The earlier staging system proposed by the American Joint Commission on Staging was inadequate to describe patient treatment groups.[33] Patients with advanced local-regional disease were grouped with patients having widespread metastases into a broad category of stage III disease and various treatment approaches attempted within this broad array of patients. Not surprisingly, there has been a diversity of clinical experience using the same treatment regimen. It appears that limiting new drug studies and comparative trials of chemotherapy to patients solely with distant metastatic disease is a more appropriate policy. The new staging system for lung cancer will make such an approach more feasible.[25] Patients with local-regional disease are subject to a large number of exclusionary criteria that may or may not make them candidates for an individual chemotherapy study. The relative degree of aggressiveness by surgeon and radiotherapist may dictate whether a patient with advanced mediastinal adenopathy is considered a candidate for an aggressive radiation approach or chemotherapy.[26] Inclusion of a significant number of patients with only mediastinal disease will skew the results if they are compared to a group of patients with bone, liver, and cutaneous metastases. Lumping these two patient groups does not permit scientific comparison between trials and should be discouraged. At the opposite extreme are patients who present with metastases to the brain. A number of large trials have included these patients on the grounds that they are "stable" following radiation therapy. While this may be true for the individual patient, it is not possible to predict which patients will experience a sudden deterioration in status as a result of progressive brain metastases. Hence this group has a generally more unfavorable outlook. Again, their inclusion in comparative clinical trials is unwarranted.

It goes without saying that patients included in randomized clinical trials should have had no prior treatment; yet, the issue of initial performance status warrants further comment. Most large groups have long since abandoned the study of chemotherapy in NSCLC patients with low performance status [Eastern Cooperative Oncology Group (ECOG) performance status (PS) 3 and 4]. However, many investigators routinely include patients with performance status 2 (confined to bed for less than half of waking hours) in major cooperative group trials. This, too, is a practice that should be discouraged. In one of the recent large ECOG trials, the issue of performance status was examined closely with respect to response and toxicity.[29] The patients who presented with performance status 2 had a response rate that was essentially identical to patients of lower performance status (PS 0 = 26 percent, PS 1 = 25 percent, PS 2 = 20 percent), but their median survival differed significantly (PS 0 = 36 weeks, PS 1 = 26 weeks, PS 2 = 10 weeks, $P = .001$). This is due almost entirely to treatment-related toxicity. In that trial of 486 patients, 92, or 19 percent, were initial PS = 2.

Nine of the twenty treatment related deaths, or 45 percent, were in this group of patients of initial PS = 2. Looked at in the other direction, 10 percent of all performance status 2 patients suffered a treatment related death.[30] Consequently, we are of the opinion that performance status 2 patients should not be included in broad phase III chemotherapy trials.

Both the ECOG and SWOG as well as Memorial Sloan Kettering Cancer Center have examined the relative contributions of specific sites of metastases and pretreatment symptoms on the outcome of patients.[12,23,27] All three series showed a consistent relationship of low performance status and male sex to a poor outcome. Each series reflected some impact of disease site or extent to survival. In the ECOG trial,[12] subcutaneous, bone, and liver metastases had an adverse effect on survival as well as pretreatment presence of bone pain, respiratory symptoms, reduced appetite, hoarseness, or the use of analgesics. The absence of many of these factors is related to relatively prolonged survival, as demonstrated in the analysis of 1-year survivors from two of the recent ECOG trials.[12] Table 18-1 summarizes the factors that appear to impact on response and survival in this group of patients. Obviously, an unbalanced number of patients with bone and liver metastases would skew the results of a comparative phase III trial. An excessive number of patients either with or without bone and liver metastases would surely impact on the ability to assess the results from a phase II trial (efficacy of therapy).

The assessment of the relative usefulness of chemotherapy for disseminated NSCLC is contingent on demonstrating a benefit in either quality or quantity of life for the patient with this disorder. This issue has led to heated discussions regarding the requirements for no treatment control groups in major trials. For many years the issue was felt to be impossible to study in the United States, where treating physicians were unwilling to place patients on a no-treatment, supportive-care-only arm. Because it was critical to assess new regimens and agents, the impact of a drug or drugs on response rates was used as a stalking horse for improved survival. For all of the previously cited reasons, the interpretation of single-arm, phase II studies is subject to a number of large variations. Consequently, we have focused on the evaluation of

Table 18-1

Prognostic Factors Related to Improved Survival for Patients with Metastatic NSCLC

Prognostically Favorable Factors	Significance P Value
Initial performance status, 0	< .0001
No distant metastasis to bone	< .0001
Sex, female	.0005
No distant metastasis to subcutaneous tissues	.006
Non-large cell histology	.011
Prior weight loss <5%	.001
No symptoms of shoulder, arm pain	.029
No distant metastasis to liver	.046

Modified from Finkelstein DM, Ettinger DS, Ruckdeschel JC: Long term survivors in metastatic non-small cell lung cancer. J Clin Oncol 4:702-709, 1986. With permission.

phase III comparative trials. While it is not of particular interest to the statistician (except as another potential prognostic factor), the presence or absence of a response to therapy is a component of the evaluation every clinician makes, both for the individual patient and in evaluating a new regimen across a group of patients. An agent that fails to cause any shrinkage of a patient's tumor (nonresponse) is of little or no interest in the armamentarium of a treating physician. Many trials have purported to demonstrate that patients who respond to therapy lived significantly longer than persons who failed to respond to therapy. While one would like to have such information to even begin the analysis of the usefulness of a regimen, the end result of too many studies was the use of this kind of responder–nonresponder comparison. There have been a number of cogent reviews discussing the inadequacy of this type of analysis.[2,16,38] There are two overriding factors involved in this. First, responders must live long enough to respond so that patients who die early in the study do not have a chance to attain a response. The responding group is therefore already preselected. Second, and probably more important, is the inability, without a control group, to ascertain whether the prolonged survival of responders is due to the therapy itself or to some previously unknown prognostic factor. While we and others have attempted to dispute this argument by citing the large number of prognostic factors already looked at, it is clear that this is a real possibility.[12] We have interpreted responder–nonresponder comparisons to mean that the regimen has at least met the basic criterion of having some activity and, when appropriate corrections are made in statistical technique, the significance of these comparisons is somewhat greater.[12,29] In particular, it would appear that even when corrected for other prognostic variables, response to therapy in itself is a significant predictor of prolonged survival.[29]

More recently a number of international trials have attempted to address this issue of a no-treatment control group. The first publication by a group in Australia consisted of a mixed group of regional and metastatic disease patients and was reported in preliminary fashion at the 1985 cancer meetings.[39] They failed to demonstrate any survival benefit in this preliminary report, but obviously further data are lacking. The National Cancer Institute of Canada, however, was able to compare vindesine plus cisplatin to CAP (cyclophosphamide, doxorubicin, and cisplatin) to a policy of supportive care only. Although difficulties were experienced with accrual, the results were presented in 1986 and demonstrate a significant survival advantage for the groups of patients who were randomized to chemotherapy.[28] In addition, it would appear that the more intensive cisplatin-containing regimen was superior to the less intensive regimen.[28] It is unlikely that these two trials will fully resolve this issue, but they at least provide reasonable evidence that patients who receive chemotherapy some benefit from it.

RESULTS OF CHEMOTHERAPY

The exploration of new agents and regimens in disseminated NSCLC has always been a high priority of physicians involved in clinical research in this area. Single agents have, by and large, had very modest effectiveness, with the impressive response rates of a handful of agents more likely due to variations in the prognostic factors for the patients making up the group than to any intrinsic activity of the drugs

Table 18-2

Recently Tested Single Agents With Some Activity in
Non-Small Cell Lung Cancer

Drug	Reference
Ifosfamide	21
Cisplatin	21
Carboplatin	4
Triazinate	7
Vinblastine	34
Vindesine	19
Etoposide	21
Mitoxantrone	35
Lonidamine	9

themselves.[21] Table 18-2 lists a number of the agents with demonstrated activity in the more contemporary trials.[7,9,19,34,35]

The phase III comparison of regimens reported active in earlier trials has been a critical need over the past few years, and most of the major regimens have now been analyzed for their relative effectiveness. Table 18-3 outlines the specific regimens that have been reported through this year in large, randomized trials. Phase II trials have

Table 18-3

Results of Recent Randomized Trials of Combination Chemotherapy for Metastatic NSCLC

Study Combinations*	Number of Patients	CR + PR (%)	Median Survival (M.)	Reference
C/A/VP	29	10.3	5.5	13
C/A/VP/PLAT	36	27.7	8.5	
VDA/PLAT	48	33.0	8.5	22
VBL/PLAT	49	41.0	12.3	
VDA/PLAT (high)	40	40.0	12.0	18
VDA/PLAT (low)	41	46.0	5.6	
VDA/PLAT	62	35.0	5.8	10
VP/PLAT	67	30.0	5.8	
VDA/VP/PLAT	62	22.0	5.6	
FU/VCR/MI	127	26.0	5.0	23
C/A/PLAT/	132	17.0	6.0	
FU/VCR/MI/C/A/PLAT	126	22.0	5.75	
C/BLEO/PLAT	112	20.0	5.5	30
A/FU/PLAT	109	17.0	5.25	
MI/VBL/PLAT	104	26.0	5.8	
C/A/PLAT	107	23.0	5.8	
VP/PLAT	124	20.0	6.5	29
C/A/MTX/PROC	115	17.0	6.25	
MI/VBL/PLAT	121	31.0	5.5	
VDA/PLAT	126	26.0	6.5	

*Abbreviations: A = doxorubicin; BLEO = bleomycin; C = cyclophosphamide; FU = 5-fluorouracil; MTX = methotrexate; MI = mitomycin C; PLAT = cisplatin; PROC = procarbazine; VBL = vinblastine; VCR = vincristine; VDA = vindesine; VP = VP 16-213 (etoposide).

suggested that high-dose cisplatin-containing regimens have more activity than do previous non-cisplatin-containing regimens.[18] Although this may be true, the analysis of EST 1581 failed to confirm a significant survival advantage and showed a significantly increased toxicity for the high dose cisplatin regimens.[29] In addition, there is no clear evidence that any of the high-dose cisplatin regimens are superior to moderate-dose cisplatin-containing regimens.[12,29] Nonetheless, the degree of activity seen with moderate- and high-dose cisplatin-containing regimens does appear higher than earlier combinations that did not include these compounds.

CURRENT RECOMMENDATIONS FOR USE OF CHEMOTHERAPY

The analysis of these large group trials has demonstrated that virtually all responses occur within the first 6–12 weeks of initiating therapy, although the duration with which these responses last may be a function of a more prolonged period to attain response.[12] In addition, no one has observed a survival benefit from chemotherapy for nonresponding patients. Consequently, the suggestion made by Minna and colleagues that patients in good performance status be given a trial of chemotherapy (two courses) would appear to be warranted.[10,13,18,23,24] The extent of response after two cycles can be measured against the degree of toxicity. In those patients who show an improved quality of life, there is little doubt that continuing chemotherapy would be beneficial. For the patients who achieve a response at high price relative to toxicity, the issue is less clear and must be individualized. The absence of response after two cycles, with or without significant toxicity, suggests little or no usefulness for the chemotherapy regimen employed. Given the nature of this disease, there is no indication that continuing therapy will be of any value. Therefore, we analyze patients for response after two cycles of therapy, and if they have shown some degree of response they are continued on therapy if toxicity permits. Patients with minor regressions that have not yet reached a true partial response (50 percent reduction in size) may be considered for additional courses of chemotherapy, as the analysis of 1-year survivors in the ECOG trials demonstrated that slower response was correlated with prolonged duration of response.[12,30]

NEW APPROACHES TO CHEMOTHERAPY OF DISSEMINATED NSCLC

The search for new agents continues unabated. Previous phase I and II trials were designed on the basis of work from highly responsive mouse cancers. These previously performed phase I and II trials have contributed little to the identification of new agents in this disease.[11,36] With the development of both small cell and non-small cell cell lines,[15,32] the NCI is examining the policy of exploring in vitro responsiveness of these generally refractory cell lines to chemotherapeutic agents and moving effective drugs into clinical trial in an expedited fashion. The relative success of such an approach has yet to be established, but the first drugs are now coming into clinical study.

It is now possible to isolate and grow a reasonable proportion of NSCLCs in vitro and/or to establish them under the renal capsule of cyclosporine treated mice.[3,20,31,37] Each of these techniques leads to the ability to examine, in a prospective fashion, the relative chance of success for that particular agent. These techniques are not yet well worked out for combinations of drugs, and none of the procedures has been demonstrated to be ready for direct and routine clinical usage. Nonetheless, this approach should be available within the next few years.

Finally, the understanding of the growth requirements for small cell anaplastic lung cancer has led to the description of bombesin, the amphibian analogue of human gastrin releasing peptide, as an autocrine growth factor for small cell lung cancer.[8] A novel approach that will inhibit this growth factor is an anti-bombesin antibody that has entered clinical trials. The results of this anti-bombesin antibody in animal models show significant cytolysis.[8] Further description of the growth requirements of NSCLC may allow identification of appropriate growth factors whose action can be interfered with and ultimately lead to therapeutic benefit for the patient.

ACKNOWLEDGMENT

The expert secretarial assistance of Ms. Gina Centanni is gratefully acknowledged.

REFERENCES

1. Aisner J, Hansen HH: Commentary: Current status of chemotherapy for non-small cell lung cancer. Cancer Treat Rep 65:979-986, 1981

2. Anderson JR, Cain KC, Gelber RD: Analysis of survival by tumor response. J Clin Oncol 1:710-719, 1983

3. Bennett JA, Pilon VA, MacDowell RT: Evaluation of growth and histology of human tumor xenografts implanted under the renal capsule of immuno-competent and immune-deficient mice. Cancer Res 45:4963-4969, 1985

4. Bonomi P, Menta C, Ruckdeschel J, et al: Phase II-III trial of mitomycin-vinblastine-cisplatin (MVP); vinblastine-cisplatin (VP); MVP alternating with cyclophosphamide-adriamycin-methotrexate-procarbazine (MVP/CAMP); CBDCA followed by MVP and CHIP followed by MVP in patients with metastatic non-small cell (NSCLC): An ECOG study. Proc Am Soc Clin Oncol 6:177, 1987

5. Cancer Patient Survival, Report Number 5, DHEW Publ No NIH 77-992, 1977

6. Carney DN, Gazdar AF, Bepler G et al: Establishment and identification of small cell lung cancer cell lines having classic and variant features. Cancer Res 45:2913, 1985

7. Creech RH, Mehta CR, Cohen M, et al: Results of a phase II protocol for evaluation of new chemotherapeutic regimens in patients with inoperable non-small cell lung carcinoma (EST 2575, generation I). Cancer Treat Rep 65:431-438, 1981

8. Cuttitta F, Carney DN, Mulshine JL, et al: Bombesin-like peptide can function as an autocrine growth factor in human small cell lung cancer. Nature 316:823-826, 1985

9. DeGregorio M, Kokron O, Scheiner W: Phase II study of lonidamine in inoperable non-small cell lung cancer. Proceedings of the 13th International Congress of Chemotherapy, Vienna 248:97-99, 1983

10. Dhingra HM, Valdivieso M, Carr DT, et al: Randomized trial of three combinations of cisplatin with vindesine and/or VP-16-213 in the treatment of advanced non-small cell lung cancer. J Clin Oncol 3:176-183, 1985

11. Driscoll JS: The preclinical new drug research program of the National Cancer Institute. Cancer Treat Rep 68:63-76, 1984

12. Finkelstein DM, Ettinger DS, Ruckdeschel JC: Long term survivors in metastatic non-small cell lung cancer. J Clin Oncol 4:702–709, 1986

13. Fuks JZ, Aisner J, Van Echo DA, et al: Randomized study of cyclophosphamide, doxorubicin and etoposide (VP16-213) with or without cis-platinum in non-small cell lung cancer. J Clin Oncol 1:295–301, 1983

14. Gazdar AF, Carney DN, Nau MM, et al: Characterization of variant subclasses of cell lines derived from small cell lines having distinctive biochemical, morphological and growth properties. Cancer Res 45:2924, 1985

15. Gazdar AF, Carney DN, Russell EK, et al: Establishment of continuous, clonable small cell carcinomas of the lung cultures having amine precursor uptake and decarboxylation properties. Cancer Res 40:3502, 1980

16. Glatstein E, Makuch RW: Illusion and reality: Practical pitfalls in interpreting clinical trials. J Clin Oncol 2:488–497, 1984

17. Gould VE, Warren WH, Memoli VA: Neuroendocrine neoplasms of the lung. Light microscopic, immunohistochemical and ultrastructural pattern, in Becker KL, Gazdar AF (eds): The Endocrine Lung in Health and Disease. Philadelphia, Saunders, 1984, p 406

18. Gralla RJ, Casper ES, Kelsen DP, et al: Cisplatin and vindesine combination chemotherapy for advanced carcinoma of the lung: A randomized trial investigating two dosage schedules. Ann Intern Med 95:414–420, 1981

19. Gralla RJ, Raphael BG, Golbey RB: Phase II evaluation of vindesine in patients with non-small cell carcinoma of the lung. Cancer Treat Rep 63:1343–1346, 1979

20. Griffen TW, Bogden AE, Reich SD, et al: Initial clinical trials of the subrenal capsule assay as a predictor of tumor response to chemotherapy. Cancer 52:2185–2192, 1983

21. Joss RA, Cavalli F, Goldhirsch A, et al: New agents in non-small cell lung cancer. Cancer Treat Rev 11:205–216, 1984

22. Kris MG, Gralla RJ, Kalman LA, et al: Randomized trial comparing vindesine plus cisplatin with vinblastine plus cisplatin in patients with non-small cell lung cancer, with analysis of methods of response assessment. Cancer Treat Rep 69:387–395, 1985

23. Miller TP, Chen T, Coltman CA, et al: Effect of alternating combination chemotherapy on survival of ambulatory patients with metastatic large cell and adenocarcinoma of the lung. J Clin Oncol 4:502–508, 1986

24. Minna JD, Higgins GA, Glatstein EJ: Cancer of the lung, in DeVita VT Jr, Hellman S, Rosenberg SA (eds): Cancer: Principles and Practice of Oncology, 2d ed. Philadelphia, Lippincott, 1985, pp 507–597

25. Mountain CF: A new international staging system for lung cancer. Chest 89:225–233S, 1986

26. Mulshine JL, Glatstein E,.Ruckdeschel, JC: The treatment of non-small cell lung cancer. J Clin Oncol 4:1704–1715, 1986

27. O'Connell JP, Kris MG, Gralla RJ, et al: Frequency and prognostic importance of pre-treatment clinical characteristics in patients with advanced non-small cell lung cancer treated with combination chemotherapy. J Clin Oncol 4:1604–1614, 1986

28. Rapp E, Arnold A, Ayoub J, et al: A comparison of best supportive care to two regimens of combination chemotherapy in the management of extensive non-small cell lung cancer (NSCLC)—a report of a Canadian multicentre trial. Proc Am Soc Clin Oncol 6:168, 1987

29. Ruckdeschel JC, Finkelstein DM, Ettinger DS, et al: A randomized trial of the four most active regimens for metastatic non-small cell lung cancer. J Clin Oncol 4:14–22, 1986

30. Ruckdeschel JC, Finkelstein DM, Mason BA, et al: Chemotherapy for metastatic non-small cell bronchogenic carcinoma: EST 2575, generation V-A randomized comparison of four cisplatin-containing regimens. J Clin Oncol 3:72–79, 1985

31. Ruckdeschel JC, Gazdar AF, Carney DN, et al: The use of human cancer cell lines for in vitro chemosensitivity testing. Proc Am Assoc Cancer Res 26:367, 1985

32. Ruckdeschel JC, Oie HK, Gazdar AF: In vitro characterization on non-small cell lung cancer, in Hansen HH (ed): Lung Cancer: Basic and Clinical Aspects. Boston, Martin Nijhoff, 1985, p 49

33. Staging of Lung Cancer, 1979. American Joint Committee for Cancer Staging and End-Results Reporting. Task force on lung cancer [Mountain CF (chairman), Carr DT, Marini N, et al]. Chicago; also Manual for Staging of Cancer 1978, pp 59-64; Chicago, American Joint Committee for Cancer Staging and End-Results Reporting, 1978

34. Shulman P, Budman DR, Vinciguerra V: Phase II study of divided dose vinblastine in non-small cell bronchogenic carcinoma. Cancer Treat Rep 66:171-172, 1982

35. Valdivieso M, Umasawasdi T, Spitzer G: Phase II clinical study of dihydroxyanthracene-dione (DHAD) in patients (pts) with advanced lung cancer (ALC). Proc Am Assoc Cancer Res 23:145, 1982

36. Venditti JM: Preclinical drug development: Rationale and methods. Semin Oncol 8:349-361, 1981

37. Weisenthal LM, Marsden JA, Dill PI, et al: A novel dye exclusion method for testing in vitro chemosensitivity of human tumors. Cancer Res 43:749, 1983

38. Weiss GB, Bunce H, Hokanson JA: Comparing survival of responders and non-responders after treatment: A potential source of confusion in interpreting cancer clinical trials. Controlled Clin Trials 4:43-52, 1983

39. Woods RL, Levi JA, Page J, et al: Non-small cell lung cancer: A randomized comparison of chemotherapy with no chemotherapy. Proc Am Soc Clin Oncol 4:177, 1986

Azhar M. Awan
Ralph R. Weichselbaum

_____ **19** _____

The Role of Radiation Therapy in Stage III$_{M_1}$ Non-Small Cell Lung Cancer

Radiation therapy plays an important role in the management of patients with metastatic non-small cell lung cancer (NSCLC). The majority of the individuals who have stage III M_1 disease will require radiation at some point in the course of the disease for relief of any one of several symptoms. Radiotherapeutic intervention does not prolong survival. The aim of therapy in these individuals is to palliate specific symptoms in an attempt to improve the quality of life. In this chapter we will delineate the role of radiation therapy in treating the primary tumor site in the chest as well as sites of distant metastases in patients with stage III M_1 lung cancer.

PALLIATION OF CHEST SYMPTOMS

Individuals with metastatic disease may have symptoms at either the primary tumor site in the chest or at distant sites. Some symptoms may develop prior to the use of any systemic therapy, and the patient must be evaluated prior to systemic treatment to assess whether local radiation should be administered first. If there are no pressing circumstances that require immediate radiation, systemic therapy can be initiated with close follow-up of the patient. However, there are some circumstances where specific problems such as impending bronchial obstruction, hemoptysis, tracheal or esophageal compromise, or superior vena caval obstruction may require more urgent initiation of radiotherapy. In the patient who is asymptomatic in the chest, there is controversy regarding the early use of radiotherapy.[3,17] It is our opinion that radiotherapy for the asymptomatic patient should be delayed until symptoms develop that require palliation. Prophylactic chest irradiation should be reserved for the rare individual who is prone to noncompliance and who is in danger of being lost to follow-up.

The goal of radiotherapy in chest symptom palliation is to provide an adequate dose in as short a time as possible to achieve the symptom relief necessary. In those patients with a survival of only a few months, protracted radiotherapy should be

LUNG CANCER: A COMPREHENSIVE TREATISE
ISBN 0-8089-1876-1

Table 19-1
Symptom Relief Achieved by
Thoracic Irradiation

Symptom	Response (%)
Superior vena caval obstruction	86
Hemoptysis	84
Pain (brachial plexus)	73
Pain (chest)	61
Dyspnea	60
Atelectasis	23
Vocal cord paralysis (hoarseness)	6

Modified from Slawson RG, Scott RM: Radiation Therapy in
bronchogenic carcinoma. Radiology 132:175-176, 1979. With
permission.

avoided so that they do not spend a significant percentage of their remaining lives undergoing treatment. A commonly used dose schedule is 3000 rads in 10 fractions over 2 weeks. In certain instances, depending on the status of the patient and the treatment site in the chest, dose schedules such as 2000 rads in five fractions over a 1 week period may be employed. Table 19-1 illustrates the frequency of symptomatic relief for a number of chest symptoms. For example, vocal cord paralysis secondary to recurrent laryngeal nerve involvement rarely is reversible. Atelectasis secondary to bronchial obstruction has only about a 25 percent chance for successful treatment with radiation therapy. The longer the duration of lobar or total lung collapse, the less likely the chance of reexpansion by the use of radiotherapy. Laser excision of endobronchial lesions with or without the use endobronchial brachytherapy is an alernative to external beam radiation for bronchial obstruction.[15,24] Symptoms such as hemoptysis, dyspnea, and pain have a very good chance of achieving symptomatic relief with external beam radiation.

Management of Superior Vena Caval Obstruction (See Chapter 27)

Obstruction of the flow of blood from the head and the upper extremities to the right heart, secondary to the obstruction of the superior vena cava, results in a clinical entity known as the superior vena cava syndrome. Superior vena cava (SVC) syndrome can be an acute or subacute event that usually requires prompt intervention to reduce the chances of irreversible superior vena caval thrombosis, central nervous system damage or pulmonary complications. Lung cancer is a leading etiology of SVC syndrome. Approximately one-half of the cases will be related to small cell carcinomas. Malignant lymphomas are the next most common cause for SVC syndrome.[14] Benign causes of SVC syndrome include thyroid goiter, primary SVC thrombosis and in the past included complications of syphilis and tuberculosis.[14,21,23]

Superior vena caval obstruction results from either an extrinsic compression of the blood vessel by either nodal metastases or the primary tumor itself or by direct extension of disease through the vessel wall. The superior vena cava is susceptible to obstruction because of the anatomic location of the vessel in the thorax, bounded by the sternum anteriorly and the right main-stem bronchus to the right. The vessel lies posterior to the right anterior mediastinal nodes and anterior to the right paratracheal lymph nodes. Thus the vessel is highly susceptible to compression.

The most common signs and symptoms of superior vena caval obstruction are neck and thoracic vein distension, facial edema, and shortness of breath. Less common features include cyanosis, facial plethora, and upper-extremity edema. On the basis of these physical findings, the diagnosis of superior vena cava syndrome can be made on clinical grounds and disgnostic studies such as venograms avoided. The chest radiograph usually will show a superior mediastinal mass. In cases where no prior diagnosis of malignancy has been made, invasive diagnostic studies such as the bronchoscopy or mediastinoscopy will be required to establish the histopathological diagnosis. These can be pursued prior to initiation of radiation therapy in cases where the surgeon is confident of achieving hemostasis. In cases where SVC syndrome is rapidly progressive, however, urgent therapy may have to be instituted prior to obtaining a histopathological diagnosis.

In NSCLC, the treatment of choice for superior vena cava obstruction is external beam radiation. Chemotherapy can be an effective modality in small-cell lung cancer (SCLC) and lymphomas. Other forms of treatment include the use of corticosteroids, anticoagulation, and—in certain rare cases—surgery. Green and Rubin in both experimental and clinical studies showed that high dose fractions used initially are both safe and effective in reversing the signs and symptoms of SVC syndrome.[9,19] They advocated doses of 400 rads for the first three fractions. The fraction size can then be decreased to 200 rads per fraction. The radiation portal should include the mediastinal and hilar lymph nodes and the primary tumor site if it is in proximity to the hilum or mediastinum. Subjective response usually is prompt, occurring within 3–4 days. By the seventh day, over 90 percent of patients have achieved a subjective response. Objective responses such as resolution of edema, venous distention and radiographic improvement occurs between 7 and 19 days.[5] There usually is no subjective or objective response with SVC syndrome as a result of superior vena caval thrombosis. Thromboses can extend proximally to the internal jugular veins up to the base of the skull.

The prognosis for patients with NSCLC who present with superior vena cava syndrome is similar to that of inoperable lung cancer if they have a good response to initial radiation therapy and if the radiation is continued to high doses. However, the total dose delivered is dependent on the extent of intrathoracic and extrathoracic disease. In general, high-dose radiation therapy should be reserved for patients whose disease can be encompassed in one radiation portal and who have no extrathoracic disease. Patients with more extensive disease should receive therapy sufficient to ensure good response (3000–4000 rads), and therapy can then be directed to their systemic disease. Whereas systemic chemotherapy may be very effective alone or as an adjuvant in the treatment of SVC syndrome in SCLC, such therapy is of limited value as an adjunct to radiation therapy in NSCLC.

MANAGEMENT OF SKELETAL METASTASES

The most common primary tumors that metastasize to bone include: breast, lung, and prostate. Nearly half the patients with these primary tumors will develop skeletal metastases in the course of the disease. Both SCLC as well as non-small cell tumors have a high propensity to metastasize to bone.

Patients who develop bony metastases most frequently present with localized pain at the site of bony involvement. Percussion or palpation tenderness at a bony site is a reliable sign of bone involvement with tumor. Certain bony sites will produce pain on weight-bearing (e.g., femur lesions) or radicular pain (vertebral body lesions). Skeletal metastases rarely are life-threatening but can cause significant morbidity such as pain, fractures, or neurologic sequalae from nerve entrapment caused by bony destruction. Local therapy for bony metastases includes surgery and radiation therapy. Orthopedic procedures are used for treatment of pathologic fractures or for prophylactic stabilization of lesions that have the potential for producing a pathological fracture in the future. In weight-bearing bones, prophylactic pinning of the bone is recommended if greater than one-third of the cross-sectioned diameter of bone is involved with a lytic lesion.[6] Radiation therapy is employed in the treatment of painful skeletal metastases as well as treating asymptomatic lesions in sites where a pathologic fracture could occur if the disease progressed. Radiation is also used as an adjunct to an orthopedic procedure such as an open reduction and internal fixation of a pathologic fracture of the femoral neck.

The total dose of radiation and the daily fraction size used in the treatment of skeletal metastases is dependent on the extent and location of the metastatic disease. The goal of therapy is to provide symptomatic relief in as short a time as possible. Since the mechanism of pain production in skeletal metastases is the stretching of and pressure on the periosteum by tumor, a very small degree of tumor lysis can cause significant relief of symptoms. The traditional dose schedule for the treatment of bony metastases is 3000 rads in 10 fractions. However, shorter courses such as 2000 rads in five fractions and 1500 rads in five fractions may produce nearly equivalent results in half the time.[6,11] In sites where radiation of sensitive structures such as bowel and central nervous system (CNS) tissue can be avoided, one or two treatments with very high doses such as 600–800 rads, in two to three fractions may be appropriate. Such areas include the appendicular skeleton and the ribs. Patients receiving a protracted course of radiation may have symptom relief rates much higher than those receiving short-course radiation at the end of therapy. Within a few weeks, however, symptom relief is usually equivalent in both groups. In the rare instance where there is a single lesion present, high-dose protracted radiation therapy may be considered in order to ensure a more complete response and delay a local recurrence. The complete and partial response rate can vary from 40 percent to as high as 90 percent.

In contrast to the use of local radiation, more extensive and widespread disease can be treated with sequential hemibody radiation. A single fraction of 600–800 rads to the upper hemibody can be followed in after approximately 1 month time with the same dose in a single fraction to the lower hemibody.[20]. Lower hemibody radiation is tolerated quite well without any significant symptomotology, but upper hemibody radiation can result in transient nausea or vomiting. Most patients achieve a partial or complete resolution of pain that usually persists for the duration of their lifetimes. Systemic hemibody radiation generally is reserved for those patients who have widespread metastatic disease and life expectancies of approximately 2–3 months. The major subacute consequence of hemibody radiation is radiation pneumonitis, which can be significantly reduced if doses do not exceed 600 rads.[7] A transient pancytopenia similar to chemotherapy effects can also occur.

MANAGEMENT OF BRAIN METASTASES

Brain metastases are more common in adenocarcinoma and large cell carcinoma and less common in squamous cell carcinoma. Patients with brain metastases may present with symptoms of increased intracranial pressure such as headache. They may also present with seizures or local neurologic deficits. A CT scan of the brain should be obtained in lung cancer patients with obvious CNS signs or symptoms. The therapy for brain metastases is dependent on the number and location of the metastatic lesions, the patient's performance status, the status of the primary tumor site and other metastatic disease sites, and disease-free interval between the development of brain metastases and initial treatment at the primary site. Surgery may be used in solitary lesions located in favorable locations in the brain in patients who have had a long disease-free interval between primary treatment and the development of brain metastases. However, most patients are candidates only for radiation therapy. When there is evidence of increased intracranial pressure, adjunctive medical treatment is important and should be initiated prior to and concomitant with the use of radiation therapy. Such measures include the use of corticosteroids, usually dexamethasone, 8-10 mg IV initially, followed by 4-6 mg every 6 hours or IV mannitol given in bolus form. In very rare instances, surgical management such as the placement of a ventricular shunt may be necessary. In some instances, patients may be placed on anticonvulsants such as phenytoin.

Radiation therapy is an effective modality in the symptomatic treatment of overt brain metastases. Since the median survival of these patients is 3-4 months, radiation therapy should be effective and yet not protracted. Treatment strategies involving large dose per fraction irradiation have emerged as the standard form of therapy for brain metastases. Such dose schedules allow for adequate doses to be delivered in a short time, usually about 2 weeks. A high-dose protracted course of radiotherapy for brain metastases may be warranted for certain patients who have one or two lesions located peripherally and who have no or only limited extracranial disease.

Although there are several reports of the results of radiotherapy in treating brain metastases, the most extensive investigations have been performed by the Radiation Therapy Oncology Group (RTOG)[1]. The RTOG studied the use of radiotherapy in the palliation of brain metastases in two sequential phase III randomized studies. Both of these studies entered large numbers of patients (910 patients in the first study and 902 patients in the second study were evaluable); thus, these two studies contribute significantly to the data regarding brain metastases. Among the two studies, five dose schedules were evaluated: (1) 2000 rads in 1 week, (2) 3000 rads in 2 weeks, (3) 3000 rads in 3 weeks, (4) 4000 rads in 3 weeks, and (5) 4000 rads in 4 weeks.

Table 19-2 outlines the performance status and neurologic impairments that were used in the assessment of treatment response. The patients within the four neurologic function groups were considered separately in the evaluation. Patients with initial neurologic function class 1 could be evaluated only with respect to how long they remained in that class. Patients with initial neurologic function class 2 could either have remained in that class, deteriorated to a lower class, or improved completely to class 1. Patients with neurologic function class 3 could have improved to class 2 or 1.

Table 19-3 shows the percentage of patients with lung cancer who showed improvement in neurologic function in both studies. In all patients, overall response and specific neurologic symptom relief varied from 69 to 86 percent for several symptoms

Table 19-2
General Performance and Neurologic Function Classifications

Class	Description
General Performance Status	
1	Normal
2	Symptoms, but ambulatory
3	Bedridden $\leq 50\%$ of the time
4	Bedridden $> 50\%$ of the time
5	100% bedridden
Neurologic Function	
1	Able to work or perform normal activities; neurologic findings minor or absent
2	Able to carry out normal activities with minimal difficulties; neurologic impairment does not require nursing care or hospitalization
3	Seriously limited in performing normal activities; requiring nursing care or hospitalization; confined to bed or wheelchair, or having significant intellectual impairment
4	Unable to perform even minimal normal activities; requiring hospitalization and constant nursing care and feeding; unable to communicate or comatose

Adapted from Borgelt B, Gelber R, Kramer S, et al: The palliation of brain metastases: Final results of the first two studies by the Radiation Therapy Oncology Group. Internatl J Radiat Oncol Biol Phys 6:1-9, 1980. With permission.

such as headache, motor loss, seizures, and lethargy. Complete response was highest in symptomatic relief of generalized seizures (66 percent) and lowest for patients with motor loss (32 percent). Similar data were obtained in the second study, with 87 percent complete response for patients with generalized convulsions and 37 percent complete response for patients with motor loss. The results obtained were independent of the dose schedule used. The overall median survival for all patients was 18 weeks in the first study and 15 weeks in the second study. Again, no significant differences were found among the treatment schedules used. Brain metastases were reported to be the cause of death for 49 and 31 percent of patients in the first and second studies, respectively. Specifically for patients with lung cancer, the median survival was 16 weeks, which was inferior to the survival of breast cancer patients (21 weeks, $p < .001$). A significant finding for lung cancer patients was the fact that patients in whom brain was the only site of metastases and who had a controlled primary and received 4000 rads in 3 weeks had a significantly prolonged median survival of 47 weeks. The efficacy of radiation in patients with brain metastases and

Table 19-3
Percentage of Lung Cancer Patients Improving
in Neurologic Function After Cranial Irradiation

Initial Functional Class 2	Initial Functional Class 3
First study ——— 38% —————————→ 62%	
Second study —— 37% —————————→ 72%	

Modified from Borgelt B, Gelber R, Kramer S, et al: The palliation of brain metastases: Final results of the first two studies by the Radiation Oncology Group. Internatl J Radiat Oncol Biol Phys 6:1-9, 1980. With permission.

controlled primary tumor sites is currently being studied by the RTOG. Other studies initiated by the RTOG include the use of radiation therapy in combination with hypoxic cell sensitizers such as misonidazole.

MANAGEMENT OF LIVER METASTASES

A significant portion of patients with lung cancer will develop liver metastases. The prognosis of patients with liver metastases is dependent on the extent of hepatic involvement. Patients with solitary lesions have a more favorable prognosis than to those with diffuse metastatic disease. Liver metastases may be asymptomatic initially and detected on routine screening tests such as liver function tests, radionuclide scans, or CT scans. Symptoms may include pain secondary to distension of the capsule of liver, liver dysfunction leading to icterus, fatigue, generalized malaise, and nausea and vomiting.

Therapy for patients with liver metastases generally is palliative but may be curative in the rare individual who presents with a solitary metastases with controlled extrahepatic disease. Surgical resection of such a lesion may result in prolonged disease-free survival. Palliative modalities include systemic chemotherapy, radiation therapy, and in some instances, limited surgical excisions. Previously, radiation was avoided in the treatment of liver metastases because normal liver tolerance was of major concern. With the experience gained in irradiating liver in some disease such as malignant lymphomas and abdominal pelvic radiation for ovarian cancer, however liver tolerance is now known. For example, Ingold et al.[12] studied radiation hepatitis in a group of patients who underwent whole-liver irradiation in the course of treatment for ovarian carcinoma.[12] The incidence of radiation hepatitis increased above doses of 3000 rads in 3 weeks. One patient developed radiation hepatitis at 3000 rads. It should be noted, however, that if higher doses per fraction are used, the total dose of radiation should be lower than 3000 rads. Most radiation oncologists do not treat the whole liver beyond 2100–2400 rads when dose fractions of 300 rads are used. Several reports in the literature point to the efficacy of radiation in palliation of patients with liver metastases. Prasad et al. reported the experience with 27 patients treated with whole liver irradiation.[18] The most common primary site was the colon and rectum, in nine patients, followed by lung primaries in four patients. Adenocarcinoma was the most common histology, accounting for 18 patients. Of these 27 patients, 11 were referred to radiation therapy after failure to respond to chemotherapy. Only 20 of their 27 patients completed the planned therapy. Some of the 7 patients who did not complete therapy died during treatment; in others, treatment was discontinued because of rapidly deteriorating medical condition. The doses received by their 20 patients who completed therapy ranged from 1900 to 3100 rads given in 2.5–4 weeks. If all 27 patients were analyzed, 19 patients (70 percent) had symptomatic relief of pain. If the 7 patients who did not complete planned therapy were excluded from the analysis, the symptomatic improvement rate increased to 95 percent (19 out of 20 patients).

Sherman et al.[22] reviewed the experience of 55 patients undergoing palliative radiation therapy for liver metastases. This was a retrospective study with a mixture of patients, since 31 patients received concomitant chemotherapy and 14 patients were prior chemotherapy failures.[22] There were 50 evaluable patients who completed therapy. Most of the patients had primary sites in the gastrointestinal tract with only one patient treated who had a lung primary. The majority of the patients received doses of 2100–2400 rads in 300-rad fractions over a 2-week period. However, the doses delivered ranged from 1500 to 3000 rads. Of the 31 patients who received concomitant chemotherapy, 17 were treated with 5-FU alone, while the remaining 14 received multiple agents. Most patients tolerated the treatment quite well, with severe nausea and vomiting as the most serious side effect and present mostly in patients who were receiving concomitant multiagent chemotherapy. Radiation induced hepatitis was not seen in any of the patients treated. Twenty-one patients had an excellent response to therapy that was equated with complete relief of pain and at least a 51 percent reduction in liver size for a minimum of 3 months. Twenty-two patients had a satisfactory response that was equated with substantial relief of pain and a reduction in liver size of 25–50 percent. Hence almost 90 percent of the patients had good symptomatic relief of pain and liver size.

The RTOG carried out a prospective pilot study to evaluate the palliation of hepatic metastases with radiotherapy.[2] This was a nonrandomized and uncontrolled study, designed mainly to gain information on the feasibility of hepatic irradiation. At the end of the study, 103 patients were evaluable, and in 25 percent of the patients studied, lung cancer was the primary site. In this study, 55 percent of the patients achieved some relief of abdominal pain. Nausea and vomiting and fever with night sweats improved in 49 percent of the patients. The patients who had the most severe symptoms at presentation had the most frequent and dramatic response rate. In approximately 50 percent of the patients, there was reduction in the palpable hepatic mass. There were no cases of radiation-induced hepatitis in this series. This RTOG study has lent further support to the retrospective studies previously carried out and point to the efficacy of irradiation in the palliation of hepatic metastases.

MANAGEMENT OF SPINAL CORD COMPRESSION

Epidural metastasis from a lung primary is one of the most common etiologies of spinal cord compression.[4] Extradural compression of the spinal cord (or the cauda equina below the first or second lumbar vertebral bodies) is a medical emergency requiring prompt treatment in order to reverse or prevent further neurologic damage. Intramedullary spinal cord metastases are quite rare. However, the clinical presentation may be similar to that of extradural cord compression.

Spinal cord compression usually arises at a site of bony metastasis to a vertebral body. The vertebral body usually is involved extensively with tumor and may even collapse, depending on the degree of destruction present. Since the etiology in most instances is due to tumor present in the vertebral body, the majority of the extradural metastases are anterior to the spinal cord. The most common site for cord compression due to a lung primary is the thoracic spine. In one series the thoracic spine was the site for 57 percent of all lung primary epidural spinal cord compressions, compared to 38 percent in cervical spine and 5 percent in the lumbo-sacral spine. The signs and symptoms of spinal cord compression can be subtle or obvious neurologic deficits such as autonomic dysfunction resulting in bowel and bladder incontinence, paralysis, and an ascending sensory loss. Most patients present with pain localized to the area of spinal cord compression. The pain may be local or radicular in nature.

Bowel and bladder incontinence is a very poor prognostic sign indicating advanced and possibly irreversible spinal cord compression. A high index of suspicion in patients with lung cancer who present with localized vertebral body pain can lead to early diagnosis of spinal cord compression and give the patient the best possible chance for preservation of neurologic function. The definitive diagnosis is made by myelography. Preferably both lumbar and cervical punctures are performed since these indicate the extent of the cord compression. A CT scan of the affected area might also be informative for both surgical planning as well as radiotherapy planning. The use of metrizamide as the contrast for the myelogram serves also as contrast material for the CT scan.

The treatment for spinal cord compression consists of radiation therapy, surgery, or a combination of the two modalities. There is no randomized study comparing the efficacy of surgery and radiotherapy in this clinical entity. The usual surgical treatment for epidural spinal cord compression is an attempt at decompression by a laminectomy. However, most metastases are anterior to the spinal cord since they arise from the vertebral bodies; thus the surgical approach is limited in that not all gross tumor can be removed from this posterior approach. Mortality and morbidity are factors to be taken into account when considering surgery. White et al. assessed decompression laminectomy performed on 226 patients.[25] In their study, 16 percent of the patients had breast cancer, with 14 percent having lung as the primary site. The 30 day mortality from the operation was 8.7 percent. In addition, neurologic function deteriorated as a direct result of surgery in 10 percent of the patients. They had 42 patients who were ambulatory preoperatively, and 64 percent of these patients were ambulatory postoperatively. Of the remaining patients 22 percent were nonambulatory after surgery and 14 percent were paraplegic. Of 155 patients who were nonambulatory prior to surgery, 35 percent became ambulatory postoperatively, 47 percent were unchanged neurologically, and 19 percent were paraplegic. Finally, 29 of their patients were paraplegic preoperatively; of these, 10 percent became ambulatory after the surgery, 76 percent remained paraplegic postoperatively, and 14 percent had mild improvement in neurologic function. Other surgical procedures include anterior decompression and stabilization of the spine by means of Harrington rod. The surgical series reporting such procedures contained very few patients but appeared to have a promising outlook.[10,13]

Radiation plays a very important role in the management of spinal cord compression. Many patients with spinal cord compression will receive radiation at some point in the course of the disease. Patients undergoing decompression laminectomy subsequently are referred for postoperative radiation therapy since the gross disease is usually left behind after such a surgical procedure. Gilbert et al. found no difference in the results obtained by surgery followed by postoperative radiation therapy and radiation therapy alone.[8] They reported on the experience with 170 patients, 65 of whom had surgery followed by postoperative radiation. Of the patients who received radiation alone, 49 percent were ambulatory at the end of treatment, compared to 46 percent of the patients who were ambulatory after the completion of surgery and postoperative radiation therapy. The best results were obtained in patients who were ambulatory prior to either therapy. Stratification of the patients by the initial neurologic symptoms and primary tumor site did not influence the results. There was no difference among patients who had radiation alone versus radiation following a surgical procedure. Interestingly, patients with tumors that were considered less radioresponsive such as melanoma and kidney had similar outcome regardless of whether they were treated by laminectomy followed by postoperative radiation therapy or by radiation alone.

Most centers used 3000 rads in 2 weeks or 4000 rads in 4 weeks as the standard treatment for cord compression resulting from epithelial tumors such as lung cancer. We generally employ 3000 rads in 10 fractions, but at times we vary the fractionation to fit a particular clinical situation. We also recommend the use of steroids for antiedema effects. Radiation should be initiated immediately after myelographic demonstration of a cord compression. There is very little role for systemic chemotherapy as the primary form of treatment for epidural spinal cord compression resulting from a NSCLC tumor, although there has been some success using chemotherapy for chemosensitive tumors such as lymphomas. Chemotherapy can be used as an adjunctive treatment either after surgery or radiation.

Regardless of the treatment chosen for patients with spinal cord compression, prompt attention and initiation of therapy leads to best outcome. Patients who are ambulatory at the time of diagnosis have a better chance of remaining ambulatory posttreatment, with less than 10 percent who are paraplegic at diagnosis becoming ambulatory after treatment. Similarly, patients with slowly progressive disease have a better treatment outcome compared to patients who have rapidly progressive neurologic disorders. Patients with loss of bladder or bowel control have a poor prognosis compared to those who are continent. The longer the duration of loss of sphincter control, the poorer the prognosis.

Since the results of surgery and radiation are for the most part fairly similar, other factors must be considered in making a judgment as to whether a patient should undergo laminectomy or irradiation alone. These include the patient's age, medical condition, and overall prognosis, determined by the patient's overall disease status. Patients who are young and have a low disease burden elsewhere may be candidates for surgical decompression. Another factor to consider is the fact that laminectomy carries a risk of immediate mortality, whereas no such risk is present for patients undergoing radiation alone. If surgery is performed, postoperative radiation therapy is invariably indicated unless the patient has had previous radiation that would preclude further treatment.

SUMMARY

In this chapter we have outlined the role of radiation in the palliative management of patients with stage III M_1 NSCLC. Judicious use of radiation can add to the quality of life of these patients with a poor longterm outlook. In general, protracted radiation therapy should be avoided and treatment should be delivered with high fractions in as short a time as possible so that patients do not remain on treatment for prolonged periods. The goal of therapy is to achieve palliation in as short a time possible while attempting to minimize the side effects of treatment.

REFERENCES

1. Borgelt B, Gelber R, Kramer S, et al: The palliation of brain metastasis: Final results of the first two studies by the Radiation Therapy Oncology Group. Internatl Radiat Oncol Biol Phys 6:1-9, 1980

2. Borgelt BB, Gelber R, Brady LW, et al: The palliation of hepatic metastasis: Results of Radiation Therapy Oncology Group pilot study. Internatl. J Radiat Oncol Biol Phys 7:587-591, 1981

3. Brashear RE: Should asymptomatic patients with inoperable bronchogenic carcinoma receive immediate radiotherapy? No. Am Rev Resp Dis 117:411-414, 1978

4. Bruckman JE, Bloomer WD: Management of spinal cord compression. Semin Oncol 5:135-140, 1978

5. Davenport D, Ferree CL, Blake D, et al: Response of superior vena caval syndrome to radiation therapy. Cancer 38:1577-1580, 1976

6. Drew M, Dickson RB: Osseous complications of malignancy, in Lokick J (ed): *Clinical Cancer Management,* Boston, GR Hall, 1980, p 19

7. Fryer CJH, Fitzpatrick PJ, Rider WD, et al: Radiation pneumonitis: experience following a large single dose of radiation. Internatl J Radiat Oncol Biol Phys 4:931-936, 1978

8. Gilbert RW, Kim JH, Posner JB: Epidural spinal cord compression from metastatic tumor. Diagnosis and treatment. Ann Neurol 3:40-51, 1978

9. Green J, Rubin P, Holzwasser G: The experimental production of superior vena caval obstruction: Trial of different therapy schedules. Radiology 81:406-414, 1963

10. Harrington KD: The use of methylmethacrylate for vertebral body replacement and anterior stabilization of pathological fracture dislocations of the spine due to metastatic malignant disease. J Bone Joint Surg 63:36-46, 1981

11. Hendrickson FR: Strategy of palliative treatment. Internatl J Radiat Oncol Biol Phys 8:155-156, 1982

12. Ingold JA, Reed GB, Kaplan H, et al: Radiation hepatitis. Am J Radiol 93:200-208, 1965

13. Lesoin F, Kabbaj J, Debout J, et al: The use of Harrington's rods in metastic tumors with spinal cord compression. Acta Neurochir 65:175-181, 1982

14. Lokich JJ, Goodman RL: Superior vena cava syndrome. JAMA 231:58-61, 1975

15. Mendiondo OA, Dillon M, Beach, LJ: Endobronchial brachytherapy in the treatment of recurrent and bronchogenic carcinoma. Internatl J Radiat Oncol Biol Phys 9:579-582, 1983

16. Perez CA, Presant CA, Amburg AL: Management of superior vena cava syndrome. Semin Oncol 5:123-234, 1978

17. Phillips TL, Miller RJ: Should asymptomatic patients with inoperable bronchogenic carcinoma receive radiotherapy? Yes. Am Rev Resp Dis 117:405-410, 1978

18. Prasad B, Lee MS, Hendricksons FR: Irradiation of hepatic metastases. Internatl J Radiat Oncol Biol Phys 2:129-132, 1977

19. Rubin P, Ciccio S: Superior mediastinal obstruction. High daily dose for rapid decompression in carcinoma of the bronchus, in Deeley TJ (ed): Carcinoma of the Bronchus. New York, Appleton-Century-Crofts, 1971, pp 276-297

20. Salazar OM, Rubin P, Hendrickson FR, et al: Single-dose half-body irradiation for palliation of multiple bone metastases from solid tumors. Int J Radiat Oncol Biol Phys 7:723, 1981

21. Schechter MM: The superior vena cava syndrome. Am J Med Sci 227:46-56, 1954

22. Sherman DM Weichselbaum R, Order SE, et al: Palliation of hepatic metastases. Cancer 41:2013-2017, 1978

23. Silverstein GE, Gurke G, Goldberg D, et al: Superior vena caval system obstruction caused by benign endothoracic goiter. Dis Chest 56:519-523, 1969

24. Slawson RG, Scott RM: Radiation therapy in bronchogenic carcinoma. Radiology 132:175-176, 1979

25. White WA, Patterson RH, Bergland RM: Role of surgery in the treatment of spinal cord compression by metastatic neoplasm. Cancer 27:558-561, 1971

PART VI

Small Cell Lung Cancer

Eric J. Seifter
Daniel C. Ihde

_____ **20** _____

Small Cell Lung Cancer: A Distinct Clinicopathologic Entity

Small cell lung cancer (SCLC) constitutes 20–25 percent of the 140,000 annual cases of lung cancer seen in the United States.[98] If SCLC were considered a separate disease, it would rank as the seventh most common cancer in incidence and as the fourth most common cause of cancer-related deaths. The unique biological and clinical features of SCLC merit its separation from the other histologic types of bronchogenic carcinoma. The rapid rate of cell division and the early dissemination of tumor account for the abrupt clinical presentation of SCLC and the low cure rates when only local therapeutic modalities are employed. When surgery or radiation therapy are used alone to treat SCLC, the end results are the worst among the different histologic types of lung cancer (Table 20-1). Prior to the use of chemotherapy, the median survival ranged from 8 to 17 weeks and the 5-year survival was invariably less than 1 percent.[26] However, SCLC is highly responsive to combination chemotherapy alone or chemotherapy combined with radiation therapy. The use of systemic therapy has improved the median survival of patients with SCLC (median, almost 1 year) and has increased the number of long-term disease-free survivors. The high response rate of SCLC to chemotherapy contrasts sharply with the minimal responses observed to cytotoxic chemotherapy in the other histologic types of lung cancer.

This chapter will focus on the clinical and pathologic features of SCLC that necessitate a specific management approach for this histologic type of lung cancer. Improved understanding of the natural history of SCLC has shaped the current recommendations for detection, staging, and therapy.

ETIOLOGY AND PATHOGENESIS

There is a significant association of SCLC with the inhalation of tobacco smoke. A clear dose-response relationship exists between cigarette consumption and lung cancer incidence or mortality.[134] The lung cancer rate has paralleled the increased inci-

LUNG CANCER: A COMPREHENSIVE TREATISE
ISBN 0-8089-1876-1

257

Table 20-1

Overall 5-Year Survival Percentage for the Major Histologic Types of Lung Cancer

| | | 5-Year Survival Percentage | |
Histologic Type	Percent Resectable	All Cases (N = 2155)	Resected (N = 835)
Small cell	11	1	0
Squamous cell	60	25	37
Adenocarcinoma and/or large cell	38	12	27

Modified from Minna JD, Higgins GA, Glatstein EJ: Cancer of the lung, in De Vita VT, Hellman S, Rosenberg SA (eds): Principles and Practice of Oncology. Philadelphia, Lippincott, 1985, pp 507-598. With permission.

dence of cigarette smokers with a lag time of 30-40 years for both men and women.[133] People who quit smoking experience a gradual decline in the risk of lung cancer over 10-15 years before approaching the risk of nonsmokers.[37] Although SCLC rarely occurs in the absence of a smoking history, cigarette smoking is also associated with other types of lung cancer, particularly squamous cell carcinoma. Unlike adenocarcinoma, SCLC seldom arises in areas of scarred or previously diseased lung. Instead, SCLC occurs in areas of well-ventilated lung tissue.[133]

Small cell cancer is the most common histologic type of lung cancer found among uranium miners.[6] Sequential sputum cytologies in this patient group have identified a progression from metaplasia to atypia to frank carcinoma. Cigarette smoke is also an important factor in the incidence of lung cancer in these miners. Whole-body exposure to more than 200 cGy of radiation may increase the risk of lung cancer, but this association is less well founded than the increased risk in uranium miners.[133] SCLC constitutes 15-30 percent of the lung cancers reported with exposure to nickel, cadmium, arsenic, chromate, and acrylonitrile.[133] There is a strong dose-response relationship between exposure to the chloromethyl ethers and the development of SCLC, since this histologic type constitutes almost 70 percent of the lung tumors associated with these compounds.[135]

The central location of most SCLC tumors is consistent with a mechanism of chronic mucosal irritation and absorption of carcinogens, particularly at points of bifurcation in the bronchial tree. The bronchial mucosa is lined with basal cells resting on a basement membrane. Some of the basal cells are argyrophilic and contain intracytoplasmic neurosecretory granules.[9,128] These cells appear to be functional equivalents to neuroendocrine cells of other tissues, such as the islet cells of the pancreas and the Kulchitsky cells of the intestinal tract. These amine precursor uptake and decarboxylation (APUD) cells are able to synthesize and secrete polypeptide hormones such as antidiuretic hormone, adrenocorticotropic hormone (ACTH), serotonin, glucagon, calcitonin, and gastrin-releasing peptide. The finding of neurosecretory granules by electron microscopy in small cell cancer biopsy specimens is a distinctive feature of SCLC.[8] The neuroendocrine nature of these cells may explain the presence of characteristic serum biochemical markers and the numerous paraneoplastic syndromes associated with this histologic type. No other type of lung cancer has neurosecretory granules with the exception of bronchial carcinoid tumors. Bronchial carcinoids have larger and more numerous intracytoplasmic granules.[88] Although the cell of origin remains in doubt, most authors believe that SCLC derives from pulmonary epithelial cells that differentiate along a neuroendocrine path in the fetal bronchus.[43] Surface antigens on SCLC shared with other cell types of diverse function and embryologic origin (such as macrophages) do not necessarily imply a common ancestry.[14,44,118] Neuroendocrine properties are also found, to a lesser extent, in other histologic types of lung cancer.[7] This lack of biochemical specificity supports the concept that the spectrum of lung cancers arises within a common cell lineage. Identification of neuro-endocrine features may eventually prove important in predicting the clinical course of response to therapy of individual tumors.

PATHOLOGY

The pathology of SCLC is discussed extensively in Chapter 2. In this chapter we will attempt to highlight some of the important histopathologic characteristics of SCLC. Small cell tumors are most frequently found in the submucosa with a laminar separation from the overlying basement membrane.[26] The tumor may circumferen-tially stenose the bronchial lumen or occasionally can exhibit exophytic intraluminal projections. Bronchoscopy reveals swelling and congestion of the mucosa, with thick-ening of bronchial spurs and narrowing of the bronchial lumen.[26,65] The tumor has a glossy gray-white mucoid surface that frequently is hemorrhagic or necrotic. Unlike squamous cell carcinoma, central liquefaction necrosis and cavitation are rare. The tumor may extend regionally to the main-stem bronchus and trachea or travel along the lymphatic channels to the bronchial, hilar, supraclavicular, and mediastinal lymph nodes. The tumor may invade, compress, or thrombose adjacent vasculature such as the superior vena cava or the pulmonary veins. Peripheral SCLC appears circum-scribed and similar in gross appearance to carcinoid or adenocarcinoma.

A most critical feature in the management of SCLC involves confirmation of the histologic diagnosis, since the clinical approach for SCLC differs markedly from the approach for non-small cell lung cancers (NSCLCs). Adequate histologic samples or multiple well-prepared cytologic specimens often are required for diagnosis. Needle biopsies often contain inadequate amounts of material or produce crushing artifacts that obscure the histologic features.[90] Rebiopsy for more tissue samples or for better tissue processing sometimes is necessary. Despite the submucosal location of the tumor, cytologic examination of bronchial washings often is helpful in establishing a diagnosis. Neoplastic cells tend to cluster and are two to three times larger than the surrounding lymphocytes. The early dissemination of SCLC and perhaps its rapid onset account for the inability of cytologic screening programs to detect earlier stages of SCLC or to impact on the existing survival rates.[58,129]

According to a revised World Health Organization (WHO) classification of lung cancer in 1981, SCLC is divided into three subtypes: (1) the classic oat cell (lympho-cyte-like) type, which is characterized by small, round, or oval cells with darkly staining nuclei, absent or indistinct nucleoli, and scanty cytoplasm; (2) an intermediate cell type that contains larger cells with a lower nuclear:cytoplasmic ratio, and more fusi-form or polygonal nuclei; and (3) combined mixtures of SCLC with other cell types of lung cancer.[124] A tendency toward clustering and nuclear molding, a salt-and-pepper distribution of nuclear chromatin, and the presence of necrotic areas and crush artifact are evident in all subtypes of SCLC. Blinded interpretation of histologic specimens by three qualified pathologists showed agreement in distinguishing SCLC from NSCLC in over 98 percent of cases but yielded only 54 percent agreement on designation of the subtype of SCLC.[61] Ultrastructural analysis by electron microscopy cannot distinguish between the two major subtypes of SCLC; the scanty cytoplasm consists of pseudopodal processes containing membrane-bound neurosecretory granules 800–2000 Å in diameter.[88] Subtypes may vary within the same tumor in 23 percent of patients.[19] Most large clinical series demonstrate no difference in clinical presentation, response to treatment, or survival for the two major subtypes of SCLC.[19,51,62,76] Biochemical and cytogenetic studies of cell lines derived from either subtype also showed no differences.[17,90,137] Thus the distinguishing of lymphocyte-like and intermediate subtypes in SCLC appears irrelevant, given the inconsistent classification by pathologists and the lack of apparent differences in tumor biology or in the clinical course.

The intermediate type of SCLC can be misclassified as an NSCLC tumor, particularly in specimens in which the tumor is arranged either in stratifying sheets, in pseudo-ductal structures, or in areas adjacent to nests of squamous cells.[90] Difficult cases require that adequate histologic material be interpreted by a pathologist experienced with the classification and varied manifestations of SCLC. Electron microscopy or biochemical and cytogenetic analyses may also help to distinguish SCLC from NSCLC tumors. In a retrospective review of SCLC biopsy specimens, however, electron microscopic features did not identify subgroups with different therapeutic reponses to intensive systemic therapy.[28] Diagnosis by light microscopy alone was sufficient to identify lung cancer patients with a high response rate to systemic therapy. The presence of neurosecretory granules is believed to confirm that the tumor has features of an APUD cell. Scattered foci of squamous or glandular elements do not alter the diagnosis of classic or intermediate type SCLC. However, the presence of non-small cell elements in every microscopic field of the tumor suggests a "combined" SCLC. The most common combination involves intermediate SCLC with large cell elements, accounting for up to 5 percent of SCLC patients in one series.[114] These mixed small cell–large cell tumors have response rates and survivals intermediate between those expected for SCLC or NSCLC tumors alone.[62,114] The clinical features of the less common mixed small cell–squamous cell or small cell–adenocarcinoma are not well defined. Autopsies reveal that up to 33 percent of SCLC tumors exhibit changes in histology compared to initial biposy and that 25 percent develop the mixed small cell–large cell type.[1,114] This histologic type is most common after relapse from chemotherapy or at autopsy. It is unclear whether this histology represents two different tumors from the onset of clinical presentation, dual differentiation from a single progenitor cell type, differentiation of a subpopulation from the initial histologic type, or the emergence of a second primary unrelated to the first tumor. What remains clear is that the clinician needs to consider pathologic heterogeneity when evaluating a new patient with SCLC. Rebiopsy of accessible lesions resistant to therapy or new lesions at time of relapse should also be considered. The development of a second primary rather than relapse of the original tumor should be suspected particularly in patients who are long-term survivors.[29,71]

GROWTH CHARACTERISTICS AND CELL BIOLOGY

Early reports described short tumor doubling times and high tritiated thymidine pulse-labeling indices for SCLC.[83,103] These growth kinetics appeared to explain the striking chemo- and radioresponsiveness and also appeared consistent with a short duration of disease control in many patients. Further studies of clinical tumor doubling times in SCLC usually exceeded 2 months, however, and were no shorter than those for large cell carcinomas or squamous cell carcinomas.[121] This suggests that patients with low tumor burdens and slower doubling times could remain clinically disease-free up to 4–5 years prior to relapse.[12] Many factors other than kinetic characteristics may be important in determining tumor responsiveness to chemotherapy.[121]

As described previously, SCLC cell lines have features of APUD cells associated with secretion of a variety of polypeptide hormones, some of which may function as autocrine growth factors.[31] In addition, these cells are characterized by the presence of the enzymes L-dopa decarboxylase, neuron-specific enolase, and creatine kinase BB isoenzyme.[7,90] SCLC cell lines share a unique chromosomal abnormality of a deletion in chromosome 3(3p⁻).[137] SCLC cell lines are more sensitive to irradiation in vitro than are cell lines derived from other histologic types of lung cancer.[20] Monoclonal antibodies have been raised that exhibit enhanced specificity for SCLC cell lines.[32] The study of SCLC cell lines may lead to innovative therapeutic approaches for this disease. The establishment of SCLC cell lines with classic or variant biochemical and morphologic features may correlate with response rates to cytotoxic therapy among newly diagnosed patients.[18,45] The development of molecular probes to identify genes specifying drug or radiation resistance, the modulation of growth factors important in the proliferation of SCLC, the use of tumor-directed or growth-factor-directed antibodies, and the screening for new drugs active in SCLC are only a few of the novel approaches that may be tested in the near future.

CLINICAL PRESENTATION

Almost three-fourths of patients with SCLC present between the ages of 50 and 70.[101] The 10:1 male:female ratio appears to be decreasing as a result of the increased incidence of lung cancer among women.[95] The signs and symptoms of SCLC depend on the site and size of the primary tumor and the presence or absence of regional or distant metastases. With the exception of the paraneoplastic syndromes, which are relatively uncommon, the usual clinical signs are not more specific for SCLC than for any other form of lung cancer. The duration of symptoms prior to diagnosis is shorter for SCLC than for the other histologic types of lung cancer.[26] More than 80 percent of patients with SCLC report symptoms for 3 months or less, and very few are asymptomatic at time of diagnosis.[65,75] In contrast, symptoms occur for an average of 8 months prior to the diagnosis of squamous cell carcinoma, and almost one-fourth of patients with adenocarcinoma are asymptomatic at diagnosis.[26,75]

Since SCLC usually develops in a central location, patients often present with symptoms of cough, wheezing, dyspnea, hemoptysis, or chest pain. Cough is the most common symptom related to the primary tumor, affecting 75 percent of patients seen at the NCI.[26] Intermittent poorly localized chest pain occurs in one-third of patients.[26] This may result from involvement of mediastinal structures or entrapment of perivascular or peribronchial nerves.[38] The chest pain due to pleural involvement usually is more constant, severe, and localized. Symptoms of dyspnea, wheeze, or pneumonitis are reported in 20–35 percent of patients.[26] The submucosal nature of SCLC accounts for the relative infrequency of hemoptysis (about 15 percent) as compared to squamous cell carcinoma, which characteristically presents as a friable exophytic mass in the bronchial lumen.[26] Weight loss, anorexia, and fatigue occur in up to one-third of patients.

Regional extension of tumor to the mediastinum occurs almost invariably with SCLC. Matthews et al. report that among patients who underwent curative resection for SCLC and then died within 30 days from causes unrelated to tumor, 70 percent had mediastinal node or distant metastatic involvement at autopsy.[91] It is not surprising that SCLC is the most common type of lung cancer with signs and symptoms of mediastinal involvement, including superior vena caval syndrome, hoarseness, and dysphagia.[23,26] The superior vena caval syndrome is recognized by distension of arm and neck veins; swelling of the face, neck, and arm; and the presence of thoracic collateral veins in association with symptoms of dyspnea, orthopnea, cough, and syncope associated with bending. SCLC is not only the most common lung tumor associated with superior vena caval syndrome but is now the most common cause in all patients.[3] Contrary to popular opinion, there is minimal evidence in the literature to suggest that invasive diagnostic procedures carry an undue risk of morbidity in this situation.[3] Consequently, a histologic diagnosis should be obtained in an expeditious manner prior to the application of definitive therapy. Chemotherapy alone appears to be as effective as chemotherapy combined with radiotherapy in resolving superior vena caval obstruction due to SCLC.[126]

Hoarseness results from involvement of a recurrent laryngeal nerve (usually in the left thorax because of the longer course of the nerve) or from a lesion along the course of the vagus nerve. When of short duration, vocal cord paralysis may be reversed with response to chemotherapy and/or radiotherapy. Dysphagia usually results from extrinsic compression by mediastinal nodes or tumor invasion of the esophageal wall. Signs and symptoms due to pericardial involvement rarely occur at presentation. However, the risk for tamponade makes this a potential medical emergency. Early suggestive signs include cardiomegaly, new-onset congestive heart failure, or new electrocardiographic abnormalities (such as an arrhythmia). Physical findings include pulsus paradoxus, distant heart sounds, friction rub, or Kussmaul's sign (distention of neck veins during inspiration).

Early dissemination of tumor is a feature of SCLC (Table 20-2).[13] Patients may present with signs and symptoms related to distant metastases located in almost any organ of the body. At time of diagnosis, two-thirds of patients have one or more clinically detectable metastatic sites, including the bones in 35 percent; liver in 25 percent; bone marrow in 20 percent; central nervous system (CNS) in 10 percent; and lymph nodes, subcutaneous tissue, or pleura in 10 percent.[68] At autopsy, almost all

Table 20-2
Frequency of Distant Metastases by Histologic Type of Lung Cancer

	Frequency of Distant Metastases (%)				
	SCLC	Squamous Cell	Adenocarcinoma	Large Cell	Reference
Autopsy within 30 days of curative resection	63	17	40	14	91
Clinical presentation	60	33	33	33	82
Autopsy series	96	54	82	86	89

patients will have involvement of hilar and mediastinal nodes, and more than half will have involvement of the bone, liver, adrenal glands, pancreas, contralateral lung, abdominal lymph nodes, and CNS.[26,89] In only 4 percent of these patients will the tumor remain limited to the thorax. CNS involvement is more frequent in SCLC than in other cell types of lung cancer, and in the absence of preventive therapy, the incidence appears to increase with lengthening survival.[107,109] CNS disease may manifest as intracranial metastases, intramedullary metastases, carcinomatous leptomeningitis, or epidural spinal cord compression.[105,111,115] Symptoms of impending spinal cord compression include localized or radicular back pain and motor or sensory nerve deficits. Lhermitte's sign, an electrical shock sensation in the spine induced by sudden flexion of the neck, may occur after treatment with radiotherapy.

Several paraneoplastic syndromes appear to be specifically associated with SCLC. The syndrome of inappropriate antidiuretic hormone secretion (SIADH) manifests as hyponatremia, decreased serum osmolarity, increased urine osmolality with urine sodium loss, or abnormal excretion on a standard water load test.[27] While fluid restriction, demeclocycline, urea, and lithium carbonate have been used for symptomatic treatment, definitive control results from a response to combination chemotherapy and/or radiotherapy.[46,50] Cushing's syndrome is associated with overproduction of adrenocorticotropic hormone (ACTH). Ectopic ACTH production is not suppressed by high-dose dexamethasone and is not increased after treatment with metyrapone. However, definitive control of the tumor will alleviate the symptoms. Elevated plasma concentrations of polypeptide hormones occur much more frequently than do the corresponding clinical syndromes.[48,53,55] Several polypeptide hormones such as gastrin-releasing peptide (bombesin) and calcitonin are not associated with any evident clinical syndromes. Some of these polypeptides, as well as several associated enzymes such as creatine kinase BB isoenzyme and neuron-specific enolase, have been employed as markers of tumor response to therapy. An extensive discussion of biomarkers in SCLC is presented in Chapter 21.

The Eaton-Lambert or myasthenic syndrome is a neurologic complication specifically associated with SCLC. Patients complain of proximal muscle weakness that improves with exercise. Electromyographic abnormalities correspondingly improve with repetitive nerve stimulation. Guanidine has been utilized for symptomatic therapy, and treatment of the underlying tumor occasionally has reversed the symptoms. As with other types of lung cancer, SCLC has been associated with carcinomatous neuromyopathies and cerebellar degeneration.[15] Recognition of these paraneoplastic syndromes is evident in less than 10 percent of patients, while the symptoms of locoregional extension predominate the clinical presentation.[15]

Scattered case reports describe extrapulmonary SCLC, which often is confused with atypical carcinoids or poorly differentiated carcinomas. Arising in many different organ systems, these tumors span a spectrum from an indolent carcinoid tumor to a rapidly dividing tumor with a tendency for early systemic spread.[41] Tumor markers or paraneoplastic syndromes may be evident. Many of these tumors respond to chemotherapy and/or radiotherapy.

Radiologic Presentation of Intrathoracic Tumor

A central tumor mass is the most common radiologic picture since more than 80 percent of patients with SCLC have involvement of the mainstem or lobar bronchi.[97]

Proximal obstruction may lead to atelectasis, postobstructive pneumonitis, or pleural effusion. A partial obstruction is heralded by a localized wheeze and confirmed on expiratory chest x-ray, where the affected segment remains inflated despite expiration.[26] Atelectasis is suggested by elevation of the hemidiaphragm, shift of the fissures and the mediastinum, and compensatory expansion of the uninvolved segments. The tendency for early metastasis results in frequent involvement of the hilum and mediastinum. Mediastinal adenopathy and lack of cavitation tend to distinguish SCLC from squamous cell carcinoma, which also presents in a central location. Mediastinal involvement is noted in up to 80 percent of cases by CT scan.[56] A radiologic "sunburst" appearance emanating from the primary tumor mass may result from rapid lymphatic and vascular invasion. A discrete peripheral tumor mass is evident in 20-30 percent of patients.[97,101] Less than 5 percent of patients successfully undergo complete surgical excision prior to chemotherapy and/or radiotherapy.[123] Most of these patients have small peripheral tumors and appear to have a particularly favorable prognosis with regard to long-term survival.[42,96,110,122] Multiple pulmonary nodules are seen in less than 10 percent of patients, while pleural effusions are noted in 10-20 percent.[97,101] Positive cytopathology is obtained by thoracentesis in 40-70 percent of pleural effusions.[84,119] Pleural biopsy or pleuroscopy increases this yield to cases when the malignant nature of the effusion requires confirmation.[119,136]

Computerized tomography (CT) of the chest provides better definition of intraparenchymal and mediastinal masses, allowing easier radiation treatment planning to involved areas.[56,108] However, chest CT scans show significant agreement with chest radiographs in most cases, especially in the absence of pulmonary fibrosis or prior pulmonary disease.[47] Chest CT scans may be most useful in designing radiotherapy ports and in assessing early chest relapse.[3,47] Other tests for mediastinal disease, such as percutaneous or transbronchial biopsies, mediastinoscopy, or ^{67}Ga scanning, are utilized when patients are evaluated for curative resection of the primary tumor. While the primary tumor almost invariably visualizes on gallium scan, mediastinal metastases are identified in only 60-80 percent of cases, and extrathoracic metastases are noted in less than 10 percent of cases.[11] Other investigators have had better success with gallium scans in initial staging.[10,35] Magnetic resonance imaging is currently under investigation.

Chest x-rays are the most common test used for assessing response, yet complete resolution of radiographic abnormalities often does not occur even in patients with a prolonged complete remission. Previous pulmonary disease, radiation fibrosis, and residual changes from atelectasis, pneumonitis, or pleural fibrosis may contribute to radiographic defects. When diagnostic accuracy is assessed by autopsy findings, chest radiographs more accurately detect lesions in the lung parenchyma and mediastinum than in the pleura or hilum.[22] Fiberoptic bronchoscopy may help to confirm complete response, particularly in cases where tumor is not evident or evaluable on chest radiographs. Of SCLC patients designated as complete responders radiologically, 25-33 percent will demonstrate residual endobronchial tumor on bronchoscopy.[65]

STAGING EVALUATION

In view of the high rate of regional or distant spread in SCLC, it is not surprising that staging procedures frequently detect metastatic disease.[13] Even apparently localized disease requires aggressive combination chemotherapy to address systemic micrometastases. It is unclear whether elaborate staging protocols to assess the extent of dissemination in SCLC provide any more than prognostic information. Tailoring therapy by extent of disease may or may not improve overall survival. However, staging procedures are used in most institutions to identify patients with seemingly localized disease when therapy depends on stage, assess the degree of response to therapy, visualize sites of relapse or unresponsive disease, and assess a patient's prognosis and ability to tolerate therapy.

In 1974 the American Joint Committee on Cancer Staging and End Results Reporting proposed a detailed tumor, nodes, and metastases (TNM) staging system for lung cancer.[102] This staging system concentrates on the size and location of the primary tumor and the extent of regional spread. These surgically oriented criteria are most appropriate for NSCLC. Over 85 percent of SCLC patients present with advanced (stage III) disease, which is defined as extensive or locally invasive primary tumor, mediastinal node involvement, or the presence of metastatic disease. The prognosis of SCLC patients appeared independent of stage in this system, with a 2-year survival of 5 percent in all three stages.[102] Prior to the use of combination chemotherapy, even the few patients able to undergo curative resection showed no survival advantage by TNM staging, with a median survival of 5 months for resected or unresected patients.[101] However, more recent studies suggest that TNM staging predicts improved survival for resectable patients with SCLC.[96,122,123]

Most clinical studies employ a two-stage classification first described by the Veterans Administration Lung Cancer Study Group, which divides unresectable SCLC into categories of limited and extensive disease.[140] Limited disease is defined as tumor confined to one hemithorax and its regional lymph nodes and tolerably encompassed in a single radiation portal, while tumor extending beyond these limits denotes extensive disease. Investigators disagree on the extent of regional involvement which defines limited disease. Authors variably include or exclude patients with ipsilateral and/or contralateral supraclavicular nodes[24,39,85] and patients with ipsilateral pleural effusions.[84,87,112] The number and types of staging procedures also impact on the staging system, as more thorough staging will result in a higher percentage of patients designated with extensive disease. The extent of staging should be considered when comparing trials from different institutions; shifting limited disease patients to the extensive disease category will improve the therapeutic results for both groups.[67] Most therapeutic trials have not employed chest CT for defining limited or extensive stage. Table 20-3 lists the frequency of limited disease patients from a number of large series with over 100 patients. About 40 percent of patients are designated limited disease at diagnosis. Most studies consistently show higher rates of complete response and prolonged survival for limited disease patients over those with extensive disease.[13,81,86] Even for untreated patients, the median survival time with limited and extensive disease was 3.1 and 1.4 months, respectively.[117]

Table 20-4 lists the various staging procedures that have been employed for patients with SCLC. In the late 1980s, it still remains debatable whether specific therapy based on extent of tumor dissemination is required, particularly the additional use of radiotherapy for limited-disease patients. When treatment is not affected by stage, special scans should be obtained only in situations with a high probability of a positive result in order to document evaluable tumor lesions. Outside of a clinical trial setting, simple screening tests are recommended initially, followed by special scans

Table 20-3

Frequency of Limited Disease in Large Series of Systematically Staged Patients with SCLC

Number of Patients	Frequency of Limited Disease		Staging Procedures	Reference
	(No.)	(%)		
375	101	27	Chest x-ray, bone marrow, liver/brain/bone scans	86
241	73	30	Chest x-ray, bone marrow, liver/bone scans	87
225	115	51	Chest x-ray, bone marrow, liver/brain/bone scans	94
337	166	49	Chest x-ray, bone marrow, liver biopsy	54
109	44	40	Chest x-ray, bone marrow, liver/brain/bone scans, chest tomography, bronchoscopy	4
357	172	48	Chest x-ray, bone marrow, liver/brain/bone scans	40
162	56	34	Chest x-ray, bone marrow, liver/brain/bone scans	33
252	103	41	Chest x-ray, bone marrow, liver/brain/bone scans, liver biopsy, bronchoscopy	71
2058	830	40		

Modified from Ihde DC: Staging evaluation and prognostic factors in small cell lung cancer, in Aisner J (ed): Lung Cancer. New York, Churchill Livingston, 1985, pp 241-268. With permission.

only if preliminary tests are positive. Chest x-ray, history, physical examination, and routine biochemical blood tests should be performed on all patients. Abnormal liver function tests or hepatomegaly should prompt the use of a radionuclide liver-spleen scan. A radionuclide bone scan should be performed with an elevated alkaline phosphatase or symptoms of bone pain. An abnormal neurologic history or examination may suggest the use of a brain CT scan. The value of routine screening with head CT scans has not been established in asymptomatic patients.[30,72] Bone marrow examination may allow pathologic documentation of extensive disease in the absence of metastases to other sites.[52] Additional staging procedures for the mediastinum are needed if the primary tumor is deemed potentially resectable. For patients with inevaluable tumor on chest radiograph, fiberoptic bronchoscopy often documents endobronchial tumor that can be followed serially to assess response. These staging recommendations for patients outside of clinical trials are summarized in Table 20-4. However, different clinical settings and therapeutic options will modify these standard recommendations for staging procedures.

Reevaluation of initially positive sites of disease allows for documentation of tumor response or progression. For patients with limited or extensive disease, previous sites of involvement are the first to herald relapse of disease unless radiotherapy has been administered.[86] The development of CNS metastases is a clear exception, particularly for patients who do not receive prophylactic cranial irradiation. Recommendations for the timing of restaging during and after chemotherapy depend on the therapeutic philosophy of the institution, the cost and availability of the procedures, and the investigatory interests of the physicians.

Table 20-4

Staging Procedures and Frequency of Distant Metastases

Procedure	Recommended Use Outside of Clinical Trials	Approximate Percent Positive at Presentation
Intrathoracic Tumor		
Chest x-ray	Routine	95
Chest tomograms	Special situations	—
Chest CT scan	Special situations or radiotherapy planning	—
Thoracentesis/pleural biopsy/pleuroscopy	Pleural effusion	—
Fiberoptic bronchoscopy	Evaluable tumor absent on chest x-ray or to document complete response	85
Mediastinoscopy	Prior to surgical resection	—
Gallium-67 scan	Special situations	—
Bone Metastases		
Marrow aspiration/biopsy	Routine if no other obvious extensive disease documented*	20
Radionuclide bone scan	Elevated alkaline phosphatase and/or symptoms of bone pain	25-40
Skeletal x-rays	Positive bone scan	—
Peripheral blood examination	Routine	—
Central Nervous System Metastases		
Brain CT scan	Suggestive neurologic history or examination†	10
Radionuclide brain scan	Special situations	—
Lumbar puncture with cytology	Special situations	—
Myelography	Suggestive neurologic history or examination	—
Hepatic Metastases		
Liver function tests	Routine	60-75
Radionuclide liver scan	Abnormal liver function tests or hepatomegaly*	20-30
Liver CT scan	Abnormal liver function tests or hepatomegaly*	20-30
Ultrasound	Special situations	—
Liver biopsies	Special situations‡	—
Other Sites		
Abdominal CT scan	Special situations	—
Laparotomy	Special situations	—
Lymph node biopsy or aspiration	For enlarged nodes	15-30
Subcutaneous nodule biopsy	For palpable nodules	5-10

Modified from Ihde DC: Staging evaluation and prognostic factors in small cell lung cancer, in Aisner J (ed): Lung Cancer. New York, Churchill Livingston, 1985, pp 241-268. With permission.

*Routine when treatment affected by stage.

†Routine screening for asymptomatic patients not established.

‡In the absence of other extensive disease and if therapy differs for limited and extensive disease patients: (1) normal liver scan and abnormal liver function tests; (2) abnormal liver scan and normal liver function tests.

Bone Metastases

Conventional bone marrow examination reveals infiltration of malignant tumor in approximately 20 percent of patients at initial presentation.[51,69] Marrow involvement often is associated with other evidence of extensive disease[69] but, as mentioned previously, may easily confirm the presence of dissemination in the initial screening process.[59] Bone marrow evaluation consists of an aspirate smear, needle biopsy with touch preparation, and clot sections of the aspirate. A touch preparation may reveal tumor when an aspirate is unobtainable because of a "dry tap." Although the superior yield of marrow aspiration over that of biopsy is not confirmed universally,[51,69] both procedures appear complementary in detection of tumor.[59] Marrow examination usually is performed at the posterior iliac crest, although other sites, such as the sternum, have been employed.[49] In one study, bilateral bone marrow biopsies increased the diagnostic yield by 30 percent over a unilateral examination.[60] The improved detection probably correlates with the increased amounts of marrow tissue available for analysis.

The marrow biopsy often demonstrates new bone formation and myelofibrotic changes in association with tumor cells, findings that also typify marrow infiltration with breast or prostate carcinoma. This histologic picture may account for the osteoblastic changes occasionally seen on bone radiographs in patients with SCLC.[69,106] Thrombocytopenia and/or leukoerythroblastic changes (the presence of circulating immature myeloid or erythroid elements) specifically suggest marrow involvement in SCLC.[51,69] However, the blood smear is normal in most cases of marrow infiltration, suggesting a low sensitivity in detecting the presence of tumor.

Other techniques for identifying marrow tumor are being tested in patients with SCLC. Monoclonal antibodies that react against surface antigens of SCLC have been applied for detection of bone marrow metastases. The proportion of patients recognized as having marrow involvement was increased from 45 percent to 72 percent in a series of 33 patients at the Dana Farber Cancer Institute.[127] However, there is no proof that the monoclonal antibodies are specifically identifying tumor cells. The finding of marrow infiltration in most patients confirms the concept of early dissemination in SCLC. Increased sensitivity of detection will allow identification of favorable and unfavorable prognostic groups and monitoring of subclinical tumor response to therapy. Improved identification and purging of tumor cells from marrow by use of monoclonal antibodies may be applicable to autologous marrow reinfusion studies.[127]

Radionuclide bone scans are more sensitive than skeletal x-rays in identifying osseous metastases.[79] Improvement or worsening of abnormalities on follow-up scans correlate 70 percent of the time with extraosseous tumor changes. Because of false-positive findings from benign bone disease, it seems prudent to designate a scan as abnormal only when there are two or more definitely positive abnormalities not explained by a benign condition. Bone scans should not serve as the sole determinant for therapeutic decisions but should, rather, alert the clinician to the need for follow-up. Skeletal x-ray surveys are rarely productive and radiographs should be used principally to confirm or exclude potential metastatic sites identified by bone scan.

Bone metastases are the most frequent site of metastasis, found in up to 40 percent of patients at presentation and are the only evident site of organ involvement in 10 percent of patients.[79] Positive scans occasionally occur in the absence of symptoms or of abnormal alkaline phosphatase levels. However, the presence of bone scan abnormalities does correlate with elevated enzyme levels and with marrow involvement.[79] Retrospective analysis of 112 cases suggests that bone scans and bone marrow biopsies identify independent patterns of bony metastases.[80] Both procedures are complementary in the assessment of bony involvement with SCLC. The probability of extraosseous metastatic sites increases with more frequent bone scan abnormalities.[79]

Hepatic Metastases

Pretreatment staging with radionuclide liver scan and percutaneous liver biopsy reveals liver metastases in 28 percent of patients.[68] After treatment with chemotherapy and/or radiotherapy, the liver is a site of relapse in up to 80 percent of patients at autopsy.[99] Hepatic metastases appear to correlate with widespread disease in various other sites.[38,68,69] The radionuclide liver scan is the most frequently employed test for liver involvement despite its inability to visualize lesions less than two centimeters in diameter. The radionuclide scan is usually negative in the absence of hepatomegaly or elevated liver function tests.[139] Clearly defined defects can be followed serially to assess response to therapy. CT scans of the liver appear to detect mass lesions at least as frequently as do radionuclide scans.[56] The value of ultrasound imaging remains to be investigated. By themselves, liver function test abnormalities [including lactate dehydrogenase, alkaline phosphatase, serum glutamate oxaloacetate transaminase (SGOT), and bilirubin] are too frequently falsely positive to allow specific identification of liver metastases. However, in one series patients with elevations in several tests had positive liver biopsies on peritoneoscopy in up to 70 percent of cases, while very few patients (<10%) had liver involvement in the presence of completely normal liver function tests.[38,104] Pathologic confirmation requires liver biopsy by peritoneoscopy or by percutaneous aspiration (blind or scan-directed). Peritoneoscopic biopsy is the most sensitive method of detection of liver metastases short of laparotomy and has been proposed as an initial staging test to replace radionuclide scans and liver function tests.[38] On peritoneoscopy, tumor can be visually identified in 90 percent of patients with positive biopsies.[38]

In a study of 157 consecutive patients at the National Cancer Institute, liver metastases were detected in 26 percent.[104] Radionuclide and CT liver scans were equally accurate, concurring with liver biopsy in 87 percent of patients. Only 7 (9 percent) out of 81 patients with a negative liver scan and two or fewer abnormal liver function tests had a positive biopsy. In contrast, 21 (88 percent) out of 24 patients with a positive liver scan and one or more abnormal liver function tests had a positive biopsy. Peritoneoscopic staging should be reserved for patients with no other metastatic sites who either have a normal liver scan with more than one abnormal liver function test or an abnormal liver scan.[104] This scenario assumes that treatment would be affected by the demonstration of extensive stage solely in the liver. Less than 10 percent of presenting patients would require peritoneoscopic biopsy according to these criteria. The need for pathologic proof of liver involvement is usually investigational since all patients ultimately receive combination chemotherapy. The presence of liver involvement is a poor prognostic sign regardless of therapy.[68]

CNS Metastases and Metastases to Other Sites

As previously discussed, CNS disease may present as intracranial metastases, intramedullary metastases, carcinomatous leptomeningitis, or epidural spinal cord compression in up to 10 percent of patients at initial presentation.[30,109] CNS metastases produce significant morbidity and may limit the survival of patients who relapse in the CNS after complete remission.[13] Once diagnosed, metastases may recur at various sites in the CNS. When prophylactic cranial irradiation is not applied, 50-80 percent of patients surviving two years will develop brain metastases, the frequency of tumor increasing with lengthening survival.[77,109,116] Autopsy studies confirm involvement of multiple CNS sites.[63] Since carcinomatous leptomeningitis may coexist with epidural compression, a cerebrospinal fluid specimen obtained at myelography should always be sent for cytopathologic analysis. Risk factors for development of CNS metastases during therapy include multiple metastatic sites of disease, liver and bone marrow metastases, and failure to achieve complete remission.[109] In contrast to the findings in acute lymphocytic leukemia, it is unclear whether prophylactic cranial irradiation significantly improves overall survival while decreasing the frequency of CNS relapse.[16,130] Since most patients who develop CNS disease have concomitant progressive systemic disease or have never attained a complete remission, their survival is not affected by the CNS involvement. Prophylactic cranial irradiation may be most beneficial for patients who achieve complete response and have prognostic features associated with the development of CNS metastases (i.e., stage of disease or involvement of liver, bone marrow, or bone).[116]

Neurologic examination, radionuclide brain scans, and head CT scans were performed at diagnosis and sequentially in 153 consecutive patients at the National Cancer Institute.[30] CT scans were superior to radionuclide scans in detecting metastases in patients with or without neurologic symptoms. CT scans were positive in 6 percent of asymptomatic patients at diagnosis and 13 percent of asymptomatic patients after systemic therapy.[30] Survival after therapeutic cranial irradiation was similar for asymptomatic and symptomatic patients. Head CT scans should be employed routinely in SCLC patients with neurologic symptoms or signs, or in patients with prior CNS involvement. Screening asymptomatic patients with radionuclide or CT scans at presentation will identify 6 percent of patients with CNS involvement.

Intra-abdominal dissemination of SCLC to the pancreas, adrenal glands, or retroperitoneal nodes usually is inapparent clinically. Abdominal CT reveals lesions in these areas that respond in concert with other sites in approximately 20 percent of newly diagnosed patients.[66,132] Abdominal CT was performed as part of the initial staging evaluation in 77 patients with SCLC at the National Cancer Institute.[66] Positive scans were obtained in patients already known to have extensive disease, altering the stage in only 10 percent of cases. Serial abdominal CT scans provided useful therapeutic information not suggested by other staging procedures in only three of 45 patients.[66] Although radioisotopic scanning of the adrenal glands with ^{131}I-iodocholesterol may reveal metastases, other procedures provide adequate staging information for most SCLC patients.[113] Gallium scans employing a tomographic scanner may help to identify hepatic and lymphatic metastases but have been reported to fail in detecting brain or bone lesions.[10] Exploratory laparotomy identified liver or nodal tumor in 6 out of 11 cases of SCLC, but this procedure is recommended only in exceptional circumstances.[100]

PROGNOSTIC FACTORS

Stage of disease is a dominant prognostic factor for SCLC in both untreated patients[140] and patients receiving combination chemotherapy with or without chest irradiation.[4,64,85,94] Patients with limited disease demonstrate a superior response rate and improved survival when identical treatment is applied to all stages. A few studies report only improved survival with no change in response for stage.[87] It should be recalled that more intensive staging efforts will seemingly improve treatment results within a given stage by transferring patients with almost undetectable metastatic disease into the extensive disease category.[67]

Performance status is an important prognostic variable alone and within each stage.[68,86,94] Performance status is also linked to stage as impaired ambulation correlates with greater likelihood of extensive disease.[68,85] A worsening performance status is associated with increased involvement of distant metastatic sites, suggesting that impaired ambulation reflects an increased tumor burden.[68] Multivariate analysis of blood tests indicates that patients with low values for albumin (<3.4 g/dl) and for hemoglobin (<12.8 g/dl) have a worse survival, and that these two laboratory parameters compensated for performance status as a prognostic factor.[25] The use of objective criteria, such as a low serum sodium, to replace the more subjective performance status requires further confirmation.[125]

Weight loss is an independent prognostic factor for untreated[140] and for treated[36] patients, especially for more ambulatory patients with a lower tumor burden. Development of progressive disease on combination chemotherapy is also an extremely poor prognostic variable, with a median survival of 8 weeks in patients relapsing on systemic therapy.[86] Thus, stage of disease, performance status, weight loss, and history of prior chemotherapy are definitely established prognostic factors for SCLC. They affect response rates and overall survival, and always should be specified in clinical trials. Any other proposed prognostic factors will need to provide information equivalent or superior to these four established factors.

Hepatic metastases and CNS involvement appear to have an unfavorable impact even within the extensive disease category.[16,68,92] Bone marrow involvement also portends a shorter survival, even though the tolerance to chemotherapy is only mildly impaired.[59,69] However, bone involvement on radionuclide scan or x-rays that is the only site of extensive disease confers no worse a prognosis than limited disease, probably partly as a result of falsely positive scans. Soft-tissue metastases as the sole form of extensive disease also have a favorable prognosis.[68] Tumor burden may also correlate with response and survival. Some investigators find that patients with single sites of extensive disease do better than those with multiple organ involvement,[68,70] but others have not confirmed this finding.[2] Tumor volume as estimated from CT scan measurements appears to correlate with survival in one study.[57] Regression rates calculated from estimated tumor volumes also predict subsequent survival; faster regression correlates with a smaller tumor volume and an increased median survival.[78,138]

As previously described, with the exception of the small cell–large cell variant, histologic subtype of SCLC does not appear to be a prognostic factor in most but not all reports.[19,34,51,114] Impaired immune status as assessed by delayed hypersensitivity skin testing correlates with shortened survival, particularly in patients with a good performance status and low tumor burden.[73] Among patients with limited disease, supraclavicular node involvement,[68,86] ipsilateral pleural effusions,[68,84] and superior vena cava syndrome[131] do not appear to affect prognosis. A clinically evident paraneoplastic syndrome may confer a worse prognosis, but this needs to be confirmed by multivariate analysis.[57,92] Investigators disagree on whether women[51,68,92,93] and younger patients[51,68,92] live longer than do other SCLC patients. Discontinuation of cigarette smoking prior to diagnosis[74] and resection of the primary tumor in limited-stage patients[42,96,110,122,123] appear to have a favorable prognosis. In fact, resectable patients may do as well even if tumor is not resected.

Biomarkers are discussed in detail in Chapter 21. The use of biomarkers to provide prognostic information is still investigational. Although carcinoembryonic antigen (CEA), ACTH, neuron-specific enolase, neurophysins, and antidiuretic hormone have been studied, when several markers are monitored in conjunction with careful clinical evaluation, the markers provide no information beyond that obtained by standard staging methods.[5] A recent multivariate analysis found that prognostic groupings based solely on performance status, serum alkaline phosphatase, serum sodium, and serum albumin were superior to the limited or extensive disease staging in predicting survival.[125] Absence of an elevated CEA independently predicts improved response and overall survival in a retrospective review of 180 patients.[120] Another study suggests that serum creatine phosphokinase BB isoenzyme also has independent prognostic value, with correlation of elevated levels with tumor dissemination, decreased response, and worse survival.[21]

CONCLUSION

In comparison with the other types of lung cancer, SCLC is a distinct clinicopathologic entity. The striking responsiveness to chemotherapy and radiotherapy clearly distinguishes this histologic type of lung cancer. Despite this sensitivity, long-term survivors are the exception rather than the rule. It is sobering to consider that the popularity of cigarette smoking in this century has clearly catapulted lung cancer to the forefront of oncologic problems. Prevention will ultimately be the most cost-effective means of controlling this disease. Until then, new therapeutic and diagnostic strategies will be based on our greater understanding of the natural history and biology of this tumor.

REFERENCES

1. Abeloff MD, Eggleston JC: Morphologic changes following therapy, in Greco FA, Oldham RK, Bunn PA Jr (eds): Small Cell Lung Cancer. Orlando, FL, Grune & Stratton, 1981, pp 235–259
2. Abeloff MD, Ettinger DS, Order SE, et al: Intensive induction chemotherapy in 54 patients with small cell carcinoma of the lung. Cancer Treat Rep 65:639–646, 1981
3. Ahmann FR: A reassessment of the clinical implications of the superior vena caval syndrome. J Clin Oncol 2:961–969, 1984
4. Aisner J, Whitacre M, Van Echo DA, et al: Combination chemotherapy for small cell carcinoma of the lung: continuous versus alternating noncross-resistant combinations. Cancer Treat Rep 66:221–230, 1982
5. Aroney RS, Dermody WC, Aldenderfer P, et al: Multiple sequential biomarkers in monitoring patients with carcinoma of the lung. Cancer Treat Rep 68:859–866, 1984
6. Auerbach O, Saccamanno G, Kuschner M, et al: Histologic findings in the tracheobronchial tree of uranium miners and non-miners with lung cancer. Cancer 42:483–489, 1978

7. Baylin SB, Gazdar AF: Endocrine biochemistry in the spectrum of human lung cancer: Implications for the cellular origin of small cell carcinoma, in Greco FA, Oldham RK, Bunn PA Jr. (eds): Small Cell Lung Cancer. Orlando, FL, Grune & Stratton, 1981, pp 123-143

8. Bensch KJ, Corrin B, Pariente R, et al: Oat cell carcinoma of the lung. Its origin and relationships to bronchial carcinoid. Cancer 22:1163-1172, 1968

9. Bensch KJ, Gordon GB, Miller LR: Studies on the bronchial counterpart of the Kulchitsky (argentaffin) cell and innervation of bronchial glands. J Ultrastruct Res 12:655-686, 1965

10. Bitran JD, Bekerman C, Pinsky S: Sequential scintigraphic staging of small cell carcinoma. Cancer 47:1971-1975, 1981

11. Brereton HD, Line B, Londer HN, et al: Gallium scans for staging small cell lung cancer. JAMA 240:666-667, 1978

12. Brigham, Bunn PA Jr., Minna JD, et al: Growth rates of small cell bronchogenic carcinomas. Cancer 42:2880-2886, 1978

13. Bunn PA, Cohen MH, Ihde DC, et al: Advances in small cell bronchogenic carcinoma. Cancer Treat Rep 61:333-342, 1977

14. Bunn PA Jr, Linnoila I, Minna JD, et al: Small cell lung cancer, endocrine cells of the fetal bronchus, and other neuroendocrine cells express the Leu-7 antigenic determinant present on natural killer cells. Blood 65:764-768, 1985

15. Bunn PA, Minna JD: Paraneoplastic syndromes, in DeVita VT, Hellman S, Rosenberg SA (eds): Principles and Practice of Oncology. Philadelphia, Lippincott, 1985, pp 1797-1842

16. Bunn PA, Rosen ST: Central nervous system manifestations of small cell lung cancer, in Aisner J (ed): Lung Cancer. New York, Churchill Livingston, 1985, pp 287-305

17. Carney DN, Broder L, Edelstein M, et al: Experimental studies of the biology of human small cell lung cancer. Cancer Treat Rep 67:27-35, 1983

18. Carney DN, Gazdar AF, Bepler G, et al: Establishment and identification of small cell lung cancer cell lines having classic and variant features. Cancer Res 45:2913-2923, 1985

19. Carney DN, Matthews M, Ihde DC, et al: Influence of histologic subtype of small cell carcinoma of the lung on clinical presentation, response to therapy and survival. J Natl Cancer Inst 65:1225-1230, 1980

20. Carney DN, Mitchell JB, Kinsella TJ: In vitro radiation and chemotherapy sensitivity of established cell lines of human small cell lung cancer and its large cell morphologic variants. Cancer Res 43:2806-2811, 1983

21. Carney DN, Zweig MH, Ihde DC, et al: Elevated serum creatine kinase BB levels in patients with small cell lung cancer. Cancer Res 44:5399-5403 1984

22. Chak LY, Paryani SB, Sikic BI, et al: Diagnostic accuracies of clinical studies in patients with small cell carcinoma of the lung. J Clin Oncol 1:290-294, 1983

23. Cohen MH: Signs and symptoms of bronchogenic carcinoma, in Straus MJ (ed): Lung Cancer: Clinical Diagnosis and Treatment. Orlando, FL, Grune & Stratton, 1977, pp 85-94

24. Cohen MH, Ihde DC, Bunn PA, et al: Cyclic alternating combination chemotherapy for small cell bronchogenic carcinoma. Cancer Treat Rep 63:163-170, 1979

25. Cohen MH, Makuch R, Johnston-Early A, et al: Laboratory parameters as an alternative to performance status in prognostic stratification of patients with small cell lung cancer. Cancer Treat Rep 65:187-195, 1981

26. Cohen MH, Matthews MJ: Small cell bronchogenic carcinoma: A distinct clinicopathologic entity. Semin Oncol 5:234-241, 1978

27. Comis RL, Miller M, Ginsberg SJ: Abnormalities in water homeostasis in small cell anaplastic lung cancer. Cancer 45:2414-2421, 1980

28. Copple B, Wright SE, Moatamed F: Electron microscopy in small cell lung carcinomas. J Clin Oncol 2:910-916, 1984

29. Craig J, Powell B, Muss HB, et al: Second primary bronchogenic carcinomas after small cell carcinoma—report of two cases and review of the literature. Am J Med 76:1013-1020, 1984

30. Crane JM, Nelson JM, Ihde DC, et al: A comparison of computed tomography and radionuclide scanning for detection of brain metastases in small cell lung cancer. J Clin Oncol 2:1017-1024, 1984

31. Cuttitta F, Carney DN, Mulshine J, et al: Bombesin-like peptides can function as autocrine growth factors in human small cell lung cancer. Nature 316:823-826, 1985

32. Cuttitta F, Rosen S, Gazdar AF, Minna JD: Monoclonal antibodies that demonstrate specificity for several types of human lung cancer. Proc Natl Acad Sci (USA) 78:4591-4595, 1981

33. Daniels JR, Chak LY, Sikic BI, et al: Chemotherapy of small cell carcinoma of the lung: a randomized comparison of alternating and sequential combination chemotherapy programs. J Clin Oncol 2:1192-1199, 1984

34. Davis S, Stanley KE, Yesner R, et al: Small cell carcinoma of the lung: Survival according to histologic subtype. Cancer 47:1863-1866, 1981

35. DeMeester TR, Golomb HM, Kirchner P, et al: The role of gallium-67 scanning in the clinical staging and preoperative evaluation of patients with carcinoma of the lung. Ann Thorac Surg 28:451-463, 1978

36. DeWys WD, Begg C, Lavin PT, et al: Prognostic effect of weight loss prior to chemotherapy in cancer patients. Am J Med 69:491-497, 1980

37. Doll R, Peto R: Mortality in relation to smoking: 20 years' observations on male British doctors. Br Med J 2:1525-1536, 1976

38. Dombernowsky P, Hirsch F, Hansen HH, et al: Peritoneoscopy in staging of 190 patients with small-cell anaplastic carcinoma of the lung with special reference to subtyping. Cancer 41:2008-2012, 1978

39. Eagan RT, Maurer LH, Forcier RJ, et al: Small cell carcinoma of the lung: Staging, paraneoplastic syndromes, treatment, and survival. Cancer 33:527-532, 1974

40. Feld R, Evans WK, DeBoer G, et al: Combined modality induction therapy without maintenance chemotherapy for small cell carcinoma of the lung. J Clin Oncol 2:294-304, 1984

41. Fer MF, Levenson RM, Cohen MH, Greco FA: Extrapulmonary small cell carcinoma, in Greco FA, Oldham RK, Bunn PA (eds): Small Cell Lung Cancer. Orlando, FL, Grune & Stratton, 1981, pp 301-325

42. Friess GG, McCracken JD, Troxell ML, et al: Effect of initial resection of small cell carcinoma of the lung: A review of Southwest Oncology Group Study 7628. J Clin Oncol 3:964-968, 1985

43. Gazdar AF: The biology of endocrine tumors of the lung, in Becker KL, Gazdar AF (eds): The Endocrine Lung in Health and Disease. Philadelphia, Saunders, 1984, pp 448-459

44. Gazdar AF, Bunn PA, Minna JD, et al: Origin of human small cell lung cancer. Science 229:679, 1985

45. Gazdar, AF, Carney DN, Nau MM, et al: Characterization of variant subclasses of cell lines derived from small cell lung cancer having distinctive biochemical, morphological, and growth properties. Cancer Res 45:2924-2930, 1985

46. Greco FA, Hainsworth J, Sismani A, et al: Hormone production and paraneoplastic syndromes, in Greco FA, Oldham RK, Bunn PA (eds): Small Cell Lung Cancer. Orlando, FL, Grune & Stratton, 1981, pp 177-223

47. Griffin CA, Lu C, Fishman EK, et al: The role of computerized tomography of the chest in the management of small cell lung cancer. J Clin Oncol 2:1359-1365, 1984

48. Gropp C, Havemann K, Scheuer A: Ectopic hormones in lung cancer patients at diagnosis and during therapy. Cancer 46:347-354, 1980

49. Guttierrez AC, Vincent RG, Sandberg AA, et al: Evaluation of sternal bone marrow aspiration for detection of tumor cells in patients with bronchogenic carcinoma. J Thorac Cardiovasc Surg 77:392-395, 1979

50. Hainsworth JD, Workman R, Greco FA: Management of the syndrome of inappropriate antidiuretic hormone secretion in small cell lung cancer. Cancer 51:161-165, 1983

51. Hansen HH, Dombernowsky P, Hirsch FR: Staging procedures and prognostic features in small cell anaplastic bronchogenic carcinoma. Semin Oncol 5:280-287, 1978

52. Hansen HH, Muggia FM: Staging of inoperable patients with bronchogenic carcinoma with special reference to bone marrow examination and peritoneoscopy. Cancer 30:1395-1401, 1972

53. Hansen M, Hammer M, Hummer L: Diagnostic and therapeutic implications of ectopic hormone production in small cell carcinoma of the lung. Thorax 35:101-106, 1980

54. Hansen M, Hansen HH, Dombernowsky P: Long-term survival in small cell carcinoma of the lung. JAMA 244:247-250, 1980

55. Hansen M, Hansen HH, Hirsch FR, et al: Hormonal polypeptides and amine metabolites in small cell carcinoma of the lung, with special reference to stage and subtypes. Cancer 45:1432-1437, 1980

56. Harper PG, Houang M, Spiro SG, et al: Computerized axial tomography in the pretreatment assessment of small cell carcinoma of the bronchus. Cancer 47:1775-1780, 1981

57. Harper PG, Souhami RL, Spiro SG, et al: Tumor size, response rate, and prognosis in small cell carcinoma of the bronchus treated by combination chemotherapy. Cancer Treat Rep 66:463-470, 1982

58. Heelan RT, Melamed MR, Zaman MB, et al: Radiologic diagnosis of oat cell cancer in a high-risk screened population. Radiology 136:593-601, 1980

59. Hirsch F, Hansen HH, Dombernowsky P, et al: Bone marrow examination in the staging of small cell anaplastic carcinoma of the lung with special reference to subtyping. Cancer 39:2563-2567, 1977

60. Hirsch FR, Hansen HH, Hainau B: Bilateral bone marrow examination in small cell anaplastic carcinoma of the lung. Acta Path Microbiol Scand 87:59-62, 1979

61. Hirsch FR, Matthews MJ, Yesner R: Histopathologic classification of small cell carcinoma of the lung. Cancer 50:1360-1366, 1982

62. Hirsch FR, Østerlind K, Hansen HH: The prognostic significance of histopathologic subtyping of small cell carcinoma of the lung according to the classification of the World Health Organization—a study of 375 consecutive patients. Cancer 52:2144-2150, 1983

63. Hirsch FR, Paulson OB, Hansen HH, et al: Intracranial metastases in small cell carcinoma of the lung. Cancer 51:529-533, 1983

64. Ihde DC: Staging evaluation and prognostic factors in small cell lung cancer, in Aisner J (ed): Lung Cancer. New York, Churchill Livingston, 1985, pp 241-268

65. Ihde DC, Cohen MH, Bernath AM, et al: Serial fiberoptic bronchoscopy during chemotherapy for small cell carcinoma of the lung: Early detection of patients at high risk for relapse. Chest 74:531-536, 1978

66. Ihde DC, Dunnick NR, Johnston-Early A, et al: Abdominal computed tomography in small cell lung cancer: Assessment of extent of disease and response to therapy. Cancer 49:1485-1490, 1982

67. Ihde DC, Hansen HH: Staging procedures and prognostic factors in small cell carcinoma of the lung, in Greco FA, Oldham RK, Bunn PA (eds): Small Cell Lung Cancer. Orlando, FL, Grune & Stratton, 1981, pp 261-283

68. Ihde DC, Makuch RW, Carney DN, et al: Prognostic implications of stage of disease and sites of metastases in patients with small cell carcinoma of the lung treated with intensive chemotherapy. Am Rev Resp Dis 123:500-507, 1981

69. Ihde DC, Simms EB, Matthews MJ, et al: Bone marrow metastases in small cell carcinoma of the lung: Frequency, description, and influence on chemotherapeutic toxicity and prognosis. Blood 53:677-686, 1979

70. Jacobs SA, Santicky MJ, Stoller RG: A comparison of survival in subsets of patients with extensive small cell carcinoma of the lung. Proc Am Soc Clin Oncol 21:455, 1980

71. Johnson BE, Ihde DC, Bunn PA, et al: Patients with small cell lung cancer treated with combination chemotherapy with or without irradiation: data on potential cures, chronic toxicities, and late relapses after a five to eleven-year follow-up. Ann Intern Med 103:430-438, 1985

72. Johnson DH, Windham WW, Allen JH, et al: Limited value of CT brain scans in the staging of small cell lung cancer. Am J Radiol 140:37-40, 1983

73. Johnston-Early A, Cohen MH, Fossieck BE, et al: Delayed hypersensitivity skin testing as a prognostic indicator in patients with small cell lung cancer. Cancer 52:1395-1400, 1983

74. Johnston-Early A, Cohen MH, Minna JD, et al: Smoking abstinence and small cell lung cancer survival: an association. JAMA 244:2175-2179, 1980

75. Kato Y, Ferguson TB, Bennet DE, et al: Oat cell carcinoma of the lung. Cancer 23:517-524, 1969

76. Knop RH, Bunn PA Jr.: Management of small cell lung cancer, in Phillips TL, Pistenma DA (eds): Radiation Oncology Annual, 1983. New York, Raven Press, 1984, pp 65-104

77. Komaki R, Cox JD, Whitson W: Risk of brain metastases from small cell carcinoma of the lung related to length of survival and prophylactic irradiation. Cancer Treat Rep 65:811-814, 1981

78. Lenhard RE, Woo KB, Abeloff MD: Predictive value of regression rates following chemotherapy of small cell carcinoma of the lung. Cancer Res 43:3013-3017, 1983

79. Levenson RM, Sauerbrunn BJL, Ihde DC, et al: Small cell lung cancer: Radionuclide bone scans for assessment of tumor extent and response. Am J Roentgenol 137:31-35, 1981

80. Levitan N, Byrne RE, Bromer RH, et al: The value of the bone scan and bone marrow biopsy in staging small cell lung cancer. Cancer 56:652-654, 1985

81. Livingston RB: Small cell carcinoma of the lung. Blood 56:575-584, 1980

82. Livingston RB: Lung cancer, in Stein JH (ed): Internal Medicine, 2d ed. Boston, Little, Brown, 1987, pp 1132-1135

83. Livingston RB, Ambus U, Geoger SL, et al: In vitro determinations of thymidine^{-3}H labeling index in human solid tumors. Cancer Res 34:1376-1380, 1974

84. Livingston RB, McCracken JD, Trauth CJ, et al: Isolated pleural effusion in small cell lung carcinoma: favorable prognosis. Chest 81:208-211, 1982

85. Livingston RB, Moore TN, Heilbrun L, et al: Small cell carcinoma of the lung: combined chemotherapy and radiation. Ann Intern Med 88:194-199, 1978

86. Livingston RB, Trauth CJ, Greenstreet RL: Small cell carcinoma: Clinical manifestations and behavior with treatment, in Greco FA, Oldham RK, Bunn PA (eds): Small Cell Lung Cancer. Orlando, FL, Grune & Stratton, 1981, pp 285-300

87. Lowenbraun S, Bartolucci A, Smalley RV, et al: The superiority of combination chemotherapy over single agent chemotherapy in small cell lung carcinoma. Cancer 44:406-413, 1979

88. MacKay B, Osborne BM, Wilson RA: Ultrastructure of lung neoplasms in lung cancer, in Straus MJ (ed): Lung Cancer: Clinical Diagnosis and Treatment. Orlando, FL, Grune & Stratton, 1977, pp 71-84

89. Matthews MJ: Problems in morphology and behavior of bronchopulmonary malignant disease, in Israel L, Chahinian AP (eds): Lung Cancer: Natural History, Prognosis, and Therapy. Orlando, FL, Academic Press, 1976, pp 23-62

90. Matthews MJ, Hirsch FR: Problems in the diagnosis of small cell carcinoma of the lung, in Greco FA, Oldham RK, Bunn PA Jr. (eds): Small Cell Lung Cancer. Orlando, FL, Grune & Stratton, 1981, pp 35-50

91. Matthews MJ, Kanhouwa S, Pickren J, et al: Frequency of residual and metastatic tumor in patients undergoing curative surgical resection for lung cancer. Cancer Chemother Rep Part 3, 4:63-67, 1983

92. Maurer LH, Pajak TF: Prognostic factors in small cell carcinoma of the lung: A Cancer and Leukemia Group B Study. Cancer Treat Rep 65:767-774, 1981

93. Maurer LH, Pajak T, Eaton W, et al: Combined modality therapy with radiotherapy, chemotherapy, and immunotherapy in limited small cell carcinoma of the lung: A Phase III Cancer and Leukemia Group Study. J Clin Oncol 3:969-976, 1985

94. Maurer LH, Tulloh M, Weiss RB, et al: A randomized combined modality trial in small cell carcinoma of the lung: Comparison of combination chemotherapy-radiation therapy versus cyclophosphamide-radiation therapy, effects of maintenance chemotherapy and prophylactic whole brain irradiation. Cancer 45:30-39, 1980

95. Meigs JW: Epidemic lung cancer in women. JAMA 238:1055, 1977

96. Meyer JA, Comis RL, Ginsberg SJ, et al: Phase II trial of extended indications for resection in small cell carcinoma of the lung. J Thorac Cardiovasc Surg 83:12-19, 1982

97. Miller WE: Roentgenographic manifestations of lung cancer, in Straus MJ: Lung Cancer: Clinical Diagnosis and Treatment. Orlando, FL, Grune & Stratton, 1977, pp 129-136

98. Minna JD, Higgins GA, Glatstein EJ: Cancer of the Lung, in DeVita VT, Hellman S, Rosenberg SA (eds): Principles and Practice of Oncology. Philadelphia. Lippincott, 1985, pp 507-598

99. Mira JG, Livingston RB, Moore TN, et al: Influence of chest radiotherapy in frequency and patterns of relapse in disseminated small cell lung carcinoma. Cancer 50:1266-1272, 1982

100. Mirra AP, Elias J, Miziara A, et al: Exploratory laparotomy in the detection of abdominal metastases of primary lung cancer. Internatl Surg 66:141-143, 1981

101. Mountain CF: Clinical biology of small cell carcinoma: Relationship to surgical therapy. Semin Oncol 5:272-279, 1978

102. Mountain CF, Carr DT, Anderson WAD: A system for the clinical staging of lung cancer. Am J Roentgenol 120:130-138, 1974

103. Muggia FM, Krezoski SK, Hansen HH: Cell kinetics studies in patients with small cell carcinoma of the lung. Cancer 34:1683-1690, 1974

104. Mulshine JL, Makuch RW, Johnston-Early A, et al: Diagnosis and significance of liver metastases in small cell carcinoma of the lung. J Clin Oncol 2:733-741, 1984

105. Murphy KC, Feld R, Evans WK, et al: Intramedullary spinal cord metastases from small cell carcinoma of the lung. J Clin Oncol 1:99-106, 1983

106. Napoli LD, Hansen HH, Muggia FM, et al: The incidence of osseous involvement in lung cancer, with special reference to the development of osteoblastic changes. Radiology 108:17-21, 1973

107. Newman SJ, Hansen HH: Frequency, diagnosis, and treatment of brain metastases in 247 consecutive patients with bronchogenic carcinoma. Cancer 33:492-496, 1974

108. Norlund JD, Byhardt RW, Foley WD, et al: Computed tomography in the staging of small cell lung cancer: Implications for combined modality therapy. Internatl J Radiat Oncol Biol Phys 11:1081-1084, 1985

109. Nugent JL, Bunn PA, Matthews MJ, et al: CNS metastases in small cell bronchogenic carcinoma: increasing frequency and changing pattern with lengthening survival. Cancer 44:1885-1893, 1979

110. Osterlind K, Hansen M, Hansen HH, et al: Treatment policy of surgery in small cell carcinoma of the lung: Retrospective analysis of a series of 874 consecutive patients. Thorax 40:272-277, 1985

111. Pedersen AG, Bach F, Melgaard B: Frequency, diagnosis, and prognosis of spinal cord compression in small cell bronchogenic carcinoma: A review of 817 consecutive patients. Cancer 55:1818-1822, 1985

112. Petrovich Z, Ohanian M, Cox J: Clinical research on the treatment of locally advanced lung cancer. Cancer 42:1129-1134, 1978

113. Qurashi MA, Costanzi JJ, Balachandran S: Iodocholesterol adrenal scanning for the detection of adrenal metastases in lung cancer and its clinical significance. Cancer 48:714-716, 1981

114. Radice PA, Matthews MJ, Ihde DC, et al: Clinical behavior of "mixed" small cell/large cell bronchogenic carcinoma compared to "pure" small cell subtypes. Cancer 50:2894-2902, 1982

115. Rosen ST, Aisner J, Makuch RW, et al: Carcinomatous leptomeningitis in small cell lung cancer: A clinicopathologic review of the National Cancer Institute experience. Medicine 61:45-53, 1982

116. Rosen ST, Makuch W, Lichter AS, et al: The role of prophylactic cranial irradiation in preventing central nervous system metastases in small cell lung cancer. Am J Med 74:615-624, 1983

117. Roswitt B, Patno ME, Rapp R: The survival of patients with inoperable lung cancer: A large-scale randomized study of radiation therapy versus placebo. Radiology 90:688-697, 1968

118. Ruff MR, Pert CB: Small cell carcinoma of the lung: Macrophage-specific antigens suggest hemopoietic stem cell origin. Science 205:1034-1036, 1984

119. Salyer WR, Eggleston JC, Erozan YS: Efficacy of pleural needle biopsy and pleural fluid cytopathology in the diagnosis of malignant neoplasm involving the pleura. Chest 67:536-539, 1975

120. Sculier JP, Feld R, Evans WK, et al: Carcinoembryonic antigen: A useful prognostic marker in small cell lung cancer. J Clin Oncol 3:1349-1354, 1985

121. Shackney SE, Straus MJ, Bunn PA Jr: The growth characteristics of small cell carcinoma of the lung, in Greco FA, Oldham RK, Bunn PA Jr (eds): Small Cell Lung Cancer. Orlando, FL, Grune & Stratton, 1981, pp 225-234

122. Shepherd FA, Ginsberg RJ, Feld R, et al: Reduction in local recurrence and improved survival in surgically treated patients with small cell lung cancer. J Thorac Cardiovasc Surg 86:498-506, 1983

123. Shields TW, Higgins GA, Matthews MJ, et al: Surgical resection in the management of small cell carcinoma of the lung. J Thorac Cardiovasc Surg 84:481-488, 1982

124. Sobin LH, Yesner R: Histologic typing of lung tumors, in International Histologic Typing of Tumors. Geneva, World Health Organization, 1981

125. Souhami RL, Bradbury I, Geddes DM, et al: Prognostic significance of laboratory parameters measured at diagnosis in small cell carcinoma of the lung. Cancer Res 45:2878-2882, 1985

126. Spiro SG, Shah S, Harper PG, et al: Treatment of obstruction of the superior vena cava by combination chemotherapy with and without irradiation in small cell carcinoma of the bronchus. Thorax 38:501-505, 1983

127. Stahel RA, Mabry M, Skarin AT, et al: Detection of bone marrow metastasis in small cell lung cancer by monoclonal antibody. J Clin Oncol 3:455-461, 1985

128. Tateishi R: Distribution of argyrophilic cells in adult human lungs. Arch Pathol 96:198-202, 1973

129. Tockman MS, Frost JK, Stitik FP, et al: Screening and detection of lung cancer, in Aisner J (ed): Lung Cancer. New York, Churchill Livingston, 1985, pp 25-40

130. Van Hazel GA, Scott M, Eagan RT: The effect of CNS metastases on the survival of patients with small cell cancer of the lung. Cancer 51:933-937, 1983

131. VanHoutte P, DeJager R, Lustman-Marechal J, et al: Prognostic value of the superior

vena cava syndrome as the presenting sign of small cell anaplastic carcinoma of the lung. Eur J Cancer 16:1447-1450, 1980

132. Vas W, Zylak CJ, Mather D, Figueredo A: The value of abdominal computed tomography in the pretreatment assessment of small cell carcinoma of the lung. Radiology 138:417-418, 1981

133. Weiss W: Small cell carcinoma of the lung: Epidemiology and etiology, in Greco FA, Oldham RK, Bunn PA Jr (eds): Small Cell Lung Cancer. Orlando, FL, Grune & Stratton, 1981, pp 1-34

134. Weiss W, Boucot KR, Seidman H, et al: Risk of lung cancer according to histologic type and cigarette dosage. JAMA 222:799-801, 1972

135. Weiss W, Moser RL, Auerbach O: Lung cancer in chloromethyl ether workers. Am Rev Resp Dis 120:1031-1037, 1979

136. Weissberg D, Kaufman M, Zurkowski Z: Pleuroscopy in patients with pleural effusion and pleural masses. Ann Thorac Surg 29:205-208, 1979

137. Whang-Peng J, Kao-Shen CS, Lee EC, et al: A specific chromosomal defect associated with human small cell lung cancer: Deletion 3p(14-23). Science 215:181-182, 1982

138. Whitley NO, Fuks JZ, McCrea ES, et al: Computed tomography of the chest in small cell lung cancer: Potential new prognostic signs. Am J Radiol 141:885-892, 1984

139. Wittes RE, Yeh SDJ: Indications for liver and brain scans: screening tests for patients with oat cell carcinoma of the lung. JAMA 238:506-507, 1977

140. Zelen M: Keynote address on biostatics and data retrieval. Cancer Chemotherapy Rep (Part 3) 4:31-42, 1973

David H. Johnson
F. Anthony Greco

_____ **21** _____

Biomarkers in Small Cell Lung Cancer

Small cell lung cancer (SCLC) accounts for approximately 25 percent of the newly diagnosed bronchogenic carcinomas each year and is unique among the lung cancers because of its clinical behavior and its exquisite sensitivity to chemotherapy.[31,37,49,69] Currently up to 90 percent of SCLC patients will experience an objective response to therapy and perhaps as many as 10–15 percent will survive disease-free for 3 or more years.[49,69] These results are in stark contrast to our ability to treat this malignancy prior to 1970, when median survivals ranged from 6 to 12 weeks and fewer than 2 percent of patients survived for more than 2 years.[49,69] However, since about 1978 very little additional progress has been made in the management of SCLC.[69] In fact, despite impressive overall response rates and improved median survivals, the majority of patients continue to die of their disease.[49] Several reasons have been proposed for this apparent plateau of therapeutic progress, not the least of which is the inadequacy of the current rather crude staging system.[49] It has been suggested that an improved ability to detect micrometastases could potentially lead to better treatment results since currently available therapy could be employed at a theoretically more optimum point, that is, when tumor burden is minimal and therefore presumably more susceptible to chemotherapy.[29] To this end, many investigators have focused on evaluating newer methods of assessing the status of patients with SCLC. Because management of other chemosensitive neoplasms (e.g., germ cell neoplasms, gestational choriocarcinoma) has been improved through the use of tumor markers, it is believed that similar improvement could be obtained in SCLC management if an adequate marker or markers were available. SCLC is known to be associated with a plethora of ectopically produced peptides [38,65,82] (Table 21-1). In addition, recent studies investigating the cellular biology of SCLC have identified several characteristic enzymes produced by this neoplasm.[13,66] Potentially all or some of these tumor products represent possible biomarkers.

Under _ideal_ circumstances, a tumor marker should satisfy the following criteria:[62]

1. It should be produced only by tumor cells.
2. Its concentration in blood or urine should reflect the extent of disease

LUNG CANCER: A COMPREHENSIVE TREATISE
ISBN 0-8089-1876-1

present, and its measurement should be sufficiently sensitive to detect micro-scopic or subclinical disease.

3. Its assay should be convenient, inexpensive, and accurate.
4. It should occur with sufficient frequency to make its measurement worth-while.

In clinical practice, no currently available tumor marker completely fulfills these crite-ria. Indeed, most substances purported to be "tumor markers" are invariably found to lack complete specificity and are typically not sensitive enough to accurately monitor therapeutic response or to predict recurrence.[49,62] Nevertheless, under appropriate circumstances, some markers such as carcinoembryonic antigen (CEA), B-human chorionic gonadotropin (B-HCG), and α-fetoprotein (A-FP) have proven useful in the management of specific malignancies.[62] For this reason, the quest for a tumor marker useful in the management of SCLC continues.

Assuming an adequate biomarker was identified, it could prove useful in several ways, such as providing for (1) initial detection and diagnosis of the neoplasm, (2) determination of recurrent disease, (3) evaluation of response, and (4) a better under-standing of the biological nature of the malignancy by evaluating changes in marker level during the course of therapy. Even if a substance possessed some of these characteristics, it could prove useful in the management of certain cancers.

This chapter will review recent studies aimed at evaluating some of the many peptides and enzymes associated with SCLC as biomarkers. When possible, sensitivity and specificity will be addressed. We will attempt to put into perspective the clinical usefulness of each marker.

POLYPEPTIDES (ACTH, ADH, CALCITONIN)

Although the association of pulmonary malignancies with certain hormonal syn-dromes has been recognized for more than 50 years, the nature of this association did not become clear until the 1960s.[9,64] Subsequently, all lung neoplasms, but especially SCLC, have been found to be associated with many "ectopically" produced hormones (Table 21-1). Because of the association of SCLC with multiple peptides, it was hoped that one or perhaps several of these substances would prove useful as a biomarker of SCLC.[9,38,82] The peptides most extensively evaluated in this regard include adreno-corticotropin (ACTH), vasopressin or antidiuretic hormone (ADH), and calci-tonin.[9,32,38] Each of these peptides has been evaluated for its frequency of elevation at diagnosis (Table 21-2), its diagnostic value, its relationship to tumor burden, the ability

Table 21-1
Protein Products Associated
with Small Cell Lung Cancer

ACTH	MSH	LH
ADH	Bombesin	Serotonin
Calcitonin	HCG	Neurophysins
CRF	HGH	Renin
FSH	HPL	PTH

Table 21-2
Frequency of Elevated Peptides at Diagnosis in SCLC

ACTH	ADH	Calcitonin	Reference
22/75 (29%)	25/75 (33%)	48/74 (65%)	39
15/50 (30%)	—	26/54 (48%)	33
—	9/54 (17%)	22/54 (41%)	32
—	9/25 (36%)	10/27 (37%)	47
37/125 (30%)	43/154 (28%)	106/209 (51%)	

to predict and mirror clinical response and relapse (Table 21-3), and its prognostic value (Table 21-4).

ACTH

Plasma ACTH levels are elevated in 10-40 percent of SCLC patients depending on the specificity of the assay employed, the timing of specimen collection, and the nature of the control population.[32,33,39,40,42] When previously untreated SCLC patients are evaluated, approximately 30 percent demonstrate elevations of biologically active ACTH.[32,39] Studies reporting a lower incidence usually have included treated as well as untreated individuals.[32,38] Groups who have measured the biologically *inactive* form of ACTH (i.e., "big" ACTH) have found a higher incidence of abnormal pretherapy ACTH in SCLC but typically report a higher frequency of abnormal ACTH levels in non-small cell lung cancers (NSCLC) as well.[26,43,44,81,97,104] Thus an elevated ACTH will not distinguish between SCLC and NSCLC (Table 21-5). Additionally, some nonmalignant processes occasionally are accompanied by elevated ACTH levels.[104]

Attempts to enhance the discriminatory ability of ACTH by means of the dexamethasone suppression test have proven unsuccessful since both false-positive and false-negative results have been reported.[9,32,38,39,97] The dexamethasone suppression test thus does not appear to enhance the diagnostic capability of ACTH determinations.[38]

Table 21-3
Pretreatment Peptide Levels; Prediction of Response

Marker		Number of Patients Responding/Total	Ratio	P Value
ACTH	Normal	30/43	.70	> .2
	Elevated	12/18	.67	
CT	Normal	12/20	.60	> .2
	Elevated	30/41	.73	
SIADH	Absent	30/41	.73	> .2
	Present	12/20	.60	
All 3 normal		6/10	.60	> .2
> 2 abnormal		16/23	.73	

Modified from Hansen J, Hammer M, Hummer L: Diagnostic and therapeutic implications of ectopic hormone production in small cell carcinoma of the lung. Thorax 35:101-106, 1980.

Table 21-4

Relationship of Pretreatment Peptide Levels to Survival

Marker		Median Survival (Days)	P Value	Number Alive >1 Year
ACTH	Normal	325	>.05	17/44 (39%)
	Elevated	298		8/18 (44%)
CT	Normal	357	>.05	9/21 (43%)
	Elevated	262		15/40 (38%)
SIADH	Absent	360	>.05	18/41 (44%)
	Present	260		6/21 (29%)
All normal		363	>.05	6/11 (55%)
>2 abnormal		262		9/24 (38%)

Modified from Hansen J, Hammer M, Hummer L: Diagnostic and therapeutic implications of ectopic hormone production in small cell carcinoma of the lung. Thorax 35:101-106, 1980.

Hansen and co-workers were unable to demonstrate a correlation between pretreatment ACTH levels and stage.[40] Likewise, changes in ACTH levels do not correlate well with clinical response.[40] Although patients with an elevated pretreatment ACTH level experience a fall in ACTH with remission in most cases, a similar correlation is lacking in those with *normal* pretreatment levels.[38-40] In relapsing patients, ACTH levels are even potentially misleading as levels increase in fewer than 50 percent of patients experiencing a recurrence of disease.[38,39]

Although an elevated pretreatment plasma ACTH per se does *not* appear to portend a worse survival when compared to individuals with normal pretreatment levels,[38,40] (Table 21-4), some investigators have reported poorer survival rates among SCLC patients exhibiting *clinical* symptoms of Cushing's syndrome.[1,10] These reports conflict with our experience at Vanderbilt University, as some of our patients with Cushing's syndrome due to ectopic ACTH production have survived for nearly 2 years (unpublished data).

Table 21-5

Relationship of Lung Cancer Cell Type to Ectopic Hormone Production

Hormone	Number Elevated/Total		
	SCLC	SqCCA*	AdenoCa†
ACTH	39/190	0/36	5/20
	(36%)	(0%)	(25%)
ADH	61/264	0/18	4/14
	(23%)	(0%)	(25%)
Calcitonin	115/226	27/137	20/60
	(51%)	(20%)	(33%)

Modified from Bondy (12) PK: The pattern of ectopic hormone production in lung cancer. Yale J Biol Med 54:181-185, 1981.
*Squamous cell lung cancer.
†Adenocarcinoma of the lung.

ADH

Inappropriate secretion of ADH (i.e., SIADH) has been reported in up to 75 percent of SCLC patients at diagnosis. The frequency of SIADH depends on how patients are tested for it.[32,38,40] In contrast, the clinical symptoms of SIADH are less frequent.[32,38,54] Our group has found immunoreactive ADH to be increased in 17–33 percent of patients with SCLC[32,36,54] (Table 21-2). Groups reporting higher incidences of SIADH have either employed water-loading (to enhance the degree of abnormality), measured urinary ADH levels, or simply evaluated patients for hyponatremia without actually measuring ADH levels.[16,34]

The presence of inappropriate ADH secretion does *not* correlate with stage at diagnosis; nor is there an obvious association with histologic subtype of SCLC. Some investigators have reported an increased frequency of SIADH in patients with extensive SCLC or with involvement of certain metastatic sites.[32,42,54,56] We found that bone marrow involvement was more common among patients with SCLC and SIADH, whereas Lokich found a higher incidence of CNS involvement.[54,56] Nevertheless, the presence of SIADH does not appear to adversely influence survival rate (Fig. 21-1). This observation is in agreement with that reported by Hansen et al.[40] (Table 21-4). Souhami et al. reported that hyponatremia at diagnosis adversely influenced survival rate; however, it is not apparent that all patients actually had SIADH.[94]

Levels of ADH fall to normal or near normal, and symptoms of SIADH typically resolve in the course of therapy.[32,40,54] Patients with relapsed SCLC generally will have elevated ADH levels and SIADH; however, there are numerous instances when this does not occur.[32,38,39,40,54] Also, the elevations of ADH at relapse frequently are modest and usually occur when the recurrent disease is readily evident.[32,36,38,54] Elevated ADH level or SIADH rarely precedes the clinical detection of recurrent SCLC.[54,103]

Calcitonin

Serum calcitonin has been reported to be abnormal in approximately 40–60 percent of SCLC patients [32,39,40,63,90,91] (Table 21-2). Pentagastrin stimulation does not substantially alter the frequency of abnormal pretreatment values.[41] As with

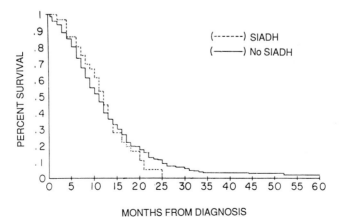

Fig. 21-1. Survival with or without SIADH.

ACTH and ADH, variation in the reported incidence appears to be related to method-ology and the type of control population. Again, elevated calcitonin levels are not unique to SCLC but can be found in NSCLC also (Table 21-5). Although very high levels of calcitonin (consistent with those reported in medullary thyroid carcinoma) frequently have been reported in SCLC, there is no consistent correlation with the calcitonin level and the stage of SCLC.[32,39-41,63] Shappino et al. reported that an elevated pretreatment calcitonin level correlated with the presence of liver metas-tases;[90] others have failed to confirm this observation.[32,40] Typically, raised pretreat-ment calcitonin levels will fall to normal or near normal with response to chemother-apy.[32,39,40] In contrast to ACTH and ADH, calcitonin may be a useful predictor of recurrent SCLC prior to the onset of clinical relapse.[32,39] Several groups of investiga-tors have reported elevated calcitonin levels in up to 90 percent of patients with SCLC prior to the clinical determination of recurrent disease.[32,39] There appears to be no difference with respect to response or survival rate on the basis of an elevated versus normal pretreatment calcitonin level[32,38-40] (Tables 21-3 and 21-4).

From the data presented, it appears that ACTH, ADH, and calcitonin, either individually and collectively, are inadequate biomarkers of SCLC.[39,49] All three lack specificity and do not correlate with the extent of disease, and changes in serum levels do not correlate well with changes in disease status to prove clinically useful.[32,38] Even in the case of calcitonin, which appears capable of reflecting early relapse of SCLC, the increments in calcitonin are modest in most instances.[32,38,40] Additionally, calci-tonin may be elevated (false-positive) at a time when the tumor is regressing in size.[38] Therefore, the routine measurement of ACTH, ADH, and calcitonin does not appear to be beneficial in the management of patients with SCLC.

It should be stressed that ectopic production of ACTH by a lung neoplasm has been convincingly demonstrated only in SCLC and carcinoids.[92] Likewise, ADH secretion is virtually confined to SCLC. Consequently, the presence of either Cush-ing's syndrome or SIADH in a patient with a lung tumor would argue strongly for the diagnosis of SCLC. Because of the infrequency of these clinical syndromes, however, fewer than 10 percent of patients can be expected to be diagnosed in this manner.

CARCINOEMBRYONIC ANTIGEN

Carcinoembryonic antigen (CEA) was first described in 1965 by Gold and Freed-man.[28] CEA is really a family of related glycoproteins with considerable heterogeneity of the carbohydrate portion but a uniform protein component. Although CEA is located on the cell surface of many normal tissues, including colon and liver, its biologic function remains unclear. CEA levels may be elevated in the absence of malignancy such as in nonmalignant hepatic, gastrointestinal, and pulmonary dis-eases. Smokers tend to have slightly higher CEA levels when compared to nonsmok-ers. The common denominator for increased plasma levels of CEA in the absence of cancer appears to be a breakdown in the anatomic barrier between an epithelial surface and its underlying tissues (i.e., disruption of the basement membrane).

CEA has been evaluated as a possible biomarker in a variety of malignan-cies,[21,58,95,98] and recently several investigators have explored its usefulness in the management of SCLC.[30,57,63,88,100,105] Because virtually all SCLC patients have a smoking history, levels of greater than 5-6 ng/ml are considered to be abnormal in

Table 21-6
CEA Elevation at Diagnosis in Small Cell Lung Cancer

Total Patients*		Pretreatment CEA >5 ng/ml		Reference
42	LD = 14	20 (48%)	3 (21%)	99
	ED = 28		17 (61%)	
85	LD = 44	37 (44%)	6 (13%)	30
	ED = 41		31 (76%)	
61	LD = 29	32 (52%)	13 (45%)	57
	ED = 32		19 (59%)	
180	LD = 97	61† (34%)	22 (23%)	88
	ED = 83		39 (47%)	
368		150 (41%)	44 (24%)	
			106 (58%)	

*LD = limited disease; ED = extensive disease.
†CEA >6 ng/ml.

this population.[30,57,88,100,105] Using the latter value as a cutoff point, between 35-50 percent of SCLC patients have been found to have elevated pretreatment CEA levels (Table 21-6). Typically, elevated levels tend to be more common among patients with extensive-stage disease, especially when multiple metastases are present.[30,57,88,99] Goslin et al reported that no patient with limited disease had a pretreatment CEA of greater than 10.1 ng/ml and that *all* patients with pretreatment values of greater than 50 ng/ml had hepatic metastases.[30] Sculier et al has confirmed that *markedly elevated* pretreatment CEA levels (i.e., >50 ng/ml) are more common among patients with liver involvement (8/42 vs 9/138; $P = 0.04$) but are not confined to the latter group.[88] Indeed, five patients with limited disease were found to have pretreatment CEA greater than 50 ng/ml.[88] Thus, although CEA levels tend to reflect tumor burden, no clear pattern emerges with respect to a particular metastatic site (Table 21-7).

Table 21-7
Correlation of Pretreatment CEA Level with Specific Metastatic Sites

Site	CEA	Goslin et al[30]	Lokich[57]	Sculier et al.[88]
Liver	Normal	2/23 (9%)	5/14 (36%)	22/42 (52%)
	Abnormal	21/23 (91%)	9/14 (64%)	20/42 (48%)
	>50 ng/ml	12/23 (52%)	6/14 (43%)	8/42 (19%)
Bone	Normal	4/11 (36%)	7/13 (54%)	21/36 (58%)
	Abnormal	7/11 (64%)	6/13 (46%)	15/36 (42%)
	>50 ng/ml	—	—	—
Bone marrow	Normal	3/5 (60%)	—	13/24 (54%)
	Abnormal	2/5 (40%)	—	11/24 (46%)
	>50 ng/ml	2/5 (40%)	—	3/24 (13%)
CNS	Normal	3/5 (60%)	—	2/4 (50%)
	Abnormal	2/5 (40%)	—	2/4 (50%)
	>50 ng/ml	—	—	1/4 (25%)

Table 21-8

Association of Pretreatment CEA Level with Response to Treatment

Response	Pretreatment CEA Level		P Value	Reference
	Normal	Elevated		
Overall	17/21 (81%)	16/20 (80%)	> .5	99
	97/112 (87%)	42/57 (74%)	.054	88
Complete	10/21 (48%)	6/20 (30%)	< .05	99
	52/112 (46%)	8/57 (14%)	.00003	88

Patients with elevated pretreatment CEA levels are no less likely to obtain an objective response to chemotherapy than are patients presenting with normal pretreatment values[30,57,88,100] (Table 21-8). However, both Waalkes et al. and Sculier et al. reported that *complete* responses are statistically more common among patients with normal pretreatment CEAs[88,100] (Table 21-8). Furthermore, Waalkes et al. noted that among patients with *extensive-stage* disease, *no* complete responses were obtained in those with a pretreatment CEA level above 15 ng/ml, whereas 40 percent with levels below 15 ng/ml achieved a complete remission.[100]

Waalkes et al. found that pretreatment CEA levels failed to predict survival outcome and that initial stage was more important in this regard.[100] Median survival for patients with raised CEA levels was 12 months, versus 14 months for those with levels below 5 ng/ml ($P > .3$) (Table 21-9). The higher complete response rate seen in extensive-stage patients with a pretreatment CEA below 15 ng/ml translated into an improved median survival compared to patients with CEA above 15 ng/ml, but this difference was also not statistically significant (12 months vs. 6 months; $P = .09$). In contrast, Sculier et al reported that patients with a normal pretreatment CEA enjoyed a statistically superior median survival compared to those with raised levels (12.2 months vs 8.8 months; $P = .0007$)[88] (Table 21-9). Of interest, this finding proved to be *independent* of pretreatment ECOG performance status and stage—features generally considered to be most predictive of prognosis in SCLC. No patient with an elevated pretreatment CEA experienced a prolonged survival, whereas 11 patients with normal pretherapy values survived more than 2.5 years.[88]

Most investigators have found an excellent correlation between changes in CEA levels and the clinical course of SCLC. Goslin et al. reported that among patients with raised pretreatment CEAs, a response was always accompanied by a fall in the CEA level[30] (Table 21-10). Similar results have been reported by Lokich[57] and Waalkes et al.[100] Likewise, responding patients with abnormal pretreatment CEA levels almost always experienced a rise in the CEA value at relapse[30,100] (Table 21-10). Waalkes et al. found that in nearly 60 percent of cases, the rise in CEA *preceded* clinical recognition of recurrence by an average of three months.[100] Patients with normal pretreat-

Table 21-9

Association of Pretreatment CEA Level with Survival Rate

Median Survival (Months)		P Value	Reference
Normal CEA	Elevated CEA		
14.0	12.0	> .3	99
12.2	8.8	.0007	88

Table 21-10
Correlation of CEA with Clinical Status of SCLC

CEA Decrease at Remission	CEA Increase Prior to or Simultaneous with Relapse	Reference
23/29 (73%)	21/27 (78%)	99
22/22 (100%)*	44/55 (80%)	30
5/8 (63%)†	5/5 (100%)	57

*Includes only patients with elevated pre-treatment CEA.
†Includes only patients with pre-treatment cea >20 ng/ml

ment CEAs were less likely to experience an increase in plasma CEA with recurrence (10/21).[30] Interestingly, Goslin et al. noted that of 11 relapsing patients with *no* change in plasma CEA, 7 (64 percent) recurred *locally* without developing evidence of extrathoracic metastases before death.[30] In contrast to responding patients, nonresponding patients experienced a progressive rise in plasma CEAs in most cases.[30,57,100]

In summary, plasma CEA is elevated (i.e., >5 ng/ml) in about 50 percent of untreated SCLC patients. Clearly, CEA lacks both sensitivity and specificity for SCLC. Although high pretherapy CEA levels are more common in patients with extensive-stage disease, levels only roughly correlate with tumor extent. Markedly elevated levels (i.e., >50 ng/ml) are found primarily in patients with hepatic metastases but are not diagnostic of liver involvement. High levels occasionally are seen in patients with limited-stage disease. Pretreatment CEA levels appear to be helpful in estimating the possibility of achieving a complete remission and in this respect may be a useful tool for stratifying patients entering randomized treatment trials. However, further evaluation is needed. Serial CEA determinations tend to mirror the clinical status of patients with elevated pretherapy levels, falling with remission and increasing with recurrence. A rise in plasma CEA may antedate clinical recognition of recurrence by several weeks to months and may be useful in determining when salvage therapy is to be started. Patients with apparently local recurrence and normal CEA levels may be the most appropriate candidates for salvage therapy aimed specifically at intrathoracic disease (i.e., radiotherapy and/or surgery) since preliminary data indicate that these patients die primarily without extrathoracic spread.[30]

CREATINE KINASE BB

Trace amounts of the brain isoenzyme of creatine kinase (CK-BB) can be found in normal serum and may be markedly elevated in patients with a variety of neoplasms including SCLC.[17,84,109] Coolen and colleagues were the first to report that CK-BB was increased in SCLC. In their study, 16 out of 39 patients with various malignancies were found to have elevated CK-BB levels.[17] Twelve of the abnormal levels were found in patients with SCLC, only one of whom had a CNS metastasis. Six patients with small cell carcinoma (3 with a lung primary; 3 with an esophageal primary) had normal CK-BB levels. Notably, in most instances, the *total* serum CK levels were within normal limits. Of these 18 patients, 8 had already received either chemotherapy or radiotherapy when CK-BB was evaluated; therefore, the incidence of pretreatment CK-BB elevation cannot be determined.

More recently Carney et al. evaluated the value of CK-BB determinations in 105 newly diagnosed and untreated SCLC patients.[14] Their patients were staged in the usual manner; 42 were found to have limited disease, while 63 had extensive-stage disease. Previously these investigators had found the mean CK-BB level to be 3.4 ng/ml in healthy adult volunteers. Although 95 percent of normal adults had levels of less than 6.2 ng/ml, a value greater than 10 ng/ml was considered abnormal.[109] Overall, only 27 out of 105 (26 percent) had a raised pretreatment CK-BB (range: 11–522 ng/ml) including 1 out of 42 (2 percent) with limited disease and 26 out of 63 (41 percent) with extensive-stage disease. These investigators did not find an association between an elevated CK-BB and metastatic disease in any specific site. In fact, only 4 out of 11 patients with brain metastasis had elevated CK-BB levels. However, as the number of metastatic sites increased, the frequency of elevated CK-BB levels also increased. Among patients with elevated CK-BB levels, those with the higher levels tended to have the greatest number of metastatic sites of disease (Table 21-11). Survival rate of patients with a raised pretreatment CK-BB was worse than that of individuals with normal levels (13 months vs 5 months; $P > .001$). This relationship held true even when the analysis was made *after* adjusting for the number of metastatic sites, indicating that both the CK-BB level and the number of metastatic sites represent independent variables that correlate with survival.

Serial CK-BB evaluations were reported for only a small number of patients. Of 12 extensive-disease patients responding to chemotherapy (5 CR: [5, complete response (CR); 7, partial response (PR)], 10 demonstrated a normalization or near normalization of serum CK-BB at the time of restaging. One nonresponding patient demonstrated a rise in CK-BB. Among patients experiencing a relapse, previously normal CK-BB levels were found to increase. Four patients remained disease-free at the time of the report, and all four had normal CK-BB levels.

These data indicate that CK-BB isoenzymes may provide some useful prognostic information in SCLC patients with extensive disease. Like the other markers, however, CK-BB provides little diagnostic information because of its lack of sensitivity and specificity.[84,109] Although CK-BB determination has provided a diagnostic clue to SCLC in certain unique circumstances, it cannot be recommended as a routine stag-

Table 21-11
Serum CK-BB Levels in SCLC

	Patient No.	Abnormal CK-BB	CK-BB Level Mean + SE (ng/ml)
LD	42	1	33.7 ± 0.5
ED			
1 met*	31	6	15.5 ± 6.39
2 mets	18	6	43.9 ± 32.06
3 mets	8	6	43.0 ± 12.87
≥ 4 mets	8	8	82.9 ± 36.57

Modified from Carney DN, Zweig MH, Ihde DC, et al: Elevated serum creatine kinase BB levels in patients with small cell lung cancer. Cancer Res 44:5399–5403, 1984.
*Metastasis.

ing test at this time.[49,52] Like CEA, CK-BB may be a useful tool for stratifying exten-sive-stage patients entering clinical trials since it does appear to provide useful prog-nostic information.

NEUROPHYSINS

Neurophysins are low-molecular-weight single-chain proteins normally produced by neurons of the hypothalamus.[61,72,73] Neurophysins are part of the precursor struc-ture of vasopressin and oxytocin and act as carrier molecules for these hormones.[73] Their close association with some of the peptides known to be produced ectopically by SCLC led investigators at Dartmouth Medical School to evaluate neurophysins as possible markers of SCLC.[72,73] Prior to undertaking this evaluation, these investiga-tors had extensively studied neurophysin kinetics in normal human plasma, using radioimmunoassays they had developed.[73] Normal values for both vasopressin-hu-man neurophysin (73 ± 5 pg/ml) and oxytocin-human neurophysin (283 ± 30 pg/ml) (VP-HNP and OT-HNP, respectively) were established.[73] An elevated value was defined as a level three times the mean for normal subjects in the absence of any conditions known to affect neurophysin release or renal clearance (e.g., estrogen is a strong stimulus for the release of OT-HNP).

In a recent update, North et al. reviewed the results in 151 SCLC patients, 103 of whom had serial determinations of HNP.[73] Overall, 64 percent (96/151) had elevated pretreatment HNP levels (i.e., "secretors" of HNP) and an additional 13 percent (19/51) had levels two to three times the normal mean (i.e., "possible secretors"). The remaining patients had normal HNP levels (nonsecretors). Among the HNP secretors, 72 patients (48 percent) produced VP-HNP, 45 (30 percent) produced OT-HNP, and 22 (15 percent) produced both VP-HNP and OT-HNP. The overall incidence of abnormal levels was the same in men and women and in those with intermediate cell subtype and oat cell subtype. Neurophysin levels were more commonly elevated in patients with extensive disease (82 percent) versus limited disease (40 percent) (Table 21-12). However, North et al. speculated that this difference was not solely elated to tumor burden but rather represented an inherent difference in cells with a proclivity for metastasis as compared to cells less inclined to spread.[40] They support their position by pointing out that neurophysin levels do not necessarily increase serially in relapsing patients. In fact, nonsecretors rarely, if ever, develop elevated HNP levels, or as they

Table 21-12
Neurophysins in SCLC

Stage	Total Patients	Number Elevated HNP
Limited	42	17 (40%)
Extensive	61	50 (82%)
All	103	67 (65%)

Modified from Maurer LH, O'Donnell JF, Kennedy S, et al: Human neurophysins in carcinoma of the lung: Relation to his-tology, disease stage, response rate, survival, and syndrome of inappropriate antidiuretic hormone secretion. Cancer Treat Rep 67:971-976, 1983.

Table 21-13

Pretreatment Neurophysin Status and Prognosis

	Limited Disease		Extensive Disease	
HNP Secretory Status	Response (CR*)	Median Survival	Response (CR)	Median Survival
Secretor	89% (65%)	9.3 mo	36% (8%)	6.1 mo
Possible secretor	100% (22%)	10.0 mo	50% (50%)	5.8 mo
Nonsecretor	76% (63%)	9.5 mo	44% (11%)	6.5 mo

Modified from North WG, Maurer LH, Valtin H, et al: Human neurophysins as potential tumor markers for small cell carcinoma of the lungs: Application of specific radioimmunoassays. J Clin Endocrin Metab 51:892–896, 1980.
*Percent complete response.

put it, "once a nonsecretor (of HNP) always a nonsecretor."[73] Indeed, recent data from Johns Hopkins would appear to support the concept of differing clinical behavior based on the presence or absence of various paraneoplastic phenomena.[20]

Although patients with nonsecreting tumors generally maintained normal HNP levels regardless of their clinical status, there appeared to be an excellent correlation between clinical status and HNP levels among the SCLC patients categorized as secretors (i.e., those with elevated pretreatment levels). All patients achieving a partial or complete response had a concomitant decrease (two to thirtyfold) in the previously elevated HNP level. Patients failing to respond to therapy typically experienced a progressive rise in plasma HNP level. Among patients achieving a partial or complete response, relapse was often heralded by a significant (i.e., >1.4 times) rise in the remission HNP level that *always* preceded clinical recognition of relapse by 3–12 weeks.[73] There has been only one "false-positive" increase in HNP to date among the 103 patients undergoing serial evaluation (although a non-tumor-related condition could have been responsible since no data on pathologic confirmation were given). Median survival, complete, and overall response rates were not statistically different between secretors, possible secretors, and nonsecretors of HNP (Table 21-13).

As is true of the various other peptides associated with SCLC, neurophysins are not specific for SCLC, and elevations can be found in patients with NSCLC (Table 21-14). In general, the HNP levels are lower in patients with NSCLC, and statistically, if

Table 21-14

Neurophysins in NSCLC

Cell Type*	Total	Number of Patients with Elevated NP
SqCCa	29	4 (14%)
AdenoCa	17	5 (29%)
LCCa	10	2 (20%)

Modified from Maurer LH, O'Donnell JF, Kennedy S, et al: Human neurophysins in carcinoma of the lung: Relation to histology, disease stage, response rate, survival, and syndrome of inappropriate antidiuretic hormone secretion. Cancer Treat Rep 67:971–976, 1983.
*Abbreviations: SqCCA = squamous cell carcinoma; AdenoCa = adenocarcinoma; LCCa = large cell carcinoma.

one uses cutoff values of 300 pg/ml for VP-HNP and 1100 pg/ml for OT-HNP, very few NSCLC patients will exceed these levels.[73] Nevertheless, the measurement of neurophysins does not appear to be a useful discriminatory test for SCLC.

NEURON-SPECIFIC ENOLASE

Enolase is a glycolytic enzyme present in all human cells that catalyzes the conversion of 2-phosphoglycerate to phosphoenol pyruvate.[59] There are three dimeric isoenzymes consisting of alpha, beta, or gamma subunits. One of these isoenzymes (gamma-gamma) was initially detected in neurons and at one time was thought to be found exclusively in these cells; hence the name "neuron-specific enolase" (NSE).[59,87] However, NSE has now been demonstrated to reside in a variety of endocrine tissues, including neuroendocrine neoplasms.[80,87,96] The cells of these endocrine tissues share many common biochemical and cytologic features with neurons and may also share a common embryologic derivation from the neuroectoderm. In view of these similarities, numerous investigators have recently evaluated NSE as a possible biomarker of SCLC based on the known neuroendocrine features of the latter.

Marangos and co-workers at the National Institute of Health (NIH) were the first to demonstrate high levels of NSE in the supernatants of SCLC cell cultures.[60] Using a rabbit antisera raised against human NSE,[75] these same investigators subsequently reported that 68 percent of 94 previously untreated SCLC patients had elevated serum NSE levels when compared to healthy adult controls.[12] NSE levels were raised more often in patients with extensive-stage disease, and especially in patients with multiple sites of involvement. Among extensive-stage patients, NSE levels tended to correlate well with tumor burden. Of 21 responding patients with elevated pretreatment NSE levels, 20 (95 percent) demonstrated a fall in serum NSE level at the time of restaging. Significantly, *all* complete responders normalized their serum NSE value. Nine of 11 relapsing patients had had a raised pretreatment NSE that fell with response and then increased with relapse. Two of these 11 patients had had normal pretherapy NSE levels but nevertheless demonstrated a rise in the NSE level with relapse. Thus all 11 relapsing patients experienced an increase in NSE at the time of recurrence. Four patients were in sustained remission at the time of the report, and all had normal NSE levels. Pretreatment NSE levels did *not* prove predictive of response or survival.

This report was followed by several others that have confirmed and expanded on these initial observations.[2,4,23,47,74] These studies have demonstrated that 65–75 percent of SCLC patients will have raised pretreatment NSE levels (65–69) (Table 21-15). Typically, patients with extensive-stage disease are more likely to present with abnormal pretreatment values (80–90 percent). We and others have found that pretreatment NSE levels fairly accurately reflect tumor burden in extensive-stage patients as judged by correlation with number of involved metastatic sites (Fig. 21-2).[2,4,23,47,74]

Serial NSE levels have proven useful in monitoring the clinical course of SCLC patients as levels tend to decrease with response and rise with relapse.[2,4,12,23,47] We obtained serial NSE determinations in 57 patients, 50 of whom responded to chemotherapy.[47] Forty (80 percent) of the responding patients demonstrated a fall in serum NSE toward normal. Of the 7 patients with progressive disease, 5 (71 percent) had further increases in NSE, while 30 out of 35 (86 percent) relapsing patients were found to have increasing NSE levels, some up to 3 months in advance of clinical

Table 21-15
Pretreatment NSE Levels in SCLC

Upper Limit of Normal (ng/ml)	Limited Stage	Extensive Stage	Total	Reference
12	15/38 (39%)	49/56 (87%)	64/94 (68%)	12
7.5	—	—	13/20 (65%)	4
20	23/39 (59%)	45/54 (83%)	68/93 (73%)	47
12	34/48 (71%)	54/55 (98%)	88/103 (85%)	23
25	24/48 (50%)	50/55 (91%)	74/103 (72%)	23
16	6/16 (38%)	22/27 (81%)	28/43 (65%)	2
13.5	25/38 (66%)	34/39 (87%)	59/77 (77%)	18

recognition of relapse[47] (Fig. 21-3). NSE levels may vary somewhat during remission, but both we and Cooper et al. found that a sustained NSE elevation in an otherwise disease-free patient is a harbinger of relapse.[18,47] In some instances, relapse has occurred in the face of a persistently normal NSE, including cases in which previously abnormal pretreatment values had normalized.[47] In some such instances the patient has been found to have a NSCLC at relapse, however, suggesting that a clinically

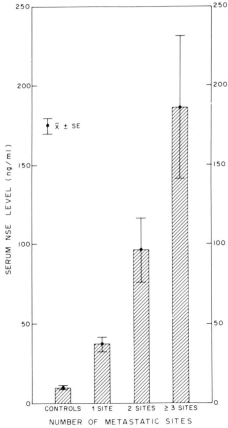

Fig. 21-2. NSE levels relative to number of metastatic sites.

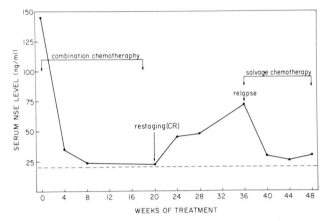

Fig. 21-3.   Serial NSE levels during and after chemotherapy.

relapsing SCLC patient with a normal NSE should undergo repeat biopsy to confirm the histological nature of the recurrence.[18]

  Although none of these studies had indicated that a pretreatment NSE level per se has prognostic value independent of other known prognostic features (such as stage and performance status), several interesting observations bear note. NSE determinations obtained at restaging do appear to have prognostic value.[47] For example, among 36 extensive-stage patients in our study with serial NSE determinations, 30 achieved an objective response (10 CR; 20 PR). Of those obtaining a CR, 9 out of 10 (90 percent) attained a normal NSE level (mean = 15.3 ± 1.0 ng/ml), versus 8 out of 20 (40 percent) achieving a PR (mean = 29.1 ± 4.7 ng/ml) ($P < .01$). Extensive-stage patients with normal NSE levels at restaging, regardless of whether a complete or partial remission was obtained, experienced a better median survival than did responding patients with persistently abnormal (albeit lower) NSE levels (12 months vs 9 months; $P < .001$) (Fig. 21-4). The duration of response appears to be longer in patients with normal restaging NSE levels as compared to those achieving a compara-

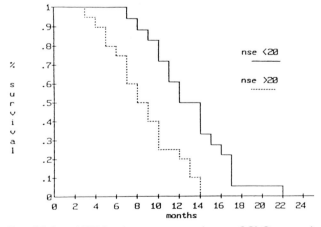

Fig. 21-4.   NSE levels in extensive-disease SCLC, normal versus raised levels at restaging.

ble clinical response, but with persistently abnormal NSE levels.[47] However, we have examined too few patients to fully verify this observation.

Akoun et al. measured serial NSE levels during a 3-day course of chemotherapy and found sharp elevations above pretreatment levels in several patients.[2] As enolase is a cytoplasmic enzyme, this finding is consistent with tumor cell lysis and subsequent release of NSE. Such a phenomenon could possibly be used to predict early during the course of treatment whether an objective response will be obtained. Of the 13 patients evaluated for release of NSE after treatment, 7 experienced increases of serum NSE to at least 100 ng/ml within 72 hours, all of whom achieved an objective response. Only one of six patients with an acute rise in NSE below 100 ng/ml responded objectively. Similar findings have been reported by Cooper et al.[18] and have been observed by us as well (unpublished data).

Although NSE levels are strikingly different in the supernatants of cultured SCLC and NSCLC cell lines[12,60], NSE can be demonstrated by immunoperoxidase technique in both NSCLC and SCLC.[35,50,85,86,90] Thus it is not surprising that serum NSE is elevated in some individuals with NSCLC.[35,50,85,86,90] If a relatively low cutoff value is used, approximately 10-25 percent of NSCLC patients will have an elevated pretreatment NSE level[4,23] (Table 21-16). However, if a higher NSE value (25 ng/ml) is used, the number of NSCLC patients with elevated NSE levels is reduced to under 10 percent while the number of SCLC with abnormal levels remains greater than 70 percent.[23] Similarly, if patients with nonmalignant lung conditions are tested, a small number will be found to have raised NSE levels[18,23] (Table 21-17).

To summarize, NSE is elevated in the serum of a majority of SCLC patients. Pretreatment levels tend to reflect overall tumor burden but are not specific for any particular metastatic site. Response rates and overall survival rate are not influenced by pretreatment NSE levels. However, normalization of previously elevated levels at the time of restaging portends a better survival, at least among patients with extensive stage disease. Serial NSE levels tend to mirror the clinical course of disease, falling with remission and rising with relapse. The latter may precede clinical recognition of recurrence by up to 12 weeks in as many as 65-75 percent of patients. Acute elevations of NSE occurring within 72 hours of initiation of chemotherapy may be useful in predicting response, but further study is required to confirm this observation. Unfortunately, NSE lacks specificity and therefore cannot be used as a screening test and, like CEA, occasionally is elevated in nonmalignant conditions. Nevertheless, NSE appears to be a useful monitor of therapy in SCLC and may best be used to determine the completeness of response.

Table 21-16
NSE Levels in Non-Small Cell Lung Cancer

Upper Limit of Normal (ng/ml)	Number NSCLC	Reference
7.5	6/54 (11%)	4
12	13/51 (25%)	23
25	4/51 (8%)	23
16	2/14 (14%)	2
13.5	16/94 (17%)	18

Table 21-17
NSE Levels in Conditions Other than SCLC (Normal < 13 ng/ml)

Condition	Total Number	< 13 ng/ml	13-25 ng/ml	25-50 ng/ml	> 50 ng/ml
Blood donors	33	31 (94%)	2 (6%)		
NSCLC	94	78 (83%)	9 (95%)	3 (3%)	4 (4%)
Lung metastases	10	8 (80%)	2 (20%)		
Benign lung lesions	11	10 (91%)	1 (9%)		
Pneumonia	20	13 (65%)	6 (30%)	1 (5%)	
Benign GI or liver disease	45	38 (84%)	7 (16%)		
Breast or GI cancer with liver metastasis	20	17 (85%)	3 (15%)		
Metastatic prostate cancer	42	31 (74%)	8 (19%)	3 (7%)	
SCLC LD	38	13 (34%)	9 (24%)	11 (29%)	5 (13%)
SCLC ED	39	5 (13%)	4 (10%)	12 (31%)	18 (46%)

Modified from Cooper EH, Splinter TAW, Brown DA, et al: Evaluation of a radioimmunoassay for neuron specific enolase in small cell lung cancer. Br J Cancer 52:333-338, 1985.

BOMBESIN

Moody and co-workers have recently described the presence of bombesin, a tetradecapeptide originally isolated from frog skin, in the supernatant of cultured small cell lung cancer cell lines.[25,67,68] Although bombesin-like immunoreactivity has been detected in numerous mammalian tissues (including human fetal and neonatal but not adult lung), very low to absent levels have been found in cultured non-small cell cancer cell lines.[25,67] This apparent qualitative difference has prompted some investigators to evaluate plasma levels of bombesin as a biomarker in patients with SCLC.[48,79,107] We found plasma bombesin-like activity raised in only 5 percent of 31 untreated patients (10 limited-stage; 21 extensive-stage).[48] Pert and Schumacher found plasma bombesin raised in six SCLC patients with limited-stage disease and three with extensive-stage disease.[79] However, raised bombesin levels were also detected in six patients with malignancies other than SCLC. Median bombesin levels were 33 ± 17 and 38 ± 12 pg/200 μ plasma in limited SCLC and NSCLC malignancies, respectively. Very high bombesin levels (median = 640 ± 72 pg/200 μ) were detected only in patients with extensive disease.[79] In contrast, Wood and co-workers found normal (< 10 pmol/1) levels of plasma bombesin in all 31 SCLC patients that they evaluated, 10 of whom had extensive disease.[107]

On the basis of these preliminary reports, therefore, it does not appear that plasma bombesin will be a useful plasma tumor marker. However, bombesin may be a very useful marker for CNS disease. Parenthetically, bombesin does appear to be an autocrine factor for SCLC and is potentially exploitable as a therapeutic target.[19]

DETECTION OF CNS METASTASES

Approximately 10 percent of SCLC patients will have CNS involvement at diagnosis; the majority will have accompanying neurologic symptoms and will be readily diagnosed on clinical grounds alone.[31,49,69] Over the course of treatment many more patients will develop CNS metastases, especially if prophylactic cranial irradiation (PCI) is not employed.[49,69] In addition, the improved median survival of SCLC patients has allowed "new" manifestations of the disease to come to light, one of the most troubling of which is an increased incidence of carcinomatous meningitis.[49,83] Treatment aimed at decreasing these troublesome problems is currently under study.[49] Although the incidence of CNS metastasis is clearly decreased by the inclusion of PCI in the treatment plan, several investigators have recently begun to question the wisdom of routinely employing PCI, especially in view of its apparent long-term sequelae.[22,45] Thus, any means that would enhance the ability to detect subclinical CNS disease would presumably improve selection of appropriate candidates for treatment aimed at the CNS (radiotherapy, intrathecal medication, or both). It was hoped that the enhanced sensitivity of CT scanners might improve the ability to detect neurologically asymptomatic CNS disease. At most, however, only 3-9 percent of neurologically asymtomatic SCLC patients will be found to have an occult CNS metastasis by head CT scan; therefore, the "routine" head scanning of neurologically asymptomatic patients does not appear to be cost-effective.[49] Similarly, the diagnosis of carcinomatous meningitis that depends on the demonstration of malignant cells in the CSF cytologically can be extremely difficult, often requiring multiple lumbar punctures. Even then it is often necessary to make the diagnosis inferentially by relying on nondiagnostic pleocytosis, low glucose, high protein, and/or raised intracranial pressure. Newer and more sensitive techniques thus are needed to help diagnose and verify the presence of CNS disease. For this reason, some investigators have begun to investigate the measurement of CSF biomarkers to assist in detection of CNS metastases at an earlier point.[76-78]

Because NSE appears very promising as a serum biomarker in SCLC, CSF NSE levels have been investigated as a potential marker of CNS disease. In a recent study, Pedersen et al. measured CSF NSE levels in 47 SCLC patients.[76] Of the 26 patients proven to have CNS involvement by head CT scan or autopsy findings, 18 (69 percent) had a raised (i.e., > 11 ng/ml) NSE level.[76] Only 10 percent (1/10) without CNS involvement proved to have an abnormal level. The mean CSF NSE for those with tumor involvement was nearly three times that of patients without CNS disease (25.15 vs 7.03 ng/ml; $P < 0.01$). NSE levels tended to correlate with the amount of CNS involvement in that patients with multiple parenchymal lesions had higher NSE values than did patients with only a few or solitary metastases (mean: 74.5 vs 13.1 ng/ml). There were 11 patients with equivocal CNS findings by CT scan or autopsy, 4 (36 percent) of whom had raised NSE levels (mean = 11.0 ng/ml). Four out of five (80 percent) patients with carcinomatous meningitis had abnormal NSE levels.

In a more recent report, Pederson and co-workers evaluated a panel of potential markers including bombesin, CK-BB isoenzyme, calcitonin, and NSE.[77] Their results are shown in Table 21-18. Both bombesin and NSE appear to be sensitive for detecting parenchymal CNS lesions, whereas these two markers plus CK-BB are all highly sensitive indicators of carcinomatous meningitis—even superior to CSF cytology. All three markers have a false-positive rate of equal to or below 11 percent.[77] Patients

Table 21-18
CSF Bombesin, Creatine Kinase BB, Calcitonin, and
Neuron-Specific Enolase as Markers of CNS Metastases in SCLC

Site	Elevated (%)			
	Bombesin	CK-BB	Cal*	NSE
CNS parenchyma	67	47	50	67
Carcinomatous meningitis	91	88	53	90
Negative	14	0	11	9
Equivocal	30	30	13	47

Modified from Pedersen AG, Becker K, Marangos P, et al: Bombesin (BM), creatine
kinase BB (CK-BB), calcitonin (C), and neuron-specific enolase (NSE) in the cerebrospinal fluid (CSF) as a marker of CNS metastases and meningeal carcinomatosis (MC) in
small cell lung cancer (SCLS). Proc Am Assoc Cancer Res 26:146, 1985.
*Calcitonin.

with equivocal CNS findings had up to a 47 percent incidence of an abnormal marker. No data were given on the symptomatic status of the patients studied; consequently, it is unclear if any of these markers proved helpful in uncovering asymptomatic disease.

Pedersen et al have also compared CSF CK-BB and β-2-microglobulin as markers of CNS involvement.[78] β-2-Microglobulin was chosen because it had previously been shown to be a useful indicator of CNS disease in lymphoma.[51] CSF CK-BB was raised ($>0.4 \mu/l$) in 15 out of 17 (88 percent) patients with carcinomatous meningitis, in 5 out of 26 (19 percent) with parenchymal lesions, and in none of 26 patients without CNS disease. CK-BB proved to be superior to total CK, CSF protein, and CSF LDH levels as a discriminator of carcinomatous meningitis. β-2-Microglobulin, however, was unable to distinguish patients with or without CNS disease.

These data seem to indicate that CSF CK-BB, NSE, and bombesin are potentially useful in identifying patients with carcinomatous meningitis. However, it is unknown whether these markers (either singly or in combination) will prove helpful in identifying patients with asymptomatic parenchymal disease or if they will provide prognostic information.

OTHER BIOMARKERS

Numerous other substances are being actively investigated as possible biomarkers of SCLC including neurotensin;[27] chromogranin;[3,85] protein-bound carbohydrates such as mannose and fucose;[99] urinary polyamines, including putrescine, spermidine, and spermine;[106] α-1-acid glycoprotein;[24] and β-2-Microglobulin;[71] as well as more commonly measured serum enzymes such as lactate dehydrogenase.[15] In addition to plasma or serum determinations, immunoperoxidase demonstration of some or many of these tumor products has been used as a means of distinguishing SCLC from NSCLC in particularly anaplastic lung tumors with varying degrees of success.[7,53,85,101] The expression of neural intermediate filaments by SCLC and not NSCLC is particularly noteworthy in this respect.[53] A specific chromosomal defect *del* 3p (14,23) is said to be unique for SCLC and may represent yet another means of distinguishing SCLC from NSCLC.[102] However, some investigators have been unable to verify these data.[108] Amplification of the C-*myc* oncogene is commonly found in SCLC cell lines, but recent data suggest that this phenomenon may be unique to in vitro cells.[46,55] Consequently, the routine determination of gene amplification may not afford any diagnostic assistance, although therapy may be influenced, as cells with C-*myc* amplification appear less sensitive to treatment.[13] Interestingly, SCLC has recently been found to express the Leu-7 antigenic determinant commonly found in natural killer cells and thus may represent yet another method of distinguishing lung cancer histologic types.[11] Finally, the emergence of monoclonal antibodies specific for SCLC will no doubt improve diagnostic accumine and may lead to the early detection of subclinical amounts of tumor.[8,106] All of these areas deserve continued investigation.

CONCLUSIONS

Small cell lung cancer cells are "biologically active" and have been associated with many tumor products. The search for a clinically useful marker remains obviously important. Many of the tumor products reviewed above demonstrate a heterogeneity of expression; therefore, it is unlikely that any *one* of these potential markers will be used exclusively as a management tool.[6,49,94] More probably two or more of these substances will be used as a panel of markers to follow the clinical course of individual patients much like α-fetoprotein and β-HCG are used in the management of germinal neoplasms. However, our results in a small study evaluating three markers (NSE, ADH, and calcitonin) was not particularly promising.[48] In fact, NSE proved superior to the panel of markers both in its ability to mirror the clinical status of patients and in its capability of predicting relapse. Similar disappointing results were reported by Aroney et al.[5] Nevertheless, the findings that pretreatment CEA and CK-BB levels may provide prognostic information and that restaging NSE values may help to predict response duration all warrant further study, and investigation of known "markers" should continue, as well as a search for new potentially useful markers.

REFERENCES

1. Abeloff MD, Trump DL, Baylin SB: Ectopic adrenocorticotropin (ACTH) syndrome and small cell carcinoma of the lung-assessment of clinical implications in patients on combination chemotherapy. Cancer 48:1082–1087, 1981
2. Akoun GM, Scarna HM, Milleron BJ, et al: Serum neuron-specific enolase. A marker for disease extent and response to therapy for small-cell lung cancer. Chest 87:39–43, 1985
3. Angeletti RH, Hickey WF: A neuroendocrine marker in tissues of the immune system. Science 230:89–90, 1985
4. Ariyoshi Y, Kato K, Ishiguro Y, et al: Evaluation of serum neuron-specific as a tumor marker for carcinoma of the lung. Gann 74:219–225, 1983
5. Aroney RS, Dermody WC, Aldenderfer P, et al: Multiple sequential biomarkers in monitoring patients with carcinoma of the lung. Cancer Treat Rep 68:859–866, 1984
6. Baylin SB, Weisburger WR, Eggleston JC, et al: Variable content of histaminase

l-DOPA decarboxylase and calcitonin in small-cell carcinoma of the lung. Biologic and clinical implications. New Engl J Med 299:105-110, 1978

7. Bergh J, Esscher T, Steinholtz L, et al: Immunocytochemical demonstration of neuron-specific enolase (NSE) in human lung cancers. Am J Clin Pathol 84:1-7, 1985

8. Bernal SD, Mabry M, Stahel RA, et al: Selective cytotoxicity of the SMl monoclonal antibody towards small cell carcinoma of the lung. Cancer Res 45:1026-1032, 1985

9. Bondy PK: The pattern of ectopic hormone production in lung cancer. Yale J Biol Med 54:181-185, 1981

10. Bondy PK, Gilby ED: Endocrine function in small cell undifferentiated carcinoma of the lung. Cancer 50:2147-2153, 1982

11. Bunn PA, Linnoila I, Minna JD, et al: Small cell lung cancer, endocrine cells of the fetal bronchus, and other neuroendocrine cells express the Leu-7 antigenic determinant present on natural killer cells. Blood 65:764-768, 1985

12. Carney DN, Marangos PJ, Ihde DC, et al: Serum neuron-specific enolase: A marker for disease extent and response to therapy of small-cell lung cancer. Lancet 1:583-585, 1982

13. Carney DN, Broder L, Edelstein M, et al: Experimental studies of the biology of human small cell lung cancer. Cancer Treat Rep 67:27-35, 1983

14. Carney DN, Zweig MH, Ihde DC, et al: Elevated serum creatine kinase BB levels in patients with small cell lung cancer. Cancer Res 44:5399-5403, 1984

15. Cohen MH, Makuch R, Johnston-Early A, et al: Laboratory parameters as an alternative to performance status in prognostic stratification of patients with small cell lung cancer. Cancer Treat Rep 65:187-195, 1981

16. Comis RL, Miller M, Ginsberg SJ: Abnormalities in water homeostasis in small cell anaplastic lung cancer. Cancer 45:2414-2421, 1980

17. Coolen RB, Progay DA, Nosenchuk JS, et al: Elevation of brain-type creatine kinase in serum from patients with carcinoma. Cancer 44:1414-1418, 1979

18. Cooper EH, Splinter TAW, Brown DA, et al: Evaluation of a radioimmunoassay for neuron specific enolase in small cell lung cancer. Br J Cancer 52:333-338, 1985

19. Cuttitta F, Carney DN, Mulshine J, et al: Bombesin-like peptides can function as autocrine growth factors in human small-cell lung cancer. Nature 316:823-826, 1985

20. de la Monte SM, Hutchins GM, Moore GW: Paraneoplastic syndromes and constitutional symptoms in prediction of metastatic behavior of small call carcinoma of the lung. Am J Med 77:851-857, 1984

21. Dent PB, McCulloch PB, Wesley-James O, et al: Measurement of carcinoembryonic antigen in patients with bronchogenic carcinoma. Cancer 42:1484-1491, 1978

22. Ellison N, Bernath A. Kane P, et al: Disturbing problems of success: Clinical status of long-term survivors of small cell lung cancer (SCLC). Proc Am Soc Clin Oncol 1:149, 1982

23. Esscher T, Steinholtz L, Bergh J, et al: Neurone specific enolase: A useful diagnostic serum marker for small cell carcinoma of the lung. Thorax 40:85-90, 1985

24. Ganz PA, Baras M, Ma PY, et al: Monitoring the therapy of lung cancer with α-1-acid glycoprotein. Cancer Res 44:5415-5421, 1984

25. Gazdar AF, Carney DN, Moody T, et al: Expression of peptide and other markers in cell lines (CL) of small cell lung carcinoma (SCLC) having classic (SCLC-c) and variant (SCLC-v) morphologies. Proc Am Assoc Cancer Res 25:217, 1984

26. Gerwititz G, Yalon RS: Ectopic ACTH production in carcinoma of the lung. J Clin Invest 53:1022-1032, 1974

27. Goedert M, Reeve JG, Emson PC, et al: Neurotensin in human small cell lung carcinoma. Br J Cancer 50:179-183, 1984

28. Gold P, Freedman SO: Demonstration of tumor-specific antigens in human colonic

carcinomata by immunologic tolerance and absorption techniques. J Exp Med 121:439-466, 1965

29. Goldie JH, Coldman AJ: The genetic origin of drug resistance in neoplasms: Implications for systemic therapy. Cancer Res 44:3643-3653, 1984

30. Goslin RH, Skarin AT, Zamchech N: Carcinoembryonic antigen: A useful monitor of small cell lung cancer. JAMA 246:2173-2176, 1981

31. Greco FA, Oldham RK: Small-cell lung cancer. New Engl J Med 301:355-358, 1979

32. Greco FA, Hainsworth J, Sismani A, et al: Hormone production and paraneoplastic syndromes, in Greco FA, Oldham RK, Bunn PA (eds): Small Cell Lung Cancer. Orlando, Fl, Grune & Stratton, 1981 pp 177-223

33. Gropp C, Harverman K, Schener A: Ectopic hormones at diagnosis and during therapy. Cancer 46:347-354, 1980

34. Haefliger JM, Dubied MC, Vallotton MB: Excretion journaliere de l'hormone antidiuretique lors de carcinome bronchique. Schweiz Med Wschr 107:726-732, 1977

35. Haimoto H, Takahashi Y, Koshikawa T, Nagura H, Kato K: Immunohistochemical localization of γ-enolase in normal human tissues other than nervous and neuroendocrine tissues. Lab Invest 52:257-263, 1985

36. Hainsworth JD, Workman R, Greco FA: Management of the syndrome of inappropriate antidiuretic hormone secretion in small cell lung cancer. Cancer 51:161-165, 1983

37. Hande KR, DesPrez RM: Current perspectives in small cell lung cancer. Chest 85:669-677, 1984

38. Hansen M: Clinical implications of ectopic hormone production in small cell carcinoma of the lung. Dan Med Bull 28:221-236, 1981

39. Hansen M, Hammer M, Hummer L. ACTH, ADH, and calcitonin as markers of response and relapse in small cell carcinoma of the lung. Cancer 46:2062-2067, 1980

40. Hansen J, Hammer M, Hummer L: Diagnostic and therapeutic implications of ectopic hormone production in small cell carcinoma of the lung. Thorax 35:101-106, 1980

41. Hansen M, Hansen HH, Tryding N: Small cell carcinoma of the lung: Serum calcitonin and serum histaminase (diamine oxidase) at basal levels and stimulated by pentagastrin. Acta Med Scand 204:257-261, 1978

42. Hansen M, Hansen HH, Hirsch FR, et al: Hormonal polypeptides and amine metabolites in small cell carcinoma of the lung with special reference to stage and subtypes. Cancer 45:1432-1437, 1980

43. Hauger-Klevene JH: Asymptomatic production of ACTH. Radioimmunoassay in squamous cell, oat cell and adenocarcinoma of the lung. Cancer 22:1262-1267, 1968

44. Imura H. Matsukura S, Yamamoto H, et al: Studies on ectopic ACTH-producing tumors. Cancer 35:1430-1437, 1975

45. Johnson BE, Ihde DC, Bunn PA, et al: Patients with small-cell lung cancer treated with combination chemotherapy with or without irradiation. Data on potential cures, chronic toxicities, and late relapses after a five-to eleven-year follow-up. Ann Intern Med 103:430-438, 1985

46. Johnson BE, Nau M, Gazdar A, et al: Amplification of myc oncogenes is less common in small cell lung cancer patients tumors than in small cell lines. Proc Am Soc Clin Oncol 5:16, 1986

47. Johnson DH, Marangos PJ, Forbes JT, et al: Potential utility of serum neuron-specific enolase levels in small cell carcinoma of the lung. Cancer Res 44:5409-5414, 1984

48. Johnson DH, Hande KR, Marangos PJ, et al: Serum neuron-specific enolase (NSE), a possible biomarker for small cell lung cancer (SCLC). Proc Am Assoc Cancer Res 25:156, 1984

49. Johnson DH, Greco FA: Small cell carcinoma of the lung. CRC, Critical Reviews Oncol Hematol 4:303-336, 1986

50. Kato K, Ishiguro Y, Ariyoshi Y: Enolase isoenzymes as disease markers: Distribution of

three enolase subunits (alpha, beta, and gamma) in various human tissues. Dis Markers 1:213-220, 1983

51. Koch TR, Lichtenfeld KM, Wiernik PH: Detection of central nervous system metastasis with cerebrospinal fluid beta-2-microglobulin. Cancer 52:101-104, 1983

52. Kurtz KJ, Nielsen RD: Serum creatine kinase BB isoenzyme as a diagnostic aid in occult small cell lung cancer. Cancer 56:562-566, 1985

53. Lehto VP, Stenman S, Miettinen M, et al: Expression of a neural type of intermediate filament as a distinguishing feature between oat cell carcinoma and other lung cancers. Am J Pathol 110:113-118, 1983

54. List A, Johnson DH, Hainsworth JD, et al: The syndrome of inappropriate secretion of antidiuretic hormone in small cell lung cancer. Proc Am Soc Clin Oncol 4:63, 1985

55. Little CD, Nau MM, Carney DN, et al: Amplification and expression of the c-myc oncogene in human lung cancer cell lines. Nature 306:194-196, 1983

56. Lokich JJ: The frequency and clinical biology of the ectopic hormone syndromes of small cell carcinoma. Cancer 50:2111-2114, 1982

57. Lokich JJ: Plasma CEA levels in small cell lung cancer: Correlation with stage, distribution of metastases, and survival. Cancer 50:2154-2156, 1982

58. Lokich JJ, Zamcheck N, Lowenstein M: Sequential carcinoembryonic antigen levels in the therapy of metastatic breast cancer: A predictor and monitor of response and relapse. Ann Intern Med 89:902-906, 1978

59. Marangos PJ, Polak JM, Pearse AGE: Neuron-specific enolase: A probe for neurons and neuroendocrine cells. Trends Neurosci 5:193-196, 1982

60. Marangos PH, Gzadar AF, Carney DN: Neuron specific enolase in human small cell carcinoma cultures. Cncer Lett 15:67-71, 1982

61. Maurer LH, O'Donnell JF, Kennedy S, et al: Human neurophysins in carcinoma of the lung: Relation to histology, disease stage, response rate, survival, and syndrome of inappropriate antidiuretic hormone secretion. Cancer Treat Rep 67:971-976, 1983

62. McIntire KR: Tumor markers, in deVita VT, Hellman S, Rosenberg SA (eds): Cancer Principles & Practice of Oncology. Philadelphia, Lippincott, 1985, pp 375-388

63. McKenzie CG, Evans IMA, Hillyard CJ, et al: Biochemical markers in bronchial carcinoma. Br J Cancer 36:700-707, 1977

64. Meador CK, Liddle GW, Island DP, et al: Cause of Cushing's syndrome in patients with tumors arising from "nonendocrine" tissue. J Clin Endocrinol 22:693-703, 1962

65. Merrill WW, Bondy PK: Production of biochemical marker substances by bronchogenic carcinomas. Clin Chest Med 3:307-320, 1982

66. Minna JD, Carney DN, Cuttitta F, et al. Clinical, cellular, and molecular biology of lung cancer, in Salmon SE, Jones SE (eds): Adjuvant Therapy of Cancer IV. Orlando, FL, Grune & Stratton, 1984, pp 167-182

67. Moody TW, Pert CB, Gazdar AF, et al: High levels of intracellular bombesin characterize human small-cell lung cancer. Science 214:1246-1248, 1981

68. Moody TW, Russell EK, O'Donohue TL, et al: Bombesin-like peptides in small cell lung cancer: Biochemical characterization and secretion from a cell line. Life Sci 32:487-493, 1983

69. Morstyn G, Ihde DC, Lichter AS, et al: Small cell lung cancer 1973-1983: Early progress and recent obstacles. Internatl J Radiat Oncol Biol Phys 10:515-539, 1984

70. Mulshine JL, Cuttitla F, Bibro M, et al: Monoclonal antibodies that distinguish non-small cell from small cell lung cancer. J Immunol 131:497-502, 1983

71. Nissen MH, Plesner T, Rorth M: Modification of β2-microglobulin in serum from patients with small cell carcinoma of the lung—correlation with the clinical course. Clinica Chemica Acta 141:41-50, 1984

72. North WG, Maurer LH, Valtin H, et al: Human neurophysins as potential tumor markers for small cell carcinoma of the lung: Application of specific radioimmunoassays. J Clin Endocrin Metab 51:892-896, 1980

73. North WG, Maurer LH, O'Donnell JF: The neurophysins and small cell lung cancer, in Greco FA (ed): Biology and Management of Lung Cancer. Boston, Martinus Nijhoff, 1983, pp 143–169

74. Pahlman S, Esscher T, Bergh J, et al: Neuron-specific enolase as a marker for neuroblastoma and small-cell carcinoma of the lung. Tumor Biol 5:119–126, 1984

75. Parma AM, Marangos PJ, Goodwin FK: A more sensitive radioimmunoassay for neuron-specific enolase suitable for cerebrospinal fluid determinations. J Neurochem 36:1093–1096, 1981

76. Pedersen AG, Marangos P, Gazdar A, et al: Neuron-specific enolase (NSE) in the cerebrospinal fluid (CSF) as a marker of CNS metastases in small cell lung cancer (SCLC). Proc Am Soc Clin Oncol 3:7, 1984

77. Pederson AG, Becker K, Marangos P, et al: Bombesin (BM), creatine kinase BB (CK-BB), calcitonin (C), and neuron-specific enolase (NSE) in the cerebrospinal fluid (CSF) as a marker of CNS metastases and meningeal carcinomatosis (MC) in small cell lung cancer (SCLC). Proc Am Assoc Cancer Res 26:146, 1985

78. Pederson AG, Bach FW, Nissen M, et al: Creatine kinase BB and β-2-microglobulin as markers of CNS metastases in patients with small-cell lung cancer. J Clin Oncol 3:1364–1372, 1985

79. Pert CB, Schumacher UK: Plasma bombesin concentrations in patients with extensive small cell carcinoma of the lung. Lancet 1:509, 1982

80. Prinz RA, Marangos PJ: Use of neuron-specific enolase as a serum marker for neuroendocrine neoplasms. Surgery 92:887–889, 1982

81. Ratcliff JG, Podmore J, Stack BHR, et al: Circulating ACTH and related peptides in lung cancer. Br J Cancer 45:230–236, 1982

82. Richardson RL, Greco FA, Oldham RK, et al: Tumor products and potential markers in small cell lung cancer. Semin Oncol 5:253–262, 1978

83. Rosen ST, Aisner J, Makauch RW, et al: Carcinomatous leptomeningitis in small cell lung cancer: A clinicopathologic review of the National Cancer Institute experience. Medicine 61:45–53, 1985

84. Rubery ED, Doran JF, Thompson RJ: Brain-type creatine kinase BB as a potential tumor marker—serum levels measured by radioimmunoassay in 1015 patients with histologically confirmed malignancies. Eur J Cancer Clin Oncol 18:951–956, 1981

85. Said JW, Vimmadalal S, Nash G, et al: Immunoreactive neuron-specific enolase, bombesin, and chromogranin as markers for neuroendocrine lung tumors. Hum Pathol 16:235–240, 1985

86. Schmechel DE:γ-Subunit of the glycolytic enzyme enolase: Nonspecific or neuron specific? Lab Inves 52:239–242, 1985

87. Schmechel D, Marangos PJ, Brightman M: Neurone-specific enolase is a molecular marker for peripheral and central neuroendocrine cells. Nature 276:834–836, 1978

88. Sculier JP, Feld R, Evans WK, et al: Carcinoembryonic antigen: A useful prognostic marker in small-cell lung cancer. J Clin Oncol 3:1349–1354, 1985

89. Shappino AP, Carter S, Ellison M, et al: Plasma calcitonin in small cell lung cancer: prognostic significance. Br J Cancer 48:881–882, 1983

90. Sheppard MN, Corrin B, Bennett MH, et al: Immunocytochemical localization of neuron specific enolase in small cell carcinomas and carcinoid tumours of the lung. Histopath 8:171–180, 1984

91. Silva OL, Broder LE, Doppman JL, et al: Calcitonin as a marker for bronchogenic cancer. Cancer 44:680–684, 1979

92. Skrabanek P, Powell D: Unifying concept of nonpituitary ACTH-secreting tumors. Evidence of common origin of neural-crest tumors, carcinoids, and oat-cell carcinomas. Cancer 42:1263–1269, 1978

93. Sorenson GD, Pettengill OS, Brinck-Johnson T, et al: Hormone production by cultures of small-cell carcinoma of the lung. Cancer 47:1289-1296, 1981

94. Souhami RL, Bradbury I, Geddes DM, et al: Prognostic significance of laboratory parameters measured at diagnosis in small cell carcinoma of the lung. Cancer Res 45:2878-2882, 1985

95. Sugarbaker PH, Zamcheck N, Moore FD: Assessment of serial carcinoembryonic antigen (CEA) assays in postoperative detection of recurrent colon cancer. Cancer 38:2310-2315, 1976

96. Tapia FJ, Polak JM, Barbosa AJA, et al: Neuron-specific enolase is produced by neuroendocrine tumours. Lancet 1:808-811, 1981

97. Upton GV, Amatruda TT. Evidence for the presence of tumor peptides with corticotropin-releasing-factor-like activity in the ectopic ACTH syndrome. New Engl J Med 285:419-424, 1971

98. Vincent RG, Chu TM, Fergen TB, et al: Carcinoembryonic antigen in 228 patients with carcinoma of the lung. Cancer 36:2069-2076, 1975

99. Waalkes TP, Abeloff MD, Ettinger DS, et al: Serum protein-bound carbohydrates and small cell carcinoma of the lung. Correlations with extent of disease, tumor burden, survival, and clinical response categories. Cancer 52:131-139, 1983

100. Waalkes TP, Abeloff MD, Woo KB, et al: Carcinoembryonic antigen for monitoring patients with small carcinoma of the lung during treatment. Cancer Res 40:4420-4427, 1980

101. Walts AE, Said JW, Shintaku IP, et al: Chromogranin as a marker of neuroendocrine cells in cytological material—an immunocytochemical study. Am J Clin Pathol 84:273-277, 1985

102. Whang-Peng J, Kao-Shan CS, Lee EC, et al: Specific chromosome defect associated with human small-cell lung cancer: Deletion 3p(14-23). Science 215:181-182, 1982

103. Willis RE: Ectopic ADH production before clinical recognition of small cell carcinoma of the lung. South Med J 73:1415-1416, 1980

104. Wolfsen AR, Odell WA: ProACTH: Use for early detection of lung cancer. Am J Med 66:765-772, 1979

105. Woo KB, Waalkes P, Abeloff MD, et al: Multiple biologic markers in the monitoring of treatment for patients with small cell carcinoma of the lung. The use of serial levels of plasma CEA and serum carbohydrates. Cancer 48:1633-1642, 1981

106. Woo KB, Waalkes TP, Abeloff MD, et al: Urinary polyamines for evaluating the course of disease for patients with small cell carcinoma of the lung. Cancer 52:1684-1690, 1983

107. Wood SM, Wood JR, Ghate, et al: Is bombesin a tumour marker for small-cell carcinoma? Lancet 1:690-691, 1982

108. Wurster-Hill DH, Cannizzaro LA, Pettengill OS, et al: Cytogenetics of small cell carcinoma of the lung. Cancer Genetics Cytogen 13:303-330, 1984

109. Zweig MH, Van Steirteghem AC: Assessment by radioimmunoassay of serum creatine kinase BB (CK-BB) as a tumor marker: Studies in patients with various cancers and a comparison of CK-BB concentrations to prostate acid phosphatase concentrations. J Natl Cancer Inst 66:859-862, 1981

Joseph Aisner

_____ **22** _____

Chemotherapy for Small Cell Carcinoma of the Lung

Small cell carcinoma of the lung (SCCL) is a unique histological form of lung cancer constituting 25–30 percent of the more than 130,000 new cases of lung cancer seen in the United States annually.[28] SCCL is clinically and pathologically differentiated from the other types of lung cancer by its high labeling index and rapid doubling time and clinically by its rapid growth, early metastases, and exquisite sensitivity to both chemotherapy and radiotherapy.[35] In part because of unique characteristics and responsiveness, SCCL has received considerable attention in laboratory and clinical studies, and some changes in the natural history of this disease have been achieved by treatment. Without treatment, the median duration of survival is 4–12 weeks,[73] depending on stage; there are no long-term survivors, and few patients live beyond a year. Surgery, even among patients with disease confined to the thorax and potentially resectable, has no impact on the survival from this disease.[92] Radiotherapy to the chest for patients with only intrathoracic disease improves survival, however, there are essentially no long-term survivors.[55] In the early 1970s combination chemotherapy was applied with initial success and resulted in a prolonged median survival for all patients and a few patients who were long-term survivors.[22] This therapeutic step resulted from the recognition that SCCL is a disseminated disease.

SCCL IS A SYSTEMIC DISEASE

With careful staging, slightly less than one-half of the patients (approximately one-third) will be found to have tumor clinically confined to the chest, with or without mediastinal or ipsilateral supraclavicular nodes. This is defined as limited disease.[97] With the exception of ipsilateral pleural effusions, all disease extending beyond the confines of the limits mentioned above is considered extensive disease.[97] The limited–extensive staging system has considerable prognostic importance since patients with limited disease have a higher complete response (CR) frequency, a longer median survival, and nearly all long-term survivors are found in this group.[97] Improvements in staging technology can also exert an apparent improvement in outcome as those previously considered to have limited disease are shifted to the group with extensive disease, resulting in an improvement in outcome for both groups. Thus analysis of results must be considered in light of the staging evaluation. This consideration is important since further improvements in technology are likely to refine the staging system. Initial studies at the University of Maryland Hospital and University of Maryland Cancer Center (UMCC) have shown that the computerized tomographic (CT) scanner may afford prognostic information which may help to further refine the staging system.[90,113]

The vast majority of the patients with so-called limited disease have bulky local and regional lymph node involvement, rendering the disease locally advanced (stage III) and technically unresectable.[97] Historically, even among the few patients with very limited disease who were selected for surgical resection, there was a high rate of early death. Necropsies in this series showed residual disease and widespread metastases.[83] Thus even in this very limited disease group there were no apparent cures with surgery alone.[83,92] It has been suggested, on the basis of a coin lesion study,[65] that when SCCL presents as an isolated lesion ($T_1N_0M_0$), surgical resection may be adequate. Even in this rare early presentation, however, and in contrast to coin lesions with other histologies, the majority of patients will eventually die of disseminated disease. Chest irradiation to all areas of involvement in limited disease did not produce any long-term survivors;[55] these patients died from widespread metastatic disease, and the metastases formed early in the course of the disease. Thus the early metastatic presentation in the majority of patients (nearly two-thirds) and the pattern of treatment failure in limited disease[8] has led to the general recognition that SCCL is a systemic disease process regardless of our ability to document all metastatic sites.

SCCL has a high propensity for involving nearly all major organs. The sites of metastatic disease at presentation in the group with extensive disease is shown in Table 22-1. As can be seen, a large percentage of patients have involvement of bone, liver, bone marrow, adrenal glands, and central nervous system (CNS). At presentation, when patients have overt metastatic disease (in contrast with micrometastatic disease), multiple organ systems tend to be involved, and single-site metastases are less common.[27,68] In autopsy series virtually all patients have involvement of multiple organs,[84]

Table 22-1
Sites of Involvement of
SCCL at Presentation

Site	Percent
Lung	95
Regional lymph nodes	95
Pleura	10
Liver	25
Bone	30
Bone marrow	25
Adrenal gland*	15
Brain	14
Other	15

*Based on CT scan evaluations.

and this provides further testimony to the ability of this SCCL to produce early widespread metastases. The recognition that SCCL is a disseminated disease led to the general acceptance that chemotherapy is the cornerstone of treatment for this disease.[7] All other therapies, if applicable, must be considered adjunctive to the systemic chemotherapy.[3] Adjunctive radiotherapy, for example, is designed to enhance local control and is thus not logically applied to patients with extensive disease as the disease has already spread beyond the confines of a local area. At the present time, local control is not the major issue for patients with limited disease since the majority of patients in whom radiotherapy has achieved local control will eventually develop distant metastases.[8] The current therapaeutic strategy is therefore to enhance systemic control of this disease; once achieved, local control will certainly become a very important issue.

THERAPEUTIC OPTIONS AND STRATEGIES

Surgery

With the recognition and the systemic nature of this disease, surgery was abandoned as an initial curative modality.[92] There has, however, been a resurgence in the interest of surgery both for very limited disease (stage I or II) or following a debulking by chemotherapy[88,104] (see Chapter 24). The role of surgery after a chemotherapy debulking is currently under prospective evaluation by the Lung Cancer Study Group. Careful analysis of patients eligible for such an approach, however, has already shown that only a minority of patients will be eligible for surgical resection after chemotherapy debulking[54] and that such patients are highly selected.[54,105]

Radiotherapy

Radiotherapy to the chest, for limited disease, was the first treatment modality to produce significant improvement in the median survival[55] and thus became the standard treatment approach. Irradiation of all the disease within the chest as the initial therapy, however, potentially allows distant micrometastases to grow. Because of the rapid doubling time of SCCL[93] and the relatively long time needed to deliver chest irradiation, radiotherapy can no longer be justified as the sole initial modality of treatment. Radiotherapy has, however, become an important part of combined modality treatment utilizing both chemotherapy and radiotherapy[20] (see Chapter 23). Whole-brain irradiation is the treatment of choice for CNS metastases[20] and is generally advocated as a prophylactic measure to prevent metastases from becoming overt in the CNS.[17,76]

Chemotherapy

Chemotherapy is the currently available systemic treatment that stands as the cornerstone of initial treatment regardless of stage of disease. A considerable literature has developed on the chemotherapy of SCCL. An overview of these data would allow for certain conclusions regarding the application of this treatment modality for SCCL:[7] (1) combination chemotherapy is more effective than single agents—thus, multiple agent combinations are necessary to produce maximal effect; (2) combinations should be based on active single agents, each given maximally—where possible, drug synergy should be sought; and (3) dose is an extremely important feature of treatment. Virtually every study of chemotherapy for SCCL has suggested or demonstrated a dose-response relationship regardless of the interpretation of the author. The higher-dose regimens, where such issues were studied, either had the higher complete response frequency or the greater number of long-term survivors or both. In order to maximize dose, however, one must be willing to accept a certain degree of toxicity. Thus, where dose has been maximized, one will predictably see severe and life-threatening toxicity in up to 20 percent of the treated patients and lethal toxicity (predominantly in the poor-performance-status patients) in up to 5 percent of the population. These toxicity guidelines are necessary to achieve so-called state-of-the-art results in response and survival.[7]

Since dose is important, one might reason that ultra-high-dose chemotherapy with bone marrow rescue would have some advantage over more conventional doses of chemotherapy and argue that such studies have not yet demonstrated a significant advantage for ultrahigh dose.[100,110,111] There are, however, certain problems in the interpretation of some of these high-dose chemotherapy regimens. In some studies, patients with previously treated disease in relapse were chosen for treatment. Such a strategy is likely to fail to show improvement since this is a tumor where multiple drug resistance emerges rapidly and is a profound and confounding problem. In some instances the wrong agents were chosen. For example, the dose response for cyclophosphamide probably approaches plateau between 1.0 and 1.5 gm/m^2,[24] making higher doses of cyclophosphamide unlikely to produce greater benefit. In nearly all such studies, there were too few patients to make meaningful interpretations of the dose-response relationship. Some reported data suggest a very steep dose-response relationship for appropriately chosen drugs and patients. In one such study, Greco et al. demonstrated that etoposide when given in high dose with autologous bone marrow transplantation can produce response frequencies similar to combination chemotherapy.[60] Further studies building on these observations continue to suggest a steep dose-response relationship.[71]

Bimodality Therapies

SCCL is sensitive to both chemotherapy and radiotherapy; thus the application of both modalities is logical. Chemotherapy would thus be directed at the systemic disease and radiotherapy, in limited disease, would be directed at control of bulk disease in the chest. Radiotherapy to control areas of bulky disease would seem appropriate in view of the data from other successfully treated tumors such as Hodgkin's disease.[86] Nearly all studies of bimodality therapy have shown that local control is enhanced with the application of radiotherapy to the regional tumor.[3,8,20] A typical pattern of treatment failure after single or bimodality treatments is shown in Table 22-2. Survival, however, is either not changed or minimally altered.[3] Thus, multiple studies have sought to identify the role of adjunctive radiotherapy in the treatment of limited disease SCCL. In general, these studies can be divided into those in which chest irradiation was given between courses of chemotherapy (sandwiched), allowing time for recovery of toxicities, and studies in which the two modalities were given concurrently or in very close proximity. Analyses of the randomized studies

Table 22-2
Recurrence After CR

Treatment	Frequency (%) of Relapse in		
	Chest Only	Chest + Other Sites	Other Sites
RT alone	5	5	90
RT + CT	20	20	60
CT alone	33	33	33

Abbreviations: CR = complete response; RT = radiotherapy;
CT = chemotherapy.

clearly shows that when radiotherapy is given in a sandwich approach between
courses of chemotherapy, there is no survival benefit for the bimodality over chemotherapy alone. In the randomized studies in which radiotherapy was given concurrently with chemotherapy and compared to the same chemotherapy alone, there is a
small but consistent advantage of approximately 5-10 percent for the bimodality.[3,20,25,98,99] There are however two necessary generalizations regarding the bimodality approach: (1) in order to apply both modalities concurrently dosage modifications
to each modality were usually necessary; and (2) the application of radiation therapy
and chemotherapy concurrently in these bimodality studies is approximately equivalent to the best of the chemotherapy-alone studies where chemotherapy was administered maximally.[3] Thus chest irradiation in many of these studies took the place of
additional chemotherapy. Since tumor response to radiotherapy is also dose-related, it
would seem logical to apply both modalities maximally. There is only one study in
which both modalities were administered maximally.[30] This study demonstrated an
enhanced response and a potential for improved survival. There was, however, unac-
ceptable toxicity in the form of esophageal fibrosis, esophageal stricture and pulmonary insufficiency. Today, with improved radiation port planning, it is technically more
feasible to apply both modalities maximally, and such studies are clearly indicated.
There is currently one such study being conducted under the auspices of the Cancer
and Leukemia Group B. Results of this study may help to define whether the application of both modalities maximally will impart a significant improvement in the long-
term survival rate.

ANTICIPATED RESULTS

In 1981 the International Association for the Study of Lung Cancer (IASLC)
convened a workshop to evaluate the state-of-the-art for the treatment and research in
SCCL. The role of the various modalities were discussed and concensus positions
were published.[7,20,97] The concensus on chemotherapy also discussed anticipated
results that were felt to be easily achievable with tolerable toxicity;[7] most of the studies
on which these expectations were based were single-institution reports. Today, the
cooperative oncology groups can routinely achieve these results. Assuming an adequate pretreatment and follow-up staging, in limited disease one would now anticipate
a complete response frequency in excess of 60 percent, a median duration of survival
of 14-15 months, and 20-25 percent of patients alive and disease-free at more than 2

Table 22-3

Prognostic Factors in SCCL

Stage (limited vs extensive)
Performance status
Weight loss
Prior chemotherapy
Sites of metastases (number, areas)
Tumor bulk
Sex*
Age*
Subhistology (small cell vs small cell/large cell).

*Not verified in all studies.

years. For extensive disease, one would anticipate a complete response frequency of 25 percent or more and a median duration of survival approaching 9 months. In both stages, the total response frequency is high (about 90 percent), but only the complete response is meaningful for survival prolongation. These results are obtained with easily tolerable combination chemotherapy or bimodality treatments. Recently, single-institution studies have begun to show some results beyond the currently anticipated results,[12] and such studies suggest that the use of synergistic combinations at maximal dose may yet produce further improvements.

A number of pretreatment factors influence these results, including performance status, weight loss, and certain visceral organ involvement such as liver, CNS, and bone marrow.[68,69,97] Age has been noted to be an important prognostic factor in some series but not in others. In our series at the UMCC, older age was associated with greater toxicity, but once response was achieved, the survival was similar to younger age groups.[102] These prognostic factors (Table 22-3) are thus also important in toxicity; patients with poor performance status, significant weight loss or increased age are most likely to experience the greatest toxicity. In the studies at UMCC, most of the lethal toxicity occurred in nonambulatory patients.[5] Infection prophylaxis with trimethoprim + sulfamethoxazol did, however, appear to reduce the incidence of neutropenic febrile episodes and hospital days on antibiotics.[43]

CHEMOTHERAPY—THE SINGLE AGENTS

Over the course of recent years a large number of antineoplastic agents have been demonstrated to have objective antitumor activity in SCCL[11,21,22,26,109] (Table 22-4). This antitumor activity is defined as a greater than 50 percent reduction in the product of the greatest cross-perpendicular dimensions of measurable disease. In addition to commercially available agents, several as yet investigational agents have been shown to have considerable antitumor activity for SCCL, including carboplatin (CBDCA),[109] and tenoposide.[21] Cisplatin is listed among the agents with activity, although the tabulated number falls below the usual threshold of 20 percent. This is due, in part, to the lack of adequate testing of cisplatin as a single agent in previously untreated patients.[11] When compared to other agents such as etoposide given to patients who were previously treated, cisplatin appears to have at least an activity equivalent to that of etoposide.[11] Furthermore, as will be discussed later, it is an

Table 22-4
Active* Agents for Small Cell Lung Cancer

Agent	Approximate Response Rate (%)*
Tenoposide (VM26)	65
Carboplatin (CBDCA)	50
Etoposide (VP16)	45
Cyclophosphamide	40
Mechlorethamine	35
Vincristine	35
Vinblastine	35
Doxorubicin	30
Methotrexate	30
Vindesine	25
BCNU	25
Methyl CCNU	25
CCNU	15
Cisplatin	15
Hexamethylmelanine	30+
Procarbazine	25+

*Does not consider dose/schedule dependency of any agent.
†Recent phase II studies have not confirmed activity.

extremely important agent in combination. Thus there are multiple agents from different drug classes with differing mechanisms of action and different and non-overlapping toxicity, which allows many permutations for combinations of chemotherapy.

Despite the number of active agents for this disease and its responsiveness to chemotherapy, there has been a paucity of new agents identified for the treatment of small cell carcinoma in recent years. This is due, in part, to the past philosophy of new drug testing in SCCL wherein new drugs were tested after patients had failed primary treatment. Although highly responsive to front-line chemotherapy, this tumor has been found to be exceptionally resistant to further chemotherapy after initial aggressive chemotherapy. For example, etoposide is a highly active single agent when given to previously untreated or minimally treated patients.[26] When given to patients who have received aggressive combination chemotherapy, the activity of etoposide is below 10 percent.[70] Furthermore, treatment with combination chemotherapy induces resistance to a broad range of chemotherapeutic agents thus indicating the induction of pleotrophic drug resistance. This pleotrophic drug resistance has produced a considerable dilemma in our philosophical approach for the testing of new drugs.

New Drug Identification

Since prior chemotherapy tends to diminish response to subsequent agents, the identification of new agents becomes a problem. Cohen et al. reviewed 97 phase II trials in SCCL and noted that only few active agents were found, but most trials were inadequate.[33] Few patients respond well to second-line chemotherapy, however, and the median survival after initial disease progression is about 3 months.[101] Several approaches have evolved as means to overcome the difficulty in new drug identification.[13] One approach would be to include new agents as part of randomized comparative trials. Such an approach, however, would require large numbers of patients and would not necessarily define the activity of the single agent, but rather its role in that given combination. Another approach might be to lower the threshold of consideration for "active" to less than 20 percent, such as to use 10 percent as the threshhold. This, however, would mean that larger numbers of patients would be exposed to drugs that have a very low order of activity. A third approach to new drug testing might be to test new drugs on those patients who achieve a stable partial response. However, the effectiveness of this approach has yet to be demonstrated. Specifically, it is not known whether new agents can be identified after initial chemotherapy has induced partial response. A lack of further response might be pleotrophic drug resistance rather then inactivity of the agent. The final approach for new drug identification has been to test new agents on previously untreated patients with extensive but stable, non-life-threatening disease. This approach would maximize the opportunity of finding new agents since the patient's tumor would not have been exposed to other chemotherapeutic agents. The difficulty with this latter approach, however, is that it is currently not certain whether treatment with an agent that has absent or low activity may preclude response to subsequent combination chemotherapy.[13] At present, many of these modalities for new drug testing are being applied and the maximal approach for new drug identification has yet to be identified. These various approaches to new drug testing, however, can be subjected to testing by prospective trial and such testing is likely to define an optimal strategy.

COMBINATION CHEMOTHERAPY

Combinations of chemotherapeutic agents with differing mechanisms of action and with differing but nonoverlapping toxicities have been effectively combined for many human diseases and have been particularly successful in SCCL. On the basis of the available active agents, as well as on agents with little or no demonstrated activity, a large number of combination chemotherapeutic regimens have been tested in small cell carcinoma of the lung (Table 22-5).* In general, drug combinations are superior to single agents,[81] and sequential studies have shown that three drugs are superior to two.[26] In some instances four drugs may be superior to three.[12,64] The most effective combination chemotherapy regimens appear to be those that incorporate etoposide either in the initial therapy or as part of a so-called crossover. Of particular importance has been the use of potentially synergistic drugs. For example, cyclophosphamide, doxorubicin, etoposide, and cisplatin are all potentially synergistic in pairs.[38,77] The two-drug combination of etoposide plus cisplatin, which has demonstrated activity in both animal and human tumor systems, has considerable activity in small cell carcinoma both as a salvage regimen behind the three-drug combination of cyclophosphamide, doxorubicin, and vincristine (CAV) as well as front-line activity.[11] The reverse is not as active; that is, CAV does not appear to have much salvage activity behind the two-drug combination of etoposide and cisplatin. Carboplatin, which has

*References 1,4,7,9,14,16,26,34,37,42,44,48-51,53,62-64,66,75,77,78,81,82 ,94,103,106,107, 114, and 115.

Table 22-5

Combinations Used in Treatment of Small Cell Lung Cancer

2 Drug	3 Drug	4 Drug	>4 Drug
AB	AVbP	CAMCc	CAMCcV
CA	CAP	CAMV	CAVEpt
CCc	CAE	CAVD	CAVHYMCcP
CE	CAV	CAVE	CAVHNVbP
CV	CME	CAVH	CAVMPr
HA	CVM	CAVM	CCcVMP
	HEM	CAMPt	
	EPT	CCcAP	
		CCcVP	

A = doxorubicin (Adriamycin); B = bleomycin; Cc = CCNU; E = etoposide; H = hexamethylmelamine; M = methotrexate; P = procarbazine; Pt = platinum; Vb = vinblastine; Bb = BCNU; C = cyclophosphamide; D = DTIC; F = fluorouracil; Hy = hydrosourea; N = nitrogen mustard; Pr = prednisone; V = vincristine. Acronyms are not necessarily those of the original authors.

also been shown to be a highly active single agent, may also be highly synergistic with etoposide.[18] The latter combination is currently the subject of considerable ongoing investigation, including optimal dose evaluation. Since there are few studies that compare the various evaluable regimens per se, specific recommendations of one regimen over another are difficult; however, several generalizations can be made: (1) within a given combination the application of the individual agents should be given in maximally tolerated dose (or very near it) as noted above, (2) etoposide is probably important as part of the induction and/or consolidating regimen, and (3) synergistic combinations may be very important in the treatment of this disease. Serial studies performed at the University of Maryland Cancer Center will serve to illustrate some generalizations for the application of combination chemotherapy.[5,12]

In 1975 we initiated a combination chemotherapy trial utilizing cyclophosphamide, adriamycin, and etoposide as shown in Table 22-6. Four sequential studies have been completed with more than 200 patients and demonstrate that this combination produced complete responses in approximately 65 percent of patients with limited disease and approximately 40 percent with extensive disease.[5,12] The median durations of survival were 15 and 9 months, respectively. Approximately 20 percent of the patients with limited disease were alive and disease-free at more than 2 years. This three-drug combination was chosen because of the possibility of multiple synergistic pairs among the three drugs. The results of this three-drug combination alone are approximately equivalent to those achieved in most bimodality studies. The toxicity was predominantly myelosuppression with a median lowest nadir of white cell count

Table 22-6

ACE Combination Chemotherapy

A = doxorubicin (Adriamycin)	45 mg/m^2 IV dl
C = cyclophosphamide	1000 mg/m^2 IV dl
E = etoposide	50 mg/m^2 IV days 1-5

of $0.9 \times 10^3/\mu l$ and the median lowest platelet count nadir in excess of $100,000\ \mu l.^{-1}$ The majority of this treatment could be delivered in an outpatient setting with approximately 20 percent of the patients having severe complications of myelosuppression (febrile episodes or infections). Slightly less than 5 percent of the patients experienced lethal toxicity, prodominantly patients who were not ambulatory.

Attempts to improve on this regimen by using alternating chemotherapies or a larger dose and continuous infusion of etoposide did not yield startling improvements. The recognition of the potential synergistic interaction of cisplatin with the other three agents[50] led to the addition of cisplatin to the combination. Cyclophosphamide was reduced by 20 percent to accommodate this addition.[12] The addition of cisplatin to this regimen produced considerably more toxicity without augmenting the response frequency, so the study was stopped to follow survival rate.[10] Updated data now suggest that there is an enhancement of the survival curve. Thus further studies are necessary to optimize utilization of this and other potentially synergistic combinations of chemotherapy.

ALTERNATING NON-CROSS-RESISTANT COMBINATION CHEMOTHERAPY

Another possible approach for optimizing the use of combination chemotherapy for SCCL was suggested from mathematical models by Goldie et al.[57,58] In this model, on the basis of behavior of some bacteria, multiple drug combinations might be combined to reduce the emergence of drug resistance. Where the toxicities of adding more drugs was prohibitive, rapid alternation of the drugs might prove useful. The alternating combinations should, in the model, be non-cross-resistant so that each combination would produce equal responses when one was used after the other. The hypothesis also assumed a constant mutation rate and a homogeneity of the cells within the tumor. The authors of the hypothesis noted that, in practice, two equal non-cross-resistant combinations would be very difficult to find. A large number of studies have been undertaken that were allegedly based on this hypothesis.[6] To date more than 50 such studies have been completed; half or more contained some form of a control group. The overall view of these studies would suggest that either alternating chemotherapies did not have a major impact on response or survival or else the best arm (or the best studies) produced results approximately equivalent to the "anticipated results" outlined above. Although some of the authors of these trials felt that their alternation improved results, the overall outcome has been disappointing with respect to its impact on survival. In general, when the initial combination was the "stronger," the alternation did not add to either response or survival, whereas in the reverse order some impact on response and survival was noted. A good example of this sequencing effect can be noted in studies that tested CAV followed by etoposide plus cisplatin and the reverse.[11]

This, however, does not suggest that the hypothesis is incorrect. Rather, these data suggest that for SCCL, the hypothesis has not been adequately tested since the original presuppositions; that is, equally effective non-cross-resistant regimens has not been demonstrated for any of the combinations used in this manner. One might conclude from these data, however, that currently one should use the most effective regimens as the initial therapy, that these regimens should be given in a maximal fashion, and that further studies may be needed to fully test the alternating chemotherapies hypothesis. Given both the number of active agents and the number of actual and potential combinations, multiple permutations are still possible. Considering the large number of studies which have attempted such alternations, however, other approaches would seem more promising.

NEWER CLINICAL APPROACHES

It is intuitively obvious that new approaches are necessary in order to improve on the results of currently available chemotherapy or bimodalities treatments. The results of studies over the last decade have clearly demonstrated that SCCL is a potentially curable disease, although only a small percentage of patients are currently rendered disease-free for more than 2 years. In some studies patients continue to have disease relapse up to 5 years,[85] further reducing the percentage of possible cures. One study noted that the continuation of smoking was a poor prognostic factor for long-term survival.[72] Considering the rapidly growing nature of this tumor, it is conceivable that late relapses may be new disease. Irrespective of this possibility, one approach that is important in the management of SCCL is to convince patients to stop smoking cigarettes. A number of clinical issues promise to provide some alterations in our therapeutic approach to SCCL.

Anticoagulants

A number of studies have demonstrated that coagulation or fibrin formation are an important component in the formation of metastases.[23,116] Alternatively, anticoagulants may have a direct cytotoxic action. Regardless of the mechanism of possible action, preliminary studies have suggested that anticoagulants may enhance response and survival in SCCL. Zacharski et al. conducted a prospectively randomized trial of chemotherapy with or without warfarin and found that the group receiving warfarin had a better response and survival.[117] There were, however, some imbalances in the two groups, with the control group not doing quite as well as would have been anticipated. In a subsequent study conducted by the Cancer and Leukemia Group B (CALGB), there was a trend in favor of the group receiving warfarin when compared to those receiving the same chemotherapy without the anticoagulant.[32] This latter study was conducted among patients with extensive disease, and thus the trend was only suggestive, but not conclusive, regarding the role of anticoagulants. On the basis of these data, the CALGB has completed a pilot study in which aggressive combination chemotherapy, chest irradiation, and anticoagulants were used together and has undertaken a randomized trial to evaluate the role of the anticoagulant, warfarin.

Consolidation or Late Intensification

Another approach toward improvement of survival rate might be to provide additional therapy after an initial response in an attempt to further reduce the residual tumor and thus augment the potential cure rate. Since the patients with complete response begin to have disease relapse at about 6 months, "late" intensification as used in this context would refer to treatment delivered at or near the 6-month period of treatment. There is some logic to this approach since there is an appreciable complete response (CR) frequency with almost two-thirds of those with limited disease in CR and virtually all of those with extensive disease in CR will eventually succumb to disease recurrence and death.

There are two basic approaches to consolidation or late intensification treatment: chemotherapy[61,67,74,80] and radiotherapy.[45,112] Preliminary data from one study conducted by the Southeastern Cooperative Oncology Group suggested that late etoposide plus cisplatin could improve the results of CAV plus chest irradiation.[61] This approach of sequencing therapies, however, may be subject to the same difficulty of interpretation as alternating chemotherapies. Another mathematical model, the Norton-Simon hypothesis,[96] suggests that late intensification with high-dose chemotherapy may offer some advantage in gaining control of the tumor when the number of tumor cells is reduced by initial chemotherapy. This approach remains to be adequately tested, however. Radiotherapy as a modality for late intensification also offers some potential rationale if used as hemibody or whole-body irradiation.[45,112] Control of tumor by irradiation is a function of dose and size such that when the tumor has been debulked with chemotherapy, radiotherapy may add to the control. Whole-body or hemibody irradiation needs further testing but has not yet shown sufficient promise to warrant routine application.

Duration of Initial Induction Treatment

Most studies have indicated that responses to chemotherapy are achieved rapidly. Cohen et al. suggested that all complete responses occurred within the first 6 weeks for patients receiving chemotherapy with cyclophosphamide, methotrexate, and CCNU (CMC)-based combinations.[36] Subsequent studies with more aggressive regimens showed that complete responses could occur up to the sixth course (18-24 weeks) of chemotherapy, but the median number of cycles to CR was still between 2 and 3.[70] The duration of the chemotherapy in most studies was, however, less clearly demarcated. Initially chemotherapy regimens were applied for up to 2 years.[2] By 2 years most of those patients whose disease was bound to relapse had done so. One study suggested that maintenance chemotherapy was useful in prolonging the duration of response and survival.[87] Subsequently, a number of studies have demonstrated that so-called state-of-the-art results could be achieved with lesser duration of chemotherapy,[52,53,75,94,115] and most regimens are now given for 6-8 months. Patients who have not achieved CR by this time are unlikely to do so, and this treatment duration appears "adequate" for those who achieved CR. This approach leaves unanswered, however, how long treatment should continue for those patients who have achieved only a partial response or for those few patients who achieved CR after the fifth or sixth cycle of chemotherapy. The question regarding the maximal duration of therapy can be tested in prospective randomized trials and is an important issue for the quality of survival. This issue, however, is difficult to test because it commits large amounts of patient resources to answer a question that will not advance the response or survival; in other words, this issue is not a question designed to further the results of therapy. The practice at the UMCC is to deliver eight courses of chemotherapy, thus giving two cycles beyond the latest seen CR. For patients who achieved only partial response

(PR), the practice is to continue chemotherapy until there is evidence of disease progression.

The Addition of More Agents

Since sequential studies have suggested that three-agent combinations are superior to two agent combinations, adding more active agents with attention to possible synergy offers another potential means for improving response frequency, duration of survival, or both. Some studies have suggested that four drug combinations are superior to three, but this did not include etoposide.[24] The UMCC study and the subsequent CALGB study of platinol, doxorubicin, cyclophosphamide, and etoposide is suggestive of an enhanced effect of four drugs,[12] but this was not a controlled study. Nevertheless, the median survivals of 15 and 11 months, respectively, in extensive disease studies are somewhat better than those considered "state of the art." The major difficulty with the addition of more agents is the increase in toxicity.[10] Whereas the three-drug ACE regimen was given predominantly on an ambulatory basis, the four-drug regimen was given predominantly on an inpatient basis. The leukopenia was more severe with the median lowest white blood cell count nadir of less than 200/μl, and there were more febrile periods during neutropenia, necessitating hospitalization and systemic antibiotics. The challenge in adding drugs to existing regimens is therefore the control of toxicity. Perhaps the toxicities may be modulated either by drug timing or rotation of agents or more likely from the technology derived from autologous bone marrow transplantation, including marrow culturing techniques and modulation of stem cells with various growth factors.

Interactions of Chemotherapy and Radiotherapy

Several of the agents used in the treatment of SCCL have considerable interactions with radiation. Some of the agents are radiomimetic and enhance the local toxicity. Doxorubicin, for example, can enhance the local toxicity within the irradiation fields and in several studies, contributed in part to the esophagitis and pneumonitis.[15,30,31,79,91] Cisplatin and probably carboplatin can act as radiation sensitizers,[46,95] and other agents also may have such properties. These interactions dictate that the timing of chemotherapy and radiotherapy be carefully evaluated when new drugs are added to a regimen in order to take advantage of drug-radiation interactions.[39] Advances in radiation portal planning have alleviated some of the overlapping toxicity problems, but care must still be exercised that drug–radiation interactions do not enhance local toxicity. The use of the chemotherapeutic agents that have some radiosensitizing activity to augment local control or to modulate the dose of radiation necessary to achieve local control has not as yet received adequate attention.

NEW APPROACHES FROM THE LABORATORY

In recent years there has been a wide proliferation of information on the biology of SCCL which distinguishes the unique nature of this tumor.[89] Permanent cell lines derived from human tumor samples provided much of this data, and such cell lines can be established, at least on a short-term basis, with considerable efficiency using serum free medium and specific growth factors.[108] These cell lines retain the biochemical properties of the original tumor. When implanted into nude athymic mice, these cell lines form tumors that are similar to the original tumor. These cell lines are unique in morphology and by the production of factors such as bombesin, dopa decarboxylase, NSE, and the BB isoenzyme of creatinine kinase.[56] Cultured SCCL cell lines may have very important clinical roles, including (1) the screening of new agents before clinical testing, (2) the identification of synergistic drug pairs and combinations, and (3) the evaluation of drug resistance.[29,40] More importantly, however, these cell lines have been and will continue to be the tools by which the biology of the disease is understood so that we might modulate the growth of this tumor in vivo. For example, some of the hormone peptides produced by SCCL cells have autostimulating effects on the growth of the tumor. Argenine vasopressin and bombesin are both produced by SCCL cells, which, in turn, have receptors for these peptides. Nanomolar quantities of these hormones can stimulate the growth of the SCCL cells. Cuttita et al. have produced a monoclonal antibody that binds bombesin and prevents the binding of this hormone to its cellular receptor.[41] This antibody inhibits the growth of SCCL cells in culture and can prevent the growth of SCCL in nude mice inoculated with SCCL cell lines. This antibody may thus prevent the regrowth of SCCL after patients have achieved CR. In a similar vane, it may be possible to capitalize on other biological properties that are unique to SCCL, such as its diminished but inducible HLA expression[47] or its unique cell surface antigen expression on two-dimensional gel electropheresis.[19] Clearly, the recognition of the biology and the modulation of growth in vitro opens entire new vistas into the treatment of SCCL and offers an optimism that a greater percentage of patients may yet be cured.

FUTURE TREATMENT STRATEGIES

The exquisite sensitivity of this tumor to chemotherapy and radiotherapy suggest strongly that bimodalities will be the important approach for initial disease debulking and local control but that additional treatments will be needed to produce a larger percentage of cures. Such a possible strategy is outlined in Figure 22-1. Initial chemotherapy in this model would be used to produce major tumor debulking and to control the micrometastases. After several courses, a local control modality such as irradiation to areas of bulk disease (or surgery for eligible patients) would be added concurrently with chemotherapy to achieve local control and maximal debulking. The dose and timing of irradiation may be a function of the chemotherapeutic agents. Prophylactic cranial irradiation would likely be part of the local control issues, but again, optimal dose has yet to be established. Late intensification may find a role following the initial debulking procedures. Finally, maintenance therapy with monoclonal antibodies directed at growth factors may allow for protracted disease control. Although such a treatment program seems fanciful at present, the exploration of its components has already begun and we can look forward to a challenging period for treatment in which the long-term survival from this previously devastating disease will continue to improve.

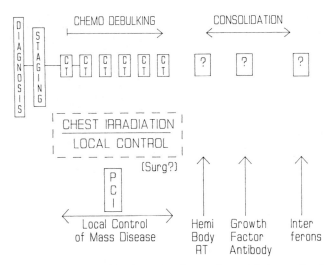

Fig. 22-1. A model schema for future clinic trials in small cell lung cancer.

REFERENCES

1. Abeloff MD, Ettinger DS, Khouri N, et al: Intensive induction therapy for small cell carcinoma of the lung. Cancer Treat Rep 63:519-524, 1979

2. Aisner J, Wiernik PH: Chemotherapy versus chemoimmunotherapy for small cell undifferentiated carcinoma of the lung. Cancer 46:2543-2549, 1980

3. Aisner J: Is combined modality treatment of small cell carcinoma of the lung necessary?, in Wernik PH (ed): Controversies in Oncology. New York, Wiley, 1982, pp 155-173

4. Aisner J, Whitacre M, Van Echo DA, et al: Combination chemotherapy for small cell carcinoma of the lung: Continuous vs. alternating non-cross resistant combinations. Cancer Treat Rep 66:221-230, 1982

5. Aisner J, Whitacre M, Van Echo DA, et al: Doxorubicin, cyclophosphamide and VP16-213 (ACE) in the treatment of small cell lung cancer. Cancer Chemother Pharmacol 7:187-193, 1982

6. Aisner J: Alternating chemotherapy for the treatment of small cell carcinoma of the lung, in Proceedings of 13th International Congress of Chemotherapy 11. Vienna, Verlag Egermann, 1983, pp 205-221

7. Aisner J, Alberto P, Bitran J, et al: Role of chemotherapy in small cell lung cancer: A Concensus Report of the International Association for the Study of Lung Cancer Workshop. Cancer Treat Rep 67:37-43, 1983

8. Aisner J, Forastiere A, Aroney R: Patterns of recurrence for cancer of the lung and esophagus. Cancer Treat Symp 2:87-105, 1983

9. Aisner J, Whitacre M, Van Echo DA, et al: Doxorubicin, cyclophosphamide and etoposide (ACE) by bolus or continuous infusion for small cell carcinoma of the lung (SCCL). Proc Am Soc Clin Oncol 2:196, 1983

10. Aisner J, Whitacre MY, Budman D, et al: Platinum (P), doxorubicin (A), cyclophosphamide (C), and etoposide (E), PACE, for small cell lung cancer (SCLC). Proc Am Soc Clin Oncol 4:181, 1985

11. Aisner J, Abrams J: Small cell lung cancer: The significance of platinol. Bristol-Meyers Oncology Division, Syracuse, New York, 1986

12. Aisner J, Whitacre MY, Abrams J, et al.: Adriamycin, cytoxan and etoposide (ACE) and platinum, adriamycin, cytoxan, etoposide (PACE) for small cell carcinoma of the lung. Semin Oncol 13 (Suppl 3):54-62, 1986

13. Aisner J: Editorial: New phase II agents as initial treatment for extensive disease small cell lung cancer. Cancer Treat Rep, in press

14. Alberto P, Berchtold W, Sonntag R, et al: Chemotherapy of small cell carcinoma of the lung: Comparison of a cyclic alternative combination with simultaneous combinations of four and seven agents. Eur J Cancer Clin Oncol 17:1027, 1981

15. Aristizabal SA, Manning MR, Miller RC, et al: Combined radiation-adriamycin effects on human skin. Front Rad Ther Oncol 13:103-112, 1979

16. Aroney RS, Bell DR, Chan WE, et al: Alternating non-cross resistant combination chemotherapy for small cell anaplastic carcinoma of the lung. Cancer 49:2449, 1982

17. Aroney RS, Aisner J, Wesley MN, et al: The values of prophylatic cranial irradiation given at complete remission in small cell lung carcinoma. Cancer Treat Rep 67:675-682, 1983

18. Atassi G, Kenis Y, Dumone P, et al: Animal screening of new platinum derivatives—studies with single agents and combinations. New Chemotherapy Drugs—Joint Meeting EORTC and NCI, 1983

19. Baylin SF, Gazdar AF, Minna JD, et al: Cell surface protein phenotype of human lung cancer in culture. Identification of common and distinguishing cell surface proteins on the membrane of different human lung cancer cell types. Proc Natl Acad Sci (USA) 79:4650, 1982

20. Bleehan NM, Bunn PA, Cox JD, et al: Role of radiation therapy in small cell anaplastic carcinoma of the lung. Cancer Treat Rep 67:11-19, 1983

21. Bork E, Hansen M, Dombernowsky P, et al: Temposide (VM-26), an overlooked highly active agent in small cell lung cancer: Results of a phase II trial in untreated patients. J Clin Oncol 4:524-527, 1986

22. Broder LE, Cohen MH, Selawry OS: Treatment of bronchogenic carcinoma. II. Small cell. Cancer Treat Rev 4:219-260, 1977

23. Brown JM: A study of the mechanism by which anticoagulation with warfarin inhibits blood-borne metastases. Cancer Res 33:1217-1224, 1973

24. Bunn PA Jr., Lichter AS, Glatstein, et al: Results of recent studies in small cell bronchogenic carcinoma and prospects for future studies, in Greco FA, Oldham RK, Bunn PA (eds): Small Cell Lung Cancer. Orlando, FL, Grune & Stratton, 1981, pp 413-446

25. Bunn PA, Cohen M, Lichter A, et al: Randomized trial of chemotherapy versus chemotherapy plus radiotherapy in limited stage small cell lung cancer. Proc Am Soc Clin Oncol 2:200, 1983

26. Bunn PA, Jr: The role of chemotherapy in small cell lung cancer, in Issell BF, Muggia FM, Carter SK (eds): Etoposide (VP-16) Current Status and New Developments. Orlando, FL, Academic Press, 1984, pp 141-161

27. Campling B, Quirt I, DeBoer G, et al: Is bone marrow examination in small cell lung cancer really necessary? Ann Intern Med 105:508-512, 1986

28. Cancer Facts and Figures 1985, American Cancer Society, New York, 1985

29. Carney DN, Gazdar AF, Minna JD: In vitro chemosensitivity of clinical specimens and established cell lines of small cell lung cancer. Proc Am Soc Clin Oncol 1:10, 1982

30. Catane R, Lichter A, Lee YJ, et al: Small cell lung cancer: Analysis of treatment factors contributing to prolonged survival. Cancer 48:1936-1943, 1981

31. Chabora BM, Hopfan S, Wittes R: Esophageal complications in the treatment of oat cell carcinoma with combined irradiation and chemotherapy. Radiology 123:185-187, 1977

32. Chahinian AP, Ware JH, Zimmer B, et al: Update on anticoagulation with warfarin on

alternating chemotherapy in extensive small cell cancer of the lung. Proc Am Soc Clin Oncol 4:191, 1985

33. Cohen EA, Gralla RJ, Kris MG, et al: Phase II studies in small cell lung cancer (SCLC): An analysis of 97 trials. Proc Am Soc Clin Oncol 4:190, 1985

34. Cohen MH, Creaven PJ, Fossieck BE, et al: Intensive chemotherapy of small cell bronchogenic carcinoma. Cancer Treat Rep 61:349-354, 1977

35. Cohen MH, Mathews MJ: Small cell bronchogenic carcinoma: A distinct clinico-pathologic entity. Semin Oncol 5:234-243, 1978

36. Cohen MH, Fossieck BE, Ihde DC, et al: Chemotherapy of small cell carcinoma of the lung: Results and concepts, in Muggia FM, Rozencweig M (eds): Lung Cancer: Progress and Therapeutic Research. New York, Raven Press, 1979, pp 559-566

37. Cohen MH, Ihde DC, Bunn PA, et al: Cyclic alternating combination chemotherapy for small cell bronchogenic carcinoma. Cancer Treat Rep 63:163, 1979

38. Corbett TH, Giowald DP, Mayo JG, et al: Cyclophosphamide-adriamycin combination chemotherapy of transplantable murine tumors. Cancer Res 35:1568-1573, 1975

39. Cox JD, Byhardt R, Komaki R, et al: Interaction of thoracic irradiation and chemotherapy on local control and survival in small cell carcinoma of the lung. Cancer Treat Rep 63:1251-1255, 1979

40. Curt GA, Carney DN, Cowan KH, et al: Unstable methotrexate resistance in human small cell carcinoma associated with double minute chromosomes. New Engl J Med 308:199-202, 1983

41. Cuttita F, Carney DN, Mulshine J, et al: bombasin-like peptides can function as autocrine growth factors in human small cell lung cancer. Nature 316:823-826, 1985

42. Dara P, Schultz MJ, Slater LM, et al: Doxorubicin, hexamethylmelamine therapy of small cell carcinoma of the lung. Cancer 48:1944, 1981

43. deJongh CA, Wade JC, Finley RS, et al: Trimethoprin/sulfamethoxazol versus placebo: A double blind comparison of infection prophylaxis in patients with small cell carcinoma of the lung. J Clin Oncol 1:302-307, 1983

44. Dillman RD, Taetle R, Seagren S, et al: Extensive disease chemotherapy and consolidation radiotherapy. Cancer 49:2003, 1982

45. Dillman RO, Seagren SL, Beauregard JC, et al: Combination chemotherapy and total body irradiation in extensive stage small cell carcinoma of the lung. Proc Am Soc Clin Oncol 2:C-745, 1983

46. Douple EB, Richmond RC, O'Hara JA, et al: Carboplatin as a potentiator of radiation therapy. Cancer Treat Rev 12 (Suppl):111-124, 1985

47. Doyle LA, Martin WJ, Gazdar AF, et al: Markedly decreased expression of class I histocompatibility antigens, protein and mRNA in human small cell lung cancer. J Exp Med 161:1135-1151, 1985

48. Eagan RT, Lee RE, Frytak S, et al: An evaluation of low dose cisplatin as part of combined modality therapy of small cell lung cancer. Cancer Clin Trials 4:267, 1981

49. Einhorn LH, Bond WH, Hornback W, et al: Long term results in combined modality treatment of small cell carcinoma of the lung. Semin Oncol 5:309-313, 1978

50. Evans WK, Osoba D, Feld R, et al: Etoposide (VP-16) and cisplatin: An effective treatment for relapse in small cell lung cancer. J Clin Oncol 3:65-71, 1985

51. Evans WK, Shepherd FA, Feld R, et al: VP-16 and cisplatin as firstline therapy for small cell lung cancer. J Clin Oncol 3:1471-1477, 1985

52. Evans WK, Shepard A, Feld R, et al: First-line therapy with VP16 and cisplatin during induction chemotherapy for small cell lung cancer. Sem Oncol 13(Suppl 3), 1986

53. Feld R, Evans WK, Coy P, et al: Canadian multicentre randomized trial comparing sequential (S) and alternating (A) administration of two non-cross resistant chemotherapy combinations in patients with limited small cell carcinoma of the lung (SCCL). Proc Am Soc Clin Oncol 3:214, 1984

54. Foster JM, Prager RL, Hainsworth JD, et al: Limited-stage small cell carcinoma (SCC): Prospective evaluation regarding the feasibility of adjuvant surgery. Proc Am Soc Clin Oncol 2:C-766, 1983

55. Fox W, Scadding JG: Medical research council cooperative trial of surgery and radiotherapy for primary treatment of small cell or oat-celled carcinoma of the bronchus. Ten year follow up. Lancet 2:62:63-65, 1973

56. Gazdar AF, Carney DN, Russel EK, et al: Establishment of continuous clonable cultures of small cell carcinoma of the lung which have aminoprecursor uptake and dicarboxylatin cell properties. Cancer Res 40:3502-3507, 1980

57. Goldie JH, Coldman AJ: A mathematical model for relating the drug sensitivity of tumors to their spontaneous mutation rate. Cancer Treat Rep 63:1727-1733, 1979

58. Goldie JH, Coldman AJ, Gudanskas GA: Rationale for the use of alternating non-cross resistant chemotherapy. Cancer Treat Rep 66:439-449, 1982

59. Greco FA, Richardson RL, Snell JD, et al: Small cell lung cancer: Complete remission and improved survival. Am J Med 66:625-630, 1979

60. Greco FA, Johnson DH, Hande KR, et al: High dose etoposide (VP16) in small cell lung cancer. Semin Oncol 12 (Suppl):42-44, 1985

61. Greco FA, Perez C. Einhorn LH, et al: Combination chemotherapy with or without concurrent thoracic radiotherapy (RT) in limited-stage (LD) small cell lung cancer (SCLC): A phase III trial of the Southeastern Cancer Study Group (SEG). Proc Am Soc Clin Oncol 5:178, 1986

62. Hansen HH, Selawry OS, Simon R, et al: Combination chemotherapy of advanced lung cancer: A randomized trial. Cancer 38:2201-2207, 1976

63. Hansen HH, Dombernnowsky P, Hansen M, et al: Chemotherapy of advanced small cell anaplastic carcinoma: Superiority of a four drug combination to a three drug combination. Ann Intern Med 89:177, 1978

64. Hansen HH, Dombernowsky P, Hansen M, et al: Chemotherapy of advanced small cell anaplastic carcinoma: Superiority of a four-drug combination to a three-drug combination. Ann Intern Med 89:177-181, 1978

65. Higgins GA, Sheilds TW, Keehn RJ: The solitary pulmonary nodule ten years follow-up of the Veterans Administration-Armed Forces Cooperative Study. Arch Surg 110:570-575, 1975

66. Hoffman PC, Weiman DS, Bitran JD, et al: Surgical resection in patients with stage III M0 small cell carcinoma of the lung. Proc Am Soc Clin Oncol 1:593, 1982

67. Humblet Y, Symann M, Bosly A, et al: Late intensification (LI) with autologous bone marrow transplantation (ABMT) for small cell lung cancer: A randomized trial. Proc Am Soc Clin Oncol 4:176, 1985

68. Ihde DC, Hansen HH: Staging procedures and prognostic factors in small cell lung cancer, in Greco FA, Oldham RK, Bunn PA (eds): Small Cell Lung Cancer. Orlando, FL, Grune & Stratton, 1981, pp 261-283

69. Ihde DC, Mukuch RW, Carney DN, et al: Prognostic implications of stage of disease and sites of metastases in patients with small cell carcinoma of the lung treated with intensive combination chemotherapy. Am Rev Resp Dis 123:500-507, 1981

70. Issell BF, Einhorn LH, Comis RL, et al: Multicenter phase II trial of etoposide in refractory small cell lung cancer. Cancer Treat Rep 69:127-128, 1985

71. Johnson DA, DeLeo MJ, Hande KR, et al: High dose (HD) cyclophosphamide (C), etoposide (E) and cisplatin (P) induction therapy in extensive-stage (ED) small cell lung cancer (SCLC). Proc Am Soc Clin Oncol 5:178, 1986

72. Johnston-Early A, Cohen MH, Minna JD, et al: Smoking abstinence and small cell cancer survival. JAMA 244:2175-2179, 1980

73. Kato Y, Fergusson TB, Bennett DE, et al: Oat cell carcinoma of the lung. A review of 13 cases. Cancer 23:517-524, 1969

74. Klastersky J, Nicaise C, Longeval E, et al: Cisplatin, adriamycin and etoposide (CAV) for remission induction of small cell bronchogenic carcinoma: Evaluation of efficacy and toxicity and pilot study of a "late intensification" with autologous bone marrow rescue. Cancer 50:652-658, 1982

75. Klastersky J, Sculier JP, Dumont JP, et al: Combination chemotherapy with adriamycin, etoposide, and cyclophosphamide for small cell carcinoma of the lung: A study by the EORTC Lung Cancer Working Party (Belgium). Cancer 56:71-75, 1985

76. Komaki R, Cox JD, Whitson W: Risk of brain metastasis from small cell carcinoma of the lung related to length of survival and prophylactic irradiation. Cancer Treat Rep 65:811-814, 1981

77. Kwiatkowski DJ, Green M, Choi N, et al: A phase II trial of cyclophosphamide, etoposide, and cisplatinum (CEP) with delayed combined chest and brain radiotherapy in previously untreated patients with limited small cell lung cancer (SCLC). Proc Am Soc Clin Oncol 5:184, 1986

78. Livingston RB, Moore TN, Heilburn B, et al: Small cell carcinoma of the lung: Combined chemotherapy and radiation. Ann Intern Med 88:194, 1978

79. Livingston RB, Mira J, Haas C, et al: Unexpected toxicity of combined modality therapy for small cell carcinoma of the lung. Internatl J Radiat Oncol Biol Phys 5:1637-1641, 1979

80. Livingston RB, Mira J: Extensive small cell lung cancer: Combined alkylators for induction with cisplatin + VP16 consolidation: A Southwest Oncology Group Study. Proc Am Soc Clin Oncol 3:210, 1984

81. Lowenbraun S, Bertolucci A, Smalley RV, et al: The superiority of combination chemotherapy over single agent chemotherapy in small cell lung carcinoma. Cancer 44:406-413, 1979

82. Markman M, Berkman A, Griffin A, et al: Intensive alternating non-cross resistant chemotherapy plus radiotherapy for small cell carcinoma. Proc Am Assoc Clin Res 23:577, 1982

83. Matthews MJ, Kanhouwa S, Pickren J, et al: Frequency of residual and metastatic tumor in patients undergoing curative surgical resection for lung cancer. Cancer Chemotherap Rep, Part 3, 4:63-67, 1973

84. Matthews MJ: Effects of therapy on the morphology and behavior of small cell carcinoma of the lung. A clinicopathologic study, in Muggia F, Rozencweig M (eds): Lung Cancer: Progress in Therapeutic Research. New York, Raven Press, 1979, pp 155-165

85. Matthews MJ, Rozencweig M, Staquet MJ, et al: Longterm survivors with small cell carcinoma of the lung. Eur J Cancer 16:527-531, 1980

86. Mauch P, Goodman R, Hellman S: The significance of mediastinal involvement in early stage Hodgkin's disease. Cancer 42:1039-1045, 1978

87. Maurer LH, Tulloh M, Weiss RB, et al: A randomized combined modality trial in small cell carcinoma of the lung. Cancer 45:30-37, 1980

88. Meyer JA, Comis RL, Ginsbery SJ, et al: The prospect of disease control by surgery combined with chemotherapy in Stage I and Stage II small cell carcinoma of the lung. Ann Thorac Surg 36:37-41, 1983

89. Minna JD: Recent advances of potential clinical importance in the biology of lung cancer. Proc Am Assoc Cancer Res 15:393-394, 1984

90. Mirvis SE, Whitley NO, Aisner J, et al: Abdominal CT in the staging of small cell carcinoma: Incidence of metastasis and effect on prognosis. Am J Radiol (in press)

91. Moore TN, Livingston R, Heilbrun L, et al: An acceptable rate of complications in combined doxorubicin-irradiation for small cell carcinoma of the lung: A Southwest Oncology Group study. Internatl J Radiat Oncol Biol Phys 4:675-680

92. Mountain CF: Biologic, physiologic and technical determinants in surgical therapy for lung cancer, in Strauss MJ (ed): Lung Cancer: Clinical Diagnosis and Treatment. Orlando, FL, Grune & Stratton, 1977, pp 88-100

93. Muggia FM, Krezoski SK, Hansen HH: Cell kinetic studies in patients with small cell carcinoma of the lung. Cancer 34:1683-1690, 1974

94. Natale RB, Shank B, Hilaris BS, et al: Combination cyclophosphamide, adriamycin, and vincristine rapidly alternating with combination cisplatin and VP-16 in treatment of small cell lung cancer. Am J Med 79:303-308, 1985

95. Nias AH: Radiation and platinum drug interaction. Internatl J Radiat Oncology Biol Phys 48:297-314, 1985

96. Norton L, Simon R: Tumor size, sensitivity to therapy, and design of treatment schedules. Cancer Treat Rep 61:1307-1317, 1977

97. Osterlind K, Ihde DC, Ettinger DS, et al: Staging and prognostic factors in small cell carcinoma of the lung. Cancer Treat Rep 67:3-9, 1983

98. Perez CA, Einhorn L, Oldham RK, et al: Preliminary report on a randomized trial of radiotherapy (RT) to the thorax in limited small cell carcinoma of the lung treated with multiagent chemotherapy. Proc Am Soc Clin Oncol 2:190, 1983

99. Perry MC, Eaton WL, Chahinian P, et al: Chemotherapy (CT) with or without radiation therapy (RT) in limited small cell cancer of the lung (SCC). Proc Am Soc Clin Oncol 5:173, 1986

100. Pico JL, Beaujean F, Debre M, et al: High dose chemotherapy (HDC) with autologous bone marrow transplantation (ABMT) in small cell carcinoma of the lung (SCCL) in relapse. Proc Am Soc Clin Oncol 2:C-806, 1983

101. Poplin EA, Asiner J, Van Echo DA, et al: CCNU, vincristine, methotrexate and procarbazine treatment of relapsed small cell lung carcinoma. Cancer Treat Rep 66:1557-1559, 1982

102. Poplin EA, Thompson B, Whitacre MY, Aisner J: Small cell carcinoma of the lung (SCCL): Influence of age on treatment outcome. Cancer Treat Rep 71:291-296, 1987

103. Schabel FM Jr, Trader MW, Laster WR, et al: Cis-dichlorodrammineplatinum (II): Combination chemotherapy and cross-resistance studies with tumors of mice. Cancer Treat Rev 63:1459-1473, 1979

104. Shields TW, Higgins GA, Matthews MJ, et al: Surgical resection in the management of small cell carcinoma of the lung. J Thorac Cardiovasc Surg 84:481-488, 1982

105. Shepperd FA, Ginsberg R, Evans WK, et al: "Very limited" small cell lung cancer (SCLC)—results of non-surgical treatment. Proc Am Soc Clin Oncol 3:223, 1984

106. Sierocki JS, Golbey RB, Wittes RE: Combination chemotherapy for small cell carcinoma of the lung (SCLC). Proc Am Soc Clin Oncol 19:352, 1978

107. Sikic BI, Chak LY, Reynolds RD, et al: Alternating chemotherapy regimens utilizing seven and nine drugs in extensive small cell lung cancer. Proc Am Soc Clin Oncol 1:C-578, 1982

108. Simms E, Gazdar AF, Abrams P, et al: Growth of human small cell carcinoma of the lung in serum-free growth factor supplemental medium. Cancer Res 40:4356-4363, 1980

109. Smith IE, Harland SJ, Robinson BA, et al: Carboplatin: A very active new cisplatin analog in the treatment of small cell lung cancer. Cancer Treat Rep 69:43-46, 1985

110. Souhami RL, Harper PG, Linch D, et al: High dose cyclophosphamide with autologous marrow transplantation as initial treatment of small cell carcinoma of the bronchus. Cancer Chemother Pharmacol 8:31-34, 1982

111. Spitzer G, Dicke KA, Litam J, et al: High-dose combination chemotherapy with autologous bone marrow transplantation in adult solid tumors. Cancer 45:307-314, 1980

112. Urtasun RC, Eelch A, Bodner D: Hemibody radiation, an active therapeutic modality for the management of patients with small cell lung cancer. Internatl J Radiat Oncol Biol Phys 9:1575-1578, 1983

113. Whitley NO, Fuks JZ, McCrae E, et al: Computerized tomography of the chest in small cell lung cancer: Staging follow-up and prognostic factors. Am J Radiol 141:885-892, 1984

114. Wittes RE, Hoptan S, Hilaris B, et al: Oat cell carcinoma of the lung. Cancer 40:653, 1977
115. Woods RL, Levi JA: Chemotherapy for small cell lung cancer (SCLC): A randomized study of maintenance therapy with cyclophosphamide, adriamycin and vincristine (CAV) after remission induction with cisplatinum (CIS-DDP), VP-16-213 and radiotherapy. Proc Am Soc Clin Oncol 3:214, 1984
116. Zacharski LR, Henderson WG, Rickles FR, et al: Rationale and experimental design for the VA Cooperative study of anticoagulation (Warfarin) in the treatment of cancer. Cancer 44:732–741, 1979
117. Zacharski LR, Henderson WG, Rickles FR, et al: Effect of warfarin on survival in small cell carcinoma of the lung. JAMA 245:831–835, 1981

Allen S. Lichter
Daniel C. Ihde

23

The Role of Radiation Therapy in the Treatment of Small Cell Lung Cancer

Radiation therapy plays a vital role in the treatment of small cell lung cancer (SCLC). Currently, uses for radiation in SCLC include:

1. Limited disease—local thoracic irradiation
2. Extensive disease—local thoracic irradiation; irradiation of sites of disseminated disease
3. Prophylactic irradiation to areas at high risk for dissemination, especially brain
4. Wide-field irradiation—hemibody or whole-body treatment
5. Palliation of local chest symptoms; treatment of metastatic disease

This chapter will summarize the current status of radiation therapy in each of these five major areas.

RADIATION THERAPY IN LIMITED-STAGE SMALL CELL LUNG CANCER (SCLC)

Over the years it has been found most appropriate to stage small cell lung cancer into two large groups, limited versus extensive disease[60] (see Chapter 20, section on staging evaluation). While some definitions vary slightly, many researchers exclude patients with pericardial or pleural effusions from the category of limited disease. All other patients are classified as having extensive disease. It is in limited disease that the use of radiation therapy has had its greatest impact and is of potential curative benefit.

It has long been recognized that SCLC is uniquely sensitive to radiation. Studies of the radiation responsiveness of lung cancer by cell type confirm this fact.[110] While non-small cell lung cancers (NSCLCs) respond to radiation approximately 30–50 percent of the time, SCLC has a response rate of greater than 90 percent.[110] These clinical observations have been further documented through laboratory investigation.

LUNG CANCER: A COMPREHENSIVE TREATISE
ISBN 0-8089-1876-1

In work on established cell lines from SCLC, Morstyn and colleagues have shown that these cell lines have almost no shoulder and very low extrapolation numbers for their radiation survival curves[95] (Fig. 23-1). These data indicate that SCLC lung cancer has a poor ability to accumulate and repair sublethal damage and is quite sensitive to irradiation, precisely matching clinical observation. Furthermore, it has been a well known clinical observation that recurrent SCLC following treatment with chemotherapy is far less responsive to treatment than primary untreated disease.[56,98] Cell culture data have also demonstrated this effect.[16] When SCLC lines "convert" to a large cell morphology, radiation sensitivity of these cells changes dramatically (Fig. 23-2). This morphologic change correlates with establishment of a large shoulder on the radiation cell survival curve and a higher extrapolation number, indicating a greater degree of radiation resistance. While this conversion to large cell morphology is associated with amplification of the C-myc oncogene,[76] it is not clear whether this oncogene amplification is directly related to the change in radiation sensitivity.

In the 1960s it was appreciated that untreated SCLC had a median survival of 6–10 weeks.[45] It was also appreciated that surgical therapy was seldom effective in curing SCLC. The resectability rate for SCLC was lower than that of other lung cancer types, and few patients were long-term survivors despite the fact that a "complete" resection of tumor had taken place. It was theorized that radiation therapy, while likely not a curative modality in SCLC because of the propensity of this tumor for widespread dissemination, nonetheless might be able to substitute for surgery. In this manner, patients could be saved the morbidity and expense of aggressive chest surgery while potentially not suffering a decrease in median survival or long-term survival. A study comparing radiation versus surgery was performed in the United Kingdom by the Medical Research Council.[4,89] In total, 144 limited-stage patients were randomly allocated to surgery or radiation therapy. The median survival time was superior for the radiated group, establishing radiation therapy as the local treatment of choice for SCLC. However, the long-term survival in either the surgery or radiation treatment arm of the trial was less than 2 percent, once again confirming the systemic nature of SCLC.

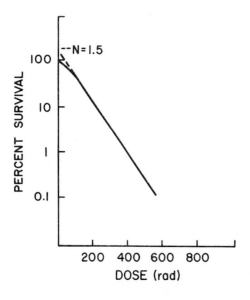

Fig. 23-1. Radiation survival curve for a typical SCLC cell line. The small shoulder and low extrapolation number (N) indicate a poor ability to accumulate and repair sublethal radiation damage.

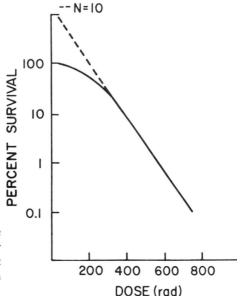

Fig. 23-2. Radiation survival curve for the large cell variant of SCLC. The large shoulder and high extrapolation number indicate that this cell line is far less sensitive to radiation than the typical small cell line.

It should be noted that with the uniform application of modern detailed staging procedures, a highly selected group of SCLC appears to be emerging for whom surgical therapy does seem beneficial. Patients with limited-stage disease without mediastinal involvement (fewer than 10 percent of all limited stage cases) can be surgically resected with reasonable expectation of 2-year survival.[120] Whether chemoradiotherapy without surgical resection would produce similar survival rates in these clinically operable patients is possible but unproven.[118]

At about the same time that radiation was becoming established as superior to surgery in the treatment of SCLC, the first clinical trials of chemotherapy in lung cancer were taking place. In the late 1960s, the Veteran's Administration Lung Cancer Study Group observed that a nine week course of cyclophosphamide more than doubled the survival of treated SCLC patients, in marked contrast to its lack of efficacy in other types of lung cancer.[50] In the early 1970s, a number of active drugs for the treatment of SCLC were identified and combinations of these drugs were employed. Combination chemotherapy proved markedly superior to single-agent chemotherapy, and complete clinical responses to treatment using chemotherapy alone were seen with regularity.[11,24] Soon thereafter, chemotherapy was combined with radiation and a number of trials were performed comparing combined modality therapy against radiation treatment alone. These studies are summarized in Table 23-1. In every study the combined modality treatment proved superior. In two recent studies, when combination chemotherapy was applied only at the time of failure following radiation, the 2-year survival was inferior when compared to a group treated with initial combined modality therapy.[101,116,117] Thus it has been conclusively established that SCLC is a systemic disease and is not amenable to treatment with radiation therapy alone; all patients should receive systemic therapy as part of their initial treatment. In patients who are elderly and infirm, aggressive combination chemotherapy may not be tolerable but modest doses of combination or perhaps single-agent chemotherapy can still

Table 23-1

Trials of Radiotherapy Alone versus Radiotherapy Plus Chemotherapy

Number of patients	Median Survival (Weeks)		1-Year Survival (%)		Reference
	XRT	XRT + Drug	XRT	XRT + Drug	
41	21	41	NS*	NS	8
58	NS	NS	19	23	17
75	24	39	20	30	55
236	25	43	18	34	88
25	18	50	44	70	84
57	48	34	36	38	101
68	21	38	30	28	103

*Not stated.

be applied. The stepwise progression of response rates, median survival, 1-year survival, and long-term survival for treatment for SCLC through the 1960s and 1970s is summarized in Table 23-2.

SCLC was so sensitive to effects of aggressive combination chemotherapy that, as noted in Table 23-2, response rates and median survival of patients treated with drugs alone approached the figures that could be achieved when combined radiation and chemotherapy were employed. Some investigators used these results to conclude that radiotherapy might not be required at all for the treatment of SCLC.[23,25,131] Subsequently, there has been considerable debate regarding the proper role of radiation therapy in the treatment of SCLC. Several retrospective reviews of SCLC treatment series have been performed.[1,9,11,15,77,94,121] These reviews have indicated that radiotherapy can be combined with aggressive chemotherapy with acceptable toxicity. However, the toxicity of combined modality therapy is clearly higher than that for chemotherapy alone or radiation alone, especially in terms of acute esophageal, pulmonary, and hematologic toxicity.[10,18,39,44,93,124] Yet, toxicity in long-term (>2 years) survivors appears similar in patients treated with chemotherapy alone or with combined modality therapy.[63] The retrospective analyses have indicated that median survival times are similar in patients treated with chemotherapy alone or with combined modality therapy but that long-term survival is greater in patients treated with combined modality therapy, especially if one considers only limited-disease patients.[11]

Table 23-2

Advances In The Treatment Of Small Cell Lung Cancer

Treatment	Complete Response Rate (%)	Median Survival (Weeks)	1-Year Survival (%)	2-Year Survival Disease-Free (%)
None	—	10	5	0
Resection (limited stage)	20	20	15	1
Radiation (limited stage)	35	25	25	2
Chemotherapy				
Single agent (extensive stage)	2	20	15	0
Combination (limited + extensive)	50	45	45	5
Combined radiation plus				
chemotherapy	50	45	45	10–15

Several points need to be emphasized concerning the conclusions of retrospective reviews of SCLC patients. The first concerns the use of median survival as an indicator of therapeutic effectiveness. In a disease where the pathologically confirmed complete response rate is not much greater than 50 percent, median survival may be a poor indicator of the effectiveness of treatment.[43] Since patients with partial response invariably die of their disease, the median survival of two groups of patients whose complete response rate is a hypothetical 49 percent would likely be similar. However, one treatment may produce more long-term survivors than the other treatment. It is only through an analysis of long-term survival that one could appreciate this difference (Fig. 23-3). Therefore, one should study the entire survival curve when judging the effectiveness of a therapy. An overemphasis on the median survival time may miss a quantifiable improvement in the effectiveness of therapy.

Many retrospective analyses are subtly biased in favor of combined modality therapy because of patient selection factors. For example, some retrospective reviews suggest that local chest failure is less frequent with combined modality treatment.[100,108] However, this conclusion could be critically dependent on the aggressiveness of the chemotherapy. Poor-quality chemotherapy combined with chest irradiation could lead to local chest control but early systemic relapse. If aggressive therapy had been employed, patients might have remained in systemic control long enough to reveal chest failures despite local radiation. Furthermore, when a patient fails systemically, thorough restaging of the primary site seldom is done, thus potentially overestimating the percentage of intrathoracic control.

Combined modality treatment may be favored as a result of other selection factors. Since combined modality treatment is more toxic, it often is administered to patients with better performance status. Performance status is the major prognostic indicator of survival time in SCLC,[60] and a retrospective nonrandomized study comparing combined modality to drug treatment alone may be comparing a more favorable group of patients with a less favorable group of patients.

Finally, retrospective reviews may cite a promising early result from a retrospective series that later fails to sustain the high level of response and survival. Table 23-3

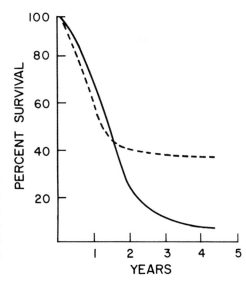

Fig. 23-3. Two hypothetical survival experiences for different treatments for SCLC. The median survival for both treatments is 15 months, yet one treatment produces far more long-term survivors, illustrating the potential problems of relying too heavily on median survival figures to evaluate efficacy of therapy.

Table 23-3
Sequential Reports of Clinical Trials in Small Cell Lung Cancer

Institution	Treatment	Survival (%)			
		1st Report	2d Report	3d Report	Final Report
NCI[23]	Chemotherapy	29			11
Medical College of Wisconsin[12,13]	Combined CT-RT	66			12
NCI[18,64,65,67]	Combined CT-RT	90	50	40	18

outlines three clinical experiences that looked extremely promising in early reports but later appeared to be less effective. If these later reports are omitted from retrospective reviews, an overly optimistic outlook for one treatment or the other could be produced. The factors that might lead to biased outcomes of retrospective reviews of radiotherapy results in SCLC are:

1. Differing ways of staging limited versus extensive therapy.
2. Differing ways of assessing complete response.
3. Differing ways of assessing site of treatment failure. Distant failure frequently may result in discontinuation of search for local failure.
4. If not randomized, selection bias usually favoring the radiation group.
5. For chemotherapy; problems due to different drugs, intensities of treatment, schedules, and duration of therapy.
6. For radiation; problems due to different dose-time fractionation, field sizes, and uses of shielding.

These problems with retrospective reviews of different series in the treatment of SCLC are encountered in most series. The best way to eliminate such biases from reporting of results in SCLC is to perform prospective randomized trials. Over the last several years, such trials have produced a great deal of the important clinical data that have formed the foundation for current treatment policies in SCLC. These trials are discussed below.

RANDOMIZED TRIALS COMPARING CHEMOTHERAPY WITH OR WITHOUT RADIATION IN THE TREATMENT OF LIMITED-STAGE SCLC

The most reliable information indicating whether radiation therapy improves the local control and survival of patients with limited-stage SCLC come from prospective randomized clinical trials. To date, seven studies have been reported in the literature, five in abstract form and two with more detailed publications. The studies are summarized in Table 23-4. In the three trials that commented on the percentage of complete response, combined modality treatment proved superior. This improvement in complete response rate has been noted in other single-institution nonrandomized trials.[81] Median survival was almost identical for the five trials that commented, ranging between a 1- and a 6-week difference. Only the trial from the Southeastern Cancer Study Group (SEG) showed a superior median survival for combined modality versus chemotherapy. In terms of local chest control, all studies that commented on this

Table 23-4

Randomized Trials Comparing Effect of Chemotherapy on Local Control and Survival of
Limited-Stage SCLC Patients

Number of patients	Complete Response (%)		Median Survival (Weeks)		Local Failure (%)		Reference
	CT	CT + RT	CT	CT + RT	CT	CT + RT	
154	NS*	NS	48	42	NS	NS	35
84	NS	NS	64	63	67	32	42
129	NS	NS	—47—		CT 2 × CT-RT		49
216	48	63	49	60	52	36	100
368	34	50	53	58	29	11	102
32	NS	NS	48	46	NS	NS	123
74	49	78	52	71	75	31	57, 74

*Not stated.

factor showed that combined modality treatment reduces the frequency of chest failure from nearly 60 percent to approximately 30 percent. Finally, in terms of overall survival, only the SEG study has concluded that combined modality treatment is superior to chemotherapy alone.

The two trials that have been published in more detail deserve further comment. The SEG trial ran from 1978 to 1982.[100] All patients were treated with two cycles of cytoxan (1000 mg/m^2 IV), adriamycin (40 mg/m^2 IV), and vincristine (1 mg/m^2 IV) (CAV) as noted in the schema of Figure 23-4. All patients who showed evidence of response or stable disease were then randomized to receive brain irradiation only or to receive brain irradiation in conjunction with chest irradiation. Radiation treatment was accomplished in three separate courses that alternated with cycles of CAV. The brain received 3600 rads in three 1200-rad courses of five fractions each. The chest was treated to the initial prechemotherapy tumor volume. The entire mediastinum, contralateral hilum, and supraclavicular nodes were included in the field. Initially, 300-rad fractions were utilized to deliver 1500 rads in each of the first two courses. The final 1000 rads in five fractions were given to a reduced field, encompassing only the primary tumor and ipsilateral hilum. A posterior spinal cord block was allowed in the small boost field if the cord dose was going to exceed a total of 4000 rads.

Following the conclusion of the three radiation courses, patients received an additional two cycles of CAV and then were evaluated for response. Any patient who

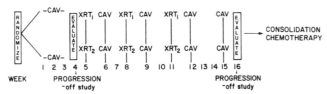

Fig. 23-4. Treatment schema for the Southeastern Cancer Group protocol (78 Lun 328) comparing chemotherapy alone to chemotherapy plus chest irradiation. CAV = cyclophosphamide, adriamycin, vincristine, XRT$_1$ = brain radiation, XRT$_2$ = brain and chest radiation.

had a complete or partial response was started on consolidation chemotherapy, which consisted of three cycles of VP16 and hexamethylmelamine.

All patients had limited disease and were staged in a routine fashion. A total of 304 patients were randomized into the study; 13 were found to be ineligible, leaving 291 eligible patients. At the time of publication, 25 percent of the patients (73) were considered inevaluable, leaving 218 patients fully evaluable for response and failure analysis. All 291 patients were evaluable for survival analysis.

Results from this trial show an improvement in median survival for combined modality patients—60 weeks compared to 49 weeks for those treated with chemotherapy alone. The actuarial survival of the entire population of 291 patients showed that chemotherapy alone produced a 19 percent 2-year survival versus 28 percent with combined modality treatment ($p = .03$). In 126 patients who underwent consolidation therapy, the 2-year survival for the chemotherapy group was 23 percent and the combined modality group, 40 percent. The survival curve for the radiated patients given consolidation was statistically superior to the group given chemotherapy alone ($p = .04$).

Further evidence of the effect of local chest irradiation in this trial can be obtained by analyzing the complete response rate and the incidence of local chest failure between the two arms of the study. After two cycles of CAV chemotherapy, approximately 20 percent of the entire population had a complete response as determined by chest x-ray. After six chemotherapy courses, which would have included radiotherapy in the combined modality arm, 48 percent of the CAV patients had a complete response versus 62 percent of the combined modality group ($p = .05$). Analysis of failure as based on chest x-ray alone showed that 52 percent of patients treated with CAV had radiographic evidence of a chest recurrence versus 36 percent of those patients receiving combined modality treatment ($p = .03$).

While improvements in local tumor control, complete response frequency, and survival may be obtained with the addition of chest irradiation, many studies have reported that combined modality therapy is associated with a substantial increase in toxicity. Interestingly, the SEG trial did not reproduce those results and showed virtually no difference in toxicity between the two treatment arms (Table 23-5). It is possible that several short courses of radiation alternating with chemotherapy can be effectively administered without increasing the toxicity of therapy compared to drug treatment alone.

This trial provides important information that supports the concept that chest irradiation forms an important part of the treatment of limited-disease SCLC. Gains in local tumor control and long-term survival are relatively modest but were obtained without a significant increase in toxicity. The unorthodox radiation therapy in this trial deserves additional study. It may be that combinations of short courses of radiation alternating with short courses of chemotherapy provide useful benefit without increased toxicity.

The National Cancer Institute trial began in late 1977 and has recently concluded accrual. All patients begin induction chemotherapy with a 6-week program of cyclophosphamide, methotrexate, and lomustine (CCNU) (CMC regimen). From weeks 7-12, vincristine, doxorubicin (Adriamycin; by Pharmitalia), and procarbazine (VAP regimen) are administered. After week 12, CMC doses are reduced, and alternating 6-week cycles of CMC and VAP are given until week 48. Complete responders receive prophylactic cranial irradiation (2400 rad/eight fractions/2 weeks) at week 13 or 25.

Table 23-5

Toxicity of Combined Modality versus Chemotherapy Alone in The SEG Trial

	Complications (%)			
	Chemotherapy (103 patients)		Chemotherapy + Radiation (115 patients)	
	Moderate	Severe/Life-Threatening	Moderate	Severe/Life-Threatening
Hemoglobin	11	11	23	13
Granulocytes	17	51	16	54
Platelets	6	1	7	5
Esophagitis	41	16	44	20
CNS	12	7	13	4

Data taken from Perez CA, Einhorn L, Oldham RK, et al: Randomized trial of radiotherapy to the thorax in limited small-cell carcinoma of the lung treated with multiagent chemotherapy and elective brain irradiation: A preliminary report. J Clin Oncol 2:1200-1208, 1984.

Half of the patients are randomized to receive chest irradiation in a schedule of 4000 rads in 15 fractions in 3 weeks beginning within 3 days of the initiation of induction chemotherapy. This radiotherapy schedule was selected since our past experience suggested that more than 3000 rads in 3 weeks was necessary to reliably assure control of chest tumor.[18] Randomization occurred only after the patient was simulated for irradiation, in order to ensure that all patients entered on study were acceptable candidates for this aggressive irradiation program. During irradiation, patients were resimulated after 5 and 10 fractions, and treatment portals were reduced if tumor shrinkage has occurred. This policy was intended to minimize damage to uninvolved lung tissue. A posterior spinal cord block is placed after 2400 rads. All radiation was given with 4- or 6-MV linear accelerators.

After the first 74 patients were randomized, median time from study entry was over 3 years. Complete response rates were 78 percent with bimodality treatment and 49 percent with chemotherapy alone ($p = .02$).[57] Actuarial disease-free survival was also significantly superior in the combined modality arm, with an estimated 35 percent of patients free of cancer at 2-4 years, compared to only 13 percent with chemotherapy alone ($p = .02$).[57] Freedom from initial tumor progression in the chest in complete responders, the only group in whom local control might be expected to affect survival, was greatly improved ($p = .001$) and estimated at 55 percent at 3 years, compared to 15 percent in chemotherapy-only patients.[32] A trend in overall survival ($p = .07$) in favor of the combined modality group was present and would have been more striking if the four out of five deaths beyond 3 years on the combined modality treatment not due to SCLC (three deaths from pathologically documented NSCLC and one from cardiovascular disease) had been excluded.[57]

Treatment-related toxicities were considerably greater when this chest irradiation regimen was added to combination chemotherapy. Myelosuppression during induction chemotherapy and esophageal toxicity were significantly more severe with combined modality treatment.[74] Probably most worrisome, however, was severe pulmonary toxicity, defined as diffuse bilateral infiltrates extending beyond radiation portals and requiring hospital admission; this occurred in 28 percent of patients given chemotherapy and irradiation but in only 5 percent of those receiving chemotherapy alone ($p = .017$). Pulmonary biopsies, obtained in 11 out of 13 patients, never revealed any evidence of an infectious agent. Eight patients died of this complication, including five who were in clinical complete remission. This frequency and severity of pulmonary dysfunction was much greater than would be expected with irradiation alone and is almost certainly a specific complication of the combined modality program that was utilized.[10] Clearly, a radiation schedule that could retain the antitumor effects of this regimen while diminishing or eliminating pulmonary damage would be useful.

How should the sometimes conflicting results of the prospective randomized trials evaluating the benefits of added chest irradiation in limited-stage SCLC be reconciled? It is clear that many combined modality regimens are not associated with improved survival, and chest irradiation that does not utilize a specific published program should not be regarded as obligatory in the management of this disease. Other regimens, including at least two that have been tested in randomized studies, however, do appear to yield modest survival gains, particularly in long-term survival. Heterogeneity of chemotherapy and radiotherapy programs undoubtedly account for the varied outcome of randomized trials, and clinical investigative efforts to find the method of integrating these two forms of therapy that are associated with the highest therapeutic index are critically important. It is humbling, however, to recall that even the most optimistic reported results suggest only an approximate 20 percent improvement in intermediate-term survival with added chest irradiation. Since limited-stage disease comprises only one-third of all cases of SCLC, this implies that thoracic radiotherapy currently benefits only 6-7 percent of patients in terms of prolongation of survival. Development of better forms of systemic treatment remains the major factor needed to increase the number of SCLC patients who can potentially be cured.

TOWARD AN OPTIMAL METHOD OF DELIVERING RADIATION THERAPY IN SCLC

Volume Requiring Treatment

Over the past decade, the volume requiring treatment in SCLC has become reasonably standard. The primary tumor is irradiated with a 1-2-cm margin. Additionally, both hilar areas, the entire mediastinum, and usually the supraclavicular nodes are treated. In some cases, the supraclavicular portion of the field is omitted when these nodes are palpably negative and the primary tumor is located in the inferior lung fields. Failure to irradiate the proper volume when treating SCLC can result in increased numbers of chest failures. When Perez and colleagues,[101] reporting for the Southeastern Cancer Study Group, analyzed treatment technique, they found that 69 percent of patients (9/13) irradiated without inclusion of the contralateral hilum or portions of the mediastinum had intrathoracic treatment failure. This contrasted with a chest failure rate of only 33 percent (13/40) when patients had adequate thoracic tumor volumes treated. This difference was statistically significant ($p = .026$). White and colleagues analyzed similar data from the Southwest Oncology Group.[129] Looking at patients who achieved a complete response, the local chest failure rate was 34 percent when an adequate chest volume was treated. This failure rate escalated to 69 percent in patients in whom there was a major violation of either radiation dose or radiation volume. The difference between these two failure rates was statistically significant ($p = .042$). When treating SCLC with radiation, careful attention must be paid to designing an adequate portal of treatment. Lapses in technique can result in an increased failure rate.

While it is desirable to completely irradiate all tumor and nodal areas, efforts must be made to reduce treatment of unnecessary areas of lung as much as possible. All fields should be custom-shaped, using poured blocks. If substantial tumor shrinkage is taking place during treatment, a resimulation with a reduction in the treatment volume can be beneficial in preserving intact lung. This is especially important in patients who have extremely large volumes that must be treated, especially in the setting of atelectasis or pulmonary collapse.

It has been the experience in most studies that when adequate radiation portals are utilized, chest failures occur within the confines of the treated volume, suggesting insufficient dose rather than insufficient tumor coverage as the cause of failure. However, some interesting reports are emerging that contradict this point of view and suggest that chest failures outside the radiated portals are more common than previously appreciated. Mira and Livingston reported on 17 patients with limited-stage SCLC who were treated with combined modality therapy.[91] Seven of these patients had recurrent disease in the chest following thoracic irradiation, and five of these seven had their recurrence outside the radiation portal, presenting as peripheral lung masses or malignant pleural effusion. These authors then analyzed failure patterns in Southwest Oncology Group (SWOG) trials for extensive-stage SCLC.[92] With chemotherapy, the primary site was the most common site of relapse. The addition of chest radiotherapy caused failures to shift outside the radiated volume, toward the periphery of the lung. A possible explanation for this failure pattern stems from the fact that patients in these two studies were initially treated with chemotherapy. Subsequent radiation was applied to the tumor volume that was apparent *after* chemotherapeutic response had taken place. Therefore, radiation given to these reduced volumes may have missed some chemotherapy-resistant tumor cells and thus allowed these resistant cells to repopulate, producing a tumor recurrence outside the irradiated volume. On the basis of these data, virtually all trials now give radiation to the original volume of the tumor, regardless of the degree of chemotherapeutic response.

Holoye and colleagues describe 31 patients (14 limited-stage and 17 extensive-stage) who were irradiated following a complete response to chemotherapy.[54] A total of 3750 rads in 3 weeks was delivered to the primary site and mediastinum. The treatment portals encompassed the extent of disease prior to chemotherapeutic intervention. The spinal cord dose was maintained below 2750 rads, although the technique for doing this was not specified. In these 31 patients, 20 recurred in the chest. Only 5 patients recurred within the field of radiation, however, and 15 recurred outside the radiation field. Of nine patients who presented with a pleural effusion, seven subsequently failed in the pleura (78 percent).

It seems clear that not all chest failures following radiation represent inability of the radiation to sterilize tumor. Clearly, some of these failures represent microscopic extension of disease outside the irradiated volume. It is interesting that the San Antonio,[91] SWOG,[92] and Holoye[54] studies all administered the radiation following chemotherapy. This may further encourage the use of radiation therapy quite early in the treatment course of SCLC. Alternatively, if radiation is to be used after many months of chemotherapy, some of the treatment may have to be given to the entire pleural cavity.

Dose–Time Fractionation

In early trials of radiation therapy for the treatment of lung cancer, it was noted that SCLC was the most responsive of lung tumors and that complete disappearance of tumor occurred in over 50 percent of the patients.[110] It was generally believed that this rapid response and high complete response rate meant that SCLC could be controlled with relatively low doses of radiation, in the order of 2500–3000 rads conventionally fractionated. To some extent this concept was accurate in the prechemotherapy era. Median survival times were in the order of a few months and a modest dose of radiation would control the local tumor, during which time the patient would rapidly succumb to widespread systemic metastases. As chemotherapy became more effective in controlling or delaying the onset of distant disease, however, median survival times increased and local chest failure following radiation became quite common. In fact, local chest failure following radiation continues to be a major problem in the treatment of SCLC, with over 30 percent of irradiated patients experiencing a local chest failure in modern studies.

In an effort to determine whether local chest recurrence was a function of dose, several retrospective series have been published. Choi and Carey reported an 88 percent local control rate with 4800 rads to the chest, a 79 percent control rate with 4000 rads, but only a 60 percent control rate with 3000 rads.[22] The local control was evaluated at 4 months following treatment, however, and probably does not reflect what long-term local control would be following these doses of radiation. The Southwest Oncology Group noted a complete response rate of 32 percent in patients receiving 3000 rads of chest radiation versus a 57 percent complete recovery (CR) rate with 4500 rads.[129] These differences were statistically significant ($p = .029$), suggesting the value of higher dose.

Kreisman and colleagues pointed out that fewer chest failures were seen if 3000 rads were given in 10 fractionations versus 15 fractions, again suggesting the value of higher dose.[70] Catane et al.[18] and Cox and colleagues[26] both showed improved local control as radiation dose was increased.

The improved local control that may result from higher doses of thoracic irradiation must be balanced against the increased toxicity that such treatment may produce. To date, no study has been performed to specifically sort out the question of optimal dose of radiation in SCLC. While several reviews and international symposia have commented on the lack of such prospective information, Bergsagel and Feld[7] are probably correct in saying that such specific radiation questions as optimal dose will likely never be definitively answered. In order to study radiation dose, a trial would have to control for fractionation, timing, and sequencing of the radiation. The chemotherapy would have to be held constant, including maintenance therapy and intensity of chemotherapy. While one may then be able to arrive at an answer concerning ideal dose for that specific set of parameters, if any of the parameters are changed, a new dose study would need to be performed. Thus the concept of optimal dose radiation will likely never be completely resolved. It is the general practice in radiation oncology, however, to deliver a maximum dose to the tumor volume limited only by the tolerance of normal structures. For SCLC, normal tolerance usually is defined by esophagus or lung. In a previous NCI study, modest increases of radiation from 3000 to 4500 rads dramatically increased the rate of complications.[18] This effect occurred in the setting of concurrent chemotherapy. While the dose–complication curve is not nearly as steep when radiation and chemotherapy are given in a sequential fashion, the desire to give high doses of radiation must be tempered by the increased complications that result from such efforts.

One method to give higher doses of radiation without increasing complications might be through the use of superfractionated radiotherapy. Such an approach recently was reported by Hudson and colleagues.[53] They irradiated patients after one or two cycles of chemotherapy to a total dose of 5000 rads. However, the radiation was given in 100-rad fractions two or three times daily; 2000 rads were delivered to the mediastinum and primary along with the liver. The final 3000 rads were delivered to reduced fields in the chest. In total, 27 patients with limited-stage disease were treated. A 75 percent (20/27) rate of complete response was seen. While this represents no obvious improvement over other combined modality protocols, it remains to be seen whether this aggressive dose of radiation, which was well tolerated, produces better long-term local control, fewer chest failures, and less pulmonary toxicity.

Timing and Sequencing of Radiation with Chemotherapy

The issues surrounding the integration of radiation therapy into combined modality programs involving chemotherapy, and at times, surgery, are complex. Three major issues must be addressed: whether radiation should (1) be given concurrently with chemotherapy or sequentially following chemotherapy, (2) begin initially with the start of chemotherapy or be delayed for weeks or months, and (3) be delivered in a continuous fashion or be given as a split course.

The issues outlined above are largely unresolved at this point. Many studies have given chemotherapy concurrently with radiation. The NCI study described previously[57,74] employed concurrent treatment, and the current SWOG protocol has adopted that method of treatment as well.[122] In contrast, the trial previously reported from the SEG has used radiation after two cyles of drug.[100] Holoye et al. have used the radiation following the completion of all chemotherapy.[54] there has only been one trial that has attempted to address the question of timing of radiation. The Cancer and Acute Leukemia Group B (CALGB) treated limited-stage patients with either concurrent radiation and chemotherapy beginning on day 1 or concurrent radiation therapy beginning after two cycles of drug.[102] No differences were apparent in an early report of this trial.

A good case can be made to support either initial or sequential use of radiation. In support of delayed treatment, one may argue that the only patients likely to be cured of SCLC are those in whom all systemic micrometastases are eradicated through the use of chemotherapy. Such patients are most likely to be found within the subset of patients who have a complete response in the chest to chemotherapy. A patient who has only a partial response in the thorax is more likely to have only a partial response in areas of systemic micrometastases. Thus one could argue that radiation should be delayed until chemotherapy response has been determined. Patients who have had a complete response could then be aggressively irradiated, while those who have had less than a complete response could be watched until symptoms of chest disease require palliation.

Several arguments could be made against the above outlined philosophy. There is little question that the addition of radiation to chemotherapy as part of initial treatment produces a higher rate of complete response. It is from the subset of complete responders that all long-term survivors are found. To increase the percentage of initial complete responders may thus be the most important advantage of radiation. This argument derives further support from data of Looper and colleagues.[81] In studying patients who were treated with chemotherapy alone versus combined modality, they found that complete responders to either program had identical survival rates. The combined modality group had twice as many complete responders, however, and consequently had an overall survival advantage. It may also be argued that patients who achieve a rapid complete response in the thorax with the use of combined modality therapy have less tumor burden remaining and less chance to continually reseed sites of distant metastases with tumor cells that might be acquiring chemotherapy resistance as treatment continues. Finally, patients who have only a partial response to chemotherapy probably are not best served by observation but rather by immediate radiation. Most partial responders in the thorax will eventually progress in that area and will need local treatment. There is now a significant amount of information to suggest that partial responders may be "converted" to complete response status with the use of chest radiation and that this change in tumor status may lead to extended survival. White et al. showed that 38 percent of patients who are in partial response or stable disease following chemotherapy could be converted to complete response (CR) through the use of chest radiation.[129] Feld et al. showed that 11 percent of complete responders in a recently conducted trial achieved a CR only after their partial response to chemotherapy was irradiated.[38] Mira, reporting for the Southwest Oncology Group,[90] analyzed 133 patients who had less than a complete response to chemotherapy. In 35 percent (65 patients), response status was improved following thoracic irradiation. Surprising is the fact that patients who achieved a complete response following chest irradiation had a longer median survival than did those who achieved a CR after initial chemotherapy (97 vs 67 weeks, $p = .004$). It thus appears that patients who achieve a partial response to chemotherapy may benefit from immediate treatment with radiation. Some of those patients will become complete responders, and some of those patients may achieve long-term survival.

There has been no direct comparison of continuous versus split-course radiation in the treatment of SCLC. In general, continuous courses of high-dose radiation have proven advantageous in other types of lung cancer when compared to split-course treatment.[27] The NCI group as well as others have favored a continuous radiation course. However, issues of continuous versus split-course treatment become virtually inseparable from issues of concurrent versus sequential treatment and initial versus delayed treatment. Since a continuous course of radiation may take at least 3 and up to 6 weeks, it is difficult to rationalize stopping all chemotherapy to give a course of radiation during the middle of drug treatment. Thus one must irradiate concurrently with chemotherapy as has been done at the NCI[57,74] and is currently being performed by the Southwest Oncology Group[122] or one must delay radiation until chemotherapy has been completed as has been reported by the group at the Medical College of Wisconsin.[13,54]

Those groups wanting to give radiation sequentially with chemotherapy but not waiting until all chemotherapy has been delivered have been administering radiation in a split course. Short cycles of radiation can be delivered in between chemotherapy cycles. This technique has been used in studies from the Southeastern Cancer Study Group,[100] the CALGB,[86] and others. An interesting report on alternating radiation and chemotherapy comes from Arriagada and colleagues.[5] Much like the SEG, they administered three short courses of radiation interspersed between cycles of chemotherapy. They treated 28 patients with 4500 rads in three 1500-rad courses and then treated an additional 35 patients with 5500 rads, increasing the dose to 2000 rads in the first two cycles of radiation. With bronchoscopic confirmation, the CR rate exceeded 85 percent and relapse-free survival was approximately 35 percent at 2 years with acceptable toxicity.

In summary, the issues of timing and sequencing of radiation remain largely unresolved. The authors favor the administration of radiation early in the course of treatment. With early administration of radiation, the complete response rate is maximized and some patients who would have been partial responders to chemotherapy can be converted to CR status. Whether such early radiation, if given, should be in a continuous course concurrent with the chemotherapy or should be in a split course sequential with the chemotherapy cannot be definitely resolved at this time. According to current data, it is uncertain whether it is justified to simply observe patients who have achieved a partial response to chemotherapy alone, and such patients should receive consideration for chest radiotherapy.

The Use of CT Scans in Radiotherapy of SCLC

CT scanning is playing an important role in treatment planning in radiation therapy.[73,75] There is little question that the use of CT scans in SCLC can better stage the disease both inside and outside the thorax. A variety of studies have shown that adenopathy in the upper mediastinum and subcarinal area is better demonstrated by CT than by conventional radiographic techniques.[46,48,72]

Some interesting aspects concerning the staging of SCLC are coming to light with the use of CT. Holoye et al. investigated 55 patients with SCLC.[54] They were staged with conventional radiographic studies and also with CT scans of the chest and abdomen. Using conventional tests, 27 patients had limited disease and 23 patients had extensive disease. CT revealed 11 limited-stage patients, however, who actually had occult extensive-stage disease. Five patients had pleural or pericardial effusion, and six had intraabdominal metastases. If one looks at response rates, there was a 78 percent CR rate in the limited-disease group and a 35 percent CR rate in the extensive-disease group when conventional definitions were used. When the new "CT definition" of stage was employed and 11 patients were shifted from the limited to the extensive disease category, the response rates increased to 88 percent CR in the limited-disease patients and 44 percent CR in the extensive-disease patients. Information of this nature will lead to some difficult decisions regarding future clinical studies and reporting of results. By "stage shifting" the patients, one can make results look better then they would have been by use of standard radiographic techniques. It may be that in the future, papers will have to report their data as Holoye and colleagues have done, using both CT and non-CT definitions of stage of disease.

With CT data as a basis for treatment planning, SCLC should be approachable with more sophisticated treatment techniques than have heretofore been employed. In most clinical trials, simple AP-PA ports have been used to encompass the radiographic image on the chest x-ray and simulator film. Spinal cord shielding has been done with the use of a posterior cord block, which, at times, can shield mediastinal tumor. The shielding of mediastinal disease by a posterior cord block may have adverse consequences on the local control of lung cancer.[119] Eaton et al. analyzed local control in a CALGB small cell trial as a function of spinal cord shielding.[36] Of 56 limited-stage cases, the local failure rate was 37.5 percent in those cases where shielding reduced the dose to any portion of the mediastinum to less than 4200 rads, but only 13 percent where the dose was greater than 4200 rads ($p = .04$). With CT data, one can now gauge the location of tumors within the chest cavity with more accuracy. This should allow for the incorporation of oblique portals into the overall treatment plan. The spinal cord can then be shielded without the need to block potential sites of tumor, and normal uninvolved lung can be spared treatment that would be unnecessarily received if AP-PA ports are used exclusively. Furthermore, future directions in radiotherapy treatment planning will incorporate corrections for the reduced density of lung into the treatment plan. Since lung is only one-fifth as dense as soft tissue, it transmits more radiation than the equivalent thickness of soft tissue. Virtually all treatment planning in radiation therapy is performed while assuming unit density throughout the body. For most treatment sites such an assumption is not without validity; however, in the thorax it can lead to serious dosimetric inaccuracy. Several studies have been performed to underscore this point.[87,99,126] Radiotherapists will have to come to grips with their newly discovered ability to appreciate inhomogeneity difference between tissues, display these differences and their influence on treatment plans, and then take such dosimetric information into account when planning a course of radiation treatments to the thorax.

THE ROLE OF RADIATION THERAPY IN EXTENSIVE-STAGE SCLC

The role of radiotherapy in extensive-stage SCLC is considerably less defined than its role in limited-stage disease. A large retrospective literature review showed that response rates, median survival, and 2-year disease-free survival were identical in patients treated with combined modality therapy versus chemotherapy alone in extensive-stage disease.[11] Since the CR rate in extensive stage SCLC is still in the range of 20–30 percent, and since the cause of death in most extensive-disease patients is rapidly progressive systemic disease, it is not surprising that the addition of a local treatment modality would fail to have an impact on survival. Until better systemic therapy is found to control disseminated tumor, it is unlikely that any local modality will play a prominent role in extensive-stage patients. The CALGB has conducted a randomized study in extensive-stage disease comparing chemotherapy with or without thoracic irradiation. No differences were found in response rates or median survival between the groups.[21]

It should be recognized that local chest failure in extensive-stage SCLC remains a problem. In a recent SWOG analysis,[78] in half of the chemotherapy responders and two-thirds of the complete responders, initial relapse occurred in the chest. Initial relapse was confined exclusively to systemic sites in only 29 percent. These data contrast with earlier SWOG data where chest radiation was used and only 20 percent of patients had an initial chest failure.[92] These data would suggest that when better systemic therapy is developed, local thoracic irradiation might play an important role in extensive-stage disease.

One effort to increase the effectiveness of systemic therapy has been the attempt to irradiate all sites of metastatic disease in patients with extensive-stage SCLC. The first report of this "systemic" radiotherapy was performed at Stanford.[3] In this study, 12 patients were treated with chemotherapy and whole-brain irradiation while 13 patients received identical treatment along with radiation therapy directed to all sites of metastatic disease excluding bone marrow. Two to three cycles of chemotherapy were first administered, and then each site of extensive disease was irradiated, one at a time. As a result of this long sequence of radiation, the median interval between the start of radiation and the reinstitution of chemotherapy was 66 days. There was no difference in survival between the group receiving radiation or the group receiving chemotherapy alone. The small number of patients in this study and the long interval off chemotherapy, however, would make it almost impossible to detect a difference in this population of patients. The Working Party for the Therapy of Lung Cancer also conducted a randomized trial in extensive-disease patients (Protocol 7222).[130] In this trial, 70 patients were treated with chemotherapy alone while 48 patients were treated with chemotherapy plus radiation to the chest and abdomen. Overall response rate was greater for the combined modality group (55 vs 31 percent; $p = .05$), but there was no difference in median survival time or overall survival. The Southwest Oncology Group treated extensive-disease patients with five cycles of chemotherapy; 94 patients then went on to receive "consolidation" radiation therapy to the chest, brain, and liver.[79] Within this group of 94, 16 additional patients attained CR status and 7 obtained PR status following radiation. An additional 24 patients, however, progressed during radiation. Overall, 79 percent of the patients still relapsed in sites of previous disease, indicating that radiation was not effective in preventing relapse in extensive-disease patients.

The NCI also studied irradiation to all sites of known disease in extensive-stage SCLC.[58,59] In this study, 29 patients began treatment with chemotherapy and 10 met the eligibility criteria for irradiation as part of a "late intensification" program. To be eligible for late intensification treatment, patients had to have a CR or PR with a negative bone marrow examination and a performance status that allowed them to be ambulatory greater than 50 percent of the time. Of the 10 eligible patients, 2 refused the irradiation and 8 were treated. Therapy consisted of autologous marrow harvest, 2000 rads in five fractions over 5 days to all sites of initial tumor excluding bone marrow, high-dose VP16 and cyclophosphamide, followed by marrow reinfusion. No maintenance treatment was given. Five patients were treated following a PR to initial chemotherapy, and one of these patients achieved a CR. However, this patient relapsed after only 3 months. Two patients remained partial responders and quickly showed signs of progressive disease, and two patients died without achieving hematopoietic recovery. Three patients were treated while they were in complete response, and all three relapsed at 4, 9, and 15 months respectively after the conclusion of intensive therapy.

The role of radiotherapy in extensive-stage SCLC remains in doubt. While this therapy likely reduces the number of initial chest failures, the overall response rate, median survival, and long-term survival is not affected by this treatment because of the high rate of systemic relapse. Radiation to sites of extensive disease has yet to be proven effective. While further research is ongoing, outside the context of a clinical trial there is no rule for routine radiation therapy in the treatment of extensive-stage SCLC. Palliation of symptomatic sites and administration of prophylactic cranial irradiation are employed on a case-by-case basis.

PROPHYLACTIC CRANIAL IRRADIATION

With increases in the median survival of SCLC, brain metastases became an all too frequent occurrence. Nugent et al. showed that 10 percent of SCLC patients presented with detectable CNS disease but that up to 80 percent of surviving SCLC patients would develop brain metastasis by 2 years.[97] It was Hansen in 1973 who suggested that prophylactic cranial irradiation (PCI) may lead to a reduced incidence of CNS failure much as it did in childhood leukemia.[47] Over the past decade it has become clear that PCI indeed reduces the incidence of brain metastasis.[115] Table 23-6 reviews randomized trials testing the value of PCI. Overall CNS failures were reduced from 20 to 6 percent with PCI treatment. Additional nonrandomized studies confirm these figures.[4,69,107] The studies by Aroney et al.[4] and Rosen et al.[107] showed that no patient receiving PCI had an initial relapse from complete response in the brain. It must be emphasized, however, that while PCI can change the pattern of relapse in SCLC, it has not affected overall survival in any study reported to date. If better systemic therapy can control micrometastatic disease, PCI may become an important factor in the curability of SCLC.

There is some debate regarding which patients are candidates for PCI, when it should be given, and what the ideal dose should be. While some investigators have suggested that all patients should receive PCI from day 1 of therapy,[69] other investigators disagree. In an analysis of patients from the NCI,[107] prevention of brain relapse was achieved only in patients who had a complete response to therapy. Patients who were partial responders had a brain relapse rate that was similar regardless of whether they received PCI, suggesting that active systemic disease simply reseeds the brain if the patient survives long enough. The NCI has recommended that PCI be withheld for the first 6-12 weeks until a restaging is performed and response status ascertained. Only patients in CR at that point should be treated.

The tolerance of the whole brain to radiation is between 5000 and 6000 rads. Countless patients with primary brain tumors or brain metastases have received this dose with little toxicity. It has now become clear, however, that a much smaller dose of radiation when combined with chemotherapy may produce CNS changes that can be profound. The first indication that these changes were taking place stemmed from studies performed on children with acute leukemia who received cranial irradiation.

Table 23-6
Randomized Trials of PCI in Small Cell Lung Cancer

Number of patients	CNS Relapse Rate (%)		P Value	Reference
	PCI	PCI		
29	0	36	.02	2
54	0	16	.05	6
45	17	24	NSS*	29
111	8	13	NSS	51
29	0	27	.05	61
163	4	18	.009	85
229	5	20	.0008	115

*Not statistically significant.

Learning disabilities and personality changes were noted.[96,106] Currently, a large number of studies have documented neurologic impairment in long-term survivors of SCLC treated with PCI and chemotherapy.[19,30,71,80,113,128] In the NCI experience, CNS damage was seen in patients treated with high-dose chemotherapy alone,[80] and this has certainly been the case in patients treated for acute leukemia. Thus it is unclear as to how much of the neurologic dysfunction is attributable to PCI, how much to chemotherapy, and how much to a combination of the two treatments. Until this question is resolved, it is prudent to keep the dose of PCI down to the lowest level possible. At the NCI, 2400 rads was delivered in eight fractions over 2 weeks and appeared to be effective. In addition, study of patients remaining free of cancer for 2-10 years revealed that those patients receiving this cranial radiotherapy program during maintenance chemotherapy were much less likely to exhibit abnormal mental status examinations or abnormal neuropsychological test results than were patients given PCI in a schedule with a higher dose per fraction or during induction chemotherapy.[62] Other institutions have found 2500 rads in 10 fractions acceptable.[68] It is possible that even lower doses, would be safe although confirmation of this will entail additional study.

HEMIBODY OR WHOLE-BODY IRRADIATION IN THE TREATMENT OF SCLC

Following successful therapy of lymphoma with total body irradiation[20] and palliation of widespread metastatic disease with hemibody irradiation,[40] investigators began to use wide-field therapy in the treatment of SCLC, a radioresponsive tumor. Possibly the first reports of this type of therapy were due to Salazar et al.[109,111] In his original work, six patients with advanced SCLC were treated with sequential upper and lower hemibody treatment. There were five responses (1 CR; 4 PR) sufficiently encouraging to prompt a larger study. In the second report, 9 patients with extensive-stage SCLC who had achieved a PR with chemotherapy (cyclophosphamide and CCNU) were treated with 600 rads upper hemibody irradiation and 2000 rads local-field irradiation, followed by maintenance chemotherapy. Of these 9 partial responders, 5 became complete responders with the radiation. Two patients survived beyond 1 year, and there was no difficulty in resuming maintenance chemotherapy after the radiation.

This study was performed with low doses of chemotherapy, and the logical next step was to apply the same type of radiation with high-dose chemotherapy. Twelve patients were treated,[83] three of whom were complete responders with chemotherapy alone and an additional three who achieved complete response status following the radiation. Two nonresponders achieved a partial response following radiation. However, the combination of hemibody treatment plus aggressive chemotherapy was poorly tolerated. Only 2 of 12 patients could receive maintenance chemotherapy. In 7 patients relapse occurred in the chest, and median survival time was 9 months for the overall group and 12 months for the eight patients who had limited-stage disease. One patient died of radiation pneumonitis, and five patients required hospitalization following the hemibody treatment because of acute toxicity.

A more successful trial of hemibody treatment plus chemotherapy was reported by Powell and colleagues.[104] In this study, 24 limited-disease patients were treated with CAV chemotherapy plus local radiation. Following this, 600 rads was given sequentially to upper and lower hemibody ports. Of 23 evaluable patients with limited disease, 12 achieved a CR (52 percent) and eight achieved PR (35 percent), with an overall response rate of 87 percent. Median response duration was 9.9 months for all patients and 15.2 months for the complete responders. No radiation pneumonitis was noted, and esophageal complications as well as thrombocytopenia were manageable. This study shows that it may be possible to integrate hemibody irradiation into a program of conventional chemotherapy. The overall results of this limited experience, however, appear no better than those of other aggressive combined modality protocols without HBI.

Two groups have reported the treatment of SCLC using HBI without chemotherapy. Urtasun and colleagues treated 30 patients with 800 rads of upper and lower hemibody radiation plus 3500 rads to the local thoracic tumor.[125] Overall response rate was 87 percent, with a complete response rate of 47 percent. Response duration was disappointingly short for these patients, however, spanning only 117 days for all patients and 70 days for those with an extensive disease. Patients who relapsed had a great deal of difficulty tolerating chemotherapy. A concurrent randomized group was treated with standard combination chemotherapy plus local chest radiation. Response rates and overall survival were identical for the conventional treated group and the HBI group. Interestingly, 37 percent of patients (8/30) undergoing upper hemibody irradiation developed a CNS recurrence, indicating that a single dose of 800 rads was not sufficient to prevent CNS relapse. Hemibody irradiation (HBI) in this study was an active form of therapy with a very short response duration.

Results of Eichhorn et al.[37] are similar to those of Urtasun. In Eichhorn's study, 42 patients were treated with upper and lower HBI along with local chest radiation. The CR rate to this therapy is reported as 100 percent. Of 35 patients who underwent autopsy at time of death, however, only 12 showed no evidence of thoracic tumor and only 5 showed freedom from distant metastases. Toxicity became acceptable when the HBI technique was shifted from a lateral set of fields to opposed anterior-posterior, and when the 800-rad treatment was divided into a 600-rad treatment in the morning then a 200-rad treatment in the afternoon. In the group treated with the less toxic protocol, median survival was 14.3 months. As with the Urtasun study, HBI was seen to be an active modality in this trial. The poor rate of local chest control and the high rate of occult systemic disease, however, indicate that HBI alone is unlikely to be a curative modality in SCLC. Continued research efforts to determine how this therapy can be integrated into conventional chemotherapy protocols is warranted.

Low-dose fractionated total-body irradiation (TBI) has also been studied in SCLC. Three studies have been reported, two in which the TBI was used along with systemic chemotherapy[14,33] and one where it was used in conjunction with local chest irradiation.[105] When TBI was used with systemic chemotherapy, no additional responders were seen after TBI administration and there was no suggestion that TBI enhanced the results over what was obtained with the chemotherapy alone. In the study where TBI was used instead of chemotherapy, 30 patients were treated, 12 with extensive disease and 18 with limited disease. In the limited-disease group, 16 had a complete response with a median duration of response of nearly 12 months. However, 15 of the 16 complete responders relapsed. All 12 patients with extensive disease showed rapid disease progression. The study indicates that TBI may be able to delay systemic recurrence in limited-disease patients but probably is less effective than chemotherapy in preventing systemic relapse.

In general, there is no suggestion that TBI plays a role in the treatment of SCLC. In contrast, HBI appears to be an active agent, especially when combined with thoracic irradiation. When HBI is used as the sole systemic agent, however, response duration is short. This clearly indicates that HBI should be integrated with systemic chemotherapy for optimal results. Efforts directed toward achieving this integration such as fractionated hemibody irradiation, probably deserve study.

PALLIATIVE RADIOTHERAPY IN SCLC

Since the majority of patients with SCLC fail systematically, palliation of symptomatic deposits of tumor forms an important part of the treatment of patients with this disease. The principles of palliation of bone metastases and spinal cord-meningeal metastases are common to most tumor types and will not be discussed. There are two specific sites where palliation of SCLC has unique factors that separate it from other lesions: (1) brain metastases and (2) obstruction of the superior vena cava (SVC syndrome).

Brain metastases will be found on presentation in 10-15 percent of patients with SCLC,[97] will escalate to 25-30 percent during treatment if PCI is not employed (Table 23-6), and will be found in 40-60 percent of patients at autopsy.[52] Radiotherapy is employed to treat brain metastases in SCLC in three clinical situations: (1) brain metastases found at presentation, (2) brain metastases found during treatment or follow-up in the absence of previous PCI, or (3) brain metastases found following delivery of PCI.

When brain metastases are discovered at presentation, survival is dependent on whether the brain is the sole site of extensive disease or whether it is present with other sites of involvement. In an NCI review, 10 patients with brain as the only initial extensive site had a median survival of 10 months, in contrast to three months in 12 patients who had intracranial spread plus widespread disease.[31] Of these 22 patients, 9 achieved a complete response to 3000-4400 rads of radiation. All survivors eventually relapsed in the brain, however, suggesting the need for higher doses. At least 5000 rads in 5 weeks with consideration for a cone-down boost should be given to patients who present with brain metastases as the sole site of metastatic spread.

Brain metastases developing after presentation have a prognosis similar to those presenting with intracranial spread; about 10 months median survival if the brain is a sole site and 3 months if it is not.[31] Overall, responses to radiotherapy in patients with brain metastases occur in 50-70 percent of patients.[28,31] However, about 20 percent of patients with brain metastases will die before or during radiation treatment, and an additional 10-20 percent will die of causes directly related to CNS disease following radiation.[28,31,97] When there is a brain metastasis seen after PCI, we have palliated such cases with an additional 3000 rads in 3 weeks, which has been well tolerated and can provide short-term symptomatic improvement.

Obstruction of the superior vena cava can occur in 7-10 percent or more of patients with SCLC.[34,82,127] While most patients with SCLC do not have the acute-onset of life-threatening SVC,[114] symptoms such as edema, dyspnea when recumbent, and venous obstruction that can lead to thrombosis frequently are present[112] and require prompt treatment. In general, symptoms respond rapidly to either radiation or chemotherapy, and there is little reason to alter one's general treatment approach to

SCLC in the face of SVC syndrome.[34,82,127] When a patient relapses with SVC syndrome following treatment, radiation or reirradiation should be offered.

SUMMARY

SCLC is the most radioresponsive of all lung tumors. Because of the systemic nature of this disease, however, radiation must be combined with systemic chemotherapy to produce optimal effect. In limited-stage SCLC, combinations of radiation and chemotherapy appear to produce the best results with increased numbers of complete responders, increased permanent local control of the primary tumor, and probably modest gains in overall survival. Methods for integrating radiation and chemotherapy are numerous and varied. The three most common approaches include (1) a continuous course of radiation beginning on day 1 of chemotherapy, (2) a continuous course of radiation beginning after chemotherapy has concluded, and (3) split-course radiation with two or three short courses of treatment interdigitated between cycles of chemotherapy. It has not demonstrated that anyone of these methods is superior to another. Ideally, different approaches of integrating combined modality therapy should be tested prospectively in randomized trials.

Prophylactic cranial irradiation definitely reduces the frequency of brain metastases and appears to reduce dramatically the number of patients who manifest brain metastases as a first sole sign of relapse. The treatment is not free of toxicity, and the dose of PCI should be kept as low as possible. The authors recommend that PCI be delayed for 6-12 weeks until response status can be determined. At that time, only complete responders should receive the therapy as partial responders can simply reseed the brain following PCI. However, other institutions have successfully employed PCI as part of initial therapy in all patients. PCI has, to date, shown no influence on overall survival in any group of patients with SCLC.

Extensive-stage SCLC does not warrant the use of radiation therapy, except for the use of PCI in complete responders and palliative radiotherapy to symptomatic sites. Radiation in extensive-stage SCLC remains a subject for clinical investigation.

Hemibody irradiation has shown responses in both limited- and extensive-stage SCLC. When HBI is used as a sole modality of treatment, however, response duration frequently is short and relapse rates are high. Integration of HBI with systemic chemotherapy is possible and will be the subject of active clinical research protocols in the future.

REFERENCES

1. Aisner J, Alberto P, Bitran J, et al: Role of chemotherapy in small cell lung cancer: A consensus report of the International Association for the Study of Lung Cancer Workshop. Cancer Treat Rep 67:37-43, 1983
2. Aisner J, Whitacre M, Van Echo DA, et al: Combination chemotherapy for small cell carcinoma of the lung: Continuous vs alternating non-cross resistant combinations. Cancer Treat Rep 66:221-230, 1982
3. Alexander M, Glatstein, EJ, Gordon DS, et al: Combined modality treatment for oat cell carcinoma of the lung: A randomized trial. Cancer Treat Rep 6:1-6, 1977

4. Aroney RS, Aisner J, Wesley MN, et al: The value of prophylactic cranial irradiation given at complete remission in small cell lung cancer. Cancer Treat Rep 67:675-682, 1983

5. Arriagada R, Le Chevalier T, Baldeyrou P, et al: Alternating radiotherapy and chemotherapy schedules in small cell lung cancer, limited disease. Internatl J Radiat Oncol Biol Phys 11:1461-1467, 1985

6. Beiler DD, Kane RC, Bernath AM, et al: Low dose elective brain irradiation in small cell carcinoma of the lung. Internatl J Radiat Oncol Biol Phys 5:941-945, 1979

7. Bergsagel DE, Feld R: Small-Cell lung cancer is still a problem. J Clin Oncol 2:1189-1191, 1984

8. Bergsagel DE, Jenkin FDT, Pringle JD, et al: Lung cancer: clinical trial of radiotherapy alone vs radiotherapy plus cyclophosphamide. Cancer 30:621-627, 1972

9. Bleehen NM, Jones DH: The role of radiotherapy in the management of small cell bronchogenic carcinoma, in Recent Results in Cancer Research, Vol 97, Berlin, Springer-Verlag, 1985, pp 116-126

10. Brooks BJ Jr, Seifter EJ, Walsh TE, et al: Pulmonary toxicity with combined modality therapy for limited stage small cell lung cancer. J Clin Oncol 4:200-209, 1986

11. Bunn PA, Ihde DC: Small cell bronchogenic carcinoma: A review of therapeutic results, in Livingston RB (ed): Lung Cancer, Vol I, The Hague, Martinus Nijhoff, 1981, pp 169-208

12. Byhardt RW, Cox JD: Is chest radiotherapy necessary in any or all patients with small cell carcinoma of the lung? Yes. Cancer Treat Rep 67:209-215, 1983

13. Byhardt RW, Cox JD, Holye PY, et al: The role of consolidation irradiation in combined modality therapy of small cell carcinoma of the lung. Internatl J Radiat Oncol Biol Phys 8:1271-1276, 1982

14. Byhardt RW, Cox JD, Wilson JF, et al: Total body irradiation vs chemotherapy as a systemic adjuvant for small cell carcinoma of the lung. Internatl J Radiat Oncol Biol Phys 5:2043-2048, 1979

15. Carney DN, Minna JD: Small cell cancer of the lung. Clinics Chest Med 3:389-398, 1982

16. Carney DN, Mitchell JB, Kinsella TJ: In vitro radiation and chemotherapy sensitivity of established cell lines of human small cell lung cancer and its large cell morphological varients. Cancer Res 43:2806-2811, 1983

17. Carr DT, Childs DS, Lee RE: Radiotherapy plus 5-FU compared to radiotherapy alone for inoperable and unresectable bronchogenic carcinoma. Cancer 29:375-380, 1972

18. Catane R, Lichter A, Lee YJ, et al: Small cell lung cancer: Analysis of treatment factors contributing to prolonged survival. Cancer 48:1936-1943, 1981

19. Catane R, Schwade JG, Yarr I, et. al.: Follow-up neurological evaluation in patients with small cell lung carcinoma treated with prophylactic cranial irradiation and chemotherapy. Internatl. J Radiat. Oncol 7:105-109, 1981

20. Chaffey, J.T., Rosenthal, D.S., Molong, W.C., Het al: Total body irradiation as treatment for lymphosarcoma. Internatl. J Radiat. Oncol Biol Phys 1:399-406, 1976

21. Chahinian AP, Comis RL, Maurer LH, et al: Small cell anaplastic carcinoma of the lung: The Cancer and Leukemia Group B experience. Bull Cancer (Paris) 69:79-82, 1982

22. Choi CH, Carey RW: Small cell anaplastic carcinoma of lung: Reappraisal of current management. Cancer 37:2651-2657, 1976

23. Cohen MH: Is thoracic radiation necessary for patients with limited-stage small cell lung cancer? No. Cancer Treat Rep 67:217-221, 1983

24. Cohen MH: Treatment of small cell lung cancer: progress, potential and problems. Internatl J Radiat Oncol Biol Phys 6:1079-1082, 1980

25. Comis RL: Small cell carcinoma of the lung. Cancer Treat Rev 9:237-258, 1982

26. Cox JD, Byhardt RW, Wilson JF: Dose-time relationship and the local control of small cell carcinoma of the lung. Radiology 128:205-207, 1978

27. Cox JD, Eisert DR, Komaki R, et al: Patterns of failure following treatment of apparently localized carcinoma of the lung, in Muggia F, Rozencweig M, (eds): Lung Cancer: Progress in Therapeutic Research. New York, Raven Press, 1979, pp 279-288

28. Cox JD, Komaki R, Byhardt RW, et al: Results of whole-brain irradiation for metastases from small cell carcinoma of the lung. Cancer Treat Rep 64:957-961, 1980

29. Cox JD, Petrovich Z, Paig C, et al: Prophylactic cranial irradiation in patients with inoperable carcinoma of the lung. Cancer 42:1135-1140, 1978

30. Craig J, Jackson D, Moody D: Prospective evaluation of changes in computerized cranial tomography in patients with small cell carcinoma treated with chemotherapy and cranial irradiation (Abstr). Proc Am Soc Clin Oncol 3:224, 1984

31. Crane J, Lichter A, Ihde D, et al: Therapeutic cranial radiotherapy (RT) for brain metastases in small cell lung cancer (SCLC) (Abstr). Proc Am Assoc Cancer Res 24:145, 1983

32. deVita VT, Lippman M, Hubbard SM, et al: The effect of combined modality therapy on local control and survival. Internatl J Radiat Oncol Biol Phys, in press

33. Dillman RO, Seagren SL, Taetle R: Failure of low-dose, total-body irradiation to augment combination chemotherapy in extensive-stage small cell carcinoma of the lung. J Clin Oncol 4:242-246, 1983

34. Dombernowsky P, Hansen HH: Combination chemotherapy in the management of superior vena caval obstruction in small-cell anaplastic carcinoma of the lung. Acta Med Scand 204:513-516, 1978

35. Dombernowski P, Hansen HH, Hansen M, et al: Treatment of small cell anaplastic bronchogenic carcinoma: Results from 2 randomized trials (Abstr). II World Conference on Lung Cancer, Copenhagen. Amsterdam; Excerpta Medica, 1980, p 149

36. Eaton WL, Maurer H, Glicksman A, et al: The relationship of infield recurrences to prescribed tumor dose in small cell carcinoma of the lung (Abstr). Internatl J Radiat Oncol Biol Phys 7:1223, 1981

37. Eichhorn HJ, Huttner J, Dalluge KH, et al: Preliminary report on "one-time" and high dose irradiation of the upper and lower half-body in patients with small cell lung cancer. Internatl J Radiat Oncol Biol Phys 9:1459-1465, 1983

38. Feld R, Evans WK, DeBoer G, et al: Combined modality induction therapy without maintenance chemotherapy for small cell carcinoma of the lung. J Clin Oncol 2:294-304, 1984

39. Feld R: Complications in the treatment of small cell carcinoma of the lung. J. Clin Oncol 2:294-304, 1984

40. Fitzpatrick PJ, Rider WD: Half-body radiotherapy. Internatl J Radiat Oncol Biol Phys 1:197-207, 1976

41. Fox W, Scadding JG: Medical Research Council comparative trial of surgery and radiotherapy for primary treatment of small-celled or oat-celled carcinoma of bronchus. Ten-year follow up. Lancet 2:63-65, 1973

42. Fox FM, Tattersall MHN, Woods RL: Radiation therapy as an adjuvant in small cell lung cancer treated by combination chemotherapy: A randomized study (Abstr). Proc Am Soc Clin Oncol 22:502, 1981

43. Glatstein E, Makuch RW: Illusion and reality: Practical pitfalls in interpreting clinical trials. J Clin Oncol 2:488-497, 1984

44. Goodman GE, Miller TP, Manning MM, et al: Treatment of small cell lung cancer with VP-16, vincristine, doxorubicin, cyclophosphamide (EVAC) and high-dose chest radiotherapy. J Clin Oncol 8:483-488, 1983

45. Green RA, Humphrey E, Close H, Patno ME: Alkylating agents in bronchogenic carcinoma. Am J Med 46:516-525, 1969

46. Griffin CA, Lu C, Fishman EK, et al: The role of computed tomography of the chest in the management of small-cell lung cancer. J Clin Oncol 2:1359-1365, 1984

47. Hansen HH: Should initial treatment of small cell carcinoma include systemic chemo-
     therapy and brain irradiation? Cancer Chemother Rep 4:239-241, 1973
48. Harper PG, Houang M, Spiro SG, et al: Computerized axial tomography in the pretreat-
     ment assessment of small cell carcinoma of the bronchus. Cancer 47:1775-1780, 1981
49. Harper PG, Souhami RL, Spiro SG, et al: Chemotherapy with and without radiotherapy
     in small cell carcinoma of the lung (SCCL) (Abstr). Proc Am Assoc Cancer Res 24:151,
     1983
50. Higgins GA Jr: Use of chemotherapy as an adjuvant to surgery for bronchogenic carci-
     noma. Cancer 30:1383-1387, 1972
51. Hirsch FR, Hansen HH, Paulson OB, et al: Development of brain metastases in small
     cell anaplastic carcinoma of the lung, in Kay J, Whitehouse J (eds): CNS Complications
     of Malignant Disease. New York, Macmillan, 1979, pp 175-184
52. Hirsch FR, Paulson OB, Hansen HH, et al: Intracranial metastases in small cell carci-
     noma of the lung: Correlation of clinical and autopsy findings. Cancer 50:2433-2437,
     1982
53. Hudson DI, Malaker K, Meikle AL, et al: Pilot studies of superfractionated radiotherapy
     and combination chemotherapy in limited oat cell carcinoma of the bronchus. Internatl J
     Radiat Oncol Biol Phys 10:1941-1945, 1984
54. Holoye PY, Libnoch JA, Anderson T, et al: Combined methotrexate and high-dose
     vincristine chemotherapy with radiation therapy for small cell bronchogenic carcinoma.
     Cancer 55:1436-1445, 1985
55. Host H: Cyclophosphamide (NSC-26271) as adjuvant to radiotherapy in the treatment
     of unresectable bronchogenic carcinoma. Cancer Chemother Rep Part 3, 4:161-164,
     1973
56. Ihde DC, Bilek FS, Cohen MH, et al: Response to thoracic radiotherapy in patients with
     small cell carcinoma of lung after failure of combination chemotherapy. Radiology
     132:443-446, 1979
57. Ihde DC, Bunn PA, Lichter AS, et al: Randomized trial of chemotherapy with or without
     adjuvant chest irradiation in limited stage small cell lung cancer, in Jones SE, Salmon SE
     (eds): Adjuvant Therapy of Cancer, Vol IV. Orlando, FL, Grune & Stratton, 1984, p
     147
58. Ihde DC, Deisseroth AB, Lichter AS, et al: Late intensive combined modality therapy
     followed by autologous bone marrow infusion in extensive stage small cell lung cancer.
     J Clin Oncol 4:1443-1454, 1986
59. Ihde DC, Lichter AS, Deisseroth AB, et al: Late intensive combined modality therapy
     with autologous bone marrow infusion in extensive stage small cell lung cancer, in Spitzy
     KH, Karrer K (eds): Proceedings of the 13th International Congress of Chemotherapy.
     Vienna, Verlang H Egermann, 1983, pp 281-288
60. Ihde DC, Makuch RW, Carney DN, et al: Prognostic implications of stage of disease and
     sites of metastases in patients with small cell carcinoma of the lung treated with intensive
     chemotherapy. Am Rev Resp Dis 123:500-507, 1981
61. Jackson DV, Richards F, Cooper MR, et al: Prophylactic cranial irradiation in small cell
     carcinoma of the lung. A randomized study. JAMA 237:2730-2733, 1977
62. Johnson BE, Becker B, Goff WB, et al: Neurologic, neuropsychologic, and computed
     cranial tomography scan abnormalities in 2- to 10-year survivors of small cell lung
     cancer. J Clin Oncol 3:1659-1667, 1985
63. Johnson BE, Ihde DC, Bunn PA, et al: Small-cell lung cancer patients treated with
     combination chemotherapy with or without irradiation: Data on potential cures, chronic
     toxicities and late relapses from a five to eleven year follow-up. Ann Intern Med
     103:430-438, 1985
64. Johnson RE, Brereton HD, Kent CH: "Total" therapy for small cell carcinoma of the
     lung. Ann Thorac Surg 25:510-515, 1978

65. Johnson RE, Brereton HD, Kent CH: Small cell carcinoma of the lung: Attempt to remedy causes of past therapeutic failure. Lancet 2:289-291, 1976

66. Kemeny MM, Block LR, Braun DW, et al: Results of surgical treatment of carcinoma of the lung by stage and cell type. Surg Gynecol Obstet 147:865-871, 1978

67. Kent CH, Brereton HD, Johnson RE: "Total" therapy for oat cell carcinoma of the lung. Internatl J Radiat Oncol Biol Phys 2:427-432, 1977

68. Komaki R, Byhardt RW, Anderson T, et al: What is the lowest effective biologic dose for prophylactic cranial irradiation? Am J Clin Oncol (CCT) 8:523-527, 1985

69. Komaki R, Cox JD, Holoye PY, et al: Changes in the relative risk and sites of central nervous system metastasis with effective combined chemotherapy and radiation therapy for small cell carcinoma of the lung. Am J Clin Oncol 6:515-521, 1983

70. Kreisman H, Wolkove N, Cohen C, et al: Multifocal relapse after concurrent chemotherapy and radiotherapy of small cell lung cancer. Cancer 50:873-876, 1982

71. Lee JS, Lee YY, Umsawasdi T, et al: Neurotoxicity in long-term survivors of small cell lung cancer (Abstr). Proc Am Soc Clin Oncol 3:220, 1984

72. Lewis E, Bernardino ME, Valdivieso M, et al: Computed tomography and routine chest radiography in oat cell carcinoma of the lung. J Comput Assist Tomogr 6:739-745, 1982

73. Lichter AS: The application of computerized tomography in radiation treatment planning, in Phillips TL, Pistenmaa DA (eds): Radiation Oncology Annual. New York, Raven Press, 1983, pp. 179-204

74. Lichter AS, Bunn PA, Jr, et al: The role of radiation therapy in the treatment of small cell lung cancer. Cancer 55:2163-2175, 1985

75. Lichter AS, Fraass BA, Fredrickson HA, et al: An overview of clinical requirements and clinical utility of CT based radiotherapy treatment planning, in Ling CC, Rogers CC, Morton RJ (eds): Computed Tomography in Radiation Therapy. New York, Raven Press, 1983, pp. 1-22

76. Little CD, Nau MM, Carney DN, et al: Amplification and expression of the c-myc oncogene in human lung cancer cell lines. Nature 306:194-196, 1983

77. Livingston RB: Small cell carcinoma of the lung. Blood 56:575-584, 1980

78. Livingston RB, Mira JG, Chem TT, et al: Combined modality treatment of extensive small cell lung cancer: A Southwest Oncology Group study. J. Clin Oncol 2:585-590, 1984

79. Livingston R, Schulman S: Radiation therapy to multiple sites as consolidation for extensive small cell lung cancer (Abstr). Proc Am Soc Clin Oncol 4:179, 1985

80. Looper JD, Einhorn LH, Garcia SA, et al: Severe neurologic problems following successful therapy for small cell lung cancer (SCLC) (Abstr). Proc Am Soc Clin Oncol 3:231, 1984

81. Looper JD, Hornback NB: The role of chest irradiation in limited small cell carcinoma of the lung treated with combination chemotherapy. Internatl J Radiat Oncol Biol Phys 10:1885-1860, 1984

82. Maddox A, Valdivieso M, Lukeman J, et al: Superior vena cava obstruction in small cell bronchogenic carcinoma: Clinical parameters and survival. Cancer 52:2165-2172, 1983

83. Mason BA, Richter MP, Catalano RB, et al: Upper hemibody and local chest irradiation as consolidation following response to high-dose induction chemotherapy for small cell bronchogenic carcinoma: A pilot study. Cancer Treat Rep 8:1609-1612, 1982

84. Matthiessen W: Controlled clinical trial of radiotherapy alone, against radiotherapy plus chemotherapy in small-cell carcinoma of the lung: Comparison of radiation damage (preliminary results). Scand J Resp Dis (Suppl) 102:209-211, 1978

85. Maurer LH, Tulloh M, Weiss RB, et al: A randomized combined modality trial in small cell carcinoma of the lung: Comparison of combination chemotherapy-radiation therapy

versus cyclophosphamide-radiation therapy, effects of maintenance chemotherapy and prophylactic whole brain irradiation. Cancer 45:30-39, 1980

86. Maurer LH, Pajak T, Eaton W, et al: Combined modality therapy with radiotherapy, chemotherapy, and immunotherapy in limited small-cell carcinoma of the lung: A phase III cancer and leukemia group B study. J Clin Oncol 3:969-976, 1985

87. McKenna WG, Yeakel K, Klink A, et al: Lung density correction in radiotherapy treatment planning: Effects seen in a group of patients with cancer of the esophagus. Internatl J Radiat Oncol Biol Phys 13:273-278, 1987

88. Medical Research Council Lung Cancer Working Party: Radiotherapy alone or with chemotherapy in the treatment of small-cell carcinoma of the lung. Br J Cancer 40:1-10, 1979

89. Miller AB, Fox W, Tall R: Five-year follow-up of the Medical Research Council comparative trial of surgery and radiotherapy for the primary treatment of small-celled or oat-celled carcinoma of the bronchus. Lancet 2:501-505, 1969

90. Mira JG, Kies MS, Chen T: Influence of chest radiotherapy in response, remission duration, and survival in chemotherapy responders in localized small cell lung carcinoma: A Southwest Oncology Group Study (Abstr). Proc Am Soc Clin Oncol 3:312, 1984

91. Mira JG, Livingston RB: Evaluation and radiotherapy implications of chest relapse patterns in small cell lung carcinoma treated with radiotherapy-chemotherapy. Cancer 46:2557-2565, 1980

92. Mira JG, Livingston RB, Moore TN, et al: Influence of chest radiotherapy in frequency and patterns of chest relapse in disseminated small cell lung carcinoma: A Southwest Oncology Group Study. Cancer 50:1266-1272, 1982

93. Moore TN, Livingston R, Heilbrun L, et al: An acceptable rate of complications in combined doxorubicin-irradiation for small cell carcinoma of the lung: A Southwest Oncology Group Study. Internatl J Radiat Oncol Biol Phys 4:675-680, 1978

94. Morstyn G, Ihde DC, Lichter AS, et al: Small cell lung cancer 1973-1983: Early progress and recent obstacles. Internatl J Radiat Oncol Biol Phys 10:515-539, 1984

95. Morstyn G, Russo A, Carney DN, et al: Heterogeneity in the radiation survival curves and biochemical properties of human lung cancer cell lines. J Natl Cancer Inst 73:801-807, 1984

96. Moss HA, Nannis ED, Poplack DG: The effects of prophylactic treatment of the central nervous system on the intellectual functioning of children with acute lymphoblastic leukemia. Am J Med 71:47-52, 1981

97. Nugent JL, Bunn PA Jr, Matthews MJ, et al: CNS metastases in small cell bronchogenic carcinoma: Increasing frequency and changing pattern with lengthening survival. Cancer 44:1885-1893, 1979

98. Ochs JJ, Tester WJ, Cohen MH, et al: "Salvage" radiation therapy for intrathoracic small cell carcinoma of the lung progressing on combination chemotherapy. Cancer Treat Rep 67:1123-1126, 1983

99. Orton CG, Mondalek PM, Spika JT, et al: Lung corrections in photon beam treatment planning: Are we ready? Internatl J Radiat Oncol Biol Phys 10:2191-2199, 1984

100. Perez CA, Einhorn L, Oldham RK, et al: Randomized trial of radiotherapy to the thorax in limited small-cell carcinoma of the lung treated with multiagent chemotherapy and elective brain irradiation: A preliminary report. J Clin Oncol 2:1200-1208, 1984

101. Perez CA, Krauss S, Bartolucci AA, et al: Thoracic and elective brain irradiation with concomitant or delayed multiagent chemotherapy in the treatment of localized small cell carcinoma of the lung. Cancer 47:2407-2413, 1981

102. Perry MC, Eaton WL, Ware J, et al: CHemotherapy with or without radiation therapy in limited small cell cancer of the lung (Abstr). Proc Am Soc Clin Oncol 3:230, 1984

103. Petrovich Z, Mietlowski W, Ohanion M, et al: Clinical report on the treatment of locally advanced lung cancer. Cancer 40:72-77, 1977

104. Powell B, Jackson D, Scarantino C, et al: Sequential hemibody radiation integrated into a conventional chemotherapy-local radiotherapy program for limited disease small cell lung cancer (Abstr). Proc Am Soc Clin Oncol 4:193, 1985

105. Qasim MM: Total body irradiation in oat cell carcinoma of the bronchus. Clin Radiol 32:37-39, 1981

106. Robinson LL, Nesbit ME, Jr, Sather HN, et al: Factors associated with IQ scores in long-term survivors of childhood acute lymphoblastic leukemia. Am J Ped Heme Oncol 6:115-120, 1984

107. Rosen ST, Makuch RW, Lichter AS, et al: Role of prophylactic cranial irradiation in prevention of central nervous system metastases in small cell lung cancer: Potential benefit restricted to patients in complete response. Am J Med 74:615-624, 1983

108. Salazar OM, Creech RH: The state of the art: Towards defining the role of radiation therapy in the management of small cell bronchogenic carcinoma. Internatl J Radiat Oncol Biol Phys 6:1103-1117, 1980

109. Salazar OM, Creech RH, Rubin P, et al: Half-body and local chest irradiation as consolidation following response to standard induction chemotherapy for disseminated small cell lung cancer. Internatl J Radiat Oncol Biol Phys 6:1093-1102, 1980

110. Salazar OM, Rubin P, Brown JC, et al: The assessment of tumor response to irradiation of lung cancer: Continuous versus split-course regimes. Internatl J Radiat Oncol Biol Phys 1:1107-1118, 1976

111. Salazar OM, Rubin P, Keller BE, et al: Systemic (half-body) radiation therapy. Internatl J Radiat Oncol Biol Phys 4:937-950, 1978

112. Scarantino C, Salazar OM, Rubin P, et al: The optimum radiation schedule in treatment of superior vena caval obstruction: Importance of Tc scintiangiograms. Internatl J Radiat Oncol Biol Phys 5:1987-1995, 1979

113. Scher H, Hilaris B, Wittes R: Long-term follow-up of combined modality therapy in small cell carcinoma of the lung (Abstr). Proc Am Soc Clin Oncol 2:199, 1983

114. Schraufnagel DE, Hill R, Leech JA, et al: Superior vena caval obstruction. Is it a medical emergency? Am J Med 70:1169-1174, 1981

115. Seydel HG, Creech RH, Pagano M, et al: Prophylactic versus no brain irradiation in regional small cell lung carcinoma. Am J Clin Oncol 8:218-223, 1985

116. Seydel HG, Creech RH, Pagano M, et al: Combined modality treatment of regional small cell undifferentiated carcinoma of the lung: A cooperative study of the RTOG and ECOG. Internatl J Radiat Oncol Biol Phys 9:1135-1141, 1983

117. Seydel HG, Creech R, Pagano M, et al: Combined modality treatment of small cell undifferentiated carcinoma of the lung: A cooperative study of the RTOG and the ECOG. Internatl J Radiat Oncol Biol Phys 7:41, 1981

118. Shepherd FA, Ginsberg R, Evans WK, et al: "Very limited" small cell lung cancer—results of nonsurgical treatment (Abstr). Proc Am Soc Clin Oncol 3:223, 1984

119. Sherman DM, Weichselbaum R, Hellman S: The characteristics of long-term survivors of lung cancer treated with radiation. Cancer 47:2575-2580, 1981

120. Shields TW, Higgins GA, Matthews MJ, et al: Surgical resection in the management of small cell carcinoma of the lung. J Thorac Cardiovasc Surg 84:481-488, 1982

121. Smyth JF, Hansen HH: Perspectives and commentaries: Current status of research into small cell carcinoma of the lung: Summary of the second workshop of the International Association for the Study of Lung Cancer (IASLC). Eur J Cancer Clin Oncol 21:1295-1298, 1985

122. Southwest Oncology Group Protocol No. 8269

123. Stevens E, Einhorn L, Rohn R: Treatment of limited small cell lung cancer (Abstr). Proc Am Soc Clin Oncol 20:435, 1979

124. Trask CW, Joannides T, Harper PG, et al: Radiation-induced lung fibrosis after treatment of small cell carcinoma of the lung with very high-dose cyclophosphamide. Cancer 55:57-60, 1985

125. Urtasun RC, Belch AR, McKinnon S, et al: Small-cell lung cancer: Initial treatment with sequential hemi-body irradiation vs 3-drug systemic chemotherapy. Br J Cancer 46:228-235, 1985

126. Van Dyk J, Keane TJ, Rider WD: Lung density as measured by computerized tomography: Implications for radiotherapy. Internatl J Radiat Oncol Biol Phys 8:1363-1372, 1982

127. Van Houtte P, DeJager R, Lustman-Marechal J, et al: prognostic value of the superior vena cava syndrome as the presenting sign of small cell anaplastic carcinoma of the lung. Cancer 16:1447-1450, 1980

128. Walker RW, Lazar RM, Gralla RJ, et al: Neuropsychological abnormalities in long-term survivors of small cell lung cancer receiving prophylactic cranial irradiation. Proc Am Soc Clin Oncol 4:187, 1985

129. White, JE, Chen T, McCracken J, et al: The influence of radiation therapy quality control on survival, response, and sites of relapse in oat cell carcinoma of the lung. Cancer 50:1084-1090, 1982

130. Wilson HE, Stanley K, Vincent RG: Comparison of chemotherapy alone versus chemotherapy and radiation therapy of extensive small cell carcinoma of the lung. J Surg Oncol 23:181-184, 1983

131. Wittes, RE, Natale RB, Sierocki JS, et al: Treatment of patients with small cell lung cancer at the Memorial Sloan Kettering Cancer Center, 1974-1979. World J Surg 5:689-694, 1981

Philip C. Hoffman

24

The Role of Surgical Resection in Management of Small Cell Carcinoma of the Lung

Small cell lung cancer (SCLC) characteristically is advanced, that is, stage III, at the time of diagnosis. Early dissemination is the rule. In the past 10 years at The University of Chicago we have treated 240 patients with stage III SCLC, 72 with stage III M_0 disease, and 168 with stage III M_1 disease.[19] During the same period we treated five patients with stage I and three patients with stage II disease. Patients thus classified as stage I and II represent only 3 percent of the total group treated. In a postmortem study of patients who died within 30 days after undergoing a "curative" lung cancer resection, Matthews and her colleagues found that 13 out of 19 (70 percent) patients with small cell carcinoma had residual cancer, almost all of whom had distant metastases.[28] Early dissemination was noted, therefore, even in the highly selected group of patients with small cell carcinoma who were even candidates for surgical resection.

Fortunately, small cell carcinoma is typically sensitive to a variety of chemotherapy drugs, and there is little disagreement among physicians who treat lung cancer that combination chemotherapy is the mainstay of treatment for this disease.[15,18] Chemotherapy has a high response rate, and median survival is predictably and significantly prolonged, especially in patients with stage III M_0 disease. Other modalities of therapy—namely, radiotherapy and surgery—are considered adjuvant. In patients with stage III M_0 disease, there is widespread use of radiation therapy to the primary tumor and mediastinum in hopes of reducing the rate of local recurrence. While this is often successful, there is controversy regarding the impact that chest radiotherapy has had on median survival.[2,4] Less controversial is the role of cranial radiation in reducing brain relapses in patients with limited disease, especially those who achieve a complete remission with chemotherapy.[37] The subject of greatest controversy, perhaps, concerns the role of surgical resection of the primary tumor, usually as part of the multimodality approach to small cell carcinoma.

This chapter will review the historical results of surgical resection in small cell carcinoma, the rationale for the resurgence of enthusiasm for surgery in recent years, and the results of recent studies that have examined the value of surgery in conjunction with chemotherapy.

HISTORICAL RESULTS OF SURGERY IN SMALL CELL LUNG CANCER

The results of historical series of surgical resection in patients with small cell cancer are quite variable. Some studies suggested a favorable outcome. Lennox et al. found a 58 percent resection rate among 275 patients with small cell cancer taken to thoracotomy and a projected 5-year survival of 10.6 percent.[22] Similarly, Taylor et al. noted a 13 percent 5-year survival among 85 patients resected.[44] Siddons reported a 34 percent 5-year survival in 38 patients.[42] Shore and Paneth reported on 63 patients undergoing thoracotomy, of whom 40 had resection; 10 (25 percent) survived for more than 5 years, including two patients who had mediastinal lymph node involvement.[41] Freise et al. reported a 5-year survival rate of 12 percent for 34 resected patients; patients with peripheral lesions who could undergo lobectomy had a 38 percent 5-year survival.[10]

By contrast, many older studies found very poor rates of resectability and survival in small cell lung cancer. Kirklin et al. noted only a 12 percent resectability rate in 121 patients and only one patient surviving five years.[21] Watson and Berg found 7 percent of patients resectable, with 2 patients of 27 (7 percent) alive 5 years, although 9 patients survived for at least 2 years.[47] Vincent et al. noted a median survival of 5.5 months for 16 patients undergoing resection and no 5-year survivors.[46] Similarly, Ashor et al. found no survivors beyond three years in 21 patients resected.[1]

One of the largest series of patients was that studied in the British Medical Research Council's trial comparing surgery with radiotherapy as the primary therapy for "operable" SCLC.[9] The 73 patients in the radiotherapy group had a median survival that was statistically significantly better than that of the surgery group, 300 versus 199 days. At 2 years, 4 percent of the surgery group was still alive, compared to 11 percent of the radiotherapy group, and the only 5-year survivors had received radiotherapy (including one patient in the surgery group who did not, in fact, undergo surgery, receiving radiotherapy instead). In the same year, Mountain reported that the median survival of 41 resected patients with small cell cancer was identical to that of 146 nonresected patients (5 months).[33] The Medical Research Council report and Mountain's report effectively dampened much of the enthusiasm for surgery in this disease. Mountain concluded that SCLC was essentially a nonsurgical disease, although left open the possibility that surgical cytoreduction, in combination with other treatment modalities, might be worthy of study.

It should be emphasized that the historical studies of surgical resection in small cell carcinoma were in patients selected as being operative candidates. Although the number of such candidates may have been somewhat higher than it would be now because of less rigorous staging evaluation in the past, the resected patients still probably represented a minority of those with this disease, since so many have obvious metastatic or extensive local (i.e., inoperable) disease at presentation. A few older studies examined the role of surgery in patients more precisely evaluated in terms of tumor, node, metastases (TNM) staging, or at least presumed staging. Higgins et al. reviewed the 10-year follow-up of 1134 patients with solitary pulmonary nodules.[14] In this group, 15 patients underwent resection with small cell carcinoma, of whom 11 had no nodal involvement and therefore had a "curative" resection. The 5-year survival of these patients was 36 percent. Mayer et al. noted seven 5-year survivors among 45 resected patients, six of whom had either T_1N_0 or T_2N_0 staging, and one had T_2N_1 disease.[29] The six survivors with negative lymph nodes represented 25 percent of patients with N_0 disease, while the one survivor with N_1 disease represented 8 percent of the patients with T_1N_1 or T_2N_1 disease. None of the nine patients with stage III disease (T_3N_0—1 patient, T_3N_1—2 patients, T_2N_2—6 patients) survived. Li et al. reported that of six patients resected, three with T_1N_0 disease were still alive at 7, 16, and 67 months, while two with T_1N_1 disease died at 13 and 43 months, and one with T_1N_2 disease died at 11 months.[24] The largest historical study with clear staging was the review by Shields et al. of the various Veterans Administration Surgical Oncology Group studies of surgery in small cell carcinoma.[40] In 132 patients surviving the postoperative period, the 5-year survival rates were as follows: T_1N_0, 60 percent, T_1N_1, 31 percent, T_2N_0, 28 percent, T_2N_1, 9 percent, T_3 or N_2, 4 percent. Two-thirds of the 5-year survivors had no lymph node involvement, and only one survivor had an involved mediastinal node. Many of the patients received postoperative chemotherapy according to the active trial at the time, and there was a suggestion of benefit, albeit not statistically significant, for prolonged cyclic chemotherapy as then used. They concluded that surgical resection was definitely indicated in T_1N_0 lesions and probably indicated in T_2N_0 and T_1N_1 lesions, but not in those with more advanced staging criteria.

RATIONALE FOR SURGICAL RESECTION AND RESULTS OF RECENT STUDIES

In the past several years, with the advent of more effective chemotherapy for SCLC, there has been some renewal of interest in the role of surgery in the management of these patients. Interest is focused in particular on the one-third of patients with disease localized in the hemithorax. Such patients commonly have complete response rates to chemotherapy of 60–80 percent.[15,34] Clearly, most of these patients relapse, since the long-term remission rate generally is less than 20 percent. In a number of series of such patients, the relapse rate at the primary site in the chest is in the range of 50–75 percent.[13,20,23,25,27] A significant number of these relapses are in the thorax exclusively, or at least initially. Thus it is theorized that if the primary tumor could be eliminated as a site of relapse, more long-term survivors would result.

This rationale for adjuvant surgery in small cell cancer was elaborated on by Meyer et al.[30,32] Based on the study of patients with stage I or II disease, they reasoned that early resection could reduce the tumor burden by many logs immediately, that is, establish a clinical complete remission immediately without causing hematologic toxicity or affecting bone marrow reserve. Resection should then be followed by a full course of aggressive chemotherapy, which would then have the advantage of dealing with a smaller tumor burden. In patients with obvious T_3 or N_2 disease, the likelihood of an incomplete excision is increased, reducing the tumor burden by only an inconsequential few logs. A complete resection, after one or two cycles of chemotherapy, with resection of as much tissue as was involved before chemotherapy, would greatly improve the chance that chemotherapy could achieve tumor control. Resection should be done earlier rather than later, before some of the effects of chemotherapy are dissipated by the development of drug resistance.[12,43] A small number of drug-resistant cells may be present in the tumor, and tumor control could be lost before significant eradication occurs. Meyer acknowledged clearly the need to assess the results of adjuvant surgery according to TNM classification, in order to define which patients can best benefit from the surgical approach.

What, then, are the recent results of surgical resection as part of combined-modality therapy for small cell lung cancer? The first consideration will be patients with stage I or II disease at presentation. Meyer et al. reported on 10 patients who underwent resection followed by chemotherapy.[31,32] Only one died from a relapse, and eight were alive more than 30 months, five of whom had survived for more than 5 years. Shepherd et al. described 35 patients who underwent resection, in 28 instances as initial treatment before chemotherapy and thoracic plus cranial radiotherapy.[38] Of these patients, 28 (80 percent) had stage I or II disease. The median survival of the group was 92 weeks, with a projected 5-year survival of 24 percent. There was no difference in survival between stage I versus stage II and III patients. Only 2 of the 15 (13 percent) relapses occurred in the chest. Surprisingly, 5 of the 21 patients (24 percent) who received prophylactic cranial radiotherapy still relapsed in the brain. Shepherd and her colleagues thus suggest that prolonged survival is achievable for some patients with limited disease when surgical resection is used as part of their treatment program.

At the University of Chicago, we have undertaken surgical resection in five patients with stage I disease (four with T_1N_0, one with T_2N_0) and three patients (all with T_2N_1) with stage II disease.[16] The stage I patients all underwent resection first, followed by chemotherapy for two cycles in two patients (one refused further treatment, one died of cardiac disease), for 12 cycles in two patients, and no chemotherapy in one (poor medical condition). Three of the patients received thoracic and cranial radiation therapy. No patient has relapsed—two died at 5 and 44 months from heart disease, two are alive and well 17 and 33 months following resection, and one has squamous cell carcinoma of the lung that was diagnosed at 65 months. The stage II patients all received 12 months of chemotherapy, as well as chest and cranial radiotherapy. Two are alive and well at 42 and 69 months, and one died of a chest wall recurrence at 35 months.

A few other reports have appeared on resection in patients with stage I and II small cell carcinoma. Marchello et al. noted four patients who underwent resection before chemotherapy, with all four alive and disease-free at 10, 12, 31, and 55 months.[26] Prager et al. prospectively evaluated patients for surgery after two to four cycles of chemotherapy.[36] Of 14 patients with clinical stage I or II disease, six went to surgery and five were pathologically confirmed as stage I or II and resected. Two died at 12 and 18 months, and three were disease-free at 15, 22, and 23 months. There were no local recurrences. Fiorentino et al. described 16 patients in stage I or II who underwent surgery followed by chemotherapy and cranial radiation: 13 of the 16 were alive at a median of eight months, too early to assess the impact of surgery.[8] Ettinger et al., in a preliminary Eastern Cooperative Oncology Group (ECOG) report, described 20 patients who underwent resection after two courses of chemotherapy.[7] Of these 20 patients, 11 were in stage I or II; 12 were disease-free at a median of 21.5 months, but the survival by stage was not stated.

On the basis of these data, as well as those from the large Veterans Administration group,[40] we can conclude that surgical resection appears to be a useful adjunct in that small minority of patients with stage I or II SCLC. Two questions, both unanswerable with present information, arise from this formulation. First, is the surgery necessary in these patients, that is, would patients with such limited disease do just as well with only chemotherapy, either with or without radiation therapy? Second, is the surgery actually "adjuvant" in this particular group of patients, or could surgery alone suffice for treatment? In other words, are the chemotherapy and radiotherapy, in fact the adjuvant modalities?

With regard to the first question, most series of combined-modality therapy in small cell carcinoma only divide patients into "limited" and "extensive" disease categories. While there are undoubtedly a few patients with stage I or II disease in these limited-disease groups, their results are not analyzed separately, and any effect specific to them would likely be diluted by the larger group of stage III M_0 patients. Recently, however, Shepherd et al. reported the results of an interesting trial of nonsurgical treatment for 33 patients with "very limited" (no demonstrable mediastinal node involvement) small cell carcinoma.[39] They were treated with chemotherapy, chest radiotherapy, and usually cranial radiotherapy; 24 of these patients relapsed, of whom 14 (58 percent) relapsed only locally. Seven were disease-free at 24–72 months, and the median survival for the group was 83 weeks, compared to 47 weeks for patients with more typical "limited" disease (i.e., including N_2). The projected 5-year survival was 23 percent, compared to 10 percent for typical limited-disease patients. Thus Shepherd introduces an important caveat concerning with whom (i.e., patients in which stage) resected patients should be compared. Nevertheless, many of the results noted above for resected stage I and II patients are better than those reported by Shepherd, suggesting that the ability to reduce thoracic relapse rate by means of resection is a critical step. Moreover, it is likely that many of the patients with "very limited" disease really have T_3 or N_2 disease, albeit not obvious clinically, making this group of patients not totally valid for comparison with surgically staged I and II patients. Thus, lacking a controlled trial comparing surgical with nonsurgical treatment in pathologic stage I and II patients, and considering the high thoracic relapse rate, one can still comfortably conclude that patients with stage I or II disease have an excellent chance of benefiting from surgical resection of the primary tumor as part of a total treatment program.

The second question is even more difficult: would surgery alone be adequate therapy for stage I or II small cell lung cancer? A few lines of evidence suggest that it might. The historical series cited early in this chapter included some with 5-year survivals in excess of 30 percent.[10,41,42] We must presume that many of those cases represented early-stage disease if they were even considered for surgical resection. The solitary nodule study noted a 36 percent 5-year survival.[14] The large VA series[40] reported substantial survival rates for such early-stage patients. All of these studies were of surgery alone, or if combined with adjuvant chemotherapy, the latter was considerably less aggressive than is typically employed today. In our group of stage I patients at the University of Chicago,[16] one had no therapy other than surgery and is alive at 65 months, and one had only two cycles of chemotherapy and is alive at 17 months. In a large series of patients reported from northwestern Washington, among a group of 15 patients with "local disease" surviving more than 2 years, 12 (80 percent) had surgery alone; among a group of 11 patients with "regional disease" surviving for more than 2 years, 4 (36 percent) had surgery alone.[6] Clearly, all of these data are uncontrolled. Considering, however, the large number of historical series indicating poor results with surgery, as well as the excellent effects of chemotherapy and radiotherapy on SCLC, it would be exceedingly risky to conclude that additional therapy need not be advised after resection of a stage I or II cancer.

The value of surgical resection as part of combined modality treatment of stage III M_0 small cell carcinoma is considerably more controversial. Meyer et al. studied 20 patients with stage III M_0 disease, in whom surgical resection was planned after two cycles of chemotherapy.[32] Chemotherapy was continued, and cranial radiotherapy was administered after surgery. Four patients had T_3N_1 staging; two died at 10 and 17 months from relapse (one of whom had been unresectable), and two were disease-free at 34 and 50 months. The 16 patients with N_2 staging fared considerably worse — six were not resectable for a variety of reasons and died at a median of 11 months, and the 10 who underwent resection all died from tumor relapse at a median of 12.5 months. Comis et al., from the same group as Meyer, reported on 19 patients with stage III disease in whom surgery was planned following chemotherapy.[5] Two patients with T_3N_0 disease survived for 34 and 43+ months after resection. Ten resected patients with N_2 disease lived a median of 16 months, the same as the survival of the patients who did not have surgery. Of all 17 patients with N_2 disease, three survived for more than 24 months, two of whom died at 33 and 34 months (both had had surgery), and one was disease-free at 46 months (not resected). Of note was that 80 percent of the relapses in resected patients were distant only, suggesting that surgical resection did reduce the local relapse rate even if it did not influence survival. Meyer and Comis both concluded that surgical resection was not supported in patients with N_2 disease.

Shepherd et al. suggested that even certain patients with N_2 disease might benefit from surgical resection.[38] As noted before, patients with stage II and III disease had survival similar to those with stage I disease. The six patients in that series with T_2N_2 disease had a mean survival of 88 weeks, two of whom had not recurred. Valdivieso et al. also suggested some value to surgical resection in stage III patients, although it is not clear which patients exactly were stage III in relation to surgical benefit.[45] In a large Southwest Oncology Group study of 262 patients treated with chemotherapy and radiotherapy, 15 had had initial surgical resection.[11] The resected patients had a median survival time and 2-year survival rate significantly better than the nonresected patients (25 vs 10.5 months and 44 vs 13.7 percent respectively). The relapse rate in the chest was considerably lower in the resected group (13.7 vs 56 percent). Unfortunately, no staging data on the resected patients were available, so it is not certain whether the initially resected patients were, in fact, stage III. Davis et al. also noted improved survival for resected patients, regardless of stage (e.g., 38 percent 2-year survival for resected patients with "regional" disease compared with 10 percent for nonresected patients).[6] Again, however, precise staging data were not available.

In the Prager et al. prospective study of 40 patients evaluated for surgery after several chemotherapy cycles, only 3 of the original 25 patients with stage III disease were ultimately resectable.[36] One died at 6 months, one was alive with recurrence at 19 months, and one (the only one with no residual tumor at operation) was disease-free at 15 months. Since most of the 40 patients of all stages originally evaluated for surgery never came to surgery or to resection, Prager et al. concluded that only a small minority of patients with small cell carcinoma would be candidates for this approach. Fiorentino et al. planned surgery after chemotherapy for 12 patients.[8] Seven actually underwent surgery; four were disease-free at 8 months, and three had relapsed. Among 16 patients with clinical stage I or II disease who underwent initial surgery before chemotherapy, 3 had relapsed, of whom 2 had had stage III pathologically at resection. Thus their data do not support surgery in stage III disease.

At the University of Chicago, we have performed surgical resections in 13 patients with stage III small cell carcinoma.[16,17] Seven patients underwent initial resection when stage III could not be conclusively documented preoperatively. All seven had T_3 or N_2 disease on pathologic examination. All received combination chemotherapy and chest and cranial radiotherapy. Only one patient is disease-free at 102 months; the other six died between 1 and 23 months. The median survival of the group was 16 months. Of interest was that four patients suffered brain relapses despite cranial radiotherapy, a feature noted by Shepherd et al. as well.[38] An additional six patients whose stage III status was documented on initial evaluation underwent surgery after two to three cycles of chemotherapy. Only one patient had no tumor at operation, two had tumor in nodes only, and three had tumor in the primary site and nodes. The median survival of these six patients was 10 months (range 6-18), and all died. Two patients died with no evidence of tumor, however—one at 6 months of a gastrointestinal hemorrhage and one at 14 months of severe pulmonary hypertension, perhaps related to therapy.[3] Among our 13 total patients, 4 had T_3N_0 or T_3N_1 disease (i.e., not N_2). Their median survival was 15.5 months, compared to 10.5 months for the nine with N_2 disease. The median survival for our 72 patients with stage III M_0 disease treated nonsurgically was 15.2 months, however.[19]

Our impression, then, is that surgical resection, even in highly selected patients, offers little to the outcome of therapy for stage III M_0 small cell carcinoma. This view is supported by a Danish study of 874 patients with small cell carcinoma.[35] In that study, a group of 33 patients who underwent resection were compared with 46 patients who were operable but who did not undergo operation (based on treatment approaches at the time). All patients received chemotherapy, often with radiotherapy. There was no difference in survival between the operated and nonoperated groups. The 2-year disease-free survivals were 12 and 13 percent, respectively. Both operated and non-operated groups had significantly better survival than did the 696 nonoperable patients. Although the study was not prospectively done, the policy of comparing resected patients with those who *could* have been resected, but were not because of the treatment philosophy for that cell type, permitted conclusions as close to a prospective analysis as can be achieved. Another facet of the study was analysis of site of relapse. The chest relapses were rare in resected patients clinically, but at autopsy the majority of patients had evidence of recurrent disease at the primary tumor site. The authors concluded that the inclusion of surgery in the treatment program for resectable small cell carcinoma does not lead to improved results over those with chemotherapy and radiotherapy.

CONCLUSIONS

Patients with small cell carcinoma who present with disease that appears clinically to be stage I or II should reasonably be considered candidates for surgical resection, probably after mediastinoscopy to rule out N_2 disease, since many studies suggest an excellent chance for long-term survival. Although the data are not certain as to whether chemotherapy and radiotherapy add to the benefit of the surgery in such early-stage patients, it seems prudent to treat patients with this combined-modality approach. Such patients clearly may have occult distant disease, and adjuvant therapy would likely be most efficacious for such minimal tumor burden.

At the present time, patients with stage III small cell carcinoma do not appear to benefit from surgical resection along with more conventional therapy. This is particularly true for patients with N_2 disease, and likely also true for patients with T_3N_0 or T_3N_1 disease. It should be noted that for most patients who relapse after surgical resection, the relapse is distant rather than local, thus representing a failure of the chemotherapy to control systemic disease. The stage III status implies a greater likelihood that distant tumor dissemination has occurred and that local measures are doomed to fail if chemotherapeutic drugs cannot eradicate distant tumor. It is possible that "adjuvant surgery" may again warrant careful study in the future if substantial survival advances with chemotherapy of small cell carcinoma occur, and yet local relapse continues to be a major problem.

REFERENCES

1. Ashor GL, Kern WH, Meyer BW, et al: Long-term survival in bronchogenic carcinoma. J Thorac Cardiovasc Surg 70:581–589, 1975
2. Bleehen NM, Bunn PA, Cox JD, et al: Role of radiation therapy in small cell anaplastic carcinoma of the lung. Cancer Treat Rep 67:11–19, 1983
3. Brooks BJ, Seifter EJ, Walsh TE, et al: Pulmonary toxicity with combined modality therapy for limited stage small-cell lung cancer. J Clin Oncol 4:200–209, 1986
4. Cohen MH: Is thoracic radiation therapy necessary for patients with limited stage small cell lung cancer? No. Cancer Treat Rep 67:217–221, 1983
5. Comis RL, Meyer J, Ginsberg S, et al: The impact of TNM stage on results with chemotherapy and adjuvant surgery in small cell lung cancer. Proc Am Soc Clin Oncol 3:226, 1984
6. Davis S, Wright PW, Schulman SF, et al: Long-term survival in small-cell carcinoma of the lung: A population experience. J Clin Oncol 3:80–91, 1985
7. Ettinger DS, Baker RR, Eggleston JC et al: Prospective evaluation of the role of surgery in limited disease small cell lung cancer. An ECOG pilot study. Proc Am Soc Clin Oncol 4:180, 1985
8. Fiorentino MV, Paccagnella A, Brandes A, et al: Combination of chemotherapy and surgery for small cell lung cancer with limited disease. Proc Am Soc Clin Oncol 4:194, 1985
9. Fox W, Scadding JG: Medical Research Council comparative trial of surgery and radiotherapy for primary treatment of small-celled or oat-celled carcinoma of bronchus. Ten-year follow-up. Lancet 2:63–65, 1973
10. Freise G, Gabler A, Liebig S: Bronchial carcinoma and long-term survival. Retrospective study of 433 patients who underwent resection. Thorax 33:228–234, 1978
11. Friess GG, McCracken JD, Troxell ML, et al: Effect of initial resection of small-cell carcinoma of the lung: A review of Southwest Oncology Group Study 7628. J Clin Oncol 3:964–968, 1985
12. Goldie JH, Coldman AJ: A mathematical model for relating the drug sensitivity of tumors to their spontaneous mutation rate. Cancer Treat Rep 63:1727–1733, 1979
13. Hansen HH, Elliott JA: Patterns of failure in small cell lung cancer: Implications for therapy. Recent Results Cancer Res 92:43–57, 1984
14. Higgins GA, Shields TW, Keehn RJ: The solitary pulmonary nodule. Ten-year follow-up of Veterans Administration-Armed Forces Cooperative Study. Arch Surg 110:570–575, 1975
15. Hoffman PC, Albain KS, Bitran JD, et al: Current concepts in small cell carcinoma of the lung. CA 34:269–281, 1984

16. Hoffman PC, DeMeester TR, Little AG, et al: Surgical resection in the management of small cell carcinoma of the lung. Manuscript in preparation

17. Hoffman PC, Weiman DJ, Bitran JD, et al: Surgical resection in patients with Stage IIIM0 small cell carcinoma of the lung. Proc Am Soc Clin Oncol 1:152, 1982

18. Ihde DC: Current status of therapy for small cell carcinoma of the lung. Cancer 54:2722-2728, 1984

19. Jacobs R, Greenburg A, Bitran J, et al: A ten year experience with combined modality therapy for small cell lung carcinoma. Proc Am Soc Clin Oncol 4:185, 1985

20. Johnson RE, Brereton HD, Kent CH: "Total" therapy for small cell carcinoma of the lung. Ann Thorac Surg 25:510-515, 1978

21. Kirklin JW, McDonald JR, Clagett L, et al: Bronchogenic carcinoma: Cell type and other factors relating to prognosis. Surg Gynec Obstet 100:429-438, 1955

22. Lennox SC, Flavell G, Pollock DJ, et al: Results of resection for oat-cell carcinoma of the lung. Lancet 2:925-927, 1968

23. Levitt M, Meikle A, Murray N, et al: Oat cell carcinoma of the lung: CNS metastases in spite of prophylactic brain irradiation. Cancer Treat Rep 62:131-133, 1978

24. Li, WI, Hammer SP, Jolly PC, et al: Unpredictable course of small cell undifferentiated lung carcinoma. J Thorac Cardiovasc Surg 81:34-43, 1981

25. Livingston RB: Small cell carcinoma of the lung. Blood 56:575-584, 1980

26. Marchello B, Hammond N, Teel P, et al: Resectability of small cell lung cancer: Timing and incidence in a community setting. Proc Am Soc Clin Oncol 3:233, 1984

27. McMahon LJ, Herman TS, Manning MR, et al: Patterns of relapse in patients with small cell carcinoma of the lung treated with Adriamycin-cyclophosphamide chemotherapy and radiation therapy. Cancer Treat Rep 63:359-362, 1979

28. Matthews MJ, Kanhouwa S, Pickren J, et al: Frequency of residual and metastatic tumor in patients undergoing curative surgical resection for lung cancer. Cancer Chemother Rep 4:63-67, 1973

29. Mayer JE Jr, Ewing SL, Ophoren JJ, et al: Influence of histologic type on survival after curative resection for undifferentiated lung cancer. J Thorac Cardiovasc Surg 84:641-648, 1982

30. Meyer JA, Comis RL, Ginsberg SJ, et al: Phase II trial of extended indications for resection in small cell carcinoma of the lung. J Thorac Cardiovasc Surg 83:12-19, 1982

31. Meyer JA, Comis RL, Ginsberg SJ, et al: The prospect of disease control by surgery combined with chemotherapy in Stage I and Stage II small cell carcinoma of the lung. Ann Thorac Surg 36:37-41, 1983

32. Meyer JA, Gullo JJ, Ikins PM, et al: Adverse prognostic effect of N_2 disease in treated small cell carcinoma of the lung. J Thorac Cardiovasc Surg 88:495-501, 1984

33. Mountain CF: Clinical biology of small cell carcinoma. Relationship to surgical therapy. Semin Oncol 5:272-279, 1978

34. Niederle N, Schutte J: Chemotherapeutic results in small cell lung cancer. Recent Results Cancer Res 97:127-145, 1985

35. Osterlind K, Hansen M, Hansen HH, et al: Treatment policy of surgery in small cell carcinoma of the lung: Retrospective analysis of a series of 874 consecutive patients. Thorax 40:272-277, 1985

36. Prager RL, Foster JM, Hainsworth JD, et al: The feasibility of adjuvant surgery in limited-stage small cell carcinoma: A prospective evaluation. Ann Thorac Surg 38:622-626, 1984

37. Rosen ST, Makuch RW, Lichter AS, et al: Role of prophylactic cranial irradiation in prevention of central nervous system metastases in small cell lung cancer. Am J Med 74:615-624, 1983

38. Shepherd FA, Ginsberg RJ, Evans WK, et al: Reduction in local recurrence and improved survival in surgically treated patients with small cell lung cancer. J Thorac Cardiovasc Surg 86:498-506, 1983

39. Shepherd FA, Ginsberg R, Evans WK, et al: "Very limited" small cell lung cancer—results of nonsurgical treatment. Proc Am Soc Clin Oncol 3:223, 1984

40. Shields TW, Higgins GA Jr, Matthews MJ, et al: Surgical resection in the management of small cell carcinoma of the lung. J Thorac Cardiovasc Surg 84:481-488, 1984

41. Shore DF, Paneth M: Survival after resection of small cell carcinoma of the bronchus. Thorax 35:819-822, 1980

42. Siddons AHM: Cell type in the choice of cases of carcinoma of the bronchus for surgery. Thorax 17:308-309, 1962

43. Skipper HE: Stepwise progress in the treatment of disseminated cancer. Cancer 51:1773-1776, 1983

44. Taylor AB, Shinton NK, Waterhouse JAH: Histology of bronchial carcinoma in relation to prognosis. Thorax 18:178-181, 1963

45. Valdivieso M, McMurtrey MJ, Farha P, et al: Increasing importance of adjuvant surgery in the therapy of patients with small cell lung cancer. Proc Am Soc Clin Oncol 1:148, 1982

46. Vincent RG, Takita H, Lane WW, et al: Surgical therapy of lung cancer. J Thorac Cardiovasc Surg 71:581-591, 1976

47. Watson WL, Berg JW: Oat cell lung cancer. Cancer 15:759-768, 1962

David G. Dienhart
Paul A. Bunn, Jr.

_____ **25** _____

Patterns of Relapse in Small Cell Lung Cancer—Implications for Future Studies

Small cell lung cancer (SCLC) is a well recognized, distinct type of lung cancer, possessing a unique biologic and clinical character reflected in its high metastatic potential, rapid growth, and sensitivity to radiation and chemotherapy.[11,18] Prior to the 1970s less than 1 percent of patients were cured with standard surgical and radiotherapeutic modalities.[11] Combination chemotherapy has become the cornerstone of treatment in all patients with SCLC, and long-term survivors now approximate 6–12 percent of patients.[70] It appears that chemotherapeutic success has reached a plateau over the past several years despite increasing dose intensity, duration of therapy, alternating non-cross-resistant regimens, and late intensification.

Because current therapies fail to cure the large majority of SCLC patients, knowledge of patterns of failure is essential for the design of future clinical trials. To review SCLC failure patterns since 1977, we have selectively chosen studies that meet three important criteria: (1) provide relapse occurrence separately for limited- and extensive-stage patients, (2) provide data on relapse from complete response, and (3) provide failure patterns as initial sites of relapse. Unfortunately, this excluded many studies not making this distinction; however, a basis is formed for discussion of failure rates. An exception appears in Table 25-8 for randomized trials of prophylactic cranial irradiation; three trials were included where limited- and extensive-stage patient relapse data were examined together. Several other issues for attention include (1) initial relapse in single or multiple sites, (2) the frequency of late relapse, (3) the effect of changing relapse patterns on long-term survival and toxicity, and (4) the development of secondary metachronous non-small cell lung cancer (NSCLC) neoplasms.

RELAPSE PATTERNS IN LIMITED-STAGE PATIENTS

Stage of disease has long been an important prognostic indicator for SCLC patients. The tumor, node, metastasis (TNM) staging system has prognostic value for NSCLC patients but has not been applicable for the SCLC patient.[73] Equivalent TNM stages in SCLC are not predictive of median or long-term survival. The limited-stage and extensive-stage system for SCLC is widely utilized as developed by the Veterans Administration Lung Study Group.[107] It provides a basic staging system to study patients in clinical trials and holds some prognostic value. "Limited-stage disease" for SCLC patients generally refers to disease confined within one hemithorax, including mediastinal and supraclavicular nodes, and can be encompassed within a single radiation port. Pleural effusions and extensive pulmonary disease may exclude patients from a limited stage. "Extensive disease" refers to further dissemination, usually outside the chest. Limited-stage patients represent approximately one-third of all SCLC patients at diagnosis.

The patterns of relapse are especially important in limited-stage SCLC patients because their localized nature makes them potentially treatable with surgery and/or irradiation. Chest relapse is also important because (1) there are significant numbers of limited-stage patients, (2) adequate evaluation of the chest and tissue biopsy is possible by current clinical techniques, (3) significant numbers of patients attain complete response (CR) status following induction therapy (40–80 percent), and (4) the majority of limited-stage patients achieving CR will relapse within 18 months.

Surgical Therapy

Relapse patterns for SCLC patients treated in early surgical trials emphasize the disseminated nature of this disease and relapse at distant sites. Five year survival rates for these trials generally have been less than 1 percent.[59,100,101] The Medical Research Council in a prospective randomized trial of limited stage patients compared "radical radiotherapy" to surgical resection alone.[34] More long-term survivors appeared in the radiotherapy group at 2, 5 and 10 years, although only the mean survival durations attained statistical significance. At 10 years, there were 3 out of 73 long-term survivors in the radiation group and none in the surgical group. Although this trial showed that radiotherapy may prove potentially better for local control, relapse with disseminated disease was not prevented by either modality alone. Investigators concluded that superior systemic approaches were needed. In other attempts to improve surgical results, four randomized trials were performed with surgery and chemotherapy versus surgery and placebo.[44,58,69,93] All except one of these studies[69] demonstrated superior 2-year survival advantage in the chemotherapy arms, despite the suboptimal chemotherapeutic regimens employed.

Retrospective studies have attempted to compare the outcome of SCLC patients treated by initial surgical resection to a similar "subgroup" of patients not resected within their study having similar tumor size and stage.[36,79,92] These data favor improved local control with surgery; one study showed a longer median survival in the resected group.[36] Fries and colleagues[36] reviewed 262 Southwest Oncology Group (SWOG) limited-stage patients and found 15 who underwent initial resection (12 lobectomy, 3 pneumonectomy) prior to further intensive multimodality therapy. These resected patients were compared to a "subgroup" of 33 unresected patients with a similar tumor (single primary tumor less than 5 cm diameter) and a favorable SWOG performance status of 0 or 1. The median survival for the resected group was 25 months, compared to 10 months for the selected 33 nonresected patients. Chest relapse was diminished to 13 percent in the resected group compared to 56 percent chest relapse among 142 study patients not receiving surgery. In this retrospective review, resection demonstrated improved control of thoracic disease and the potential of prolonging survival.

Similarly, Osterlind et al. reviewed the experience of 874 patients who were treated from 1973 to 1981 in any of six clinical trials.[79] Resection were done in 15 patients (4 lobectomy, 11 pneumonectomy). A similar subset of 46 nonresected patients fulfilling the requirements for operability together with a normal mediastinoscopy served as a control group. They found a decreased incidence of chest relapse in the resected group compared to controls. However, although 3 out of 15 resected patients had clinical initial relapse at the primary site, compared to 32 out of 40 for the unresected group, autopsy data showed equivalent primary site recurrence for both groups. At autopsy, there were 12 out of 14 proven chest failures at the primary site or mediastinal nodes within the resected group, compared to 23 out of 25 in unresected patients. There were no significant differences in 2-year disease free survival or life table projections for the two groups. Other investigators have identified a "very limited" subgroup of their limited-stage SCLC patients not undergoing resection whose median survival was significantly longer,[92] suggesting that surgical selection bias must be excluded in randomized trials. Therefore the role of surgical resection cannot be determined from retrospective studies.

In a prospective trial, Comis and colleagues[19] utilized traditional TNM staging and resected stage 1 and stage 2 patients prior to CAVE (cyclophosphamide, adriamycin, vincristine, and etoposide) combination chemotherapy. In contrast, stage 3 patients received 2-4 cycles of CAVE chemotherapy prior to resection. Preliminary survival projections were encouraging for stage 1 and 2 patients. For stage 3 patients, 14 of 21 (67 percent) completed both chemotherapy and resection. However, there was no survival advantage for resected patients compared with patients not resected. As in retrospective studies, low chest relapse was found for resected patients. Similarly, other investigators have prospectively evaluated their limited stage patients to determine the fraction that may be resected,[33,103] and performed thoracotomy in 21-28 percent of patients. Although local tumor control was generally improved, no survival advantage was found for resected patients. These studies have identified limited stage patients that may be successfully resected, although the utility of surgery to improve survival remains uncertain.

The solitary pulmonary nodule represents the clearest indication for surgical resection in SCLC, producing similar 5- and 10-year survival rates to other lung cancer histologies in the Veterans Administration-Armed Forces Cooperative Study.[45] Patients with resected SCLC nodules have shown significant relapse, and trials of early chemotherapeutic regimens demonstrated some modest survival prolongation for these patients. This suggests that current adjuvant combination chemotherapy regimens following resection should be employed in all patients with resected nodules. The T_1N_0 SCLC patient is rare, however. Randomized trials would require large numbers of patients to demonstrate survival advantage. Therefore, the majority of current trials are examining adjuvant surgery in selected limited-disease patients (T_1, T_2; N_0, N_1; M_0), such as adjuvant surgical resection following combination chemotherapy regimens and preceding chest radiotherapy consolidation.

Radiation Therapy

Radiation therapy has long played a significant role in the therapy of limited-stage SCLC. After therapeutic activity was demonstrated for several chemotherapeutic

Table 25-1
Nonrandomized Trials Evaluating Chest Relapse in Limited-Stage SCLC Treated with Combined-Modality Therapy

Therapy Drugs	Radiation Dose/Fraction/Time	Number of Patients	CR (%)	MS	Number of Chest Failures from CR/No. CR (%)		Total No. Chest Failures/No. Evaluable (%)		Reference
CAV	3000/Cont/Initial 4500/Split/Delayed	36	75	NR	10/27*	37	10/27*	37	57
CAV	4500/Split/Delayed	108	41	12	9/28*	32	9/28*	32	63
CAV	3000/Cont/Initial	3	NR	NR	NR		0/3*	0	20
CAV	3000/Cont/Initial	32	90	NR	2/29*	7	2/29*	7	39
CA	3000/Cont/Delayed 4500/Split	10	80	18.5	NR		6/10*	60	68
CML	4000/Split/Delayed	55	NR	10	NR		25/109* 50/109	23 46	41†
CAV or CAVM or CVMF	3000/Cont/Delayed 4500/Split	17	NR	NR	NR		2/7*	28	71
CAE (high-dose)	3000/Split/Delayed	9	22	15	NR		1/9	11	1
CAV	2500/Cont/Delayed	66	24	10.5	NR		9/40* 20/40	22 50	32
CAD	4500/Cont/Initial	70	50	7.5	NR		11/27*	40	82
CAVEcDDP	5000/Cont/Delayed	24	83	16	NR		13/23*	57	90
EAM or CLVP/EAM	5000/Cont/Delayed	55	43	12	5/20*	25	5/20*	25	15
CAV	3000/Cont/Delayed	10	30	8.5	NR		2/10*	20	61
CVE or CAVE (high-dose)	5000/Cont/Delayed	5	60	NR	1/3*	33	1/3* 2/5	33 40	29
EVAC	5000/Cont/Delayed	33	76	19	3/25*	12	3/25*	12	37
CAV	2500/Cont/Delayed	153	52	11	NR		40/92* 64/92	43 70	31

Regimen	Dose/Fraction/Time	No. Pts	CR (%)	MS	Relapse A (n)	%	Relapse B (n)	%	Ref
LAVb	4000/Split/Initial	146	70	10.5	21/89*	24	21/89*	24	87
					40/89	45	40/89	45	
AECM or	4500/Split/Delayed	28	86	14	9/24*	37	9/24*	37	5‡
AECcDDP	5500/Split/Delayed	35	91	20	4/32*	12	4/32*	12	
CAVM	3750/Cont/Delayed	16	88	13.5	3/14*	21	3/14*	21	47
CAV alt EHM / C/E (high-dose)	5100/Split/Delayed	26	62	13	4/16*	25	4/16*	25	64
CAV alt EcDDP	5000/Cont/Delayed	24	83	18.5	6/15*	40	6/15*	40	75
							9/15	60	
AVE or CAVE CE (intens)	5000/Cont/Delayed	11	45	NR	4/5*	80	6/11*	55	88§
CAV alt EcDDP	5100/Cont/Delayed	35	65	21	1/8*	13	1/8*	13	91
							9/16	56	
C or CE (high-dose)	4000/Cont/Delayed	26	50	NR	NR		18/26*	69	97
CbE	4000/Cont/Delayed	28	29	9.5	NR		6/28*	21	96
	6000/Split						13/28	46	
		1061	56	—	82/335*	24.5	216/716*	30.2	
					101/335	30.1	315/735	42.9	

Abbreviations: Dose = dose in rads; Fraction = fractionization; Split = split course; Cont = continuous course; Time = Initial or Delayed course chest radiotherapy; C = cyclophosphamide; A = adriamycin; V = vincristine; M = methotrexate; L = lomustine (CCNU); F=5/fluorouracil; E = etoposide (VP16); D = dimethyltriazenoimidozole carboxamide (DTIC); H = hexamethylmelamine; cDDP = cis-diammine dichloroplatinum; P = procarbazine; Vb = vinblastine; Cb = carboplatin; CR = complete response = complete regression of tumor; MS = median survival in months; NR = not reported; Cont = continuous radiation therapy; Split = split course radiation therapy; Alt = alternating; Intens = intensification chemotherapy.

*Chest failure represents the initial site of relapse.

†Randomized trial between localized (primary tumor and regional nodes) radiotherapy or extensive (primary tumor, regional nodes, upper abdominal nodes, adrenals, and brain) radiotherapy. Table 25-8 reviews the PCI randomization relapse data for this trial.

‡Each trial examined chemotherapy alternating with three cycles of radiotherapy.

§Trial examined late intensification with high-dose etoposide and high-dose cyclophosphamide.

agents, several randomized trials were performed and showed superior survival for patients treated with chemotherapy combined with radiation compared to radiation alone.[7,9,50,66,84] These early trials did not address treatment with combination chemotherapy alone. As systemic chemotherapy regimens improved, the role of chest radiation became controversial.

In a large retrospective review of limited-stage SCLC patients, Bunn and Ihde found improved local control of chest disease as well as superior 2-year disease-free survival in the chemotherapy plus radiotherapy group (17 percent) compared to patients treated with chemotherapy alone (7 percent).[12] However, response rates and survival were similar in each group. Many nonrandomized trials employing chemotherapy alone produced results similar to those employing both chemotherapy and radiotherapy. Table 25-1 details cumulative chest relapse data of 25 nonrandomized trials for limited-stage SCLC patients treated with bimodality (combination chemotherapy and chest irradiation) therapy.* Of 335 patients, 82 (24.5 percent) achieving complete response status from bimodality therapy relapsed initially in the chest. There were 42.9 percent (315/735) chest failures for all evaluable patients regardless of their previously attained response status. As detailed, most of these chest recurrences were the first evidence of relapse. Although bimodality treatment generally has decreased chest relapse rates compared to combination chemotherapy or chest radiotherapy alone, chest relapse remains a frequent site for failure in limited-stage patients.

Treatment with combination chemotherapy without chest radiotherapy has been utilized in a number of trials for limited stage SCLC. Table 25-2 details seven nonrandomized trials of patients treated with combination chemotherapy alone, finding an initial chest failure rate from complete response status of 37.8 percent (17/45), and subsequently increasing to a 58.4 percent (52/89) cumulative chest relapse, including patients previously attaining less than a complete response.[1,2,14,16,17,24,29] Two trials detailed in Table 25-2 also suggest poor local chest control for treatment regimens employing chest radiation alone at induction.[20,82] In conclusion, nonrandomized studies show superior chest control for limited-stage patients with the use of bimodality therapy. However, these nonrandomized studies do not adequately address the effect on survival of additive chest radiotherapy.

Seven randomized trials in limited-stage SCLC have explored the potential advantage of the addition or exclusion of chest radiotherapy to combination chemotherapy to potentially reduce primary chest failure and improve survival. Results from these trials are provided in Table 25-3.[13,35,78,81,83,98,99] Five of these seven trials reported their chest failure patterns, and all five trials demonstrated significantly diminished chest relapse for the bimodality arms. The Cancer and Acute Leukemia Group B[83] entered the largest number of patients and also studied in a random fashion the utility of initial or delayed course chest radiotherapy. Both radiotherapy strategies proved superior to chemotherapy alone for achievement of complete response, prevention of chest relapse, and 2-year survival attainment. The delayed radiotherapy regimen was slightly superior compared to initial course radiation for each of these factors. Only the NCI reported chest failure from a complete response status and further determined chest relapse as the sole site of initial failure.[13] For the bimodality group, 5 out of 38 (13 percent) complete responders failed in the chest as the sole site

---

*References 1, 5, 15, 20, 29, 31, 32, 37, 39, 41, 47, 57, 61, 63, 64, 68, 71, 75, 82, 87, 88, 90, 91, 96, and 97.

Table 25-2
Nonrandomized Trials Evaluating Chest Relapse in Limited-Stage SCLC Treated with Combination Chemotherapy or Radiotherapy Alone

Therapy	Number of Patients	CR (%)	MS	Number of Chest Failures from CR/No. CR (%)		Total No. Chest Failures/No. Evaluable (%)		Reference
Chemotherapy								
CML	5	NR	13	NR		1/5*	20	16
CML alt	19	74	14	5/14*	36	5/14*	36	17
VAP						6/14	43	
CAE (high-dose)	11	55	15	NR		5/11*	46	1
CAV	12	100	16	8/12*	67	8/12*	67	14
EVCAcDDP	30	40	13	NR		14/27*	52	24†
						21/27	78	
CAE or	44	64	14	3/17*	17	3/17*	17	2†
CAE/LVMP				8/17	47	8/17	47	
CVE or	3	67	NR	1/2*	50	2/3*	67	29
CAVE (high-dose)				2/2	100	3/3	100	
	124	62	—	17/45*	37.8	38/89*	42.7	
				23/45	51.1	52/89	58.4	
Radiation Dose/Time/Fraction								
3000/Cont/Delayed	26	NR	5.5	NR		13/26	50	20
4500/Cont/Initial	33	30	11	NR		7/26*	27	82
						14/26	54	
	59	—	—	NR		7/26*	26.9	
						27/52	51.9	

Abbreviations: Dose = dose in rads; Fraction = fractionization; Cont = continuous course; Time = Initial or Delayed course chest radiotherapy; C = cyclophosphamide; M = methotrexate; L = lomustine (CCNU); V = vincristine; cDDP = *cis*-diammine dichloroplatinum; E = etoposide (VP16); P = procarbazine; CR = complete response = complete regression of tumor; MS = median survival in months; NR = not reported.

* Chest failure represents the initial site of relapse.

† Randomized trial evaluating PCI; data for brain relapse shown in Table 25-8.

Table 25-3

Chest Failure Rates for Randomized Trials Evaluating Combination Chemotherapy With or Without Chest Radiotherapy in Limited-Stage SCLC

Location (or name) and Year of Study	Therapy Design	Radiation Dose/Fraction/Time	Number of Patients	CR (%)	MS	P Value	2-Year Survival (%)	Total Chest Failures/No. Evaluable (%)	P Value	Reference
Indiana 1979	CAV + RT	3500/Split/Delayed	14	71	13	p > .05	NR	NR	NR	99
	CAV alone	None	18	50	11.5		NR	NR		
Australia 1980	CAV + RT	4000/Cont/Delayed	36	NR	15.5	p = .003	15	3/21* (14)	NR	35
	CAV alone	None	37	NR	14		2	9/22* (41)		
London 1984	CMAV + RT	4000/Cont/Delayed	57	NR	13	p > .05	NR	NR (NR)		98
	CMAV alone	None	73	NR	12		NR	NR (NR)		
SECSG 1984	CAV + RT	4000/Split/Delayed	149	62	14		28	29/114* (25)		81
								41/114 (36)		
	CAV alone	None	142	48	11	p = .03	19	46/102* (45)	p = .03	
								53/102 (52)		
Copenhagen 1986	CMLV + RT	4000/Split/Delayed	69	37	10.5		3	28/57 (49)	p = .005	78
	CMLV alone	None	76	46	11.5	p = .24	7	48/60 (80)		
CALGB 1987	CAEV + RT	5000/Cont/Initial	125	49	13.1		15	26*/125* (21)		83
								33/125 (26)		
	CAEV + RT	5000/Cont/Delayed	145	58	14.6	p = .0099	25	39/145* (27)	p = .0001	
								59/145 (41)		
	CAEV alone	None	129	36	13.6		8	71/129* (55)		
								88/129 (68)		
NCI 1987†	CML/VAP + RT	4000/Cont/Initial	47	81	15		28	10/38*·† (26)		13
								14/47 (30)		
	CML/VAP alone	None	49	43	11.6	p = .035	12	11/21*·† (52)	p = .001	
								33/49 (67)		
Total chemotherapy and chest RT			642	57		—	—	107/443* (24.2)	178/509 (35.0)	
Total chemotherapy alone			524	43		—	—	137/274* (50.0)	231/362 (63.8)	

Abbreviations: SECSG = Southeast Cancer Study Group; NCI = National Cancer Institute; CALGB = Cancer and Acute Leukemia Group B; RT = radiation therapy; C = cyclophosphamide; A = adriamycin; V = vincristine; M = methotrexate; L = lomustine (CCNU); P = procarbazine; E = etoposide (VP16); Dose = dose in rads; Fraction = fractionization; Split = split course; Cont = continuous course; Time = Initial or Delayed course chest radiotherapy, CR = complete response = complete regression of tumor; MS = median survival in months, NR = not reported.

* Chest failure represents the initial site of relapse.

† Only trial examining chest failure from complete response status as the initial site of relapse; representing chest alone and chest plus systemic relapse. For the combined-modality group, 5 out of 38 (13 percent) of complete responders failed in the chest as the sole site of initial relapse; while 5 out of 21 (24 percent) of complete responders treated with chemotherapy alone relapsed in the chest as the sole site of initial relapse.

of initial relapse; while 5 out of 21 (24 percent) of complete responders treated with chemotherapy alone relapsed in the chest as the sole site of initial relapse. In summary, these randomized studies demonstrate initial failure in the chest for 24.2 percent (107/443) of patients treated with bimodality treatment, compared to a 50.0 percent (137/274) initial chest relapse rate in patients receiving combination chemotherapy alone. They support the cumulative experience for treatment failures described earlier for nonrandomized studies. Additional improvements in local therapy may further reduce chest relapse, although the numbers of patients to benefit are small after considering initial chest relapse as the sole site of failure. The major problem determining survival continues to by systemic relapse.

Four of seven randomized trials demonstrated modest survival advantage for the bimodality arms.[13,35,81,83] The NCI[13] and Southeast Cancer Study Group[81] demonstrated superior overall, median, and 2-year disease-free survivals for the bimodality therapy. The Cancer and Acute Leukemia Group B study[83] showed improved survival for both arms of bimodality treatment (chemotherapy plus delayed or chemotherapy plus initial radiotherapy) compared to treatment with chemotherapy alone. The Australian[35] trial had similar median survival rates for both arms, although 2-year disease free survival was improved for the bimodality group. The average median survival was approximately 15 months for the bimodality arms in these four trials, compared to 12 months for the chemotherapy-alone-treated patients. In contrast, three trials (Indiana, London, and Copenhagen) failed to demonstrate survival advantage for bimodality treatment. A few factors may have contributed to the negative results and include: (1) small numbers of patients, (2) possible inadequate chemotherapeutic delivery, and (3) sequential use of chemotherapy and chest radiotherapy.

Toxicity was generally increased for the bimodality arms in these trials. In the NCI trial, radiation was administered initially and concurrent with combination chemotherapy.[13] This approach caused greater myelosuppression, days of fever, days of antibiotics, and increased numbers of documented infections. Moderate to severe esophagitis occurred in 31 out of 47 patients in the bimodality group and led to a greater weight loss. Severe and late pulmonary toxicity was seen in 14 patients, with 12 in the bimodality group. For five patients, pulmonary toxicity was the cause of death while in complete remission. Metachronous NSCLC tumors developed in three patients in the bimodality group, occurring at 52, 58, and 68 months from the initiation of therapy.

Optimal methods of radiation delivery remain unclear today. Investigators have suggested improved documentation of treatment plans in all clinical trials, including (1) treatment volume, (2) dose-time fractionation, (3) continuous versus split course, (4) initial versus delayed course, and (5) spinal cord shielding details.[8,13] These trials illustrate a variety of dose, fractionation and timing schedules. In a second randomized trial comparing bimodality treatment to chemotherapy alone in limited-stage SCLC patients, the Southeast Cancer Study Group has preliminarily reported a slight but not significant survival advantage for the bimodality group.[38] This trial differed for radiotherapy delivery time from their earlier study,[81] the new trial administered continuous course radiotherapy at the onset of treatment rather than delayed radiotherapy. Interestingly, two cooperative groups, the Cancer and Acute Leukemia Group B[83] and the Southeast Cancer Study Group,[81] have demonstrated superior survival advantage for delayed over initial course radiotherapy. Trials examining changes in radiotherapy delivery schedules are important; however, systemic

Table 25-4
Nonrandomized Trials Evaluating Chest Relapse in Extensive-Stage SCLC Treated with Combined-Modality Therapy

Therapy Drugs	Radiation Dose/Fraction/Time	Number of Patients	CR (%)	MS	Chest Failures from CR/ No. CR (%)		Total No. Chest Failures/ No. Evaluable (%)		Reference
CAV	3000/Cont/Initial 4500/Split/Delayed	35	40	NR	8/14*	57	8/14*	57	57
CAV	4500/Split/Delayed	250	14	5.5	NR		10/66*	15	63
CAV	3000/Cont/Initial	22	NR	10	NR		4/22	18	20
CA	3000/Cont 4500/Split	17	18	2.5	NR		3/17*	20	68
CAV or CAVM or CVMF	3000/Cont/Delayed	17†	NR	NR	NR		6/15†	40	71
CL	2000/Cont/Delayed + 600 hemibody	19	26	NR	1/5*	20	1/5*	20	86
CAV	2500/Cont/Delayed	81	10	8	NR		5/39* 17/39	13 44	32
CAVEcDDP	5000/Cont/Delayed	20	NR	12.5	NR		13/18	81	90
EAM or CLVP/ EAM	5000/Cont/Delayed	106	30	8.5	18/25*	72	18/25*,†	72	15

Regimen	Dose/course	N							
HVAC; CME alt AME	4000/Split/Delayed	29	38	9.5	6/10*·§	60	6/10*·§	60	23
CAV	3000/Cont/Delayed	11	9	10	NR		3/10‡	30	61
CAV	3000/Cont/Delayed	236	14	6.5	NR		18/75	24	72
CVE or (high-dose) CAVE	5000/Cont/Delayed	4	40	NR	0/1*	0	1/2*	50	29
							2/4	50	
EVAC	5000/Cont/Delayed	38	34	8	1/13*	8	1/13*	8	37
CAV	2500/Cont/Delayed	167	10	7.5	NR		19/98*	19	31
							44/98	45	
CAVM	3750/Cont/Delayed	34	44	10	2/15*	13	2/15*	13	47
		1086	18	—	36/83*	43.4%	74/304*	24.3	
							156/446	35.0	

Abbreviations: C = cyclophosphamide; A = adriamycin; V = vincristine; M = methotrexate; F = 5-fluorouracil; L = lomustine (CCNU); E = etoposide (VP16); cDDP = cis-diammine dichloroplatinum; P = procarbazine; H = hexamethylmelamine; dose = dose in rads; Split = split course; Cont = continuous course; Time = Initial or Delayed course chest radiotherapy; CR = complete response = complete regression of tumor; MS = median survival in months; fraction = fractionization; NR = not reported; Alt = alternating.

* Chest failure represents the initial site of relapse.

† Only 10 of 17 patients received chest radiation.

‡ All 10 patients relapsed systemically; 3 patients had concurrent chest failure.

§ All six patients with chest relapse had concurrent systemic relapse.

relapse dominates overall and directs future trials to primarily examine potential improvements in systemic treatments.

In summary, bimodality treatment in limited-stage SCLC patients has led to improved control of primary chest disease; randomized trials show that chest radiotherapy adds modest survival advantage. The central issue for chest failure is identification of the number of patients who relapse from complete remission and who relapse in the chest as the sole site of initial failure. These trials indicate that at best, 13-25 percent of limited-stage patients may benefit from further reduction of chest relapse. Although not representing a large number of limited SCLC patients, improved local control is worth exploring for these patients. More aggressive local chest radiotherapy has been at the expense of significant toxicity. The potential of improving local tumor control and survival through adjuvant surgical resection in addition to chemotherapy and radiotherapy is the subject of current randomized trials. However, systemic relapse concurrently or immediately following chest failure and at multifocal sites frequently determines survival duration. To prolong survival further, improved local measures such as delivering optimal radiotherapy, adjuvant surgical resection, or specifically targeting therapy to tumor cells must supplement improved control of systemic disease.

EXTENSIVE-STAGE RADIATION THERAPY

Trials of chest radiotherapy when added to combination chemotherapy failed to demonstrate any survival advantage for extensive-stage SCLC patients. However, there was some diminution in chest relapse rates for patients receiving bimodality treatment, as shown in Tables 25-4 and 25-5. These 16 nonrandomized trials[†] suggest overall reduced chest relapse as an initial site of relapse for extensive-stage patients treated with bimodality therapy (74/304, 24.3 percent; Table 25-4); patients treated with combination chemotherapy alone[1,2,10,14,16,17,62,72,88,96] relapsed in the chest more often as their initial failure site (224/481, 46.6 percent; Table 25-5). These data bear less importance until improved systemic approaches are developed as (1) only a few trials assessed chest recurrence from a complete response status, as fewer patients attain a complete response with extensive disease; (2) systemic relapse frequently determines survival duration in extensive-stage SCLC patients, often with multiple sites with or without chest recurrence; and (3) review of limited-stage patients in randomized trials (Table 25-3), theoretically where bimodality treatment holds the most promise, demonstrates only a modestly increased survival advantage for bimodality therapy over combination chemotherapy alone.

Two randomized trials comparing the addition or exclusion of involved field radiotherapy together with combination chemotherapy have failed to show survival benefit for the addition of radiotherapy.[104,105] In a trial by Williams et al. sites of initial relapse, complete remission rate, and median survival were unaffected by the addition of chest, hepatic, and pleural radiotherapy.[104] Similarly, Wilson and colleagues randomly added or excluded chest, whole-brain, and abdominal irradiation to combination chemotherapy.[105] They found improved partial response rates, without change in complete response or median survival status. Furthermore, the incidence of hepatic

---

[†]References 15, 20, 23, 29, 31, 32, 37, 47, 57, 61, 63, 68, 71, 72, 86, and 90.

Table 25-5

Nonrandomized Trials Evaluating Chest Relapse in Extensive-Stage
SCLC Treated with Combination Chemotherapy Alone

Therapy Drugs	Number of Patients	CR (%)	MS	Number of Chest Failures from CR/No. CR (%)		Total No. Chest Failures/ No. Evaluable (%)		Reference
CML	27	NR	8.5	NR		9/20*	45	16
CML alt	42	36	9	5/15*	33	5/15*	33	17
VAP						7/15	47	
CAE (high-dose)	34	18	9.5	NR		6/28*	21	1
CAV	19	42	NR	NR		12/19*	63	14
CAE or	65	40	10	1/20*	5	1/20*	5	2†
CAE/LVMP				6/20	30	6/20	30	
CAEM-V	365	14	7	NR		63/114*	55	72
CAVE	48	23	12	NR		2/42*	5	10
VME or	429	16	7	33/43*	77	118/195*	61	62
VAC or								
VME/VAC								
AVE or	4	75	NR	0/3*	0	1/4*	25	88‡
CAVE								
CE (intens)								
CbE	24	13	9.5	NR		7/24*	28	96
						17/24	71	
	1057	19	—	39/81*	48.1	224/481*	46.6	
				44/81	54.3	241/481	50.1	

Abbreviations: C = cyclophosphamide; M = methotrexate; V = vincristine; P = procarbazine; L = lomustine (CCNU); A = adriamycin; E = etoposide; Cb = carboplatin; CR = complete response = complete regression of tumor; MS = median survival in months; NR = not reported; Intens = intensification chemotherapy; Alt = alternating.
*Chest failure represents the initial site of relapse.
†Randomized trial evaluating PCI; data provided for brain relapse in Table 25-8.
‡Trial examined late intensification with high-dose etoposide and high-dose cisplatin.

metastases at autopsy was unchanged with the addition of abdominal irradiation when compared with the chemotherapy alone group.

The use of wide-field (upper or lower hemibody) radiation combined with local chest radiation has produced some improved response rates of short duration; the majority of studies demonstrate no survival advantage for the addition of hemibody irradiation.[65,86,102] Myelosuppression has been the dose-limiting factor for delivery of radiotherapy in this fashion.

The ultimate utility of radiation therapy in extensive-stage SCLC awaits superior systemic disease control.

CHEMOTHERAPY

Combination chemotherapy has become the primary therapeutic modality for treating both limited- and extensive-stage SCLC and is reviewed in Chapter 22.

Multiple single agents have demonstrated significant activity and provide opportunities to study potential synergistic and effective combinations. In numerous trials, superior response rates and improved survival are demonstrated for combinations of three to four drugs over one or two drug regimens.[12] The two-drug combination of etoposide and cisplatin, however, has recently equalled the induction response and survival rates of many three or four drug regimens; these two drugs are included in many current trials.[28]

Several chemotherapy delivery strategies have not yet produced a significant change in relapse rates locally or systemically and include (1) increased induction therapy intensification, (2) maintenance chemotherapy, (3) alternating non-cross-resistant regimens, and (4) late intensification schedules. Future studies should include methods for improving remission duration for patients achieving complete remission as well as examination of new approaches for systemic treatment.

Dose Intensity

Abeloff and co-workers (Tables 25-1 and 25-2) found equivalent complete response rates and survival duration for patients treated with higher-dose induction chemotherapy with cyclophosphamide, doxorubicin, and etoposide (VP16-213) compared to less intense induction regimens.[1] Patients had marked myelosuppression and mucositis, as well as three treatment-related deaths among 54 patients. Higher-dose treatment produced no significant change in chest failure patterns for this trial; chest radiotherapy was not utilized. Souhami and colleagues (Table 25-1) found no improvement in complete response, relapse occurrence, or survival duration for 26 limited-stage patients treated with high-dose cyclophosphamide with or without etoposide.[97] They found shortened survival after relapse secondary to difficulty in administering additional chemotherapy as a result of significant hematologic toxicity. Johnson et al. likewise found no improvement in median survival, or chest relapse rates for high-dose cyclophosphamide together with high-dose etoposide therapy in extensive-stage patients.[56]

Studying the potential of autologous bone marrow transplantation after high-dose therapy (cyclophosphamide, etoposide, and vincristine with or without adriamycin), Farha and co-workers demonstrated at least partial response achievement for all 14 patients but no change in chest relapse occurrence or survival over less intensive regimens.[29] Tables 25-1, 25-2, and 25-4 review their treatment results.

Thus far, additional myelosuppressive therapy with or without bone marrow rescue has not shown improved relapse free survival or survival duration.

Maintenance Therapy

Maintenance chemotherapy has not shown overall success for prevented relapse in any sites, nor lengthened survival duration. Maurer and colleagues demonstrated improved median and 2-year disease free survival for limited-stage patients attaining a complete response who were randomized to continue maintenance therapy at 6 months; however, time to recurrence was not significantly prolonged by maintenance (median duration 5.0 months for maintenance group, 3.7 months for no maintenance).[67] Similarly, two nonrandomized trials by Feld and co-workers from the Ontario Cancer Institute compared induction therapy for 4 months to maintenance treatment of 1-year duration.[31,32] The maintenance-treated[32] patients experienced a minimal reduction in chest relapse for limited- and extensive-stage patients and no significant difference for survival duration. Chest relapse data for these two trials in limited- and extensive-stage patients are detailed in Tables 25-1 and 25-4. Maintenance chemotherapy did not change chest relapse patterns or produce a significant survival advantage. Other studies by investigators from the NCI,[57] Vanderbilt,[39] and the University of Indiana[25] administering cyclophosphamide, adriamycin, and vincristine (CAV) chemotherapy and chest radiotherapy show no survival advantage regardless of chemotherapy duration for 4, 12, or 24 months, respectively.

Two preliminary randomized trials[22,106] for maintenance or no maintenance therapy for responding patients from induction showed no survival benefit for patients receiving maintenance treatment. Long-term survivorship was not increased, and there was no prevention of relapse in the maintenance treated group.

Overall, maintenance therapy has not affected chest relapse or survival in SCLC and cannot be currently recommended outside of randomized trials.

Non-Cross-Resistant Alternating Drug Regimens

The use of non-cross-resistant regimens has become an attractive combination in exploration for SCLC treatment, especially with the demonstrable tumor heterogeneity and drug sensitivity of the disease. The NCI added VAP (vincristine, adriamycin, and procarbazine) at weeks 6 to 12 after induction therapy with cyclophosphamide, methotrexate, and CCNU (CMC); increasing the overall and complete response rates, but not influencing survival.[17] Tables 25-2 and 25-5 show chest failure rates for this trial,[17] which demonstrated no improvement in primary chest disease control compared to similar regimens. Sierocki and colleagues from the Memorial Sloan Kettering Cancer Center examined alternation of two 3-drug regimens for limited and extensive SCLC patients, CAV, and bleomycin, methotrexate, and procarbazine (BMP) and administered local chest radiation to patients with less than a complete response or recurrent chest disease.[95] Median survival time was proved similar to other regimens (limited stage 11.5 months, extensive stage 7.5 months). When examining chest failure patterns in 26 patients, they found 22 out of 34 sites of initial relapse within the lungs or mediastinum.

Several investigators have utilized etoposide in alternating drug regimens. Treating 29 extensive-stage SCLC patients, Dillman and colleagues alternated cycles of cyclophosphamide, methotrexate, and etoposide (CME) with adriamycin, methotrexate, and etoposide (AME) for responders from induction therapy with hexamethylmelamine, cyclophosphamide, adriamycin, and vincristine (HCAV).[23] As shown in Table 25-4, they evaluated 10 complete responders who received chest consolidation radiotherapy while in complete remission; 6 out of 10 relapsed in lung, together with concurrent disease progression at other sites. Analyzing relapse patterns in limited disease patients, Markman et al. alternated an etoposide-containing regimen (etoposide, hexamethylmelamine, and methotrexate) with CAV.[64] Both cyclophosphamide and etoposide were given at higher than normal doses. Table 25-1 details their data, revealing 4 chest failures from 16 complete responders. However, only two relapsed solely in the chest at the primary site.

The use of etoposide with cisplatin has demonstrated significant activity for SCLC at presentation, with results similar to standard induction regimens.[28] Nonrandomized trials that alternated regimens of CAV and EcDDP (etoposide and cisplatin) at the Memorial Sloan Kettering Cancer Center demonstrated modestly improved complete response and median survival rates for limited-stage patients.[75,91] However, both trials showed similar chest failure rates to other commonly used regimens (Table 25-1). Administering etoposide and cisplatin as intensification agents immediately following induction therapy, the Southeast Cancer Study Group reported preliminary data in limited-disease patients, achieving partial or complete response, and thereafter randomized to two cycles of intensification with etoposide and cisplatin or to no intensification.[38] The intensification-treated patients demonstrated significant improved median survival, with complete remission patients achieving more durable remissions. The potential delay or change in relapse rates awaits analysis.

Several randomized trials have addressed the potential survival advantage of alternating regimens including etoposide and cisplatin alternating with CAV. In limited stage patients, Feld and coworkers[30] examined randomized treatment between sequential CAV for 3 courses followed by etoposide and cisplatin for 3 courses compared to alternating therapy with CAV and etoposide-cisplatin for 6 courses. Responding patients received prophylactic cranial irradiation and thoracic irradiation. They found no difference in complete response rate or survival between sequential or alternating methods of non-cross-resistant regimen delivery. The same group of investigators studied extensive stage patients; comparing 6 courses of CAV to 6 treatment cycles of CAV alternating with etoposide and cisplatin.[27] They found significantly higher overall and complete response attainment and superior progression free survival for patients treated with the alternating drug regimen. Overall median survival, however, was only slightly improved for the alternating group: 9.8 versus 7.8 months.

Thus far, non-cross-resistant alternating drug regimens have not added a significant survival advantage. Randomized trials of alternating regimens including etoposide and cisplatin combinations are in progress.

Late Intensification

Late-intensification regimens have not yet demonstrated improved disease control or survival attainment for SCLC patients. Similar to other treatment schemes, the ultimate value may likely be appreciated first for limited-stage patients. A group from Belgium has shown data suggesting that limited-stage patients have improved response duration when randomized to receive late-intensification chemotherapy and autologous bone marrow transplantation; long-term follow-up was incomplete.[51] Ihde and colleagues from the NCI treated extensive-stage patients with CMC (cyclophosphamide, methotrexate, and CCNU) induction, and then administered late intensification to complete and partial responders.[52] Intensification consisted of irradiation to sites of initial tumor involvement followed by high-dose cyclophosphamide and etoposide chemotherapy and autologous marrow infusion. Of 29 patients, 8 received intensification. Sites of relapse for 2 out of 3 patients in prior complete remission were identical to areas of initial involvement that received irradiation during intensification. No patient survived for 2 years, and two treatment-related deaths were recorded. Treatment with late intensification in this case produced increased toxicity without relapse prevention or survival gain.

Other trials of late intensification have not shown overall survival benefit. Its use in complete responders holds the most promise to demonstrate improved survival.

INTRACRANIAL RELAPSE AND THE ROLE OF PROPHYLACTIC CRANIAL IRRADIATION (PCI)

Central nervous system (CNS) metastases are a major problem for patients with SCLC, especially since the major chemotherapeutic agents do not cross the blood-brain barrier. Autopsy series demonstrate high CNS metastases compared to clinically evident manifestations. Nugent and colleagues confirmed CNS dissemination by showing CNS SCLC involvement in 55 out of 85 autopsied SCLC patients; 54 had intracranial disease.[77] They furthermore demonstrated an 80 percent 2-year actuarial probability of developing CNS metastasis for 209 patients retrospectively reviewed; about 10 percent of these patients had intracranial disease at diagnosis.

The utility of PCI in preventing development of intracranial SCLC metastases is clear, although it has no established value for increasing survival duration. Rosen and co-workers performed a large retrospective review of 332 SCLC patients at the NCI[85] and formed several conclusions: (1) PCI has maximum potential utility in complete responders from induction therapy; as fewer intracranial metastases and improved 2-year survival appeared for complete responders who had received PCI compared to patients not receiving PCI, although the differences were not statistically significant; (2) patients not achieving a complete response showed no significant relationship between PCI administration and development of CNS metastases; and (3) PCI did not influence the development of leptomeningeal, spinal, or epidural metastases. Their study furthermore showed CNS metastases as the first and only site of relapse from complete response status in 17 percent of patients who had not received PCI, while no patient receiving PCI relapsed solely in the CNS. To improve cure rates for SCLC, the major issue must be examination of primary CNS relapse from complete response.

A relatively small number of trials report intracranial failure data distinctly for limited- and extensive-stage patients. Tables 25-6 and 25-7 review these nonrandomized trials. Notably, among eleven trials[15,23,29,31,37,40,57,62,63,82,97] administering PCI and examining relapse from complete remission in limited- or extensive-stage disease; six of 104 (5.8 percent) limited-stage patients relapsed intracranially after complete response, and 5 out of 97 (5.2 percent) extensive-stage patients relapsed intracranially from complete response status. However, only two failures in each group of complete responders relapsed initially in the brain. For limited-stage patients who received PCI, intracranial failure increased to 11.5 percent (32/279) for all evaluable intracranial failures regardless of response status. This compares to a 32.4 percent (132/408) intracranial failure rate for evaluable limited-stage patients not receiving PCI as detailed in Table 25-7.[3,9,32,87,96]

The majority of published trials report intracranial failure rates for limited- and extensive-stage patients combined. Our review of an additional 13 nonrandomized trials administering PCI[1,4,25,43,46,47,54,60,64,68,85,90,94] and 10 nonrandomized trials not administering PCI,[1,4,14,46,49,60,61,76,85,95] combined with Tables 25-6 and 25-7, yielded the following results for limited- and extensive-stage patients together: 24 trials delivering PCI had a 8.4 percent (26/308) intracranial relapse from complete response status compared to 36.8 percent (53/144) in 15 trials without PCI. In the PCI trials there were 11.3 percent (145/1286) who had intracranial relapse regardless of response compared to 29.7 percent (306/1030) intracranial failures in non-PCI trials.

Randomized trials of PCI confirm the improved prevention of intracranial metastases. Results from each trial with its intracranial failure rates for limited and extensive

Table 25-6

Intracranial Relapse in SCLC Patients Treated with Prophylactic Cranial Irradiation

Stage	PCI Dose (Rads)	Number of Patients	CR (%)	Number of Intracranial Failures from CR/No. CR (%) Limited	Extensive	Total No. Intracranial Failures/No. Evaluable (%) Limited	Extensive	Reference
LD	2000–3000	36	75	0/27* (0)	—	0/27* (0)	—	57
ED	2000–3000	35	40	—	1/14 (7)	—	1/14 (7)	57
LD	3000	28	41	2/28* (7)	—	2/28* (7)	—	63
ED	3000	83	14	—	NR	—	9/83 (11)	63
LD	3500	53	40	NR	—	4/53 (7)	—	82
LD	3000	55	43	2/20 (10)	—	2/20 (10)	—	15
ED	3000	106	30	—	1/25 (4)	—	1/25 (4)	15
ED	2000	14	38	—	NR	—	0/14 (0)	23
ED	3000	28	24	—	NR	—	2/28 (7)	40
LD	3000	8	50	0/4* (0)	—	0/8* (0)	1/5* (20)	29
ED	3000	5	40	—	0/2* (0)	—	2/5 (40)	29
LD	4000	33	76	2/25 (8)	—	2/25 (8)	—	37
ED	4000	38	34	—	1/13 (8)	—	1/13 (8)	37
LD	2000	92	NR	NR	—	10/92* (11); 21/92 (23)	—	31
ED	2000	98	NR	—	NR	—	19/98* (19); 44/98 (45)	
ED	3000	429	16	—	2/43* (5)	—	7/195* (4)	62
LD	2000	26	50	NR	—	1/26* (4)	—	97
				2/59* (3.4); 6/104 (5.8)	2/45* (4.4); 5/97 (5.2)	13/181* (7.2); 32/279 (11.5)	27/298* (9.1); 67/475 (14.1)	

Abbreviations: CR = complete response = complete regression of tumor; PCI = prophylactic cranial irradiation; LD = limited-stage disease; ED = extensive-stage disease; NR = not reported.

*Intracranial failure represents the initial site of relapse.

Table 25-7

Intracranial Relapse in SCLC Patients not Receiving Prophylactic Cranial Irradiation

Stage	Number of Patients	CR (%)	Total No. Intracranial Failures†/No. Evaluable (%)				Reference
			Limited		Extensive		
LD	23	23	3/15*	20	—		3
			6/15	40	—		
LD	40	24	10/40*	25	—		32
			18/40	45	—		
ED	39	10	—		5/39*	13	
			—		11/39	28	
LD	236	NR	67/236	28	—		9
LD	89	70	23/89*	26	—		87
			33/89	37	—		
LD	28	29	8/28	28	—		96
ED	24	13	—		2/24	8	
			36/144*	25.0	5/39*	12.8	
			132/408	32.4	13/63	20.6	

Abbreviations: CR = complete response; NR = not reported; LD = limited-stage disease; ED = extensive-stage disease.

* Intracranial failure represents the initial site of relapse.

† These trials did not report intracranial relapse from complete response status.

stage patients are presented in Table 25-8.[2,6,21,24,41,53,67,89] Two trials demonstrated minimal decrease in intracranial relapse for PCI over non-PCI.[21,41] The remaining six trials demonstrated significantly decreased intracranial relapse by PCI. In summary, 3.4 percent (4/119) of limited- and extensive-stage SCLC patients developed intracranial relapse as an initial site of failure following PCI, while 12.2 percent (14/115) of limited- and extensive-stage SCLC patients failed intracranially initially when not given PCI. Only one trial of Aisner and colleagues randomized patients to PCI or non-PCI from complete response status.[2] There were no intracranial failures in the complete responders receiving PCI. Unfortunately, the study was discontinued before valid statistical conclusions could be determined. The small numbers of patients in this trial as well as four other randomized trials contributed largely to insignificant survival gains. The ultimate significance of intracranial failure prevention must be determined by potential survival advantage; none of these eight randomized trials show improvement in survival with PCI administration. Furthermore, the extensive-disease patients have survival duration primarily determined by systemic relapse.

PCI has been suggested to be a likely contributor to neurologic abnormalities found in long-term survivors of SCLC, including memory difficulties, gait abnormalities, intention tremors, and abnormal mental status examinations.[55] Johnson et al. reported that 15 of 20 long-term survivors on NCI protocols had neurologic complaints; 13, abnormal neurologic examinations; 12, abnormal mental status examinations; and 15, abnormal CT scans (ventricular dilatation and cerebral atrophy).[55] They found an association of increased neurologic impairment in patients receiving high-dose induction chemotherapy during PCI and for patients treated with larger radiotherapy fractions (400 vs 200–300 rads). Future randomized trials studying large

Table 25-8

Intracranial Failure Rates for Randomized Trials Evaluating Prophylactic Cranial Irradiation in SCLC

Stage	Chemo	Chest RT	PCI	Dose/Time	Total Intracranial Failure/No. Evaluable (%)				Reference
					PCI		No PCI		
LD + ED	+	+	Yes	3000/Initial	0/14*	0	—		53
LD + ED	+	+	No	None	—		1/15*	7	
							4/15	27	
LD	−	+	Yes	2000/Initial	4/24	17	—		21
LD	−	+	No	None	—		5/21	24	
LD	+	+	Yes	2400/Delayed	0/13*	0	—		6
LD	+	+	No	None	—		2/17*	12	
ED	+	+	Yes	2400/Delayed	0/10*	0	—		
ED	+	+	No	None	—		3/14*	21	
LD	+	+†	Yes	4000/Delayed	2/54*	4	—		41
					5/54	9	—		
LD	+	+‡	No	None	—		2/55*	4	
					—		7/55	13	
LD + ED	+	+	Yes	3000/Initial	3/79	4	—		67
LD + ED	+	+	No	None	—		15/84	18	
LD	+	−	Yes	3600/Delayed	2/13*,**	15	—		24§
LD	+	−	No	None	—		6/14*	43	
LD + ED	+	−	Yes	3000/Delayed	0/15*,††	0	—		2††
LD + ED	+	−	No	None	—		5/14††	36	
LD	+/−	+	Yes	3000/Initial	5/106	5	—		89
LD	+/−	+	No	None	—		24/111	22	
					4/119*	3.4	14/115*	12.2	
					19/328	5.8	71/345	20.6	

Abbreviations: Chemo = chemotherapy; PCI = prophylactic cranial irradiation; LD = limited-stage disease; ED = extensive-stage disease; RT = radiation therapy; Dose = dose in rads; Time = Initial or Delayed course chest radiotherapy.

*Intracranial failure represents the initial site of relapse.

†Radiotherapy included "extensive" treatment to primary tumor, regional nodes, brain, adrenals, and upper retroperitoneal nodes.

‡Radiotherapy included primary tumor and regional nodes only.

§Patients not receiving PCI were given a mannitol infusion concurrent with chemotherapy administration.

**Both intracranial relapses were prior to PCI administration.

††Only trial randomizing patients to PCI from complete response status.

numbers of patients randomized to PCI from a complete remission, with primary intracranial failure rates examined independently for limited and extensive stage patients, hold promise to evaluate potential survival gain for PCI.

LEPTOMENINGEAL CARCINOMATOSIS AND SPINAL CORD COMPRESSION

Leptomeningeal carcinomatosis and spinal cord compression are relatively uncommon at diagnosis of SCLC, although improved disease free survival has produced significant failure at these sites for long-term survivors. Nugent et al. demonstrated autopsy leptomeningeal involvement in 24 out of 55 cases and spinal cord tumor in 13 out of 55 cases. They found a high correlation for the presence of initial bone marrow involvement and eventual development of leptomeningeal spread ($p < .001$).

As suggested for the development of intracranial metastases, leptomeningeal spread is increased in patients responsive to therapy and achieving longer survival, analogous to sanctuary sites of disease in diffuse lymphomas or leukemias. At autopsy, Elliott and colleagues detected a 24 percent (7/29) incidence of meningeal involvement in patients previously attaining complete response status, while 10 percent (9/86) patients achieving prior partial response had meningeal metastases.[26]

The incidence of spinal cord compression in SCLC may vary from 3.5 to 14 percent.[40,80] Patients may experience significant morbidity with paraplegia, pain, and death from nerve root compression and tumor expansion.

Investigators have found that PCI does not influence the development of leptomeningeal carcinomatosis, spinal cord compression, or epidural metastases.[85] Although 3-15 percent of patients with long-term survival may develop these lesions, their appearance frequently signals the presence of other metastatic disease. The addition of high-dose methotrexate or other chemotherapeutic regimens has not significantly affected their occurrence.[47,76] Craniospinal irradiation has been suggested as a prophylactic measure; however, marrow toxicity would be significant and impair delivery of adequate systemic chemotherapy. Since these particular CNS failure sites occur rarely as a sole site of relapse, and most often with multifocal systemic relapse, studying local modalities to significantly influence their occurrence would require large numbers of patients. Current trials studying systemic treatments may more realistically affect later CNS failure.

INTRA-ABDOMINAL RELAPSE

The liver, bone and bone marrow, adrenals, upper abdominal nodes, pancreas, and kidneys are all sites of common involvement at presentation and at autopsy in SCLC patients. Many of these sites present with clinically silent lesions and therefore are not discovered by usual investigative studies.

Elliott and colleagues performed a large retrospective review of postmortem material collected from 537 SCLC patients treated on several Finsen Institute protocols from 1973 through 1981.[26] Intra-abdominal autopsy distribution for patients initially presenting with limited- versus extensive-stage disease is as follows: (1) liver, 60.5 percent (130/215) versus 73.5 percent (197/268); (2) bone and bone marrow, 44.8 percent (73/163) versus 56.2 percent (127/226); (3) adrenals, 31.6 percent (68/215) versus 35.0 percent (93/266); (4) retroperitoneal lymph nodes, 28.2 percent (51/181) versus 28.6 percent (63/220); (5) pancreas, 13.6 percent (29/213) versus 17.4 percent (46/264); and (6) kidneys, 8.1 percent (17/210) versus 16.0 percent (42/263). As may be expected when limited-stage patients fail and die of disseminated disease depicted at autopsy, the autopsy organ involvement figures are similar for limited- and extensive-stage patients. Disease was found in a significantly higher percent of autopsied patients presenting initially with extensive-stage tumor compared to limited-stage patients for the liver ($p < .01$), bone and bone marrow ($p < .05$), and the kidneys ($p < .05$).

Table 25-9
Hepatic Relapse in SCLC Treated with Combined-Modality Therapy

Stage	Chest RT	PCI	Number of Patients	CR (%)	Number of Hepatic Failures from CR/No. CR (%) — Limited		Extensive		Total No. Hepatic Failures/No. Evaluable (%) — Limited		Extensive		Reference
LD	+	+	36	75	0/27*	0	—		0/27*	0	—	—	57
ED	+	+	35	40	—		2/14	14	—		2/14	14	
LD	+	+	108	41	2/28*	7	—		2/28*	7	—		63
ED	+	+	250	14	—		NR		—		14/66*	21	
LD	−	+	30	40	0/12*	0	—		2/15*	13	—		24
LD	+	+	27	50	NR		—		8/27	30	—		82
LD	+	+	55	43	3/20	15	—		3/20	15	—		15
ED	+	+	106	30	—		9/25	36	—		9/25	36	
LD	+/−	+	8	62	2/5	40	—		3/8	37	—		29
ED	+/−	+	5	40	—		0/2*	0	—		0/5*	0	
LD	+	+	33	76	3/25	12	—		3/25	12	—		37
ED	+	+	38	34	—		7/13	54	—		7/13	54	
LD	+	+	153	52	NR		—		7/92*	8	—		31
ED	+	+	167	10	—		NR		—		14/98*	14	
LD	+/−	+/−	11	45	1/5*	20	—		2/5*	40	—		88†
ED	−	+/−	4	75	—		1/3*	33	—		1/4*	25	
LD	+	+	26	50	NR		—		14/26*	54	—		97
					3/72*	4.2	1/5*	20.0	27/193*	14.0	29/173*	16.8	
					11/122	9.0	19/57	33.3	44/273	16.1	47/225	20.9	

Abbreviations: CR = complete response = complete regression of tumor; RT = radiation therapy; PCI = prophylactic cranial irradiation; LD = limited stage disease; ED = extensive-stage disease; NR = not reported.
*Hepatic failure represents the initial site of relapse.
†Trial examined late intensification with high-dose etoposide and high-dose cisplatin.

Our clinical ability to detect liver metastases has been improved at initial staging procedures by several complementary procedures, including peritoneoscopy and hepatic biopsy, percutaneous hepatic biopsy, ultrasound, or CT scan of the abdomen. When studied sequentially at the NCI in 157 consecutive patients, peritoneoscopic hepatic biopsy following percutaneous hepatic biopsy increased the discovery of hepatic metastases from 18 to 27 patients.[74] Similarly, the Finsen Institute demonstrated complementary hepatic staging when comparing peritoneoscopic hepatic biopsy to ultrasonographic fine-needle aspiration.[42] Of 131 patients, 33 (25 percent) had hepatic SCLC involvement, with 82 percent detection of tumor by ultrasound and 76 percent by peritoneoscopic approach.

Such involved staging typically is not performed or needed at relapse of SCLC. Symptoms due to chest or from CNS relapse may more often herald relapse. However, trials that examined hepatic failures show significant eventual hepatic failure. Table 25-9 details nonrandomized trials that have studied hepatic relapse.[15,24,29,31,37,57,63,82,88,97] Only 3 out of 72 (4.2 percent) limited-stage patients in complete remission had hepatic relapse as an initial clinically detected failure site, although the numbers are small; while 16.1 percent of limited-stage and 20.9 percent of extensive-stage patients eventually relapsed in the liver.

Randomized trials examining the utility of radiation to abdominal sites including hepatic irradiation have shown no significant change in abdominal failure pattern for radiated patients over patients not irradiated. Autopsy studies confirm this finding, although Elliott and colleagues found a significant decrease in pancreatic metastases at autopsy ($p < .05$) for patients receiving prophylactic abdominal irradiation.[26] Of 29 irradiated patients, 2 had pancreatic metastases, as compared to eleven of 31 autopsied patients not receiving prophylactic irradiation; while failures in the liver, adrenals and retroperitoneal nodes were not significantly different for either group.

Intra-abdominal relapse often occurs in combination with multiple abdominal sites together with thoracic or CNS dissemination. The multifocal nature of spread has made local measures ineffective. These sites of failure strongly support the need for improved systemic measures.

CONCLUSIONS

Relapse rates in SCLC have demonstrated our treatment success and failures. Limited-stage patients demonstrated superior primary tumor control when treated with bimodality therapy, although this translates to only modest survival advantage in randomized trials when compared to combination chemotherapy alone. Optimal methods for radiation delivery, including fractionization, dose, timing, and shielding are not known. Surgery has current utility for resection of the rare $T_1N_0M_0$ SCLC, and adjuvant chemotherapy after resection will, hopefully, prolong survival in these patients. To further decrease chest relapse and potentially improve survival, a prospective randomized trial is currently evaluating adjuvant surgery following chemotherapy and prior to consolidation chest radiotherapy compared to chemotherapy and chest radiotherapy alone.

Even with improved local control, however, systemic relapse dominates extensive-stage patients and plays a major role for therapeutic failure in limited-stage patients. Radiation therapy reduction of chest failure in extensive disease has not shown survival advantage.

Optimal agents, dose intensity, maintenance regimens, alternating non-cross-resistant regimens, and late-intensification treatments are currently under study in multiple trials. Thus far, these variations have not shown a significant diminution in chest failure or improved survival advantage.

Intra-abdominal relapse occurs in significant numbers of limited- and extensive-stage patients. Clinical series underestimate its frequency at relapse, while autopsy series highlight the disseminated nature of SCLC. Radiation randomly applied to prophylactic abdominal fields and to the liver has not influenced abdominal failure patterns or survival.

Prophylactic cranial irradiation has significantly decreased morbidity for intracranial failure. While it has decreased intracranial failure in both nonrandomized and randomized trials, no survival gain has been demonstrated for patients randomly assigned to receive PCI over no cranial irradiation. PCI holds the most promise for patients achieving complete remission, as they may survive long enough to benefit. PCI has produced some increased CNS toxicity for long-term disease-free survivors; including dementia, gait disturbances, and memory loss. Sanctuary sites of SCLC appear in the leptomeninges and spinal cord and are unusual as sole sites of initial relapse.

Increased biologic understandings of SCLC growth, including growth factor stimulation, HLA expression, and demonstrable antigenic expressions, have produced potential additional therapeutic modalities, such as monoclonal antibodies. The addition of these agents holds promise to attain additional complete response, complete remission maintenance, and lengthened survival duration.

REFERENCES

1. Abeloff MD, Ettinger DS, Order SE, et al: Intensive chemotherapy in 54 patients with small cell carcinoma of the lung. Cancer Treat Rep 65:639-646, 1981
2. Aisner J, Whitacre M, Van Echo DA, et al: Combination chemotherapy for small cell carcinoma of the lung: Continuous versus alternating non-cross-resistant combinations. Cancer Treat Rep 66:221-230, 1982
3. Alexander M, Glatstein EJ, Gordon DS, et al: Combined modality treatment for oat cell carcinoma of the lung: A randomized trial. Cancer Treat Rep 61:1-6, 1977
4. Aroney RS, Aisner J, Wesley MN, et al: Value of prophylactic cranial irradiation given at complete remission in small cell lung carcinoma. Cancer Treat Rep 67:675-682, 1983
5. Arriagada R, Chevalier TL, Baldeyrou P, et al: Alternating radiotherapy and chemotherapy schedules in small cell lung cancer, limited disease. Internatl J Radiat Oncol Biol Phys 11:1461-1467, 1985
6. Beiler DD, Kane RC, Bernath AM, et al: Low dose elective brain irradiation in small cell carcinoma of the lung. Internatl J Radiat Oncol Biol Phys 5:941-945, 1979
7. Bergsagel D, Jenkin R, Pringle J, et al: Lung cancer: Clinical trial of radiotherapy alone vs. radiotherapy plus cyclophosphamide. Cancer 30:621-627, 1972
8. Bleehen NM, Bunn PA Jr, Cox JD, et al: Role of radiation therapy in small cell anaplastic carcinoma of the lung. Cancer Treat Rep 67:11-19, 1983
9. Bleehen NM, Cleland WP, Deeley TJ, et al: Radiotherapy alone or with chemotherapy in the treatment of small-cell carcinoma of the lung: The results at 36 months. Br J Cancer 44:611, 1981

10. Brower M, Ihde DC, Johnston-Early A, et al: Treatment of extensive stage small cell bronchogenic carcinoma: Effects of variation in intensity of induction chemotherapy. Am J Med 75:993-1000, 1983

11. Bunn PA Jr, Cohen MH, Ihde DC, et al: Advances in small cell bronchogenic carcinoma. Cancer Treat Rep 61:333-342, 1977

12. Bunn PA, Ihde DC: Small cell bronchogenic carcinoma: A review of therapeutic results, in Livingston RB (ed): Lung Cancer I. The Hague, Martinus Nijhoff, 1981, pp 169-208

13. Bunn PA Jr, Lichter AS, Makuch RW, et al: Chemotherapy alone or chemotherapy with chest radiation therapy in limited stage small cell lung cancer: A prospective, randomized trial. Ann Intern Med 106:655-662, 1987

14. Byhardt RW, Libnoch JA, Cox JD, et al: Local control of intrathoracic disease with chemotherapy and role of prophylactic cranial irradiation in small-cell carcinoma of the lung. Cancer 47:2239-2246, 1981

15. Chak LY, Daniels JR, Sikic BI, et al: Patterns of failure of small cell carcinoma of the lung. Cancer 50:1857-1863, 1982

16. Cohen MH, Creaven PJ, Fossieck BE Jr, et al: Intensive chemotherapy of small cell bronchogenic carcinoma. Cancer Treat Rep 61:349-354, 1977

17. Cohen MH, Ihde DC, Bunn PA Jr, et al: Cyclic alternating combination chemotherapy for small cell bronchogenic carcinoma. Cancer Treat Rep 63:163-170, 1979

18. Cohen MH, Matthews MJ: Small cell bronchogenic carcinoma: A distinct clinicopathologic entity. Semin Oncol 5:234-243, 1978

19. Comis RL: The role of surgery in small cell lung cancer: A reappraisal. Clin Oncol 4(1):141-150, 1985

20. Cox JD, Byhardt R, Komaki R, et al: Interaction of thoracic irradiation and chemotherapy on local control and survival in small cell carcinoma of the lung. Cancer Treat Rep 63:1251-1255, 1979

21. Cox JD, Petrovich Z, Paig C, et al: Prophylactic cranial irradiation in patients with inoperable carcinoma of the lung: Preliminary report of a cooperative trial. Cancer 42:1135-1140, 1978

22. Cullen MH: Maintenance chemotherapy for small cell lung cancer: A randomized controlled trial (Abstr), in Proceedings of the International Association for the Study of Lung Cancer. Copenhagen, International Association for the Study of Lung Cancer, 1984, p 43

23. Dillman RO, Taetle R, Seagren S, et al: Extensive disease small cell carcinoma of the lung. Cancer 49:2003-2008, 1982

24. Eagan RT, Creagan ET, Frytak S, et al: A case for preplanned thoracic and prophylactic whole brain radiation therapy in limited small-cell lung cancer. Cancer Clin Trials 4:261-266, 1981

25. Einhorn LH, Bond WH, Hornback N, et al: Long-term results in combined modality treatment of small cell carcinoma of the lung. Semin Oncol 5:309-313, 1978

26. Elliott JA, Osterlind K, Hirsch FR, et al: Metastatic patterns in small-cell lung cancer: Correlation of autopsy findings with clinical parameters in 537 patients. J Clin Oncol 5:246-254, 1987

27. Evans K, Murray N, Feld R, et al: Canadian multicenter randomized trial comparing standard (SD) and alternating (A) combination chemotherapy in extensive small cell lung cancer (SCLC). Proc Am Soc Clin Oncol 5:169, 1986

28. Evans WK, Shepherd FA, Feld R, et al: VP-16 and cisplatin as first-line therapy for small-cell lung cancer. J Clin Oncol 3:1471-1477, 1985

29. Farha P, Spitzer G, Valdivieso M, et al: High-dose chemotherapy and autologous bone marrow transplantation for the treatment of small cell lung carcinoma. Cancer 52:1351-1355, 1983

30. Feld R, Evans WK, Coy P, et al: Canadian multicentre randomized trial comparing

sequential (S) and alternating (A) administration of two non-cross resistant chemotherapy combinations in patients with limited small cell carcinoma of the lung (SCCL). Proc Am Soc Clin Oncol 4:177, 1985

31. Feld R, Evans WK, DeBoer G, et al: Combined modality induction therapy without maintenance chemotherapy for small cell carcinoma of the lung. J Clin Oncol 2:294–304, 1984

32. Feld R, Pringle JF, Evans WK, et al: Combined modality treatment of small cell carcinoma of the lung. Arch Intern Med 141:469–473, 1981

33. Foster JM, Preger RL, Hainsworth JD, et al: Limited-stage small cell carcinoma (SCC): Prospective evaluation regarding the feasibility of adjuvant surgery. Proc Am Soc Clin Oncol 2:196, 1983

34. Fox W, Scadding JG: Medical Research Council comparative trial of surgery and radiotherapy for primary treatment of small-celled or oat-celled carcinoma of bronchus. Lancet 2:63–65, 1973

35. Fox RM, Woods RL, Brodie GN, et al: A randomized study: Small cell anaplastic lung cancer treated by combination chemotherapy and adjuvant radiotherapy. Internatl J Radiat Oncol Biol Phys 6:1083–1085, 1980

36. Friess GG, McCracken JD, Troxell ML, et al: Effect of initial resection of small-cell carcinoma of the lung: A review of Southwest Oncology Group Study 7628. J Clin Oncol 3:964–968, 1985

37. Goodman GE, Miller TP, Manning MM: Treatment of small cell lung cancer with VP-16, vincristine, doxorubicin (adriamycin), cyclophosphamide (EVAC), and high-dose chest radiotherapy. J Clin Oncol 1:483–488, 1983

38. Greco FA, Perez C, Einhorn LH, et al: Combination chemotherapy with or without concurrent thoracic radiotherapy (RT) in limited-stage (LD) small cell lung cancer (SCLC): A phase III trial of the Southeastern Cancer Study Group (SEG). Proc Am Soc Clin Oncol 5:178, 1986

39. Greco F, Richardson RL, Snell JD, et al: Small cell lung cancer: Complete remission and improved survival. Am J Med 66:625–630, 1979

40. Hande KR, Oldham RK, Mehmet FF, et al: Randomized study of high-dose versus low-dose methotrexate in the treatment of extensive small cell lung cancer. Am J Med 73:413–419, 1982

41. Hansen HH, Dombernowsky P, Hirsch FR, et al: Prophylactic irradiation in bronchogenic small cell anaplastic carcinoma. Cancer 46:279–284, 1980

42. Hansen SW, Jansen F, Pederson NT, et al: Detection of liver metastases in small-cell lung cancer: A comparison of peritoneoscopy with liver biopsy and ultrasonography with fine-needle aspiration. J Clin Oncol 5:255–259, 1987

43. Herman TS, Jones SE, McMahon LJ, et al: Combination chemotherapy with adriamycin and cyclophosphamide (with or without radiation therapy) for carcinoma of the lung. Cancer Treat Rep 61:875–879, 1977

44. Higgins GA: Use of chemotherapy as an adjuvant to surgery for bronchogenic carcinoma. Cancer 30:1383–1387, 1972

45. Higgins GA, Shields TW, Keehn RJ: The solitary pulmonary nodule: Ten-year follow-up of Veterans Administration-Armed Forces cooperative study. Arch Surg 110:570–575, 1975

46. Hoffman PC, Golomb HM, Bitran JD, et al: Small cell carcinoma of the lung: A five-year experience with combined modality therapy. Cancer 46:2550–2556, 1980

47. Holoye PY, Libnoch JA, Anderson T, et al: Combined methotrexate and high-dose vincristine chemotherapy with radiation therapy for small cell bronchogenic carcinoma. Cancer 55:1436–1445, 1985

48. Holoye P, Libnoch J, Cox J, et al: Spinal cord metastasis in small cell carcinoma of the lung. Internatl J Radiat Oncol Biol Phys 10:349–356, 1984

49. Holoye PY, Samuels ML, Lanzotti VJ, et al: Combination chemotherapy and radiation therapy for small cell carcinoma. JAMA 237:1221-1224, 1977

50. Host H: Cyclophosphamide (NSC-26271) as adjuvant to radiotherapy in the treatment of unresectable bronchogenic carcinoma. Cancer Chemother Rep 4:161-164, 1973

51. Humblet Y, Symann M, Bosly A, et al: Late intensification (LI) with autologous bone marrow transplantation (ABMT) for small cell lung cancer: A randomized trial. Proc Am Soc Clin Oncol 4:176, 1985

52. Ihde DC, Deisseroth AB, Lichter AS, et al: Late intensive combined modality therapy followed by autologous bone marrow infusion in extensive-stage small-cell lung cancer. J Clin Oncol 4:1443-1454, 1986

53. Jackson DV Jr, Richards F, Cooper MR, et al: Prophylactic cranial irradiation in small cell carcinoma of the lung: A randomized study. JAMA 237:2730-2733, 1977

54. Jackson DV Jr, Zekan PJ, Caldwell RD, et al: VP-16-213 in combination chemotherapy with chest irradiation for small-cell lung cancer: A randomized trial of the Piedmont Oncology Association. J Clin Oncol 2:1341-1351, 1984

55. Johnson BE, Becker B, Goff WB, et al: Neurologic, neuropsychologic and computed cranial tomography scan abnormalities in 2 to 10 year survivors of small cell lung cancer. J Clin Oncol 3:1659-1667, 1985

56. Johnson DH, Wolff SN, Hainsworth JD, et al: Extensive-stage small cell bronchogenic carcinoma: Intensive induction chemotherapy with high-dose cyclophosphamide plus high-dose etoposide. J Clin Oncol 3:170-175, 1985

57. Johnson RE, Brereton HD, Kent CH: "Total" therapy for small cell carcinoma of the lung. Ann Thorac Surg 25:510-515, 1978

58. Karrer K, Pridun N, Denek H: Chemotherapy as an adjuvant to surgery in lung cancer. Cancer Chemother Pharmacol 1:145-159, 1978

59. Kirklin JW, McDonald JR, Clagett OT, et al: Bronchogenic carcinoma: Cell type and other factors relating to prognosis. Surg Gynecol Obstet 100:429-438, 1955

60. Komaki R, Cox JD, Whitson W: Risk of brain metastasis from small cell carcinoma of the lung related to length of survival and prophylactic irradiation. Cancer Treat Rep 65:811-814, 1981

61. Kreisman H, Wolkove N, Cohen C, et al: Multifocal relapse after concurrent chemotherapy and radiotherapy of small cell lung cancer. Cancer 50:873-876, 1982

62. Livingston RB, Mira JG, Chen TT, et al: Combined modality treatment of extensive small cell lung cancer: A Southwest Oncology Group Study. J Clin Oncol 2:585-590, 1984

63. Livingston RB, Moore TN, Heilbrun L, et al: Small-cell carcinoma of the lung: Combined chemotherapy and radiation: A Southwest Oncology Group Study. Ann Intern Med 88:194-199, 1978

64. Markman M, Abeloff MD, Berkman AW, et al: Intensive alternating chemotherapy regimen in small cell carcinoma of the lung. Cancer Treat Rep 69:161-166, 1985

65. Mason BA, Richter MP, Catalano RB, et al: Upper hemibody and local chest irradiation as consolidation following response to high-dose induction chemotherapy for small cell bronchogenic carcinoma—a pilot study. Cancer Treat Rep 66:1609-1612, 1982

66. Matthiessen W: Controlled clinical trial of radiotherapy alone, against radiotherapy plus chemotherapy in small-cell carcinoma of the lung: Comparison of radiation damage. Scand J Resp Dis (Suppl) 102:209-211, 1978

67. Maurer LH, Tulloh M, Weiss RB, et al: A randomized combined modality trial in small cell carcinoma of the lung. Cancer 45:31-39, 1980

68. McMahon LJ, Herman TS, Manning MR, et al: Patterns of relapse in patients with small cell carcinoma of the lung treated with adriamycin-cyclophosphamide chemotherapy and radiation therapy. Cancer Treat Rep 63:359-362, 1979

69. Medical Research Council: Study of cytotoxic chemotherapy as an adjuvant to surgery in carcinoma of the bronchus. Br Med J 2:421-428, 1971

70. Minna JD, Higgins GA, Glatstein EJ: Cancer of the lung, in DeVita VT, Hellman S, Rosenberg S (eds): Principles and Practice of Oncology. Philadelphia, Lippincott, 1985, pp 507-597

71. Mira JG, Livingston RB: Evaluation and radiotherapy implications of chest relapse patterns in small cell lung carcinoma treated with radiotherapy-chemotherapy. Cancer 46:2557-2565, 1980

72. Mira JG, Livingston RB, Moore TN, et al: Influence of chest radiotherapy in frequency and patterns in chest relapse in disseminated small cell lung carcinoma. Cancer 50:1266-1272, 1982

73. Mountain CF, Carr DT, Anderson WAD: A system for the clinical staging of lung cancer. Am J Roentgenol 120:130-138, 1974

74. Mulshine JL, Makuch RW, Johnston-Early A, et al: Diagnosis and significance of liver metastases in small cell carcinoma of the lung. J Clin Oncol 2:733-740, 1984

75. Natale RB, Shank B, Hilaris BS, et al: Combination cyclophosphamide, adriamycin, and vincristine rapidly alternating with combination cisplatin and VP-16 in treatment of small cell lung cancer. Am J Med 79:303-308, 1985

76. Neijstrom ES, Capizzi RL, Rudnick SA, et al: High-dose methotrexate in small cell lung cancer: Lack of efficacy in preventing CNS relapse. Cancer 51:1056-1061, 1983

77. Nugent JL, Bunn PA Jr, Matthews MJ, et al: CNS metastases in small cell bronchogenic carcinoma: Increasing frequency and changing pattern with lengthening survival. Cancer 44:1885-1893, 1979

78. Osterlind K, Hansen HH, Hansen HS, et al: Chemotherapy versus chemotherapy plus irradiation in limited small cell lung cancer. Results of a controlled trial with 5 years follow-up. Br J Cancer 54:7-17, 1986

79. Osterlind K, Hansen M, Hansen HH, et al: Treatment policy of surgery in small cell carcinoma of the lung: Retrospective analysis of a series of 874 consecutive patients. Thorax 40:272-277, 1985

80. Pedersen AG, Bach F, Melgaard B: Frequency, diagnosis, and prognosis of spinal cord compression in small cell bronchogenic carinoma: A review of 817 consecutive patients. Cancer 55:1818-1822, 1985

81. Perez CA, Einhorn L, Oldham RK, et al: Randomized trial of radiotherapy to the thorax in limited small-cell carcinoma of the lung treated with multiagent chemotherapy and elective brain irradiation: A preliminary report. J Clin Oncol 2:1200-1208, 1984

82. Perez CA, Krauss S, Bartolucci AA, et al: Thoracic and elective brain irradiation with concomitant or delayed multiagent chemotherapy in the treatment of localized small cell carcinoma of the lung: A randomized prospective study by the Southeastern Cancer Study Group. Cancer 47:2407-2413, 1981

83. Perry MC, Eaton WL, Propert KJ, et al: Chemotherapy with or without radiation therapy in limited small-cell carcinoma of the lung. N Engl J Med 316:912-918, 1987

84. Petrovich Z, Ohanian M, Cox J: Clinical research on the treatment of locally advanced lung cancer. Cancer 40:72-77, 1977

85. Rosen ST, Makuch RW, Lichter AS, et al: Role of prophylactic cranial irradiation prevention of central nervous system metastases in small cell lung cancer. Potential benefit restricted to patients with complete response. Am J Med 74:615-624, 1983

86. Salazar OM, Creech RH, Rubin P, et al: Half-body and local chest irradiation as consolidation following response to standard induction chemotherapy for disseminated small cell lung cancer: An Eastern Cooperative Oncology Group Pilot Report. Internatl J Radiat Oncol Biol Phys 6:1093-1102, 1980

87. Schultz HP, Overgaard M, Steenholdt S: Small cell anaplastic carcinoma of the lung: The Aarhus experience 1976-1981. Acta Radiol Oncol 23:153-158, 1984

88. Sculier JP, Klastersky J, Stryckmans P, et al: Late intensification in small-cell lung cancer: A phase I study of high doses of cyclophosphamide and etoposide with autologous bone marrow transplantation. J Clin Oncol 3:184-191, 1985

89. Seydel HG, Creech R, Pagano M, et al: Combined modality treatment of regional small cell undifferentiated carcinoma of the lung: A cooperative study of the RTOG and ECOG. Internatl J Radiat Oncol Biol Phys 9:1135-1141, 1983

90. Shank B, Natale RB, Hilaris BS, et al: Treatment of small cell carcinoma of lung with combined high dose mediastinal irradiation, whole brain prophylaxis and chemotherapy. Internatl J Radiat Oncol Biol Phys 7:469-475, 1981

91. Shank B, Scher H, Hilaris BS, et al: Increased survival with high-dose multifield radiotherapy and intensive chemotherapy in limited small cell carcinoma of the lung. Cancer 56:2771-2778, 1985

92. Shepherd FA, Ginsberg R, Evans WK, et al: "Very limited" small cell lung cancer (SCLC)—results of non-surgical treatment. Proc Am Soc Clin Oncol 3:223, 1984

93. Shields TW, Humphrey EW, Eastridge CE, et al: Adjuvant cancer chemotherapy after resection of carcinoma of the lung. Cancer 40:2057-2062, 1977

94. Sibille Y, Steyuaert J, Francis C, et al: Three-drug chemotherapy combined with radiation therapy in small cell carcinoma of the lung. Eur J Resp Dis 64:113-120, 1983

95. Sierocki JS, Hilaris BS, Hopfan S, et al: Small cell carcinoma of the lung: Experience with a six-drug regimen. Cancer 45:417-422, 1980

96. Smith IE, Evans BD, Gore ME: Carboplatin (Paraplatin; JM8) and etoposide (VP-16) as first-line combination therapy for small-cell lung cancer. J Clin Oncol 5:185-189, 1987

97. Souhami RL, Finn G, Gregory WM, et al: High-dose cyclophosphamide in small-cell carcinoma of the lung. J Clin Oncol 3:958-963, 1985

98. Souhami RL, Geddes DM, Spiro SG, et al: Radiotherapy in small cell carcinoma of the lung treated with combination chemotherapy: A controlled trial. Br Med J 288:642-646, 1984

99. Stevens E, Einhorn L, Rolin R: Treatment of limited small cell lung cancer. Proc Am Soc Clin Oncol 20:435, 1979

100. Takita H, Brugarolas A, Marabella P, et al: Small cell carcinoma of the lung, clinicopathological studies. J Thorac Cardiovasc Surg 66:472-477, 1973

101. Taylor AB, Shinton NK, Waterhouse JAH: Histology of bronchial carcinoma in relation to prognosis. Thorax 18:178-181, 1963

102. Urtasun RC, Belch A, Bodnar D: Hemibody radiation, an active therapeutic modality for the management of patients with small cell lung cancer. Internatl J Radiat Oncol Biol Phys 9:1575-1578, 1983

103. Valdivieso M, McMurtrey MJ, Farha P, et al: Prospective evaluation of adjuvant surgical resection (ASR) in small cell lung cancer (SCLC). Proc Am Soc Clin Oncol 3:220, 1984

104. Williams C, Alexander M, Glatstein EJ, et al: Role of radiation therapy in combination with chemotherapy in extensive oat cell cancer of the lung: A randomized study. Cancer Treat Rep 61:1427-1431, 1977

105. Wilson HE, Stanley K, Vincent RG, et al: Comparison of chemotherapy and radiation therapy of extensive small cell carcinoma of the lung. J Surg Oncol 23:181-184, 1983

106. Woods RL, Levi JA: Chemotherapy for small cell lung cancer: A randomized study of maintenance therapy with cyclophosphamide, Adriamycin and vincristine after remission induction with cis-platinum, VP-16-213, and radiotherapy (Abstr). Proc Am Soc Clin Oncol 3:214, 1984

107. Zelen M: Keynote address on biostatistics and data retrieval. Cancer Chemother Rep 4:31-42, 1973

PART VII

Supportive Care

James B. D. Mark
John C. Baldwin

26

Endobronchial Therapy for Unresectable Lung Cancer

The treatment of obstructing or bleeding lesions in the trachea or proximal bronchi remains a challenging and often insurmountable problem. Major airway obstruction by tumor or relatively small amounts of blood may lead rapidly to hypoxic death. While benign lesions may cause these problems, they are most frequently due to malignant neoplasms. Often, these neoplasms have recurred after surgical resection and/or external-beam radiotherapy and treatment options are limited. Surgical resection is almost always contraindicated because of proximal extent of the tumor or limited pulmonary reserve. Retreatment by external-beam radiotherapy may not be possible because radiation tolerance of intervening normal tissue would be exceeded. Even when radiation can be given, its effect generally is too slow to be useful in the circumstance of impending airway obstruction.

Until recently, endoscopic maneuvers have had little to offer because they have been principally observational rather than therapeutic. Attempts at establishing airway patency by removing tumor with biopsy forceps usually were met with bleeding and further obstruction. Frequently, patients with no systemic spread of disease faced a fatal outcome because of a relatively small tumor burden in a critical location.

The development of the laser and its adaptation for medical and endoscopic use has substantially altered this perspective. Schawlow and Towne reported stimulated emission of radiation in 1958.[35] This work led to the development of the laser (light amplification by stimulated emission of radiation). They shared the Nobel prize in physics in 1981 for this work. Adaptation of the laser for medical and specifically endoscopic use occurred quickly, and by the early 1980s, reports began to appear from this country and from abroad about the endoscopic use of lasers for treatment of endobronchial tumors and some benign processes such as strictures and papillomata. As the endoscopic application of lasers in the tracheobronchial tree has increased in frequency, the indications for and limitations of the procedure have become more clearly understood.

In an attempt to prolong the effect of laser treatment of tumors, intracavitary and interstitial methods for application of radiation sources have been adapted to endo-

LUNG CANCER: A COMPREHENSIVE TREATISE
ISBN 0-8089-1876-1

bronchial use. This technique is commonly called *brachytherapy*. This form of treatment generally is applicable to main or lobar bronchial lesions, and while tumor shrinkage is relatively slow, the duration of effect is longer than that achieved with laser ablation alone. The risk of acute complications is lower than with laser therapy. With the use of transtracheal, bronchoscopically guided placement of catheters, which can subsequently be loaded with radiation sources, local radiation therapy can be delivered to a discrete area of endobronchial or even extraluminal tumor.

LASER THERAPY

While electrocautery has been performed through the rigid bronchoscope, it generally lacks precision and efficacy in the removal of endobronchial tumors.[25] Advantages of cost and availability have been cited, but this form of therapy does not enjoy significant popularity.

The major advantage of laser ablation of endobronchial tumor is the rapidity of action. In addition to the potential complications of bleeding, perforation and fistula formation, a major limitation of laser treatment in this setting is the tendency for rapid recurrence of the tumor. Obstructions involving the upper lobes generally are poorly suited to laser ablation, and the laser beam cannot be directed toward the depth of an end the depth of an endobronchial tumor because of the hazard of perforation of the bronchial wall. Additionally, the laser is not suitable for treatment of tumor extrinsic to the bronchial lumen, which may be causing obstruction. Therefore, laser endoscopic therapy has the advantages of rapid effectiveness and repeatability, but significant disadvantages include its relatively high risk of acute complications and its short duration of effectiveness.

While relative contraindications, such as the presence of very extensive and bulky tumor, upper lobe lesions, and total luminal and significant external tumor compression have been cited, any endoscopically visible tumor is theoretically amenable to laser therapy. While much of the early experience was with laser treatment after failure of surgery and/or radiation, recent attention has been focused on the use of this modality as an initial treatment of patients with lung cancer to avoid the complications of bronchial obstruction during therapy and to reduce the tumor burden for irradiation therapy.

The neodymium-YAG laser is the one most frequently used for endobronchial treatment of tumors.[44] This instrument employs a wavelength of 1060 nm; penetration generally is between 3 and 4 mm, and tissue absorption is nonspecific. The energy source itself is large and somewhat cumbersome because of the requisite water-cooling system, but the highly efficient coagulation, the relatively poor absorption by hemoglobin, and the facility for transmission of the beam through a flexible quartz fiber make this instrument the clear choice for endobronchial treatment of lung tumors. In addition, animal studies done by Wolfe and his colleagues demonstrated the effectiveness of the laser in controlling both parenchymal bleeding and air leaks and found it to be superior to cautery or suturing.[42] While the carbon dioxide laser, first used for the treatment of respiratory papillomatosis in 1973, has the advantage of precision cutting, an awkward mirror system is still necessary for direction of the beam, and use of the flexible bronchoscope is not possible.[29,38]

Personne and his colleagues, pioneers in the use of the Nd-YAG laser for endoscopic treatment of lung tumors, strongly advocate the use of the rigid broncho-scope.[33] They cite the advantages of improved operating conditions and safety, stating categorically that "the success of laser in bronchology depends entirely upon the choice of the endoscope." Their use of anesthetic paralysis and high-frequency jet ventilation for maintenance of a completely motionless operating field lends further advantages to this technique. The ability to maintain airway patency in the presence of significant bleeding and during the extraction of charred tumor is certainly improved with the rigid bronchoscope. However, extensive favorable experience has been gained with the flexible bronchoscope in the application of Nd-YAG laser treatment, and the preference and experience of the operating surgeon will remain the overriding factors in this choice.

Ordinarily, the Nd-YAG laser is used in endobronchial therapy with 40-60 W power and with 0.3-1.0-second applications to total energies of 1000-6000 joules (watt-seconds). Dumon has suggested that in order to reduce the risk of perforation, the laser should be used at power settings not higher than 45 W.[13,14] It is exceedingly important that the laser be fired only in a direction parallel to the bronchial wall; perpendicular or angular applications substantially increase the risk of perforation.

With regard to anesthetic technique, it is important to remember that the possibility of intratracheal fire and/or explosion is enhanced by the use of high concentrations of oxygen and flammable anesthetics.[24] The latter must be entirely avoided, and inspired oxygen concentration must be kept to 0.4 or less during laser treatment. Extensive experience, now totaling several thousand patients in the literature, has suggested that with proper patient selection and careful surgical and anesthetic technique, the complication rate of laser treatment is less than 2 percent. Hemorrhage remains the most common complication. Bronchial perforation and tracheoesophageal fistula may occur. Intraoperative cardiac complications reflect the characteristics of the patient population.

This extensive experience now indicates that the great majority of patients will experience significant relief of obstruction or hemoptysis with endobronchial Nd-YAG laser treatment.[2-4,7,10,21,28,30-32,39-41,43] It remains evident that better results are achieved when the patient presents with partial rather than total obstruction of the airway by tumor. Furthermore, the improvement in airway patency is greatest in patients undergoing their first laser treatment for obstruction. Kvale and associates reported that 12 out of 13 patients with bronchogenic carcinoma had doubling of airway size and relief of obstructing symptoms with initial Nd-YAG treatment while only 22 out of 32 had the same degree of improvement after the treatment of recurrent disease.[27]

Nd-YAG laser ablation of endobronchial tumor has the major advantage of rapidity of action. The tumor is vaporized and removed within minutes. As mentioned previously, the major limitation of laser treatment of endobronchial tumor is that the tumor tends to recur rather rapidly. The laser beam cannot be directed toward the depth of the tumor because of the real hazard of perforation of the bronchial wall. It must be directed in the long axis of the bronchus, which is efficient for removal of exophytic endobronchial tumor but inadequate for total ablation of the tumor. Laser treatment may be repeated, but the tumor tends to recur more frequently after each treatment, and complications are more apt to occur each time. In addition, the patient tends to become discouraged, even depressed, knowing that treatment sessions will become more and more frequent.

Recent attention has been focused on the use of hematoporphyrin-derivative phototherapy for treatment of early bronchogenic carcinoma.[8,9,19,20] One 5 year cure has been reported with this method of treatment for squamous carcinoma.[26] This technique involves the intravenous injection of this derivative with subsequent photoradiation using the argon laser. It has been observed that small, early malignant lesions absorb such photosensitizing agents and that they can be made to fluoresce under certain conditions. Argon phototherapy in the presence of the hematoporphyrin sensitizer has cytotoxic effect through energy transfer by the hematoporphyrin and by the direct effect of the laser. While larger, obstructive cancers are best treated with high-power sources such as the Nd-YAG laser, the argon laser can be used in a complementary fashion, that is, this modality may play a role in the primary treatment of very small tumors that have not eroded through the bronchial wall.

BRACHYTHERAPY

In an attempt to prolong the effect of endobronchial treatment of tumor, intracavitary or interstitial methods of application of radiation sources have been adapted for endobronchial use.[6,15,35] This is commonly called *brachytherapy*. This method of treatment offers the opportunity for more prolonged effective treatment of endobronchial tumor. Interstitial implantation of radioactive sources is a long-standing concept, and the technique was employed with resection in 1933[18] and for unresectable lung carcinoma in 1941.[5,22,23] There has been continual improvement in radiologic and surgical technique, and a large experience with brachytherapy has now been accumulated. Principal applications have been in patients with limited pulmonary reserve and in those with unresectable tumors. Since the late 1970s, attention has focused on endobronchial radiotherapy as a means of augmenting treatment in patients who have received the maximum permissible external-beam treatment. Previous interest in permanent implantation of ^{222}Rn and ^{125}I for endobronchial lesions has been supplanted in many centers by the use of temporary intraluminal placement of ^{192}Ir sources. Schray and colleagues reported on treatment of malignant airway obstruction with the use of combination Nd-YAG laser and temporary intraluminal brachytherapy with ^{192}Ir.[36] In 1985 Seagren and colleagues reported on the use of ^{60}C source for endobronchial brachytherapy after Nd-YAG laser debulking and concluded that significant endobronchial palliation could be achieved.[37]

While reliable and stable positioning of brachytherapy catheters has been a significant problem with catheters placed transnasally or via a tracheostomy or an endotracheal tube, we recently reported on a technique for positioning the catheters below the glottis.[1] This results in diminished cough and reduced risk of dislodgement. The patient is able to breathe and eat normally during the duration of radiation treatment.

In this technique, a 7-French endobronchial catheter with a closed tip and removable inner guidewire is used. This aids in positioning of the catheter, especially in the upper lobe bronchi. A 2-3-mm transverse incision in the cricothyroid membrane can be used for direct placement of the catheter into the trachea. Alternatively, an 8-French Cook introducer may be placed percutaneously through the cricothyroid membrane and used as a sheath through which endobronchial catheter can be passed. We have also used this technique for placement of multiple endobronchial catheters.

The fiberoptic bronchoscope is passed through an endotracheal tube to guide placement of the catheters in the correct anatomic position. The line source of ^{192}Ir seeds is then loaded into the catheter with measurements providing for the length of the radiation source to be 2 cm more than the length of the tumor as determined by bronchoscopy and computerized tomography (CT). Ordinarily a dose of 2000–4000 cGy is delivered over 1–3 days. For purely endobronchial lesions, the cylindrical volume of effective radiation treatment is calculated at 5 mm from the radiation source. When significant peribronchial disease is identified, a radius up to 15 mm has been employed for dosimetric calculation. The isodose curve of ^{192}Ir is such that the hourly dose at 15 mm from the source is about one-third that at 5 mm. When the treatment has been completed, the catheter is removed and the tiny cricothyroid incision heals rapidly. Problems of prolonged air leak and bleeding have not been encountered in our experience. Hospital guidelines for radiation therapy precautions are meticulously followed.

The combination of Nd-YAG therapy with improved endobronchial brachytherapy has offered significantly better palliation than laser alone for patients with endobronchial tumor. Laser therapy provides for immediate improvement of obstruction by reopening of occluded bronchi. This immediate and dramatic relief is, however, often short-lived. In view of this fact and the documented reduced efficacy of repeat laser therapy, the addition of simultaneous placement of endobronchial catheters for brachytherapy appears to enhance and extend the efficacy of endobronchial treatment. Furthermore, the relative contraindication to laser therapy represented by tumor-related external compression of the airway is substantially obviated through the addition of local irradiation to laser endobronchial treatment. In is clear that the most effective endobronchial treatment of lung cancer in individual patients will result from skillful combination of these two evolving and complementary techniques.

PATIENT SELECTION AND TECHNIQUE

Candidates for local endobronchial treatment usually present with symptoms and signs of proximal bronchial obstruction, hemoptysis, or both. Bothersome cough may be present, along with nonspecific systemic symptoms of advancing carcinoma. Most often, these patients are know to have lung cancer and have been treated previously. Local endobronchial recurrence of tumor after external-beam radiotherapy is not uncommon. Suture or staple-line recurrence after surgical resection is less common. These tumors are most often squamous carcinoma, less frequently large cell and adenocarcinoma, and rarely oat cell carcinoma. Recurrence of the latter tumor is most often manifest by systemic spread rather than local recurrence. Preliminary evaluation includes chest x-ray, which may demonstrate atelectasis of one or more lobes or an entire lung. The urgency of the treatment depends on the patient's clinical presentation. While we have had intubated patients transferred by helicopter from another hospital who require relatively emergent treatment, there is an opportunity to do some orderly evaluation of most of these patients. Tomograms or CT scans help to delineate the location and the extent of the obstruction. Pulmonary function tests along with ventilation and perfusion lung scans before and after treatment are excellent for documenting the extent of respiratory compromise and the effectiveness of the treatment but are not necessary in most patients. Certainly one should not withhold treatment awaiting such studies if the patient needs urgent treatment. This is a situation in which the objective of treatment is to provide palliation of bothersome symptoms.

The radiotherapists are informed about the patient as soon as the surgeons become aware. It is important that the radiotherapists be in the operating room at the time of bronchoscopy and catheter placement in order to see and assess the location and extent of the tumor and participate in all treatment decisions. Of additional critical importance to the radiotherapists is the precise knowledge about any prior x-ray treatment such as when it was given, the treatment ports, dosage, and source. They must know all this history in order to plan safe and effective endobronchial treatment.

We do these procedures in the operating room under general anesthesia. Laser treatment alone may be performed under topical anesthesia, although we prefer general anesthesia in most instances, even for laser treatment. We believe that patients who are hypoxic, have major airway problems, and need intratracheal manipulation of this sort are best served by general anesthesia with good control of the airway, proper monitoring, and similar measures. In most patients, cutaneous monitoring of oxygen saturation is satisfactory. In some patients, intra-arterial catheters are used for continuous monitoring of blood pressure and intermittent sampling for blood gases.

Shapshay and Dumon are among those who recommend the rigid bronchoscope for laser bronchoscopy.[11-14,38] One cannot argue with their experience and opinion. Others, including Gelb, use the fiberoptic instrument.[16,17] We have used both and prefer the fiberoptic bronchoscope in most instances. The excellent airway control and ability to adjust the concentration of oxygen in the inspired gas is unsurpassed when endotracheal intubation and the flexible bronchoscope are used. The major disadvantage of the flexible instrument is the small viewing channel, necessitating relatively frequent cleaning of the lens if there is bleeding. Similarly, removal of debris, while usually possible by irrigation and suction with the smaller instrument, is more easily accomplished with the larger rigid bronchoscope.

The most important consideration in this or any other kind of treatment is patient safety. The laser is a powerful tool that can accomplish great good but if not used properly can cause great and sometimes irreparable harm. Each person who uses the laser has the responsibility of becoming familiar with the important principles of laser safety and following them without fail.

The trachea and bronchial tree are first assessed by visualizing all accessible bronchi. Again, the flexible bronchoscope is superior to the rigid one for this purpose. The uninvolved side usually is inspected first; then inspection and appropriate treatment of the involved area are carried out. Laser treatment can be carried out for any endobronchial tumor that can be visualized. We have found it most useful and safest for endobronchial tumors that cause high-grade but incomplete obstruction of the trachea or major bronchi. For more distal obstruction at the lobar level, the benefit of treatment is less certain to occur. We have documented this by both clinical assessment and serial pulmonary function testing and ventilation perfusion scans pre- and posttreatment in selected patients. If the obstruction is in the upper lobes, laser treatment is more dangerous. It is of critical importance that the laser beam be aimed in the long axis of the bronchus to be treated in order to avoid penetration of the bronchial wall with its attendant complications. Because the upper lobe bronchi take off at a considerable angle from the main bronchi, precise and proper aim of the beam is more difficult. The same principle holds true with placement of the brachytherapy catheter. Placement and fixation into an upper lobe bronchus may be difficult even under direct vision. With the newer steerable catheter, this difficulty may be overcome.

It should be emphasized that laser treatment must be carried out with the utmost care. Even if endobronchial tumor is visualized, if the patient's symptoms are only mild and the obstruction low grade, we do not use the laser. When it is used, we start with a relatively low setting, usually 40 W delivered in 0.5-second bursts. If things are proceeding well and visualization is excellent, we will then gradually increase the power to 50 or 55 W and the time of each application to 1 second. Prior to starting laser treatment, one should always confirm with the anesthetists that the concentration of inspired oxygen is 0.4 or less. This will help to prevent combustion or even flaming or explosion. Inspired oxygen concentration may be increased as determined by the needs of the patient during intervals between laser treatments. Clearly, good communication and cooperation between endoscopists and anesthesiologists are essential.

The end point of laser treatment is not always easy to determine. Sometimes the anesthesiologists will note that inspiratory pressures have decreased during treatment and that ventilation is more effective. Visualization of an adequate tracheobronchial channel is the best end point and the goal of laser treatment, but this is not always easy to achieve. Final tidying up can be carried out with the laser or with biopsy forceps. Then the tracheobronchial tree should be irrigated and aspirated to clear it of debris and the area reinspected for adequacy of treatment and for bleeding. The rigid instrument sometimes is more efficient for this final cleaning purpose. Total treatment is usually in the range of 1500–5000 joules.

The main disadvantage of successful laser treatment is that tumor tends to recur relatively rapidly, usually within a month or two. Treatment may be repeated as necessary; however, treatment intervals usually decrease with repeated treatment. While patients appreciate the relief of airway obstruction that laser treatment provides, they do tend to become discouraged or even depressed when they realize that another treatment may be needed in a short period of time. A second important limitation in laser treatment is that it is not applicable for patients with tracheobronchial obstruction due to extrinsic compression by tumor or tumor-bearing nodes.

The development of brachytherapy has helped to overcome both of these problems. Properly planned and administered, this type of internal radiotherapy may be used even for patients who have already received what might be considered to be the maximum allowable (or safe) dose of radiotherapy from an external-beam source. The main limitation of external-beam treatment in most patients with carcinoma of the lung is the tolerance of the normal intervening tissues such as the esophagus, spinal cord, heart, and lung.

CONCLUSION

Initial enthusiasm for most new tools in medicine is tempered by time and experience. Such is the case with the laser for treatment of endobronchial neoplasms. Control of hemoptysis and opening of proximal airways is possible in most instances. A small but real incidence of major complications is one factor that limits use of the technique. Another is the relatively short duration of effectiveness of the treatment.

Brachytherapy prolongs the duration of palliation of symptoms. The judicious combination of endobronchial laser treatment and brachytherapy will provide palliation usually lasting for several months in a selected group of patients with localized endobronchial carcinoma of the lung that is not amenable to other types of therapy.

EDITORIAL COMMENT

The important principle of this chapter is that it is now possible to safely and reasonably palliate patients endobronchially who have failed other therapies and have obstructive tumors in the proximal tracheobronchial tree. It is no longer necessary to allow all patients to die of obstructive pneumonia when, with relief, they might expect good quality of life for their remaining lifetimes.

It is not appropriate to assume that every hospital will have access to these expensive and somewhat logistically complicated modalities; however, they are available in a sufficient number of regional centers that access is possible for all patients. It should be emphasized that, particularly before complete obstruction from a proximal cancer has occurred, outpatient treatment is possible in many cases. Even when endobronchial brachytherapy is required, only a very short duration admission may be necessary.

REFERENCES

1. Allen, MD, Baldwin JC, Fish VJ, et al: Combined laser therapy and endobronchial radiotherapy for unresectable lung carcinoma with bronchial obstruction. Am J Surg 150:71–77, 1985
2. Arabian AA: Experience with the Nd:YAG laser for lung cancer. Chest 89:332–333, 1986
3. Arabian A, Spagnoto SV: Laser therapy in patients with primary lung cancer. Chest 86:519–523, 1984
4. Beamis JF, Shapshay SM: More about the YAG, editorial. Chest 87:277–278, 1985
5. Binkley JS: The role of surgery and interstitial radon therapy in cancer of the superior sulcus of the lung. Acta Unio Intermationalis Contra Cancrum 6:1200–03, 1950
6. Boedker A, Hald A, Kristensen D: A method for selective endobronchial and endotracheal irradiation. J Thorac Cardiovasc Surg 84:59–61, 1982
7. Brutinel WM, Cortese DA, McDougall JC: Bronchoscopic phototherapy with the neodymium YAG laser. Chest 86:158–159, 1984
8 Cortese DA: Endobronchial management of lung cancer. Chest 89:234S–236S, 1986
9 Cortese DA, Kinsey JH: Hematoporphyrin derivative phototherapy in the treatment of bronchogenic carcinoma. Chest 86:8–13, 1984
10. Dixon JA: Lasers in Surgery. Current Problems in Surgery. Chicago, Year Book Medical Publishers, 1984
11. Dumon JF: YAG Laser Bronchoscopy. New York, Praeger, 1985, 116 pp
12. Dumon JF, Reboud E, Meric B, et al: Bronchofibroscopie et laser YAG:Nd. Rev Fr Mal Respir 9:4–76, 1981
13. Dumon JF, Reboud E, Garbe L, et al: Treatment of tracheobronchial lesions by laser photoresection. Chest 81:278–284, 1982
14. Dumon JF, Shapshay S, Bourcereau J, et al: Principles for safety in appreciation of neodymium-YAG laser in bronchology. Chest 86:163–168, 1984

15. Eichenhorn MS, Kvale PA, Miks VM, et al: Initial combination therapy with YAG laser photoresection and irradiation for inoperable non-small cell carcinoma of the lung. Chest 89:782-785, 1986

16. Gelb AF, Epstein JD: Laser in treatment of lung cancer. Chest 86:662-666, 1984

17. Gelb, AF, Epstein JD: Nd-YAG laser in lung cancer. West J Med 140:393-397, 1984

18. Graham E, Singer JJ: Successful removal of an entire lung for carcinoma of the bronchus. JAMA 101:1371-1374, 1933

19. Hayata Y, Kato H, Konaka C, et al: Hematoporphyrin derivative and laser photoradiation in the treatment of lung cancer. Chest 81:269-277, 1972

20. Hayata Y, Kato H, Konaka C, et al: Photoradiation therapy with hematoporphyrin derivative in early and stage 1 of lung cancer. Chest 86:169-177, 1984

21. Hetzel MR, Nixon C, Edmondstone WM, et al: Laser therapy in 100 tracheobronchial tumors. Thorax 40:341-345, 1985

22. Hilaris BS: Brachytherapy in lung cancer. Chest 89:349S, 1986

23. Hilaris BS, Martini N: Interstitial brachytherapy in cancer of the lung. A 20 year experience. Internatl J Radiat Oncol Biol Phys 5:1951-56, 1979

24. Hirshman CA, Smith J: Indirect ignition of the endotracheal tube during CO_2 laser surgery. Arch Otolaryngol 106:639-641, 1980

25. Hooper RG, Jackson FN: Endobronchial electrocautery. Chest 87:712-714, 1985

26. Kato H, Konaka C, Kawate N, et al: Five year disease-free survival of a lung cancer patient treated only by photodynamic therapy. Chest 90:768-770, 1986

27. Kvale PA, Eichenhorn MS, Radke JR, Miks V: YAG laser photoresection of lesions obstructing the central airways. Chest 87:283-288, 1985

28. McDougall JC, Cortese DA: Neodymium-YAG laser therapy of malignant airway obstruction. Mayo Clin Proc 58:35-39, 1983

29. McElvein RB, Zorn GL: Indications, results, and complications of bronchoscopic carbon dioxide laser therapy. Ann Surg 199:522-525, 1984

30. Mendiondo OA, Dillon M, Beach LJ: Endobronchial brachytherapy in the treatment of recurrent bronchogenic carcinoma. Internatl J Radiat Oncol Biol Phys 9:579-582, 1983

31. Parr GBS, Unger M, Trout RG, et al: One hundred neodymium-YAG laser ablations of obstructing tracheal neoplasms. Ann Thorac Surg 38:374-381, 1984

32. Percarpio B, Price JC, Murphy P: Endotracheal irradiation of adenoid cystic carcinoma of the trachea. Radiology 128:209-210, 1978

33. Personne C, Colchen A, Leroy M, et al: Indications and technique for endoscopic laser resections in bronchology. J Thorac Cardiovasc Surg 91:710-715, 1986

34. Rabie T, Wilson RK, Easley JD, et al: Palliation of bronchogenic carcinoma with 198 An implantation using the fiberoptic bronchoscope. Chest 90:641-645, 1986

35. Schawlow AL, Townes CH: Infra-red and optical masers. Phys Rev 112:1940, 1958

36. Schray MF, McDougall JC, Martinez A, et al: Management of malignant airway obstruction: Clinical and dosimetric considerations using an iridium-192 afterloading technique in conjunction with the neodymium-YAG laser. Internatl J Radiat Oncol Biol Phys 11:403-409, 1984

37. Seagren SL, Harrell JH, Horn RA: High dose rate intralumenal irradiation in recurrent endobronchial carcinoma. Chest 88:811-814, 1985

38. Shapshay SM: Use of the CO_2 laser bronchoscope for palliation of tracheobronchial malignancy airway obstruction. Chest 89:333-334, 1986

39. Toty L, Personne C, Colchen A, et al: Utilisation d'un faisceau laser YAG a conducteur souple pour le traitement endoscopique de certaines lesions tracheobronchiques. Rev Fr Mal Respir 7:475-482, 1979

40. Toty L, Personne C, Colchen A, et al: Bronchoscopic management of tracheal lesions using neodymium YAG laser. Thorax 36:175-178, 1981

41. Wieman TJ: Lasers and the surgeon. Am J Surg 151:493-500, 1986

42. Wolfe WG, Cole PH, Sabiston DC: Experimental and clinical use of the YAG laser in the management of pulmonary neoplasms. Ann Surg 199:526-531, 1984
43. Wolfe WG, Sabiston DC: Management of benign and malignant lesions of the trachea and bronchi with the neodymium-yttrium-aluminum-garnet laser. J Thorac Cardiovasc Surg 91:40-45, 1986
44. Zollinger RM: Introduction to lasers, in Surgical Practice News, May 1986

Martin D. Abeloff
David S. Ettinger

_____ **27** _____

Diagnosis and Management of Medical and Surgical Problems in the Patient with Lung Cancer

The successful application of the biologic and therapeutic principles discussed in the preceding chapters requires an understanding of the medical and surgical problems that occur as part of the natural history of lung cancer and as a consequence of treatment. An in-depth understanding of the complications of lung cancer is increasingly important in this era of complex multimodality therapy. In this chapter, the direct and indirect (paraneoplastic) effects of lung cancer will be reviewed, as well as some of the major complications of surgery, systemic chemotherapy, and radiotherapy. These manifestations of cancer will be presented according to organ systems. However, many of these syndromes result in multiorgan complications.

THORAX

In the chest, complications can be classified as either local or regional in nature. Such complications may be present as a direct effect of the primary tumor or an extension of the tumor or metastases to a specific site or as a consequence of local therapy affecting normal as well as abnormal tissue(s). In the symptomatic patient with lung cancer, it is necessary to distinguish between symptoms caused by the cancer itself or as a consequence of its treatment in order to institute appropriate therapy.

The approximate incidence of presenting local and regional signs and symptoms in patients with lung cancer is shown in Table 27-1.[76,111] Their frequency at presentation is dependent on the location (i.e., centrally or peripheral) and size of the primary tumor and whether regional metastases have occurred. Primary tumors located centrally (generally squamous or small cell carcinoma) frequently cause atelectasis and bronchial obstruction, thereby producing cough, dyspnea, hemoptysis, and wheezing. Extension of the tumor to mediastinal structures may produce chest pain, dysphagia, hoarseness, and superior vena cava (SVC) syndrome and pericardial disease. Periph-

LUNG CANCER: A COMPREHENSIVE TREATISE
ISBN 0-8089-1876-1

411

Table 27-1
Presenting Local and Regional Effects of Lung Cancer

Sign or Symptom	Frequency (%)
Cough	75
Dyspnea	45
Chest pain	40
Hemoptysis	35
Hoarseness	5
Effects of SVC obstruction	5
Wheezing	2
Dysphagia	2
Effects of brachial plexus compression	Rare
Horner's syndrome	Rare
Pericardial effusion	Rare

eral lung tumors (generally adenocarcinoma or large cell carcinoma), despite being more common than centrally located cancers, cause less local symptoms than the latter.[179] However, when peripheral lung lesions enlarge and involve the pleura, they may cause symptoms such as cough, dyspnea, and chest pain. In the case of Pancoast's tumor, the tumor involves the apex of the lung affecting the first thoracic and eighth cervical nerves, causing shoulder pain.[132]

Fever, as a presenting sign of lung cancer, is an unusual occurrence. It may be present when a lung tumor causes an obstructive pneumonitis. In addition, in epidermoid or large call undifferentiated carcinomas that cavitate and are associated with lung abscesses, fever usually is present.[176]

Spontaneous pneumothorax as a presenting sign of lung cancer is rare.[101,103] In most cases, it occurs in the presence of mass lesions; however, it also has been reported to occur in primary cavitating lung carcinoma.[93,97] Squamous cell carcinoma is the most common histologic type associated with spontaneous pneumothorax.

Since these signs and symptoms are nonspecific, pulmonary diseases other than lung cancer should be considered in the differential diagnosis. These nonmalignant diseases include tracheobronchitis, bacterial and fungal pneumonia, tuberculosis, lung abscess, bronchial adenoma, hamartoma, and pulmonary infarction. Diagnostic studies to consider are reviewed in Chapter 8.

With direct extension or metastases to the mediastinum, obstruction or involvement of the major vessels, the esophagus, the pleura, and the pericardium and nerve entrapment can occur[32] and will be discussed separately in this chapter.

Superior Vena Cava Syndrome

The SVC syndrome occurs in approximately 5 percent of patients with bronchogenic carcinoma. In small-cell carcinoma, however, the SVC syndrome occurs in about 10 percent of cases.[45] Bronchogenic carcinoma accounts for 75-85 percent of all cases of the SVC syndrome.[100]

The SVC, formed by the junction of the innominate veins, is a thin-walled vessel situated in a closed mediastinal space surrounded by lymph nodes and close to the right main-stem bronchus. This vessel is susceptible to compression by a lung cancer, therefore, particularly of the right lung.[141] SVC obstruction usually is the result of invasion or extrinsic compression of the vein with the occurrence of a secondary thrombus formation.[53,149]

The pathophysiology of the SVC syndrome involves the occurrence of the following: (1) obstruction of the SVC, (2) increase in venous pressure distal to the obstruction, and (3) development of collaterals.

The most common symptoms of the SVC syndrome at presentation are shortness of breath (>50 percent), facial swelling (edema) (43 percent), or swelling of the trunk or upper extremities (40 percent).[134] Less common symptoms occurring in approximately 20 percent of patients include cough, chest pain, and dysphagia. The most common signs of the SVC syndrome are distention of the thoracic veins (67 percent), neck vein distention (59 percent), facial edema (56 percent), and tachypnea (40 percent). Less frequent signs include cyanosis (15 percent), vocal cord paralysis (4 percent), Horner's syndrome (2 percent), and confusion.[47] As the SVC obstruction worsens, there is an increase in intracranial pressure and the appearance of glossal or laryngeal edema. If untreated, death results from either cerebral anoxia, respiratory center failure, or suffocation from edema of the glottis or tracheobronchial lumen. Over 50 percent of patients have symptoms from the SVC obstruction for less than 4 weeks prior to hospitalization. Only 20 percent will have symptoms for longer than 8 weeks.[134]

The diagnosis of the SVC syndrome in most instances can be made by the history and physical examination alone. Rarely are other diagnostic procedures such as peripheral venous pressure recordings, vena caval pressure recordings, venography, or ^{99}Tc scintiphotography needed to confirm the diagnosis.[75,90,109,128]

The condition of the patients with SVC syndrome should dictate whether pathologic proof of a cancer is necessary before appropriate therapy is instituted. This approach is justifiable since 97 percent of cases of SVC syndrome are secondary to malignant disease, with approximately 80 percent due to lung cancer. In the vast majority of cases, however, the pathologic diagnosis can be safely made prior to the initiation of therapy. Sputum cytology, bronchoscopy with biopsy, bronchial washings, and biopsy of a palpable supraclavicular node will accurately establish the diagnosis in 70 percent of patients.[134] The latter procedure, if performed, should be done with great care to minimize the risk of hemorrhage because of the collateral vessels in the vicinity. The use of mediastinoscopy and thoracotomy to establish a diagnosis should be reserved for good-risk patients in whom no other procedures can be used since these procedures are associated with increased morbidity.[24,152] Since small cell carcinoma is the most common histologic subtype of lung carcinoma associated with the SVC syndrome, a bone marrow biopsy should also be performed in an attempt to establish the diagnosis.

Antitumor therapy for the SVC syndrome consists of radiation therapy and chemotherapy. Radiotherapy is the treatment of choice for non-small cell carcinoma. Currently, the initial radiotherapy is given in high daily doses (400 rads/day).[59] Such therapy is well tolerated. After the initial high daily doses of radiation therapy, the total dose of irradiation and dose rate should be individualized based on the clinical situation. The total dose of irradiation should be in the range of 3000–5000 rads.[134]

With the development of effective combination chemotherapy in the treatment of small cell carcinoma of the lung (SCLC), chemotherapy has been used as initial therapy for the SVC syndrome due to this malignancy. Dombernowsky and Hansen, using cyclophosphamide, methotrexate, CCNU, and vincristine, reported relief of the SVC syndrome due to small cell carcinoma in 23 out of 26 patients (88 percent).[46] Resolution of symptoms occurred at a median of 7 days from the beginning of therapy. Other investigators have found similar good responses in patients treated with chemo-therapy.[85,102,145,162] The advantage for cytotoxic drugs in comparison to radiotherapy in newly diagnosed patients with SVC syndrome secondary to small cell cancer in-cludes the fact that combination chemotherapy can rapidly achieve control of this systemic disease as well as the SVC syndrome.

The effect of the SVC syndrome on survival time for patients with bronchogenic carcinoma, although not known, probably is dependent on the histologic subtype, that is, small cell versus non-small cell carcinoma. The occurrence of the SVC syndrome in small cell carcinoma does not appear to significantly affect survival time or duration of response to therapy.[67] However, SVC syndrome in non-small cell cancer is an adverse prognostic factor in that it indicates that the patient is not a candidate for surgical cure.

Pleural Effusion

The most common cause of symptomatic pleural effusion is malignancy. In 1 percent of patients, it is the presenting finding of lung cancer.[120] However, approxi-mately 50 percent of patients with lung cancer have a pleural effusion at some time during the illness.[44,56]

The pathogenesis of a malignant effusion secondary to lung cancer is either by direct invasion of the pleural space by a primary or metastatic tumor or indirectly by mediastinal lymphatic obstruction.

The mechanisms by which the malignant effusion occurs are (1) increased capil-lary permeability and (2) impaired lymphatic obstruction.

Patients with malignant pleural effusion commonly present with chest pain, dysp-nea, and cough and have increased dullness to percussion, decreased vocal fremitus, poor diaphragmatic excursion, and decreased breath sounds on physical examination. However, the most practical way for assessing the presence of pleural fluid is the chest x-ray.

Once it is established that a patient has a pleural effusion, a thoracentesis should be performed for diagnostic and therapeutic purposes. To alleviate symptoms from a pleural effusion, 1000–1500 cc of fluid can be removed rapidly. However, removal of larger amounts may cause reexpansion pulmonary edema.[138,175]

The sine qua non of a malignant pleural effusion is the presence of malignant cells in the pleural space. Cytology is the best way to establish a diagnosis of malignant pleural effusion having an overall diagnostic yield of 50–75 percent.[151,183] The chance of demonstrating that cytology from an effusion is positive for malignancy increases as more thoracenteses are performed. When cytology is combined with pleural biopsy, a diagnosis can be established in 80–90 percent of cases.[151,183]

Chromosomal analysis of cells found in the pleural effusion may indicate that an effusion is malignant.[41,54] However, such analyses are expensive and time-consuming. Other diagnostic studies used in malignant effusions include pleural fluid carcinoem-bryonic antigen, LDH, protein, amylase, pH, and glucose; however, none are spe-cific.[139,150]

The use of pleuroscopy and/or thoracotomy should be used as the final diagnos-tic procedure in patients with a pleural effusion. The former procedure has a diagnostic yield of approximately 95 percent.[180] A thoracotomy should be considered only in carefully selected patients, since it can be associated with significant morbidity and mortality.

An asymptomatic effusion in a patient with a proven lung cancer need not be specifically treated unless a diagnostic evaluation is contemplated. By effectively treating the lung cancer itself with radiation therapy or combination chemotherapy, the pleural effusion may resolve. The chances of this occurring are higher with SCLC than with NSCLC.

Symptomatic effusions usually will require local treatment. The methods employed include thoracentesis or chest tube drainage alone, intrapleural administration of sclerosing agents to obliterate the pleural space, intrapleural instillation of radioisotopes, external-beam radiotherapy, and pleurectomy.[70]

A thorocentesis, or chest tube drainage alone, can give immediate symptomatic control of a malignant pleural effusion; however, it is ineffective in preventing recurrences of the effusion.[5,51] With the former procedure, the effusion recurs in less than 4 days, while with the latter procedure it takes several weeks for the effusion to recur.

With recurrent malignant pleural effusion, chest tube drainage with instillation of sclerosing agents, such as quinacrine, nitrogen mustard, tetracycline, and bleomycin is the treatment of choice. The latter two sclerosing agents are the preferred drugs.[10,19,131,146] Prior to instilling the sclerosing agent, it is important that the chest tube drainage be less than 100 cc/day. If tetracycline is utilized as a sclerosing agent, 70 percent of patients should have relief from pleural effusion for approximately 1 month.[70] The majority of side effects associated with its administration are fever and pain. Bleomycin (60-90 units) as a sclerosing agent is 60-85 percent effective in controlling a malignant effusion. It is not myelosuppressive, and the incidence of side effects is low.

The effectiveness of radioisotopes to treat pleural effusions is less than with tetracycline or bleomycin.[70,124] Moreover, the radioisotopes are expensive and potentially hazardous.

Both external-beam radiotherapy and pleurectomy have limited use in lung cancer patients who develop a pleural effusion. Radiation therapy should be considered as treatment for hilar or mediastinal masses or endobronchial lesions if these cause inadequate pulmonary reexpansion following treatment of a malignant pleural effusion with chest tube drainage and instillation of a sclerosing agent. Pleurectomy should be limited to patients who have failed all other procedures to control an effusion, and even then, such patients should be carefully selected since the procedure is associated with an increase in morbidity and mortality.[107]

Pericardial Disease

In patients with bronchogenic carcinoma, involvement of the pericardium usually results from direct invasion by the primary tumor. Pericardial involvement rarely is discovered antemortem; however, at autopsy the heart is involved by bronchogenic carcinoma in approximately 30 percent of patients.[168]

The early diagnosis of pericardial involvement by bronchogenic carcinoma usually is difficult to make, especially since the symptomatology may be attributed to the lung cancer itself. The signs and symptoms of pericarditis secondary to malignancy are not specific for cancer but are similar to those of other causes of pericarditis. They include the following in the order of decreasing frequency: dyspnea, cough, pleural effusion, hepatomegaly, thoracic pain, orthopnea, cyanosis, venous distention, leg edema, cardiac enlargement, pulmonary rales, dysphagia, splenomegaly, and systolic murmur. Distant heart sounds, paroxysmal nocturnal dyspnea, pulsus alternans, friction rub, and paroxysmal supraventricular tachycardia are uncommon findings.[171]

Electrocardiographic (ECG) changes associated with pericardial involvement with a malignancy include sinus tachycardia, premature contractions, low QRS voltage, and nonspecific ST-T wave abnormalities. A chest x-ray may show cardiac enlargement or mediastinal widening.

Unfortunately, despite early signs and symptoms of pericardial disease, the diagnosis usually is made when there is cardiac tamponade.[18,170] Clinically, the patient has dyspnea, clouded sensorium, pulsus paradoxus, low systolic blood pressure, and dilated neck veins. The diagnosis of cardiac tamponade is associated with the following: pulsus paradoxus, Ewart's sign, total electrical alternans on ECG, and "waterbottle heart" on chest x-ray.[125,163]

Echocardiography is a simple, sensitive, and safe noninvasive method for diagnosing pericardial effusion.[116,163]

Once a diagnosis of cardiac tamponade is made, it is considered a medical emergency. Effective treatment consists of a pericardiocentesis.[87] Since pericardial fluid is likely to recur rapidly after removal, other therapeutic procedures should be considered for prolonged palliation of the cardiac tamponade. These include pleural pericardial window, indwelling pericardial catheter, and pericardiectomy.[55,99] Sclerosing agents such as tetracycline or radioactive isotopes (i.e. ^{32}P, ^{198}Au, ^{90}Y) have been instilled into the pericardial space through an indwelling pericardial catheter to control the malignant effusion.[127] External-beam irradiation has been used to treat a pericardial effusion secondary to a malignancy.[30]

Although the presence of a malignant pericardial effusion is an ominous prognostic sign, survival rates approach 1–1.5 years from the time therapy for the effusion has been initiated.[159]

Esophageal Compression

Dysphagia as a presenting symptom of a bronchogenic carcinoma is uncommon, occurring in approximately 2 percent of patients.[164] It usually is caused by invasion of the mediastinum with tumor—in particular, squamous cell and small cell carcinoma. This results in displacement or compression of the esophagus, thereby causing dysphagia.

The diagnosis usually can be established by a barium swallow radiograph. However, fluoroscopy or a cinefluoroscopic are other diagnostic studies that may be of value.

Esophageal wall invasion with or without the formation of a fistula by a primary bronchogenic carcinoma rarely occurs.[106] However, it presents a serious problem when it does. Computed tomography (CT) may assist in identification of esophageal invasion by tumor.[58]

Treatment of esophageal compression by a bronchogenic carcinoma consists primarily of radiation therapy. For small cell carcinoma, chemotherapy may be utilized. If the esophageal wall has been invaded by tumor causing a fistula between the primary lung tumor and the esophagus, surgical intervention to provide alternative methods of nutrition may be required.[165]

Nerve Entrapment

The nerves most frequently affected by bronchogenic carcinoma are the recurrent laryngeal nerve, the phrenic nerve, and the first thoracic and eight cervical nerves. These nerves may become involved as a direct extension of the primary tumors.

Hoarseness as an initial symptom of lung cancer occurs in approximately 5 percent of cases. It is due to involvement of the recurrent laryngeal nerve, causing left vocal cord paralysis, by a bronchogenic carcinoma usually situated in the left lung. The left recurrent laryngeal nerve is more frequently affected than the right since it has a greater intrathoracic course than the right.

Dyspnea can result as a consequence of phrenic nerve involvement by a lung cancer causing a paralysis of the diaphragm.[3] Classic radiographic findings consist of elevation of the hemidiaphragm.

A superior sulcus tumor extending to involve the first thoracic and eight cervical nerves cause pain in the shoulder and arm. Extension of the tumor to involve the sympathetic nerves may produce Horner's syndrome.

Complications of Thoracic Surgery

In the past, surgery as treatment for bronchogenic carcinoma was associated with a high incidence of postoperative mortality and major complications.[69,88] Probably because of better patient selection, improved surgical techniques, and better supportive care, the present-day operative mortality rate is 4 percent, while the rate of major complications is 9 percent (Table 27-2).[61,123] The postoperative course in patients undergoing surgery for bronchogenic carcinoma is uneventful in over 80 percent of cases.[123]

Approximately 90 percent of the major complications associated with surgery of lung cancer are cardiorespiratory in nature. Pneumonia and atelectasis occur in 2.5 and 2 percent of patients, respectively, while empyema with or without broncho-

Table 27-2

Complications of Surgery

Sign or Symptom	Frequency (%)
No significant complications	90
Major thoracic complications	9
Pneumonia	<3
Atelectasis	2
Empyema ± bronchopleural involvement	<1
Pulmonary fistula insufficiency	<1
Cardiac arrhythmias	1
Bleeding	<1
Major extrathoracic complications	<2
Renal failure	<1
GI bleeding	<2
Mortality	4

pleural fistula, pulmonary emboli, respiratory failure, tension pneumothorax, ventricular arrhythmia, congestive heart failure and myocardial infarction, bleeding, and ruptured esophagus occur in less than 1 percent of cases.[123] Other uncommon major complications of the surgery that are not cardiorespiratory in nature include renal failure, gastrointestinal bleeding, perforated ulcer, cerebral infarct, and femoral arterial thrombosis. Minor complications include, in decreasing order of frequency, cardiac arrhythmias (i.e., atrial flutter—fibrillation), persistent air leakage, wound infection, deep-vein thrombosis, bronchospasm, and prolonged ileus.[123]

The morbidity and mortality rate associated with surgery of lung cancer is significantly higher in patients who are elderly (70 years or older), have prior cardiac disease and/or restricted preoperative pulmonary reserve and who undergo a pneumonectomy.[123] The mortality rate appears to be highest in patients undergoing a right pneumonectomy.[68]

Surgery as a treatment option is being made available to more patients with lung cancer. This is due to earlier diagnosis of NSCLC as well as the fact that surgery is now being considered in selected patients with limited-disease SCLC. Therefore, it is important to carefully select appropriate patients for surgery. It appears that both preoperative and postoperative cardiorespiratory care, especially in the elderly patient, will decrease the risks of surgery as treatment for lung cancer.

Chest Complications of Radiation Therapy

Radiation therapy, although used to treat both primary non-small cell and small cell bronchogenic carcinoma, may be associated with acute (early) and/or chronic (late) toxicity. In order to assess the possibility of radiation therapy toxicity to a given organ, the tolerance of normal tissues to radiation must be known. The normal tissues that are usually affected by irradiation of a primary lung tumor include the skin, lung, pericardium, esophagus, and spinal cord, which are able to tolerate a total dose of radiation of 6500, 1800, 1850, 6000, and 4000 rads, respectively.[40]

The majority of side effects of radiation therapy include radiation pneumonitis-fibrosis, pericarditis, esophagitis, dermatitis, subcutaneous fibrosis, and myelitis. The latter side effect will be discussed in the section dealing with side effects affecting the CNS.

Radiation Pneumonitis-Fibrosis

Damage to the lungs by radiation has been recognized as far back as 1898, when the development of radiation pneumonitis was first described. Hines in 1922 described pulmonary fibrosis secondary to radiation.[74] The occurrence of radiation lung damage can be divided into two phases: an acute phase, at which time radiation pneumonitis develops; and a late phase, with the development of radiation fibrosis (see Chapter 5).

Factors that can potentiate the side effects of radiation include concomitant chemotherapy, previous radiation therapy, and steroid withdrawal.[65,136] Adriamycin and high-dose cyclophosphamide have also been shown to potentiate the pulmonary toxicity associated with irradiation.[50,110,172] It is known that retreatment of lung tissue with additional radiation therapy will increase the chances of a patient developing radiation pneumonitis over patients irradiated for the first time.[86] Steroid withdrawal may contribute to the appearance of pneumonitis caused by latent radiation injury.[27]

The differential diagnosis of radiation injury to the lung includes recurrence of the tumor, including lymphangitic spread and infection. Pulmonary signs and symptoms occurring 16 weeks or longer after lung irradiation with the findings of metastases elsewhere is suggestive of recurrent disease rather than radiation pneumonitis. Rapidly progressive pulmonary symptoms out of proportion to chest x-ray abnormalities is suggestive of lymphangitic spread of the lung tumor. In addition, lymphangitic spread usually is most prominent in the bases.[65] At times, infection can be difficult to distinguish from radiation pneumonitis, especially if the apices are involved. In this latter situation, tuberculosis should be considered in the differential diagnosis.[97]

The incidence of pulmonary fibrosis in patients with lung cancer is high and increases with time. The severity of the pulmonary fibrosis is variable, and although it has been reported to occur in all lung cancer patients treated with radiation therapy, significant symptoms occur in 5–30 percent of patients.[71,156] In the treatment of small cell carcinoma, utilizing combination chemotherapy (cyclophosphamide, vincristine, adriamycin, bleomycin) and chest irradiation, pulmonary fibrosis occurred in 38 percent of patients and was fatal in 23 percent of the patients treated.[50] In another study, chemotherapy (cyclophosphamide, adriamycin, vincristine) given concurrently with chest irradiation resulted in 38 percent of the patients developing pneumonitis-pulmonary fibrosis, with approximately half of these patients dying.[82] Pulmonary toxicity can be reduced to less than 5 percent when combination chemotherapy is given either sequentially with chest irradiation or concurrently when the radiotherapy is given for 10 days.[31,115]

Therapy of symptomatic radiation pneumonitis consists of administration of corticosteroids, antibiotics, and anticoagulants.[65] Once the diagnosis is suspected, prednisone 60–100 mg daily should be given until the signs and symptoms of the pneumonia are resolved, at which time the dose should be tapered slowly. Although antibiotics and anticoagulants have been used in the treatment of radiation pneumonitis, there is no substantial evidence that they are beneficial.

Radiation Pericarditis

The occurrence of radiation pericarditis as a consequence of chest irradiation as treatment for a lung cancer is relatively uncommon. A 4 percent incidence has been reported after the mediastinum has been irradiated following lung resection for bronchogenic carcinoma.[94] The radiation pericarditis appeared approximately 12 months after treatment with 4500–5000 rads from a linear accelerator in which 50 percent of the heart received the full dose of radiation. The time of onset of symptoms of the pericarditis after radiation therapy may vary from several months to several years. The incidence of radiation pericarditis following radiation therapy of lung cancer may be low because it takes time to develop and only a small percentage of patients who receive radiation therapy as treatment for their disease are still alive 12 months later.

Radiation pericarditis may be acute or chronic in nature.[33,166,167] The acute form may occur during therapy or shortly after its completion and is associated with fever, chest pain, pericardial friction rub, and ECG and chest x-ray abnormalities.[166] A pericardial effusion may be present but transient, and the patient may be asymptomatic with a self-limiting disease.[167] The chronic form may be insidious, occurring months to years after the completion of the radiation therapy. The pericardium may become thickened, causing constriction and eventually leading to cardiac tamponade.

When pericarditis develops in a patient with lung cancer who has received chest irradiation, the differential diagnosis is between radiation-induced disease versus pericardial metastasis. The cytologic examination of pericardial fluid may or may not be of help in distinguishing between the two conditions since the absence of tumor cells in the pericardial fluid does not rule out metastasis.

Corticosteroids may be of value in treating the acute form of radiation pericarditis.[17] In the chronic form, a pericardiectomy may be necessary.

Chemotherapy-Induced Pulmonary-Cardiac Toxicity

In patients with lung cancer treated with chemotherapy who subsequently develop pulmonary or cardiac symptoms, toxicity as a consequence of chemotherapy should be included in the differential diagnosis.

The three drugs used to treat metastatic lung cancer, especially NSCLC, which are implicated in causing pulmonary toxicity, are bleomycin, the nitrosoureas, and mitomycin.[7,34,129] The lung injury that occurs is pulmonary fibrosis. In addition, methotrexate has been reported to cause pneumonitis.[161]

The first symptoms of bleomycin-induced pulmonary toxicity may be a dry, hacking cough followed by dyspnea on exertion. Progressive symptoms include dyspnea at rest, tachypnea, fever, and cyanosis. On physical examination, bibasilar rales involving the lower one-third of the lung fields may be heard. As the toxicity progresses, coarse rales, rhonchi, and an occasional pleural friction rub may be heard. On chest x-ray, the early changes are fine reticular bibasilar infiltrates, which may progress to alveolar and interstitial infiltrates, and then consolidation.[7]

The incidence of bleomycin pulmonary toxicity has been reported to range from 0 to 40 percent; however, the incidence of lethal pulmonary toxicity is 1-2 percent. Although bleomycin can cause pulmonary toxicity sporadically at low cumulative doses, the risk of toxicity increases at cumulative doses above 450-500 units.

Steroids have been used to treat bleomycin pulmonary toxicity; however, there is no known effective therapy for the drug-related pulmonary fibrosis. The pulmonary toxicity of bleomycin may increase the chances of subsequent pneumonitis due to radiation therapy.[136]

Carmustine (i.e., bischloroethylnitrosourea; BCNU) is also know to cause pulmonary toxicity. The symptoms are similar to those that occur with bleomycin toxicity. The incidence of BCNU-related pulmonary toxicity is probably close to 20-30 percent. The risk of developing BCNU-related pulmonary toxicity is a function of the total, cumulative BCNU dose. Once the toxicity occurs, the outcome is variable. The mortality rate appears to be greater than 50 percent.[34]

Mitomycin has also been implicated in causing pulmonary toxicity similar to that seen with bleomycin. The incidence of this toxicity ranges from 2.8 to 12 percent. The mortality rate is high once the toxicity develops.[129]

Few chemotherapeutic drugs cause cardiac toxicity. However, the anthracyclines (i.e., doxorubicin) have cardiotoxicity as one of their major toxicities.[137,174] Electrocardiographic abnormalities associated with doxorubicin administration are a common occurrence and are not dose-related. Up to 41 percent of patients receiving the drug will manifest ECG abnormalities. The ECG abnormalities associated with doxorubicin administration are reversible and are not associated with the development of drug-induced cardiomyopathy.

The most serious cardiotoxicity associated with doxorubicin administration is drug-induced cardiomyopathy. Once it develops, the mortality rate is greater than 50 percent. The total dose of doxorubicin administered is the most significant risk factor for development of doxorubicin-induced cardiomyopathy. The incidence of cardiomyopathy is less than 1 percent in patients receiving less than 550 mg/m^2; however, in patients receiving greater than 550 mg/m^2, the incidence of cardiomyopathy is approximately 30 percent. Cardiomyopathy has been reported to develop in patients with lower cumulative doses of doxorubicin who have had prior radiotherapy to the heart.[35,113]

When doxorubicin-induced congestive heart failure occurs, the patient presents with classic signs of congestive heart failure. The heart failure may occur between 0 to 231 days after the last dose of doxorubicin (median 23 days).

No noninvasive tests are available that will be completely predictive for the development of doxorubicin-induced congestive heart failure. The role of percutaneous endomyocardial biopsies to monitor the myocardium for damage is of value but is not routinely available.

Esophagitis

Radiation esophagitis occurs when the esophagus is included in the treatment field. Often patients complain of dysphagia that is transient, starting 2 weeks after radiation therapy and lasting for 1-2 weeks. In the treatment of SCLC, mild esophagitis occurs in 5-50 percent of patients receiving sequential chemotherapy and radiation therapy.[49,98] With concurrent chemotherapy and radiation therapy, the esophagitis is more severe, occurring in 65-77 percent of patients.[28] One of the chemotherapy agents implicated in the potentiation of radiation-induced esophagitis is doxorubicin.

The esophagitis is usually treated symptomatically with viscous Xylocaine (lidocaine; by Astra Pharm., Worcester, MA). The irritated esophagus can be infected with herpes and/or candida, and such infections must be included in the differentiated diagnosis of esophagitis. Herpes infections can be treated with acyclovir, while candida esophagitis usually responds to treatment with oral Mycostatin (nystatin; by Squibb, Princeton, NJ). Esophageal stricture requiring esophageal dilatation is an uncommon problem.

Dermatitis and Subcutaneous Fibrosis

Radiation dermatitis and subcutaneous fibrosis occur in less than 5 percent of patients receiving radiation therapy as treatment for lung cancer. The low incidence is due to the use of high-energy x-ray equipment.

ABDOMEN

In patients with lung cancer, signs and symptoms referable to the abdomen are a consequence of metastatic disease, toxic effects of chemotherapy, ectopic hormone production by the tumor, and paraneoplastic tumor effects. The latter two will be discussed elsewhere.

In patients with lung cancer, the liver and adrenal glands are common sites of metastases. Less commonly involved metastatic sites include the gastrointestinal tract and the pancreas. The pancreas is affected by metastatic small cell carcinoma more than the other histologic subtype of lung cancer.

Liver involvement at the time of diagnosis has been reported in 28 percent of patients with small cell carcinoma.[77] At autopsy, however, it appears in up to 80 percent of patients.[114] Methods for detection of liver metastases include physical examination, liver function tests, radionuclide liver scan, CT scan of liver, percutaneous liver biopsy, and peritoneoscopy. Peritoneoscopy-directed liver biopsy is the most sensitive method of detecting liver metastases in patients with small cell carcinoma.[46,119]

Adrenal metastases are very common in lung cancer; however, its diagnosis often is not made until the time of autopsy since such adrenal metastases do not cause symptoms. With the CT scan, adrenal metastases are detected frequently.[1] Percutaneous thin-needle biopsy had been used to detect metastatic small cell carcinoma in normal adrenal glands.[130]

Small cell carcinoma may cause extrahepatic bilary obstruction by metastasizing to the pancreas.[81] Effective palliation of such obstruction can be achieved with combination chemotherapy. In addition, acute pancreatitis in association with small cell carcinoma with and without evidence of metastases to the pancreas has been noted.[4] The latter condition was associated with cholelithiasis, which was the probable cause of the pancreatitis and not the carcinoma. It is important to exclude common causes of pancreatitis before instituting appropriate therapy for presumed metastatic disease.

Toxicities in normal gastrointestinal tract tissue are a consequence of chemotherapy used in the treatment of bronchogenic carcinoma. The major symptoms produced are nausea and vomiting, diarrhea, and constipation.

Different chemotherapeutic agents produce varying degrees of nausea and vomiting. Drugs commonly used in the treatment of lung cancer and associated with a significant degree of nausea and vomiting are cyclophosphamide. Adriamycin (doxorubicin; by Farmitalia, Milan, Italy, also known by former generic name, adriamycin), and cisplatin. Usually, nausea and vomiting associated with chemotherapy is dose-dependent. From the time the chemotherapy is given, nausea and vomiting usually begin 1–6 hours after administration and subside within 24–36 hours. Sometimes the symptoms can persist for a week or two after a single dose of chemotherapy; however, this is the exception rather than the rule.

Antiemetic drugs can be most effective in given doses and schedules that prevent occurrences of nausea and vomiting secondary to emetogenic chemotherapy. Antiemetics commonly used include prochlorperazine (Compazine; by SK & F, Carolina, PR), thiethylperazine (Torecan; by Boehringer, Ing., Ridgefield, CT), metoclopramide (Reglan; by Robins, Richmond, VA), haldoperidol (Haldol; by McNeil, Spring House, PA), dexamethasone (Decadron; by MSD, West Point, PA or Hexadrol; by Organon, West Orange, NJ), and the investigational drug, tetrahydrocannabinol (THC).[63,95,105]

Diarrhea may occur because of mucous membrane sensitivity to the cytotoxic effects of the chemotherapy. If the diarrhea is severe, the patient may experience malabsorption and dehydration. Diarrhea is commonly associated with 5-FU administration but is uncommon with other commonly used chemotherapeutic agents.

Antidiarrheal agents such as loperamide (Imodium; by Janssen, New Brunswick,

NJ) and diphenoxylate hydrochloride (Lomotil; by Searle, Chicago, IL) decrease bowel motility. Low-residue, easily digested food or elemental diets increase absorption and decrease bowel irritation. In general, however, diarrhea is short-lived and rarely results in a protracted problem.

In patients receiving vincristine or, less commonly, vinblastine, toxicity is manifested by abdominal pain, constipation, and adynamic ileus.[143] Patients who are elderly are more susceptible to this toxicity. The symptoms usually occur within 3 days of the vinca alkaloid administration. The symptoms usually resolve over a 2-week period. Constipation should be treated prophylactically with mild laxatives and stool softeners.

Liver damage is an uncommon toxicity associated with chemotherapy. The chemotherapeutic agents used to treat lung cancer that are associated with hepatic toxicity are methotrexate and the nitrosoureas (BCNU, CCNU). Methotrexate causes fibrosis and cirrhosis, while nitrosoureas cause elevated liver enzymes.

A number of chemotherapeutic agents are metabolized by the liver. If liver function tests are abnormal, it often is necessary to decrease the dosage of certain drugs known to be excreted by the liver. Examples of these drugs are Adriamycin, vinblastine, vincristine, and etoposide.

SKELETAL SYSTEM

The skeletal system commonly is affected by lung cancer. Approximately 25 percent of all patients with lung cancer will present with bone pain reflecting distant metastases to bone.[76] The most common histologic subtype associated with bone metastasis is small cell carcinoma.

Osteolytic bone lesions are the most common type of bone metastases seen in lung cancer. Osteoblastic metastases do occur, however, particularly in small cell carcinoma.[117]

The bone scan is more sensitive than bone x-rays in detecting metastases from lung cancer. A common site of metastatic bone involvement, especially in patients with small cell carcinoma of the lung, is the vertebral column. While peripheral bone metastases distal to the elbow and knee are rare, their occurrence is usually due to lung cancer.[120] Rarely, the patient with metastatic lung cancer may present with a monoarticular arthritis commonly involving the knee followed by the hip.[122] Patients usually present with an inflamed joint and effusion with tumor cells noted in the synovial fluid.

The most frequent cause of clubbing in men is lung cancer. It occurs more frequently in patients with squamous cell carcinoma of the lung and is due in part to an increase in peripheral blood flow.

Hypertrophic pulmonary osteoarthropathy occurs in up to 12 percent of patients with lung cancer.[184] It affects mainly the long bones of the extremities and appears as a symmetrical, proliferating, subperiosteal osteitis with new bone formation. The pathogenesis of hypertrophic pulmonary osteoarthopathy is unclear.

Hypercalcemia

Hypercalcemia frequently is associated with bronchogenic carcinoma. Approximately 12 percent of patients with bronchogenic carcinoma will have hypercalcemia.[13]

It is most common in squamous cell carcinoma of the lung and least common in small cell carcinoma of the lung, despite the fact that the latter histology is most frequently associated with osseous metastasis.

The occurrence of hypercalcemia in a patient is a medical emergency since it may be life-threatening, and yet reversible if treated appropriately. Besides lung cancer, other malignancies associated with hypercalcemia include breast cancer, multiple myeloma, squamous cell carcinoma of the head and neck and esophagus, and hypernephroma. Nonmalignant causes of hypercalcemia must be considered when a patient, despite having lung cancer, has an elevated serum calcium. Such causes include hyperparathyroidism, vitamin D intoxication, hyperthyroidism, milk-alkali syndrome, immobilization, and sarcoidosis.[112] Since an elevated serum calcium could be a laboratory error, it should be repeated, if appropriate.[83]

The most common mechanism by which cancer produces hypercalcemia is as a result of bone metastases (i.e., destruction of bone mass).[118] Immobilization, dehydration, and volume depletion and the use of thiazide diuretics in the cancer patient can worsen hypercalcemia.[112] Another mechanism by which cancer causes hypercalcemia is through the production of parathyroid hormone (PTH) or a PTH-like hormone. Squamous cell lung cancers have been associated with the production of PTH.[14,15] A prostaglandin substance and a metabolite of vitamin D has been found to cause hypercalcemia in squamous cell carcinoma lung and small cell carcinoma of the lung, respectively.[154,157]

The clinical manifestations of hypercalcemia are associated primarily with effects on the gastrointestinal, cardiovascular, renal, and neuromuscular systems. The gastrointestinal effects occur early and are nonspecific, consisting of anorexia, nausea, vomiting, abdominal pain, and constipation. Ileus and pancreatitis may also occur as a consequence of hypercalcemia.

Calcium exerts a positive inotropic effect on the heart. As a consequence of this, there is a shortening of the systolic time intervals. The ECG shows shortening of the QT interval with modest elevations of serum calcium; however, with higher elevations (i.e., 16 mg/d1) of calcium, the QT interval is prolonged. In addition, hypercalcemia may cause life-threatening cardiac arrhythmias.[112]

Hypercalcemia can affect both glomerular filtration and renal tubular function. The effect on the tubular function causes polyuria and nocturia as a consequence of nephrogenic diabetes insipidus, while the glomerular dysfunction results in acidosis and azotemia. Neuromuscular abnormalities secondary to hypercalcemia include muscle weakness, apathy, depression, mental obtundation, and coma. The electroencephalogram shows the nonspecific findings of diffuse slow waves.

Symptoms can be confused with other effects of tumor, side effects of narcotics, or chemotherapy. The treatment of hypercalcemia in the lung cancer patient will depend on the serum calcium level and clinical setting. While most patients are treated, terminally ill lung cancer patients who are hypercalcemic might not be, since death associated with elevated serum calcium is relatively painless.

Asymptomatic or minimally symptomatic patients with hypercalcemia may respond to hydration alone. More symptomatic patients, besides requiring hydration, may also require diuretics, mithramycin, oral phosphates, diphosphonates, or calcitonin. Intravenous phosphates and sodium sulfate are used less commonly.

Hydration is the earliest therapeutic maneuver that should be instituted to treat hypercalcemia, since dehydration secondary to a nephrogenic diabetes insipidus-like syndrome and vomiting causes volume depletion and, therefore, aggravates the hypercalcemia.[112] Intravenous saline or half-normal saline administration is required to replace the diminshed intravascular volume.

Following adequate hydration, diuretic therapy may be indicated to enhance calcium excretion. The two diuretics used are furosemide and ethacrynic acid.[169] Thiazides should not be used since they aggravate the hypercalcemia.[48] If the above mentioned methods are not effective in lowering the serum calcium levels within 24 hours following the initiation of therapy, other drug therapy should be administered. Mithramycin, a cytoxic antibiotic, has been the drug of choice in treatment of the hypercalcemic cancer patient. It exerts its effect by inhibiting bone resorption.[135,147] The drug usually is given intravenously at a dose of 25 μg/kg body weight either as a bolus injection or over a prolonged infusion.[147] A lowering of the serum calcium is noted in 24–48 hours. Toxicities associated with mithramycin include hepatocellular necrosis, hemorrhage, renal failure, and thrombocytopenia.[112] Hypocalcemia, although rare, may occur with mithramycin administration.

Newer diphosphonates (i.e., etidronate disodium) may be useful in treating hypercalcemia. They act by inhibiting bone resorption. These drugs are administered intravenously or orally and are currently being evaluated as treatment for hypercalcemia.[84]

Other treatments of hypercalcemia include infusion of isotonic sodium sulfate, oral and intravenous phosphates, calcitonin, and glucocorticords.[29,62,96,173] Calcitonin has a rapid onset of effectiveness; however, its effect may be of short duration, although its effect on lowering serum calcium levels may be extended by the addition of glucocorticords.[16]

CENTRAL NERVOUS SYSTEM

A myriad of neurologic syndromes occur in patients with lung cancer.[25,72,73] Prior to the initiation of any therapy, a meticulous neurologic examination is essential. If neurologic signs and/or symptoms are present, metastatic disease must be differentiated from a paraneoplastic syndrome. Once antitumor therapy has been started, the differential diagnosis must include adverse effects of radiation therapy and chemotherapy. Neurologic complications of lung cancer may arise as direct or indirect effects of the tumor or as side effects of therapy, as follows:

1. Direct effects of tumor
    a. Intracranial metastases
    b. Leptomeningeal disease
    c. Spinal cord compression
2. Indirect effects of tumor
    a. Paraneoplastic syndromes
        i.   Encephalomyelitis
        ii.   Cortical cerebellar degeneration
        iii. Disorders of neuromuscular function (e.g., Eaton-Lambert syndrome)
        iv.   Disorders of muscle (e.g., dermatomyositis)
        v.   Peripheral neuropathies
    b. Thrombotic and/or embolic complications
    c. Metabolic complications (e.g., SIADH)

3. Side effects of therapy
    a. Radiation therapy
        i.   CNS syndrome associated with prophylactic cranial radiotherapy
        ii. Transverse myelitis
    b. Cytotoxic chemotherapy
        i.   CNS syndrome associated with intrathecal chemotherapy
        ii. Peripheral neuropathies secondary to systemic chemotherapy

Direct Effects of Lung Cancer

Intracranial Metastases

Brain metastases are a major cause of morbidity and mortality for patients with bronchogenic carcinoma. The relative frequencies of brain metastases correlate with the histopathologic subclassification. Autopsy and clinical studies have demonstrated an overall incidence of brain metastases in 31 percent of patients with SCLC, 29 percent in large cell carcinoma, 25 percent in adenocarcinoma, and 14 percent in squamous cell carcinoma.[124] The risk of developing brain metastases increases as survival is prolonged, from an autopsy-proven frequency of 10 percent for patients with small cell cancer living 3 or more months to 80 percent for those living 2 or more years.[126]

The majority of patients with brain metastases have neurologic symptoms and/or signs. However, recent studies have shown that routine CT scans of the brain in neurologically asymptomatic patients with small cell cancer detect brain metastases in 5 percent of patients. These patients would have been otherwise classified as limited-disease.[39]

The clinical manifestations of intracranial metastases in patients with lung cancer are similar to those of patients with other metastatic tumors. Symptoms include headache, focal weakness, seizures, change in mental status, aphasia, and ataxia. Because cerebral metastases generally are multiple, the surgical removal of such lesions rarely is indicated. Radiotherapy, however, is quite effective in providing relief of symptoms in 70–90 percent of patients with brain metastases or can be used as prophylactic therapy to prevent clinical emergence of intracranial metastases in patients at high risk.[25,37]

There is considerable controversy regarding the relative efficacy and toxicity of prophylactic or elective cranial radiotherapy versus therapeutic or symptomatic brain irradiation. The most substantial data can be found in studies of SCLC in which prophylactic cranial radiotherapy has been shown to reduce CNS relapse rate from an average of 22 to 8 percent. However, there are no definitive data that prophylactic cranial radiotherapy results in a significant increase in survival, even for patients with SCLC who achieve complete remission with systemic chemotherapy[2,9,12,78,108,155] (see Chapters 20 and 22).

In view of the lack of clear-cut impact of prophylactic cranial radiotherapy on survival, the recent identification of neurologic toxicity secondary to such therapy, and the demonstrated efficacy of radiotherapy in relieving symptoms secondary to brain metastases, some authors do not advocate the prophylactic use of such radiotherapy in SCLC. Until the role of prophylactic cranial radiotherapy (i.e., PCI; prophylactic cranial irradiation) is clarified in a prospective study with adequate sample size and stratification in which complete responders are randomized to receive or not receive prophylactic therapy, most investigators limit the use of such treatment to complete responders with SCLC. A similar argument can be made for prophylactic cranial radiotherapy in patients with large cell carcinoma and adenocarcinoma, but the data base is even more limited.[36]

Leptomeningeal Metastases

It is now well recognized that multiple areas of the neuraxis frequently are involved in patients with lung cancer (particularly SCLC) and CNS metastases. Leptomeningeal metastases have been increasingly identified as a complication of small SCLC[6,22,142] but are diagnosed much less frequently in NSCLC. Few patients have meningeal carcinomatosis at the time of diagnosis of small cell lung cancer, but actuarial analysis reveals a probability of 25 percent of developing leptomeningeal metastases over the first 3 years after diagnosis.[126]

Patients with leptomeningeal metastases generally present with symptoms and signs reflecting multiple areas of involvement of the neuraxis. Headache, cranial nerve palsies, and changes in mental status are among the common presenting clinical findings. Leptomeningeal disease often occurs in the setting of progressive systemic disease so that SCLC patients frequently have symptoms and signs referable to multiple organ systems.

A positive cerebrospinal fluid (CSF) cytology establishes the diagnosis of leptomeningeal carcinomatosis. The positive cytology frequently is accompanied by an elevated CSF protein or low CSF glucose. Multiple lumbar punctures may be required to make a cytologic diagnosis; and in approximately 15 percent of cases, a presumptive clinical diagnosis of meningeal involvement with SCLC is made on the basis of clinical findings, abnormal CSF protein, and glucose levels despite repeated negative cytologic examinations.

Since carcinomatous leptomeningitis most often occurs concomitantly with progression of SCLC in multiple other sites, the therapeutic considerations must include systemic therapy as well as treatment of the meningeal disease. Treatment options for carcinomatous meningitis include intrathecal or intraventricular chemotherapy (methotrexate, thiotepa, cytosine arabinoside), radiotherapy to sites of measurable disease, or bimodality therapy.[142] Since the results of treatment of carcinomatous meningitis in these patients as well as the ability to control relapsing disease in other sites have been disappointing, treatment that focuses primarily on relief of symptoms is often most appropriate.

Spinal Cord Metastases

Review of the origin of metastases to the spine and epidural space indicates that bronchogenic carcinoma is the most common primary tumor, accounting for 15–30 percent of cases.[20] Small cell lung cancer has the greatest propensity to metastasize to the spine, with an incidence in autopsy series of 5–13 percent and 7 percent in clinical series.[133]

Spinal cord compression is an example of a complication of lung cancer in which early detection can prevent serious neurologic dysfunction.[60,140] Pain is the most frequent and earliest symptom of spinal cord compression. Once neurologic impairment (i.e., weakness, sensory changes, loss of bowel or bladder function) occurs, the chances of reversing the symptoms and signs are greatly diminished.

Although pain is the most frequent and earliest symptom, the diagnosis of spinal cord compression usually is made when other neurologic symptoms are present. Weissman and colleagues have recently reviewed the diagnostic approach to the early identification of epidural metastases.[181] These authors have noted a high correlation between cortical disruption on spinal CT scan and epidural cord compression. For patients with back pain, normal neurologic findings, and normal or equivocal plain spine films, they recommend spinal CT scan. If one or more vertebrae with cortical disruption are demonstrated, myelography is indicated. Certainly, myelography is indicated in any lung cancer patient with back pain and abnormal neurologic findings.

A rare neurologic complication of cancer, intramedullary spinal metastases,[121] is worthy of mention in that approximately 20 percent of the reported cases have been in patients with SCLC. Signs and symptoms can be indistinguishable from those of epidural metastases. The Brown-Sequard syndrome has been reported in a number of cases, and in one series, over 50 percent of the patients had coexistent carcinomatous meningitis.[182] Myelography can be interpreted as normal, but CT scan of the spine should be helpful in making this diagnosis. Prompt initiation of radiation therapy and consideration of therapy for leptomeningeal metastases are indicated in patients with SCLC and intramedullary spinal metastases.

Indirect Effects of Tumor

The majority of neurologic signs and symptoms in patients with lung cancer are accounted for by metastatic lesions. Metabolic effects (hypercalcemia, hyponatremia, hepatic encephalopathy) also represent a common etiology of neurologic problems. Much less common are the paraneoplastic neurologic syndromes. Croft and Wilkinson reported a 7 percent incidence of neuromyopathies in cancer patients, and lung cancers were the most frequent underlying diagnoses.[38] Small cell lung cancer is by far the most frequent malignancy associated with these paraneoplastic neurologic syndromes.

Two syndromes generally associated with SCLC can be easily confused with other neurologic disorders and can be reversed with systemic therapy; these are limbic encephalopathy[21,23,104] and the Eaton-Lambert syndrome.[91,92] Limbic encephalopathy is associated with intense nonspecific inflammatory reaction in the limbic system and often the temporal lobe. The earliest feature is usually dementia, but changes in affect and bizarre behavior patterns are frequently seen. There are no specific laboratory findings in this disorder, which can be diagnosed only when CNS metastases have been ruled out. Subacute cerebellar degeneration and sensory neuropathies are often seen in association with limbic encephalopathy.[23]

The Eaton-Lambert syndrome is a variant of myasthenia gravis in which muscle strength improves with repetitive exercise and there is poor response to Tensilon (edrophonium bromide; by Hoffmann-LaRoche, Nutley, NJ). The most prominent findings are muscle weakness in the proximal muscles of the lower extremities, but dysarthria, dysphagia, diplopia, and ptosis have also been noted. Lambert and colleagues have reported that as many as 6 percent of SCLC patients have this syndrome;[92] in general, however, it is clinically recognized much less frequently than that.

Simpson has proposed that induction of excess acetylcholinesterase activity by an immunoglobulin is the mechanism involved in the Eaton-Lambert syndrome.[158] The postulated etiologies of limbic encephalopathy include viral process, elaboration of a neurotoxin by the tumor, or an autoimmune process. Autoimmune processes involving antibodies that cross-react with antigens of small cell carcinoma and neural tissues have been identified as potential pathogenetic factors not only in limbic encephalopathy but also in paraneoplastic sensory neuropathy,[64] visual dysfunction,[66] cerebellar degeneration,[79] and intestinal pseudoobstruction (Olgilvie's syndrome).[153]

Side Effects of Therapy

A variety of neurologic side effects of cytotoxic therapy have been documented particularly with drugs such as cisplatin, vinca alkaloids, and hexamethylmelamine. Transverse myelitis is also a potential complication of chest radiotherapy. Rubin and Casarett estimated that radiation myelitis will develop in 1–5 percent of patients within 5 years after a spinal cord dose of 5000 rads administered in 25 fractions in 5 weeks.[144] Improvement in treatment planning techniques have further reduced this adverse effect of radiotherapy. There is great concern regarding the neurologic consequences of prophylactic cranial radiotherapy (PCI) with or without systemic chemotherapy. It has been demonstrated that neurologic abnormalities are common in long-term survivors of SCLC treated with PCI. Johnson and colleagues reviewed the neurologic status of 20 SCLC patients who were disease-free for over 2 years.[80] Fifteen patients (75 percent) had neurologic complaints, with recent memory loss as the most common symptom. Abnormalities in neurologic examination, including gait disturbances, muscle weakness, intention tremors, and peripheral neuropathy were noted in 13 (65 percent) patients. CT scans of the brain showed ventricular dilatation or cerebral atrophy in the majority of cases, and these radiologic changes were progressive over many years. Studies have not been conducted to precisely identify the contribution of other factors (i.e., the underlying cancer, paraneoplastic syndromes, aging process) in these neurologic syndromes; nonetheless, it is clear that prophylactic cranial radiotherapy can result in deleterious effects in this elderly population. On the basis of the NCI experience, a number of investigators have suggested a means of potentially minimizing CNS toxicity by decreasing the dose fractions of radiotherapy and minimizing or eliminating systemic chemotherapy during the period of cranial radiotherapy.[80,89] In addition, it appears that magnetic resonance imaging may provide a more sensitive means for radiologically detecting and monitoring neurotoxicity in patients with lung cancer.[57]

ENDOCRINE SYMPTOMS

The endocrine manifestations of lung cancer are of considerable interest to clinicians as well as tumor biologists because these syndromes (1) provide a clue to the presence of an underlying neoplasm and frequently parallel the progression of the cancer, (2) can cause significant morbidity for the patient, and (3) provide considerable insight into the biologic behavior of cancer and the mechanisms concerned with the synthesis, packaging, and secretion of peptide hormones.[8]

Small cell lung cancer is unique among lung carcinoma and cancer in general because of its association with paraneoplastic syndromes. Even more striking is the ability of small cell cancer to produce detectable levels of peptide hormones in in vitro systems. Some small cell carcinomas have been demonstrated to produce as many as

12 hormones in vitro.[160] For a detailed review of polypeptide synthesis in SCLC, see Chapter 22, section headed "SCCL Is a Systemic Disease."

SYSTEMIC-PARANEOPLASTIC SYNDROMES

There are a number of systemic effects of cancer that are certainly not specific for lung cancer but do cause significant morbidity for patients with bronchogenic carcinoma.

Weight Loss

Weight loss is one of the most frequent and demoralizing adverse systemic effects of malignancy.[42] Although there may be mechanical (i.e., esophageal obstruction) and iatrogenic (i.e., radiotherapy and chemotherapy) etiologies of weight loss in patients with lung cancer, the precise metabolic mechanisms for anorexia and weight loss have not been elucidated.

Pretreatment weight loss has been shown to be a poor prognostic factor for patients with SCLC as well as NSCLC.[43] Decrease in survival has been shown to be associated with weight loss in patients with limited stage of lung cancer, but in patients with more advanced tumor extent, weight loss has not been shown to affect survival. Certainly, good nutritional support is an important part of the overall management schema of patients with cancer. However, there is no evidence that aggressive nutritional support will improve response rate to chemotherapy or survival in patients with lung cancer or any other neoplasm. In fact, a randomized controlled study of parenteral nutrition in patients with SCLC receiving systemic chemotherapy was reported recently. Although the group receiving parenteral nutrition had an initial, but transient, weight gain and less delays of induction chemotherapy, there were no differences in complete or partial response rates or survival between the two groups.[52]

Coagulopathy—Vascular Complications

In addition to the direct hematologic consequences of marrow invasion by tumor, there are a variety of indirect effects of solid tumors, including lung cancer on erythroid and myeloid elements, as well as platelets and coagulation factors.[177] The hypercoagulable state associated with many forms of cancer is a major cause of morbidity as a result of the clinical syndromes of migratory thrombophlebitis, disseminated intravascular coagulation, and nonbacterial thrombotic endocarditis.

Although the greatest risk of migratory thrombophlebitis (Trousseau's syndrome) may be associated with pancreatic cancer, lung cancer is the most common association because of its greater prevalence. Migratory thrombophlebitis is also frequently associated with other mucin-secreting adenocarcinomas of the gastrointestinal tract, but breast, ovarian, prostate, and other solid tumors have also been reported. The deep venous thrombosis in these patients is not only migratory but also recurrent and involves veins in unusual locations such as the upper extremities. In general, heparin therapy is recommended for thrombophlebitis associated with malignancy or for other chronic or symptomatic syndromes related to disseminated intravascular coagulation.[148] However, such patients are prone to have other organ dysfunction and must be very carefully monitored on heparin therapy. As is the case with other paraneoplastic syndromes, treatment of the underlying malignancy is the key to control of the coagulopathy.

Cutaneous Manifestations

The cutaneous manifestations of cancer have been extensively reviewed.[26] There are no cutaneous paraneoplastic syndromes that are specific for lung cancer. Dermatomyositis is a skin and muscle disorder that has been linked to underlying cancer, including lung cancer. Although only 25 percent of cases of dermatomyositis have been associated with cancer, the syndrome of heliotropic eruption and periungual telangiectasias, in conjunction with proximal symmetrical muscle weakness certainly is an indication for evaluation of the patient for a malignancy.

REFERENCES

1. Abrams HL, Siegelman SS, Adams DF, et al: Computed tomagraphy versus ultrasound of the adrenal gland: A prospective study. Radiology 143:121-128, 1982
2. Aisner J, Whiteacre M, Van Echo DA, et al: Combination chemotherapy for small cell carcinoma of the lung: Continuous versus alternating non-cross resistant combinations. Cancer Treat Rep 66:221-230, 1982
3. Alexander C: Diaphragm movements and the diagnosis of diaphragmatic paralysis. Clin Radiol 17:79-83, 1966
4. Allan SG, Bundred N, Eremin O, et al: Acute pancreatitis in association with small cell lung carcinoma: Potential pitfall in diagnosis and management. Postgrad Med J 61:643-644, 1985
5. Anderson CB, Philpott GW, Ferguson TB: The treatment of malignant pleural effusions. Cancer 33:916-922, 1974
6. Aroney RS, Dolley DN, Chan WK, et al: Meningeal carcinomatosis in small cell carcinoma of the lung. Am J Med 71:26-32, 1981
7. Aronin PA, Mahaley MS, Rudnick SA, et al: Prediction of BCNU pulmonary toxicity in patients with malignant gliomas. An assessment of risk factors. New Engl J Med 303:183-188, 1980
8. Azzopardi JG, Freeman E, et al: Endocrine and metabolic disorders in bronchial carcinoma. Br Med J 4:528-529, 1970
9. Baglan RJ, Marks JE: Comparison of symptomatic and prophylactic irradiation of brain metastases from oat cell carcinoma of the lung. Cancer 47:41-45, 1981
10. Bayley TC, Kisner DL, Sybert A, et al: Tetracycline and quinacrine in the control of malignant pleural effusions. Cancer 41:1188-1192, 1978
11. Baylin SB, Gazdar AF: Endocrine biochemistry in the spectrum of human lung cancer: Implications for the cellular origin of small cell carcinoma, in Greco FA, Oldham RK, Bunn PA (eds): Small Cell Lung Cancer. Orlando, FL, Grune & Stratton, 1981, pp. 123-143
12. Beiler DD, Kane RC, Bernath AM, et al: Low dose elective brain irradiation in small cell carcinoma of the lung. Internatl J Radiat Oncol Biol Phys 5:941-945, 1979
13. Bender RA, Hansen H: Hypercalcemia in bronchogenic carcinoma. Ann Intern Med 80:205-208, 1974
14. Benson R, Riggs L, Pickard B: Radioimmunoassay of parathyroid hormone in hypercalcemic patients with malignant disease. Am J Med 56:821-826, 1974

15. Besarab A, Caro J: Mechanisms of hypercalcemia in malignancy. Cancer 41:2276–2285, 1978

16. Binastock ML, Mundy GR: Effects of calcitonin and glucocorticords in combination in malignant hypercalcemia. Ann Intern Med 93:264–272, 1980

17. Biran S: Corticosteroids in radiation-induced pericarditis. Chest 74:96–98, 1978

18. Biran S, Hachman A, Leij IS, et al: Clinical diagnosis of secondary tumors of the heart and pericardium. Dis Chest 55:202–208, 1969

19. Bitran JD, Brown C, Desser RK, et al: Intracavitary bleomycin for the control of malignant effusions. J Surg Oncol 16:273–277, 1981

20. Black P: Metastatic tumors of the central nervous system: Spinal metastases, in Abeloff MD (ed): Complications of Cancer. Baltimore, The Johns Hopkins University Press, 1979, pp 313–356

21. Brennan LV, Craddock PR: Limbic encephalopathy as a nometastatic complication of oat cell lung cancer. Am J Med 75:518–520, 1983

22. Brereton HD, O'Donnell JF, Kent CH, et al: Spinal meningeal carcinomatosis in small cell carcinoma of the lung. Ann Intern Med 88:517–519, 1978

23. Brierly JB, Corsellis JAN, Hierons R, et al: Subacute encephalitis of later adult life mainly affecting the limbic areas. Brain 83:357–368, 1960

24. Brouchow IB, Johnson J: Obstructions of the vena cava. Surg Gynecol Obstet 134:115–121, 1972

25. Bunn PA, Rosen ST: Central nervous system manifestations of small cell lung cancer, in Aisner J (ed): Lung Cancer. New York, Churchill Livingston, 1985, pp. 287–305

26. Callen JP: Cutaneous complications of cancer, in Calabresi P, Schein PS, Rosenberg SA (eds): Medical Oncology: Basic Principles and Clinical Management of Cancer. New York, Macmillan Company, 1985, pp. 223–234

27. Castellino RA, Glatstein E, Turbow MM, et al: Latent radiation injury of lungs or heart activated by steroid withdrawal. Ann Intern Med 80:593–599, 1974

28. Catane R, Lichter A, Lee YJ, et al: Small cell lung cancer: Analysis of treatment factors contributing to prolonged survival. Cancer 48:1936–1943, 1981

29. Chak Makjian ZH, Bethune JE: Sodium sulfate treatment of hypercalcemia. New Engl J Med 275:862–869, 1966

30. Cham WC, Freiman AH, Carstens PHB, et al: Radiation therapy of cardiac and pericardial metastases. Ther Radiol 114:701–704, 1975

31. Chori CH, Carey RW: Small cell carcinoma of the lung: Reappraisal of current management. Cancer 37:2651–2657, 1976

32. Cohen MH: Signs and symptoms of bronchogenic carcinoma, in Straus, MJ (ed): Lung Cancer, Clinical Diagnosis and Treatment. Orlando, FL, Grune & Stratton, 1983, pp. 97–111

33. Cohn KE, Stewart JR, Fajardo LF, Hancock EW: Heart disease following radiation. Medicine 46:281–298, 1971

34. Comis RL: Bleomycin pulmonary toxicity, in Crooke ST, Umezawa H (eds): Bleomycin: Current status and new developments. Orlando, FL, Academic Press, 1978, pp. 279–291

35. Cortes EP, Lutman G, Wanka J, et al: Adriamycin (NSC-123127) cardiotoxicity: A clinicopathologic correlation. Cancer Chemother Rep 6:215–225, 1975

36. Cox JD, Komaki R, Byhardt RW: Radiotherapy for non-small cell cancer of the lung, in Aisner J (ed): Lung Cancer. New York, Churchill Livingston, 1985, pp. 131–154

37. Cox JD, Komaki R, Byhardt RW, et al: Results of whole brain irradiation for metastases from small cell carcinoma of the lung. Cancer Treat Rep 64:957–961, 1980

38. Croft P, Wilkinson M: The incidence of carcinomatous neuromyopathy in patients with various types of carcinoma. Brain 88:427–434, 1965

39. Cruz JM, Jackson DV, Muss HB, et al: Detection of brain metastases at diagnosis of small cell carcinoma of the lung. J Neuro-Oncol 2:67-71, 1984

40. D'Angio GJ: Early and delayed complications of therapy. Cancer 51:2515-2518, 1983

41. Dewald G, Dines DE, Weiland LH, et al: Usefulness of chromosome examination in the diagnosis of malignant pleural effusions. New Engl J Med 295:1494-1500, 1976

42. DeWys WD: Management of cancer cachexia. Semin Oncol 12:452-460, 1985

43. DeWys WD, Begg C, Lavin P, et al: Prognostic effect of weight loss prior to chemotherapy in cancer patients. Am J Med 69:491-497, 1980

44. Dollinger M: Management of recurrent malignant effusions. CA 22:138-147, 1972

45. Dombernowsky P, Hansen HH: Combination chemotherapy in the management of superior vena caval obstruction in small cell anaplastic carcinoma of the lung. Acta Med Scand 204:513-516, 1978

46. Dombernowsky P, Hirsch F, Hansen HH, et al: Peritoneoscopy in staging of 190 patients with small cell anaplastic carcinoma of the lung with special reference of subtyping. Cancer 41:2008-2012, 1978

47. Dossetor JB, Vennings EH, Beck JC: Hyponatremia associated with superior vena cava obstruction. Metabolism 10:149-161, 1961

48. Duarte CG, Winnacker JL, Becker KL, et al: Thiazide-induced hypercalcemia. New Engl J Med 284:828-830, 1971

49. Einhorn LH, Bond WH, Hornback N, et al: Long-term results in combined modality treatment of small cell carcinoma of the lung. Semin Oncol 5:309-313, 1978

50. Einhorn L, Krause M, Hornback N, et al: Enhanced pulmonary toxicity with bleomycin and radiotherapy in oat cell lung cancer. Cancer 37:2414-2416, 1976

51. Estenne M, Yernault JC, Troyer AD: Mechanism of relief of dyspnea after thorocentesis in patients with large pleural effusions. Am J Med 74:813-819, 1983

52. Evans WK, Makuck R, Clamon GH, et al: Limited impact of total parenteral nutrition on nutritional status during treatment for small cell lung cancer. Cancer Res 45:3347-3353, 1985

53. Failor HT, Edwards JE, Hodgson CH: Etiologic factors in obstruction of the superior vena cava. Mayo Clin Proc 33:671-678, 1958

54. Fraisse J, Brizard CP, Emonot A, et al: Diagnosis of malignancy by cytogenetic means in effusions (Abstr). Clin Genetics 14:288, 1978

55. Fredrickson RT, Cohen LS, Mullins CB: Pericardial windows or pericardiocentesis for pericardial effusions. Am Heart J 82:158-162, 1978

56. Friedman MA, Slater E: Malignant pleural effusions. Cancer Treat Rev 5:49-66, 1978

57. Frytak S, Franklin E, O'Neill B: Magnetic resonance imaging for neurotoxicity in long-term survivors of carcinoma. Mayo Clinic Proc 60:803-812, 1985

58. Gale ME, Brinbaum SB, Gale DR, et al: Esophageal invasion by lung cancer: CT diagnosis. J Comput Assist Tomogr 8:694-698, 1984

59. Ghosh BC, Cliffton EE: Malignant tumors with superior vena caval obstruction. NY State J Med 73:283, 1973

60. Gilbert RW, Kim JH, Posner JB: Epidural spinal cord compression from metastatic tumor: Diagnosis and treatment. Ann Neurol 3:40-51, 1978

61. Ginsberg RJ, Hill LD, Eagan RT, et al: Modern thirty-day operative mortality for surgical resections in lung cancer. J Thorac Cardiovasc Surg 86:654-658, 1983

62. Goldsmith RS, Angbar SH: Inorganic phosphate treatment of hypercalcemia of diverse etiologies. New Engl J Med 274:1-7, 1966

63. Gralla RJ, Itri LM, Pisko SE, et al: Antiemetic efficacy of high-dose metoclopramide: Randomized trials with placebo and prochlorperazine in patients with chemotherapy-induced nausea and vomiting. New Engl J Med 305:905-909, 1981

64. Graus F, Elkon KB, Cordon-Cardo C, et al: Sensory neuropathy and small cell lung cancer. Am J Med 80:45-52, 1986

65. Gross NJ: Pulmonary effects of radiation therapy. Ann Intern Med 86:81–92, 1977
66. Grunwald GB, Simmonds MA, Klein R, et al: Autoimmune basis for visual paraneoplastic syndrome in patients with small cell lung carcinoma. Lancet 1:658–661, 1985
67. Hansen HH, Dombernowsky P, Hansen MF, et al: Chemotherapy of advanced small cell anaplastic carcinoma. Superiority in a randomized trial of a 4-drug combination to a 3-drug combination. Ann Intern Med 89:177–181, 1978
68. Harmon H, Fergus S, Cole F: Pneumonectomy: Review of 351 cases. Ann Surg 183:719–722, 1976
69. Harviel JD, McNamara JJ, Straehley CJ: Surgical treatment of lung cancer in patients over the age of 70 years. J Thorac Cardiovasc Surg 75:802–805, 1978
70. Hausheer FH, Yarbro JW: Diagnosis and treatment of malignant pleural effusion. Semin Oncol 12:54–75, 1985
71. Hellman S, Kligerman MM, von Essen CF, et al: Sequelae of radical radiotherapy of carcinoma of the lung. Radiology 82:1055–1061, 1964
72. Henson RA, Urich H: Cancer and the Nervous System. Oxford, Blackwell Scientific Publications, 1982, p
73. Hildebrand J: Lesions of the Nervous System in Cancer Patients. New York, Raven Press, 1978, pp. 123–125
74. Hines LE: Fibrosis of the lung following roentgen-ray treatments for tumor. JAMA 79:720–722, 1922
75. Howard N, Pick EJ: The value of phlebography in superior vena caval obstruction. Clin Radiol 12:290–294, 1961
76. Hyde L, Hyde CI: Clinical manifestations of lung cancer. Chest 65:299–306, 1974
77. Ihde DC, Makuch RW, Carney DN, et al: Prognostic implications of stage of disease and sites of metastases in patients with small cell carcinoma of the lung treated with intensive combination chemotherapy. Am Rev Respir Dis 123:500–507, 1981
78. Jackson DV, Richards F, Cooper MR: Prophylactic cranial irradiation in small cell carcinoma of the lung. A randomized study. JAMA 237:2730–2733, 1977
79. Jaeckle KA, Greco F, Houghton A, et al: Autoimmune response of patients with paraneoplastic cerebellar degeneration to a Purkinje cell cytoplasmic protein antigen. Ann Neurol 18:592–600, 1985
80. Johnson BE, Becker B, Goff WB, et al: Neurologic, neuropsychologic, and computed cranial tomography scan abnormalities in 2 to 10 year survivors of small-cell lung cancer. J Clin Oncol 3:1659–1667, 1985
81. Johnson DH, Hainsworth JD, Greco FA: Extrahepatic biliary obstruction caused by small cell lung cancer. Ann Intern Med 102:487–490, 1985
82. Johnson RE, Brereton HD, Kent C: "Total" therapy for small cell carcinoma of the lung. Am Thorac Surg 25:509–515, 1978
83. Jordan GS, Eisenberg E, Loken HF, et al: Clinical endocrinology of parathyroid hormone excess. Recent Progr Horm Res 18:297–336, 1962
84. Jung A: Comparison of two parenteral diphosphonates in hypercalcemia of malignancy. Am J Med 72:221–226, 1986
85. Kane RC, Cohen M, Broder LE, et al: Superior vena caval obstruction due to small cell anaplastic lung carcinoma. JAMA 235:1717–1718, 1976
86. Kaplan HS, Stewart JR: Complications of intensive megavoltage radiotherapy for Hodgkin's disease. Natl Cancer Inst Monogr 36:439–444, 1973
87. Kilpatrick ZM, Chapman CB: On pericardiocentesis. Am J Cardiol 16:722–728, 1965
88. Kirsch MM, Rotman H, Behrendt DM, et al: Complications of pulmonary resection. Ann Thorac Surg 20:215–236, 1975
89. Komaki R, Byhardt RW, Anderson T, et al: What is the lowest effective biologic dose for prophylactic cranial irradiation. Am J Clin Oncol 8:523–527, 1985
90. Krishnamurthy GT, Blahd WH, Winston MA: Superior vena caval syndrome. Scin-

tophotographic evaluation of response to radiation therapy. Am J Roetgenol Radium Ther Nucl Med 117:609-614, 1973

91. Lambert EH, Eaton LM, Rooke ED: Defect of neuromuscular conduction associated with malignant neoplasms. Am J Physiol 187:612, 1956

92. Lambert EH, Rooke ED: Myasthenic state and lung cancer, in Brain WR, Norris FH Jr (eds): The Remote Effects of Cancer in the Nervous System. Orlando, FL, Grune & Stratton, 1965, pp. 67-80

93. Laurens RG Jr, Pines JR, Honig EG: Spontaneous pneumothorax in primary cavitating lung carcinoma. Radiology 146:295-297, 1983

94. Lawson RAM, Ross WM, Gold RG, et al: Post-radiation pericarditis: Report on four more cases with special reference to bronchogenic carcinoma. J Thorac Cardiovasc Surg 63:841-847, 1972

95. Lazlo J (ed): Antiemetics and Cancer Chemotherapy. Baltimore, Williams & Wilkins, 1983, pp. 1-5

96. Lazor MZ, Rosenberg LE: Mechanism of adrenal steroid reversal of hypercalcemia in multiple myeloma. New Engl J Med 270:749-755, 1964

97. Lichtenstein H: X-ray diagnosis of radiation injuries to the lung. Dis Chest 38:294-297, 1960

98. Livingston BR, Moore TN, Heibrun L, et al: Small cell carcinoma of the lung: Combined chemotherapy and radiation. Ann Intern Med 88:194-199, 1978

99. Lokich JJ: The management of malignant pericardial effusions. JAMA 224:1401-1404, 1973

100. Lokich JJ, Goodman R: Superior vena cava syndrome. JAMA 231:58-61, 1975

101. Lundgren R, Stjernberg N: Spontaneous pneumothorax as first symptom in bronchial carcinoma. Acta Med Scand 207:329-330, 1980

102. Maddox AM, Valdivieso M, Lukeman J, et al: Superior vena cava obstruction in small cell bronchogenic carcinoma. Cancer 52:2165-2172, 1983

103. Mahrajan V, Kupferer CF, Van Ordstrand HS: Pneumothorax. A rare manifestation of lung cancer. Chest 68:730-732, 1975

104. Markman M, Abeloff MD: Small cell lung cancer and limbic encephalitis. Ann Intern Med 96:785, 1982

105. Markman M, Sheidler V, Ettinger DS, et al: Antiemetic efficacy of dexamethasone: A randomized, double-blind, cross-over study with prochlorperazine in patients receiving cancer chemotherapy. New Engl J Med 311:549, 1984

106. Martini MM, Goodner JT, D'Angio GJ, et al: Tracheoesophageal fistula due to cancer. J Thorac Cardiovasc Surg 59:319-324, 1970

107. Martini N, Bains MS, Beattie EJ Jr: Indications for pleurectomy in malignant effusion. Cancer 35:734-738, 1975

108. Maurer LH, Tulloh M, Weiss RB, et al: A randomized combined modality trial in small cell carcinoma of the lung: Comparison of combination chemotherapy—radiation therapy versus cyclophosphamide—radiation therapy, effects of maintenance chemotherapy and prophylactic whole brain irradiation. Cancer 45:30-39, 1980

109. Maxfield WS, Meckstroth GR: Technetium-99m superior vena cavography. Radiology 62:913-917, 1969

110. Mayer EG, Poulter CA, Aristizabal SA: Complications of irradiation related to apparent drug potentiation by Adriamycin. Internatl Radiat Oncol Biol Phys 1:1179-1188, 1976

111. Mayer E, Maier H (eds): Pulmonary carcinoma. New York, New York University Press, 1956, p 159

112. Mazzaferri EL, O'Dorisio TM, LoBuglio AF: Treatment of hypercalcemia associated with malignancy. Semin Oncol 5:141-153, 1978

113. Minow RA, Benjamin RS, Gottleib JA: Adriamycin (NSC-123127) cardiomyopathy—

an overview with determination of risk factors. Cancer Chemother Rep 6:195-201, 1975

114. Mira JG, Livingston RB, Moore TN, et al: Influence of chest radiotherapy in frequency and patterns of relapse in disseminated small cell lung carcinoma. Cancer 50:1266-1272, 1982

115. Moore TN, Livingston R, Heilbrun L, et al: An acceptable rate of complications in combined doxorubicin-irradiation for small cell carcinoma of the lung. A Southwest Oncology Group Study. Internatl J Radiat Oncol Biol Phys 4:675-680, 1978

116. Morris AL: Echo evaluation of tamponade. Circulation 53:746-747, 1976

117. Muggia FM, Hansen HH: Osteoblastic metastases in small cell (oat-cell) carcinoma of the lung. Cancer 30-801-805, 1972

118. Muggia FM, Heinemann HO: Hypercalcemia associated with neoplastic disease. Ann Intern Med 73:281-290, 1970

119. Mulshine JL, Makuch RW, Johnson-Early A, et al: Diagnosis and significance of liver metastases in small cell carcinoma of the lung. J Clin Oncol 2:733-740, 1984

120. Mulvey RB: Peripheral bone metastases. Am J Roentgenol Radium Ther Nucl Med 91:155-160, 1964

121. Murphy KC, Feld R, Evans WK, et al: Intramedullary spinal cord metastases from small cell carcinoma of the lung. J Clin Oncol 1:99-106, 1983

122. Murray GC, Persellin RH: Metastatic carcinoma presenting as monoarticular arthritis: A case report and review of the literature. Arth Rheum 23:95-100, 1980

123. Nagasaki F, Flehinger BJ, Martini N: Complications of surgery in the treatment of carcinoma of the lung. Chest 82:25-29, 1982

124. Newman SJ, Hansen HH: Frequency, diagnosis, and treatment of brain metastases in 247 consecutive patients with bronchogenic carcinoma. Cancer 33:492-496, 1974

125. Niarchos AP: Electrical alternans in cardiac tamponade. Thorax 30:228-233, 1975

126. Nugent JL, Bunn PA, Matthews MJ: CNS metastases in small cell bronchogenic carcinoma. Cancer 44:1885-1893, 1979

127. O'Bryan RM, Talley RW, Brennan MJ, et al: Critical analysis of the control of malignant effusions with radioisotopes. Henry Ford Hosp Med J 16:3-14, 1968

128. Okay NH, Bryk D: Collateral pathways in occlusion of the superior vena cava and its tributaries. Radiology 92:1493-1498, 1969

129. Orwoll ES, Kiessing P, Paterson R: Interstitial pneumonia from mitomycin. Ann Intern Med 89:352-355, 1978

130. Pagani JJ: Normal adrenal glands in small cell lung carcinoma: CT-guided biopsy. Am J Roentgenol 140:947-951, 1983

131. Paladine W, Cunningham TJ, Sponzo R, et al: Intracavitary bleomycin in the management of malignant effusions. Cancer 38:1903-1908, 1976

132. Paulson, DL. Carcinomas in the superior pulmonary sulcus. J Thorac Cardiovasc Surg 7:1095-1102, 1975

133. Pedersen AG, Bach F, Melgaard B: Frequency, diagnosis and prognosis of spinal cord compression in small cell bronchogenic carcinoma. Cancer 55:1818-1822, 1985

134. Perez CA, Presant CA, Van Amburg A: Management of superior vena cava syndrome. Semin Oncol 5:123-134, 1978

135. Perlia CP, Gubisch NJ, Wolter J, et al: Mithramycin treatment of hypercalcemia. Cancer 25:389-394, 1970

136. Phillips TL, Wharam MD, Margolis LW: Modification of radiation injury to normal tissues by chemotherapeutic agents. Cancer 35:1678-1684, 1975

137. Praga C. Beretta G, Vigo PL, et al: Adriamycin cardiotoxicity: A survey of 1273 patients. Cancer Treat Rep 63:827-834, 1979

138. Ratliff JL, Chavez CM, Jamchuk A, et al: Reexpansion pulmonary edema. Chest 64:654-656, 1973

139. Rittgers RA, Loewenstein MS, Feinerman AE, et al: Carcinoembryonic antigen levels in benign and malignant pleural effusions. Ann Intern Med 88:631-634, 1978

140. Rodichok LD, Harper GR, Ruckdeschel J, et al: Early diagnosis of spinal epidural metastases. Am J Med 70:1181-1187, 1981

141. Rodrigues N, Straus MJ: Superior vena caval syndrome, in MJ Straus (ed): Lung Cancer, Clinical Diagnosis and Treatment. Orlando, FL, Grune & Stratton, 1983, pp 323-333

142. Rosen ST, Aisner J, Makuch RW, et al: Carcinomatous leptomeningitis in small cell lung cancer: A clinicopathologic review of the National Cancer Institute experience. Medicine 61:45-53, 1982

143. Rosenthal S, Kaufman S: Vincristine neurotoxicity. Ann Intern Med 80:733-737, 1975

144. Rubin P, Casarett GW: Clinical Radiation Pathology. Philadelphia, Saunders, 1968

145. Rubin P, Green J, Holzwasser G: Superior vena caval syndrome. Radiology 82:388-401, 1963

146. Rubinson RM, Bolooki H: Intrapleural tetracycline for control of malignant pleural effusion: A preliminary report. South Med J 65:847-849, 1972

147. Ryan WG, SChwartz TB, Perlia CP: Effects of mithramycin on Paget's disease of bone. Ann Intern Med 70:549-557, 1969

148. Sack GH, Levin J, Bell WR: Trousseau's syndrome and other manifestations of chronic disseminated coagulopathy in patients with neoplasms. Medicine 56:1-37, 1977

149. Salsali M, Cliffton EE: Superior vena cava obstruction with lung cancer. Ann Thorac Surg 6:437-442, 1968

150. Salt WB, Schenker S: Amylase—its clinical significance. A review of the literature. Medicine 55:269-289, 1976

151. Salyer WR, Eggleston JC, Erozan YS: Efficacy of pleural needle biopsy and pleural fluid cytopathology in the diagnosis of malignant neoplasm involving the pleura. Chest 67:536-539, 1975

152. Scannell JG: Etiology and surgical approaches in superior vena caval obstruction. Radiology 81:378-379, 1963

153. Schuffler MD, Baird HW, Fleming R, et al: Intestinal pseudo-obstruction as the presenting manifestation of small cell carcinoma of the lung. Ann Intern Med 98:129-134, 1983

154. Seyberth HR, Hornet P, Segre GV: Prostaglandin as mediators of hypercalcemia associated with certain types of cancer. New Engl J Med 293:1278-1282, 1975

155. Seydel HG, Creech R, Pogans M, et al: Combined modality treatment of small cell undifferentiated carcinoma of the lung. A cooperative study of the RTOG and the ECOG. Internatl J Radiat Oncol Biol Phys 9 (Suppl 1):1135-1141, 1983

156. Seydel HG, Maun J: Pulmonary fibrosis following radiotherapy for bronchogenic carcinoma and Hodgkin's disease. MD State Med J 18:61-62, 1969

157. Shigeno C, Yamamoto I, Dokoh S, et al: Identification of $1,24(R)$-Dihydroxyvitamin D_3-like bone resorbing lipid in a patient with cancer-associated hypercalcemia. J Clin Endocr Met 61:761-768, 1985

158. Simpson JA: The myasthenic (Eaton-Lambert) syndrome associated with carcinoma: Enzyme induction as a possible mechanism of paraneoplastic syndromes. Scott Med J 27:220-228, 1982

159. Smith FE, Lane M, Hudgkins PT: Conservative management of malignant pericardial effusion. Cancer 33:47-57, 1974

160. Sorenson GD, Pettengill OS, Cate CC, et al: Biomarkers in small cell carcinoma of the lung, in Aisner J (ed): Lung Cancer: Contemporary Issues in Clinical Oncology. New York, Churchill Livingston, 1985, pp. 203-241

161. Sostman HD, Matthay RA, Putman CE, et al: Methotrexate-induced pneumonitis. Medicine 55:371-388, 1976

162. Spiro SG, Shah PG, Tobias JS, et al: Treatment of obstruction of the superior vena cava by combination chemotherapy with and without irradiation in small-cell carcinoma of the bronchus. Thorax 38:501–505, 1983

163. Spodick DH: Acute cardiac tamponade. Pathologic physiology, diagnosis and management. Progr Cardiovasc Dis 10:64–96, 1967

164. Stankey RM, Roshe J, Sogocio RM: Carcinoma of the lung and dysphagia. Dis Chest 55:13–17, 1969

165. Steiger Z, Wilson RF, Leichman L, et al: Management of malignant bronchoesophageal fistulas. Surg Gynecol Obstet 157:201–204, 1983

166. Steinberg I: Effusive-constrictive radiation pericarditis: Two cases illustrating value of angiocardiography in diagnosis. Am J Cardiol 19:434–439, 1976

167. Stewart JR, Cohn KE, Fajardo LF, et al: Radiation-induced heart disease: A study of twenty-five patients. Radiology 89:302–310, 1967

168. Strauss BL, Matthews MJ, Cohen MH, et al: Cardiac metastases in lung cancer. Chest 71:607–611, 1977

169. Suki WN, Yium JJ, Von Minden M, et al: Acute treatment of hypercalcemia with furosemide. New Engl J Med 283:836–840, 1970

170. Theologides A: Neoplastic cardiac tamponade. Semin Oncol 5:181–192, 1978

171. Thurber DL, Edwards JE, Achor RWP: Secondary malignant tumors of the pericardium. Circulation 26:228–241, 1962

172. Trask CWL, Joannides T, Harper PG, et al: Radiation-induced lung fibrosis after treatment of small cell carcinoma of the lung with very high dose cyclophosphamide. Cancer 55:57–60, 1985

173. Vaughn CB, Vaitkevcius K: The effects of calcitonin in hypercalcemia in patients with malignancy. Cancer 34:1268–1271, 1974

174. Von Hoff DD, Layard NW, Base P, et al: Risk factors for doxorubicin-induced congestive heart failure. Ann Intern Med 91:710–717, 1979

175. Wagaruddin M, Bernstein A: Reexpansion pulmonary edema. Thorax 30:54–60, 1975

176. Wallace RJ, Cohen A, Awe RJ: Carcinomatous lung abscess: Diagnosis by bronchoscopy and cytopathology. JAMA 242:521–522, 1979

177. Waterbury L: Hematologic problems, in Abeloff MD (ed): Complications of Cancer. Baltimore, The Johns Hopkins University Press, 1979, pp. 121–145

178. Waterfield R: Biot respiration in superior vena caval obstruction. Guys Hosp Rep 78:305–307, 1928

179. Weiss W: The Philadelphia pulmonary neoplasm research project. Clin Chest Med 3:243–256, 1982

180. Weissburg D, Kaufman M: Diagnostic and therapeutic pleuroscopy: Experience with 127 patients. Chest 78:732–735, 1980

181. Weissman DE, Gilbert M, Wang H, et al: The use of computed tomography of the spine to identify patients at high risk for epidural metastases. J Clin Oncol 3:1541–1544, 1985

182. Weissman DE, Grossman SA: Simultaneous leptomeningeal and intramedullary spinal metastases in small cell lung carcinoma. Med Ped Oncol 14:54–56, 1986

183. Winkelmann M, Pfitzer P: Blind pleural biopsy in combination with cytology of pleural effusions. Acta Cytol 25:373–376, 1981

184. Yacoub MH: Relation between the histology of bronchial carcinoma and hypertrophic pulmonary osteorthropathy. Thorax 20:537, 1965

Index

Page numbers in *italics* indicate illustrations.
Page numbers followed by *t* indicate tables.

Abdomen
  complications involving, 421-423
  metastases to, in small cell lung cancer
    staging, 270
  relapse involving, in small cell lung cancer,
    389-391
ACE combination chemotherapy for small cell
  lung cancer, 315-316
Actinomycin-D as antitumor antibiotic, 81
Adenocarcinoma(s)
  cell lines of, 37-38
  with neurosecretory granules, 28
  pathology of, 17-21
    gross, 18
    microscopic, 18-20
    research efforts on, 20, 21
Adenosquamous carcinoma, 21-22
Adrenal glands, complications involving,
  diagnosis and management of, 422
Adrenocorticotropin (ACTH) as small cell
  lung cancer (SCLC) biomarkers,
  283-284
Adriamycin
  as antitumor antibiotic, 81-82
  with cyclophosphamide
    and etoposide for small cell lung cancer,
    315-316
    methotrexate, and procarbazine. *See*
    CAMP

  with cytoxan
    and platinum. *See* CAP
    and vincristine. *See* CAV
  in stage II adjuvant chemotherapy,
    179-180
Air embolism complicating percutaneous
  needle biopsy, 106
AJC staging system, 116-118
AJC/Zubrod Performance Scale as
  noninvasive staging technique, 120
Alkaloids, plant, pharmacology of, 80-81
Alkylating agents, pharmacology of, 77, 79
Antibiotics, antitumor, 81-82
Antibodies, monoclonal, against lung cancer-
  associated antigens, 44-45
Anti-bombesin antibody for NSCLC, 239
Anticoagulants in small cell lung cancer
  therapy, 317
Antidiuretic hormone (ADH) as small cell
  lung cancer (SCLC) biomarkers, 283*t*,
  284*t*, 285
Antigen(s)
  carcinoembryonic, as small cell lung cancer
    (SCLC) biomarkers, 286-289
  lung cancer-associated, monoclonal
    antibodies against, 44-45
Antimetabolites, pharmacology of, 79-80
Antineoplastic chemotherapeutics,
  pharmacology of, 77-81

Antitumor antibiotics, 81–82
Arterial blood gas values, preoperative, 57
Artery, pulmonary, invasion of, by T_3 tumor,
 management of, 194

Bacillus Calmette-Guerin (BCG)
 immunotherapy, intrapleural,
 adjuvant, in stage I disease, 144–145
Biliary obstruction, diagnosis and
 management of, 422
Bimodal therapy. *See also* Combined modal
 therapy
 for advanced non-small cell lung cancer,
 221–227
 early studies on, 221–222
 optimal use of, 222–223
 recent clinical trials on, 223–227
 for small cell lung cancer, 310–311
 extensive-stage, relapse patterns after,
 378–379t, 380
Biologic principles of cancer, 71–72
Biology, 35–45
 of cancer, 72–75
Biomarker(s)
 as prognostic factor in small cell lung
 cancer, 272
 in small cell lung cancer (SCLC), 281–300
 bombesin as, 297
 carcinoembryonic antigen as, 286–289
 creatine kinase BB as, 289–291
 criteria for, 281–282
 in detection of CNS
 involvement, 298–299
 neuron-specific enolase as, 293–296
 neurophysins as, 291–293
 polypeptides as, 282–286
Biopsy
 bronchoscopic, 102–103
 in detecting metastases in stage III_{M_0}
 disease, 186
 needle, percutaneous, 104–107
 in lung nodule evaluation, 137–138
 in superior sulcus tumor diagnosis, 189
 scalene node, 108
 for staging, 127, 128
 supraclavicular node, 108
Bleomycin as antitumor antibiotic, 82
Blood gas values, arterial, preoperative, 57
Bombesin in small cell lung cancer, 16, 41
 as biomarker, 297

Bone
 metastases to
 in small cell lung cancer staging, 269
 in stage III_{M_1} disease, management of,
 radiotherapy in, 245–246
 scan of
 as noninvasive staging technique, 125,
 126t, 128
 in superior culcus tumor diagnosis, 189
Brachytherapy of unresectable endobronchial
 tumor, 404–405
Brain
 irradiation of, prophylactic, in small cell
 lung cancer, 346–347
 intracranial relapse and, 385–388
 metastases to
 diagnosis and management of, 426–427
 in small cell lung cancer
 palliative radiotherapy in, 349
 relapse of, prophylactic cranial
 irradiation and, 385–388
 in stage III_{M_1} disease management of,
 radiotherapy in, 247–249
 scan of, as noninvasive staging technique,
 125, 126t
Bridges, intracellular, in squamous cell
 carcinoma, 11
Bronchiolalveolar adenocarcinoma (BAC),
 18, 27
Bronchopulmonary carcinoids, pathology of,
 24–27
Bronchoscopy
 diagnostic, 102–103
 in evaluating stage III_{M_0} disease, 106
 to re-establish airway in T_3 tumor of main-
 stem bronchus within 2 cm of carina,
 191
 in staging, 56, 126–127
Bronchus, main-stem, involvement of, within
 2 cm of carina, management of,
 191–193

Calcification, lung cancer and, 89
Calcitonin as small cell lung cancer biomarker,
 283t, 284t, 285–286
CAMP with radiotherapy for advanced non-
 small cell lung cancer, 222, 223, 224t,
 225
Cancer
 biologic principles of, 71–72
 biology of, 72–75
 viruses causing, 72

CAP
   with radiotherapy for advanced non-small
      cell lung cancer, 223, 224*t*, 225-226
   in stage II adjuvant chemotherapy,
      179-180
Carboplatin for small cell lung cancer, 312,
   314-315
Carcinoembryonic antigen (CEA)
   production of, in lung cancer, 45
   as small cell lung cancer (SCLC) biomarker,
      286-289
Carcinogens, 72
Carcinoids, bronchopulmonary
   atypical, 24-25, 26
   pathology of, 24-27
      gross, 24
      microscopic, 24-25
      research efforts on, 25-26
Carcinomatosis, leptomeningeal, in small cell
   lung cancer, 388-389
Carcinomatous neuromyopathies in small cell
   lung cancer, 263
Cardiac ejection fraction in preoperative
   evaluation in stage I disease, 139
Cardiac evaluation in preoperative evaluation
   in stage I disease, 139
Carina, T_3 tumor of main-stem bronchus
   within 2 cm of, management of,
   191-193
CAV for small cell lung cancer, 314
   limited-stage, compared to radiotherapy,
      randomized trials on, 335-336
CCNU with radiotherapy for advanced non-
   small cell lung cancer, 224
Cell cycle
   chemotherapy and, 73-74
   effects of radiation on, 63-64
Cell lines
   human lung cancer
      characteristics of, 36-38
      development of, 35
   NSCLC
      characteristics of, 37-38
      DNA content of, flow cytometric analysis
         of, 39
      SCLC, 319-320
      characteristics of, 36-37
      cloning of, in vitro soft agarose, 38-39
      DNA content of, flow cytometric analysis
         of, 39
Cellular kinetics in cancer, 73-74
Central nervous system (CNS)
   complications involving, 425-429
      from direct effects, 426-427
      from indirect effects, 426-429
      side effects of therapy as, 429
      spinal cord metastases as, 427-428
   involvement of, in small cell lung cancer,
      263
   metastases to
      as prognostic factor in small cell lung
         cancer, 272
      of small cell lung cancer
         detection of, biomarkers in, 298-299
         for staging, 269-270
Cerebellar degeneration in small cell lung
   cancer, 263
Cervical mediastinoscopy in staging N_2
   disease, 203
Chemicals in cancer etiology, 72
Chemotherapy
   adjuvant, of stage II disease, 179-180
   adjuvant, of stage III_{M_0} non-small cell lung
      cancer, 221-227
      early studies in, 221-222
      optimal use of, 222-223
      with radiotherapy
         recent clinical trials on, 223-227
   alkylating agents in, 77, 79
   antimetabolites in, 79-80
   antineoplastic agents in, 77-81
   of disseminated non-small cell lung cancer,
      233-239
      current recommendations for, 238
      new approaches to, 238-239
      patient characteristics in, 233-236
      results of, 236-238
   drug resistance in, genetic instability of
      cancer cells and, 76-77
   evaluation of, SCLC cloning in, 38-39
   principles of, 75-76
   pulmonary-cardiac toxicity from, 420-421
   of small cell lung cancer, 307-320
      combination, 314-316
      alternating non-cross-resistant, 316-317
      extensive-stage, relapse patterns after,
         381-384
         late intensification and, 384
         maintenance therapy and, 382-383
         non-cross-resistant alternating drug
          regimens and, 383-384
      future strategies for, 320, *321*
      limited-stage
         with radiotherapy, 331-333
         radiotherapy versus, randomized trials
          on, 334-338

Chemotherapy *(continued)*
  newer approaches to
    clinical, 317-318
    from laboratory, 319-320
  with radiotherapy, 310-311, 319
    sequencing of, 341-343
    timing of, 341-343
  results of, anticipated, 311-312
  with single agents, 313-314
  surgical resection as adjuvant to,
    359-366. *See also* Surgical therapy of
    small cell lung cancer
Chest
  pain in, in small cell lung cancer, 261
  symptoms in, from stage III_{M_1} disease
    palliation of, radiotherapy in,
    243-245
  wall of, invasion of, by T_3 tumor,
    management of, 186-189
  x-ray of
    in detection, 87-89, *90-91*
    in lung nodule evaluation, 137
    in postoperative follow-up, 59
    in small cell lung cancer evaluation, 264
    in staging, 56
    in superior sulcus tumor diagnosis, 189
Chlorambucil, 77
Cisplatin
  as antineoplastic agents, 82
  with cyclophosphamide, and doxorubicin.
    See CAP
  for small cell lung cancer, 312-313
Clara cells, response of, to chronic injury, 8
Classification, staging, 118-119
Clear cells in large cell carcinomas, 23
Cloning, in vitro soft agarose, 38-39
Clonogenic cell, malignant, 73
Coagulopathy, diagnosis and management
  of, 430-431
Coin lesion in stage I disease, 135-137
Coldman-Goldie hypothesis on drug
  resistance, 77
Combined modal therapy. *See also* Bimodal
  therapy
  for limited-stage small cell lung cancer,
    331-333
Complications
  abdominal, 421-423
  central nervous system, 425-429
  endocrine, 429-430
  paraneoplastic, 430-431
  skeletal, 423-425
  systemic, 430-431

  thoracic, 411-421. *See also* Thorax,
    complications involving
Computed tomography (CT)
  in detecting metastases in stage III_{M_0}
    disease, 185
  diagnostic, 94-95, *96-97, 98*
  in lung nodule evaluation, 137, 138
  as noninvasive staging technique, 121-124
  in postoperative follow-up, 59
  in radiotherapy of small cell lung cancer,
    343-344
  in small cell lung cancer evaluation, 264
  in staging, 56
    of N_2 disease, 203
  in superior sulcus tumor diagnosis, 189
Consolidation in small cell lung cancer
  therapy, 317-318
Constrictive pericardial syndrome
  complicating radiation therapy, 153
Conventional tomography, diagnostic,
  92-93, *94*
Core vesicles in small cell lung carcinoma cell
  lines, 36
Cough
  complicating radiation therapy of stage I
    disease, 153
  in small cell lung cancer, 261
  in stage I disease, 135
Cranial irradiation, prophylactic, in small cell
    lung cancer, 346-347
  intracranial relapse and, 385-388
Creatine kinase BB as small cell lung cancer
    (SCLC) biomarker, 291-293
Creatine kinase (CK) in tumors, 42-43
Cushing's syndrome in small cell lung cancer,
  263
Cutaneous manifestations, diagnosis and
    management of, 431
Cyclophosphamide, 77-79
  with adriamycin
    and etoposide for small cell lung cancer,
    315-316
    methotrexate, and procarbazine. *See*
    CAMP
  with doxorubicin
    and cisplatin. *See* CAP
    and vincristine. *See* CAV
Cytogenetics, tumor cell, 40
Cytoketatin in squamous cell carcinoma,
  12-13
Cytology, sputum, diagnostic, 100, 102
Cytosine arabinoside, 79
Cytoskeletal proteins in tumors, 43-44

Cytoxan
  with adriamycin
    and platinum. *See* CAP
    and vincristine. *See* CAV
  in stage II adjuvant chemotherapy,
    179-180

Daunomycin as antitumor antibiotic, 81-82
Death, radiobiological definition of, 63
Deoxyribonucleic acid (DNA) content of
    tumor cells, flow cytometric analysis
    of, 39
Deoxythymidine kinase (TK) in tumors, 43
Dermatitis, radiation, 152, 421
Dermatomyositis, diagnosis and management
    of, 428-429
Diagnostic methods, 87-109
  chest radiography as, 92. *See also* Chest,
    x-ray of computed tomography as,
    94-95, *96-97, 98. See also*
    Computed tomography (CT)
  conventional tomography as, 92-93, *94*
  for detection, 87-89
  magnetic resonance imaging as, 99-100,
    101, 102
  noninvasive, 89, 92-102
  sputum cytology as, 100, 102
  tissue sampling as, 102-109. *See also*
    Tissue diagnosis
cis-Diamminedichloroplatinum II as
    antineoplastic agent, 82
Diaphragm, invasion of, by T_3 tumor
    management of, 194
Diarrhea, diagnosis and management of,
    422-423
Distant metastases (M) in TNM system,
    115-116
Dose intensity of chemotherapy for extensive-
    stage small cell lung cancer, relapse
    patterns after, 382
Dose-time fractionation in radiotherapy of
    small cell lung cancer, 340-341
Dose tumor volume relationships in clinical
    radiation oncology, 149-150
Doubling times
  of non-small lung cancer cell lines, 38
  of small cell lung carcinoma cell lines, 37
Doxorubicin
  with cyclophosphamide
    and cisplatin. *See* CAP
    and etoposide for small cell lung
      cancer, 315-316
    and vincristine. *See* CAV

Drug resistance, genetic instability of cancer
    cells and, 76-77
Dysphagia
  complicating radiotherapy for stage III
    disease, 216
  in small cell lung cancer, 262

Eaton-Lambert syndrome
  diagnosis and management of, 428-429
  in small cell lung cancer, 263
Edema, pulmonary, postpneumonectomy,
    prevention of, 193
Effusion
  pericardial, complicating radiation therapy,
    153
  pleural
    diagnosis and management of, 414-415
    in T_3 tumor, management of, 195
Electron affinic agents in radiation oncology,
    66-67
Electron microscopy (EM) in diagnosis, 5-6
  of adenocarcinoma, 20
  of carcinoids, 25
  of large cell carcinomas, 23
  of small cell lung carcinoma, 16, 17
  of squamous cell carcinoma, 11
Embolism, air, complicating percutaneous
    needle biopsy, 106
Encephalopathy, limbic, diagnosis and
    management of, 428
Endobronchial therapy for unresectable lung
    cancer, 401-408
  brachytherapy in, 404-405
  laser therapy in, 402-404
  patient selection for, 405-407
  technique of, 405-407
Endocrine symptoms, diagnosis and
    management of, 429-430
Endoscopic brushing in lung nodule
    evaluation, 137
Enolase, neuron-specific
  as small cell lung cancer biomarkers,
    293-296
  in tumors, 42
Environmental risk factors, 9
Enzyme markers in tumors, 42-43
Epidermal growth factors (EGF) in non-small
    cell lung carcinomas, 42
Esophagitis, radiation, 68, 152-153, 421
  complicating radiotherapy for stage III
    disease, 216, 217t
Esophagus
  compression of, diagnosis and

Esophagus *(continued)*
    management of, 416–417
    mucosa of, desquamation of, complicating
        radiotherapy for stage III disease, 216
    stenosis of, complicating radiation therapy,
        153
Etoposide, 81
    with cyclophosphamide and adriamycin for
        small cell lung cancer, 315–316
    for small cell lung cancer, 313, 314, 315
Extrapulmonary intrathoracic structures,
        invasion of, by T_3 tumor, management
        of, 193–196
Extrapulmonary small cell lung cancer, 263

Familial risk factors, 9
Fiberoptic bronchoscopy,
        diagnostic, 102–103
Fibrosis
    pulmonary, complicating radiotherapy, 69
        for stage III disease, 216, 217t
    subcutaneous, radiation, 421
Flow cytometric (FCM) analysis of DNA
        content of tumor cells, 39
5-Fluorodeoxyuridine (5-FUDR), 79
5-Fluorouracil (5-FU), 79
Folate antagonists, 80
Forced expiratory volume in one second
        (FEV_1), preoperative, 57–58

^{67}Gallium (^{67}Ga) scanning
    as noninvasive staging technique,
        124–125, *126*
    in postoperative follow-up, 59
    in staging, 56–57
Gastrointestinal tract, complications
        involving, diagnosis and management
        of, 422–423
Gender, incidence by, 9–10
Genetic instability of cancer cells, drug
        resistance and, 76–77
Genetic risk factors, 9
Giant cells
    multinucleated, in large cell carcinomas, 23
    in squamous cell carcinoma, 11
Granules, neurosecretory, in small cell lung
        cancer specimen, 258–259
Growth factors
    in non-small cell lung carcinomas, 42
    in small cell lung carcinomas, 41

Hemibody or whole-body irradiation for small
        cell lung cancer, 347–349

Hemoptysis
    complicating percutaneous needle biopsy,
        106
    in stage I disease, 135
Hemorrhage
    complicating bronchoscopy, 103
    complicating percutaneous needle biopsy,
        106
Hepatic metastases
    as prognostic factor in small cell lung
        cancer, 271
    in small cell lung cancer staging, 269
    in stage$_{M_1}$ disease, management of,
        radiotherapy in, 249–250
High-LET radiation in radiation oncology, 67
Hilar mass, 89, *90*
Hoarseness in small cell lung cancer, 262
Horner's syndrome in superior pulmonary
        sulcus carcinoma, 211
Hypercalcemia, diagnosis and management
        of, 423–425
Hypertrophic pulmonary osteoarthropathy,
        diagnosis and management of, 423
Hypoxia complicating bronchoscopy, 103
Hypoxic cells in radiation oncology, 66–67

Immunohistochemistry (IHC) in diagnosis,
        5–6
    of adenocarcinoma, 20
    of carcinoids, 25
    of small cell lung carcinoma, 17
Immunotherapy (BCG), intrapleural,
        adjuvant in stage I disease, 144–145
Incidence, 9
    of adenocarcinomas, 17
    of carcinoids, 24
    of small cell lung carcinoma, 13
    of squamous cell carcinoma, 10
Inorganic salts as antineoplastic agents, 82
Intensification, late, in small cell lung cancer
        therapy, 317–318
Interstitial radiation, 61
Intra-abdominal metastases in small cell lung
        cancer staging, 270
Intra-abdominal relapse, in small cell lung
        cancer, 389–391
Intracellular bridges in squamous cell
        carcinoma, 11
Intracranial metastases. *See* Brain,
        metastases to
Intrapleural BCG immunotherapy, adjuvant,
        in stage I disease, 144–145

Invasive staging techniques, 126-128
Involucrin in squamous cell carcinoma, 13
Ionizing radiation, interaction of, with matter, 62
Irradiation. *See* Radiation therapy
Irradiation portals in radiotherapy
   of locally advanced stage III disease, 213-216
   of stage II disease, 168-170

Keratin
   in squamous cell carcinoma, 12-13
   in tumors, 43
Kinetics, cellular, in cancer, 73-74

Labeling index
   of non-small lung cancer cell lines, 38
Large cell carcinoma
   with neurosecretory granules, 28
   pathology of, 22-23
Laryngospasm complicating bronchoscopy, 103
Laser
   to re-establish airway in T_3 tumor of main-stem bronchus within 2 cm of carina, 191
   for unresectable endobronchial tumor, 402-404
Late intensification regimens for extensive stage small cell lung cancer, relapse patterns after, 384
Leptomeningeal carcinomatosis in small cell lung cancer, 388-389
Leptomeningeal metastases, diagnosis and management of, 427
Light microscopy (LM)
   concepts of pathology with, challenge to, 5-6
   in diagnosis
      of adenocarcinomas, 18
      of carcinoids, 24
      of large cell carcinomas, 23
      of squamous cell carcinoma, 11
Limbic encephalopathy, diagnosis and management of, 428
Liver
   complications involving, diagnosis and management of, 422, 423
   metastases to
      as prognostic factor in small cell lung cancer, 271
      in small cell lung cancer staging, 269

   in stage III_{M_1} disease, management of, radiotherapy in, 249-250
   scan of, as noninvasive staging technique, 125, 126*t*
Lobectomy
   sleeve, for stage I disease, 141-142
   for stage I disease, 140-141
   for stage II disease, 162
Lung function evaluation, preoperative, 57
Lymph nodes
   hilar, CT scanning of, diagnostic, 95, 97, 99
   mediastinal, CT scanning of, diagnostic, 95, 97, 99
   scalene, biopsy of, diagnostic, 108
   supraclavicular, biopsy of, diagnostic, 108
   in T_3 tumor, management of, 195
Lymphadenectomy, radical, for N_2 disease, 204

Magnetic resonance imaging (MRI), diagnostic, 100, 102
Marlex and methylmethacrylate for prosthesis for chest wall defect, 187-188
Matter, ionizing radiation and, interactions of, 62
Median survival as indicator of therapeutic effectiveness, 330-333
Mediastinal lymph nodes, CT scanning of, diagnostic, 95, 97, 99
Mediastinal (N_2) disease, resection of, 201-204
   indications for, 204
   prognosis in, 201-203
   staging before, 203
Mediastinoscopy
   cervical, in staging N_2 disease, 203
   in detecting metastases in stage III_{M_0} disease, 185-186
   diagnostic, 107
   in evaluation of T_3 tumor of main-stem bronchus within 2 cm of carina, 191
   preoperative, in stage I disease, 139
   for staging, 127
Medical oncology
   chemotherapy in, 75-81. *See also* Chemotherapy
   principles of, 71-82
6-Mercaptopurine, 79
Metastasis(es)
   adrenal, diagnosis and management of, 422

Metastasis(es) *(continued)*
  biology of, 74-75
  bone
    in small cell lung cancer staging, 269
    in stage III disease, management of,
      radiotherapy in, 245-246
  brain. *See* Brain, metastases to
      distant, in TNM system, 115-116
  hepatic
    as prognostic factor in small cell lung
      cancer, 271
    in small cell lung cancer staging, 269
    in stage III_{M_1} disease, management of,
      radiotherapy in, 249-250
  intra-abdominal, in small cell lung cancer
      staging, 270
  intracranial. *See* Brain, metastases to
  leptomeningeal, diagnosis and
      management of, 427
  osteoblastic, diagnosis and management
      of, 423
  pancreatic, diagnosis and management of,
      422
  spinal cord, diagnosis and management of,
      427-428
Methotrexate, 80
  with cyclophosphamide, adriamycin, and
      procarbazine. *See* CAMP
Methylmethacrylate and Marlex for prosthesis
      for chest wall defect, 187-188
Migratory thrombophlebitis, diagnosis and
      management of, 430
Miners, uranium, small cell lung cancer in,
      258
Mitomycin-C as antitumor antibiotic, 82
Monoclonal antibodies (MAs) against lung
      cancer-associated antigens, 44-45
Morphogenesis, 7-8
Mucin production in adenocarcinoma, 18, 20
Multimodality approach, 3-4
Multinucleated giant cells in large cell
      carcinomas, 23
Myasthenic syndrome in small cell lung
      cancer, 263
Myelitis, radiation, 153

N_2 disease, 201-204. *See also* Mediastinal
      (N_2) disease
Neodymium-YAG laser therapy for
      unresectable lung cancer, 402-404
Nerve(s)
  entrapment of, diagnosis and management
      of, 417

  phrenic, invasion of, by T_3 tumor,
      management of, 194-195
Neuroendocrine (NE) cells in chronically
      injured lung, 7
Neuroendocrine (NE) features, non-small cell
      lung cancer with, 27-28
Neuroendocrine (NE) tumor
  carcinoids as, 27
  small cell lung carcinoma as, 16, 17, 27
Neurofilament in small cell lung carcinoma
      lines, 43
Neurologic complications, 425-429
Neuromyopathies, carcinomatous, in small
      cell lung cancer, 263
Neuron-specific enolase (NSE)
  as small cell lung cancer (SCLC) biomarker,
      293-296
  in tumors, 42
Neurophysins (HNP) as small cell lung cancer
      (SCLC) biomarkers, 291-293
Neurosecretory granules in small cell lung
      cancer specimen, 258-259
Nitrogen mustard, 77-79
Nitroimidazoles in radiation oncology, 66-67
Nodal involvement (N) in TNM system, 115,
      116
Nodule(s), lung, 89
  clinical evaluation of, 137-138
  in stage I disease, 135-137
  synchronous, problem of, 138
Noninvasive staging techniques, 120-126
  patient evaluation as, 120
  radiography as, 120-124
  scintigraphy as, 124-126
Non-small cell lung cancer (NSCLC),
      133-253
  cell lines of
    characteristics of, 37-38
    DNA content of, flow cytometric analysis
      of, 39
  cytoskeletal proteins in, 43-44
  epidermal growth factors in, 42
  ras genes in, 40-41
  monoclonal antibodies against, 44-45
  with neuroendocrine features, 27-28
  peptide hormone production by, 42
  stage I, 133-157. *See also* Stage I non-
      small cell lung cancer
  stage II, 159-182. *See also* Stage II non-
      small cell lung cancer
  stage III_{M_0}, 183-229. *See also* Stage III_{M_0}
      non-small cell lung cancer
  stage III/stage IV, 231-253. *See also* Stage

III$_{M_1}$/stage IV non-small cell lung
  cancer
Nuclear magnetic resonance imaging in
    superior sulcus tumor diagnosis, 189
Nucleus(i), in small cell lung carcinoma, 14,
    15
  cell lines, 36-37

Occupational risk factors, 9
Oncogenes
  ras, in non-small cell lung cancer, 40-41
  in tumor cells, 40-41
Oncology
  medical, 71-82. *See also* Medical
      oncology
  surgical, 55-59. *See also* Surgical
      oncology
Orthovoltage radiation, 61
Osteoarthropathy, pulmonary, hypertrophic,
    diagnosis and management of, 423
Osteoblastic metastases, diagnosis and
    management of, 423
Osteolytic bone lesions, diagnosis and
    management of, 423

Palliative radiotherapy in small cell lung
    cancer, 349-350
Pancreas, metastases to, diagnosis and
    management of, 422
Paraneoplastic syndromes
  diagnosis and management of, 430-431
  in small cell lung cancer, 263
Parasternal exploration, 107-108
Parasternal mediastinotomy for staging, 127
Pathogenesis, 8-9
Pathology, 5-28
  of adenocarcinoma, 17-21
    gross, 18
    microscopic, 18-20
    research efforts on, 20, *21*
  of carcinoids, 24-27
    gross, 24
    microscopic, 24-25
    research efforts on, 25-26
  of large cell carcinomas, 22-23
  of small cell carcinomas, 13-17
    gross, 13-14
    microscopic, 14-16
    research efforts on, 16, *17*
  of squamous cell carcinomas, 10-13
    gross, 10
    microscopic, 10-11
    research efforts on, 12-13

Peptide hormone production
  by non-small cell lung carcinomas, 42
  by small cell lung carcinomas, 41-42
Percutaneous needle biopsy
  diagnostic, 104-107
  in lung nodule evaluation, 137-138
Performance status as prognostic factor in
    small cell lung cancer, 271
Pericardial disease, diagnosis and
    management of, 415-416
Pericardial effusion complicating radiation
    therapy of stage I disease, 153
Pericardial syndrome, constrictive,
    complicating radiation therapy of stage
    I disease, 153
Pericarditis, radiation, 419-420
  acute, 68
Pericardium, invasion of, by T$_3$ tumor,
    management of, 194-195
L-Phenylalanine mustard, 77
Phrenic nerve, invasion of, by T$_3$ tumor,
    management of, 194-195
Plant alkaloids, pharmacology of, 80-81
Platinol as antineoplastic agents, 82
Platinum
  with cytoxan and adriamycin. *See* CAP
  in stage II adjuvant chemotherapy,
      179-180
Pleural effusion
  diagnosis and management of, 414-415
  in T$_3$ tumor, management of, 195
Pleuroscopy, diagnostic, for staging, 127
Pneumonectomy
  intrapericardial, for stage I disease, 141
  for stage II disease, 162
Pneumonitis
  persistent, in stage I disease, 135
  radiation, in stage I disease, 153
    acute, 68-69
    complicating radiotherapy for stage III
        disease, 216, 217*t*
Pneumonitis-fibrosis, radiation, 418-419
Pneumothorax
  complicating bronchoscopy, 103
  complicating percutaneous needle biopsy,
      106
Podophyllotoxins, 80, 81
Polypeptide hormone production by small cell
    lung carcinomas, 41-42
Polypeptides as small cell lung cancer (SCLC)
    biomarkers, 282-286
Portals, irradiation, in radiotherapy

Portals (continued)
  of locally advanced stage III disease,
      213-216
  of stage II disease, 168-170
Postpneumonectomy pulmonary edema,
      prevention of, 193
Primary tumor (T) in TNM system, 114, 115
Procarbazine, cyclophosphamide,
      adriamycin, and methotrexate. See
      CAMP
Proteins, cytoskeletal, in tumors, 43-44
myc Proto-oncogenes in small cell lung
      carcinoma, 16, 17, 46
Pulmonary artery, invasion of, by T_3 tumor,
      management of, 194
Pulmonary edema, postpneumonectomy,
      prevention of, 193
Pulmonary fibrosis complicating radiotherapy
      for stage III disease, 216, 217t
Pulmonary function tests, preoperative, 57
  in stage I disease, 138-139
Pulmonary sulcus, superior
  carcinoma of, diagnosis and management
      of, 211-213
  tumors of, management of, 189-190
Purine antagonists, 79
Pyrimidine antagonists, 79

Race, incidence by, 9
Radiation
  in cancer etiology, 72
  damage from
      potentially lethal, repair of, 65-66
      sublethal, repair of, 64-65
  high-LET, in radiation oncology, 67
  interstitial, 61
  ionizing, interaction of, with matter, 62
  orthovoltage, 61
      superficial, 61
      supravoltage, 61
Radiation dermatitis, 421
Radiation esophagitis, 421
  complicating radiotherapy for stage III
      disease, 216, 217t
Radiation fibrosis of lung, 69
Radiation myelitis in stage I disease, 153
Radiation oncology
  biological aspects of, 62-70
  cell cycle effects of, 63-64
  clinical, dose-tumor volume relationships
      in, 149-150
  hypoxic cells in, 666-67

  normal tissue effects in, 68-70
  physics of, 61-62
  principles of, 61-70
  radiocurability and, 63
  radioresponsiveness and, 63
  radiosensitivity and, 62-63
  repair in, 64-66
  treatment planning for, 61-62
Radiation pericarditis, 419-420
Radiation pneumonitis
  acute, 68-69
  complicating radiotherapy for stage III
      disease, 216, 217t
  in stage I disease, 153
Radiation pneumonitis-fibrosis, 418-419
Radiation subcutaneous fibrosis, 421
Radiation therapy
  adjuvant, for stage II disease, 165-170,
      176-179
    future directions in, 170
    operative, 166
    postoperative, 167-168
    preoperative, 166
    prognostic factors and, 165-166
    staging before, 165
    techniques of, 168-170
  chest complications of, 418-420
  for locally advanced stage III disease,
      207-218
    complications of, 216, 217t
    dose for, 207-211
    evaluation before, 207
    future directions in, 216-218
    superior pulmonary sulcus, 211-213
    techniques of, 213-216
  for small cell lung cancer, 309, 310-311,
      319, 329-350
    with chemotherapy, 331-333
      sequencing of, 341-343
      timing of, 341-343
    chemotherapy versus, randomized trials
      on, 334-338
    cranial, prophylactic, 346-347
      intracranial relapse and, 385-388
    CT scans in, 343-344
    delivery of, toward optimal method
      of, 338-344
    dose-time fractionation in, 340-341
    extensive-stage, 344-345
    hemibody or whole-body, 347-349
    limited-stage, 329-334
      relapse patterns after, 371-377, 380

palliative, 349-350
volume requiring treatment in, 338-339
for stage I disease, 149-156
  complications of, 152-153
  dose-tumor volume relationships in,
    149-150
  experience with, 150-152
  new directions in, 153-155
  risk analysis in, 156
  side effects of, 152-153
for stage III_{M_0} disease
  chemotherapy as adjuvant to, 221-227.
    See also Chemotherapy, adjuvant, for
    stage III_{M_0} non-small cell lung cancer
  with chest wall invasion, 188-189
  of superior sulcus, 189-190
for stage III_{M_1} disease, 243-252
  in chest symptom palliation, 243-245
  in management
    of brain metastases, 247-249
    of liver metastases, 249-250
    of skeletal metastases, 245-246
    of spinal cord compression, 250-252
    of superior vena caval obstruction,
      244-245
  for superior sulcus tumors, 189-190
Radical lymphadenectomy for N_2 disease,
  204
Radiocurability, 63
Radiography
  chest. See Chest, x-ray of
  as noninvasive staging technique, 120-124
Radiologic presentation of intrathoracic small
  cell tumor, 263-264
Radionuclide scanning in staging, 56-57
Radioresponsiveness, 63
Radiosensitivity, 62-63
Relapse patterns in small cell lung cancer
  central nervous system, 385-389
  extensive-stage, 378-379t, 380-384
    after chemotherapy, 381-384
  intra-abdominal, 389-391
  limited-stage, 369-392
    after radiation therapy, 371-377, 380
    after surgical therapy, 370-371
Reoxygenation of tumor in radiation
  oncology, 67
Repair of radiation damage
  potentially lethal, 65-66
  sublethal, 64-65
Risk factors, 9
Roentgenography, chest. See Chest, x-ray of

Salts, inorganic, as antineoplastic agents, 82
Scalene node biopsy, diagnostic, 108
Scintigraphy as noninvasive staging
  technique, 124-126
Screening of asymptomatic smokers, 88-89
Skeletal system
  complications involving, 423-425
  metastases to
    in small cell lung cancer staging, 269
    in stage III_{M_1} disease, management of,
      radiotherapy in, 245-246
Skin effects of radiation therapy, 152, 421
Sleeve lobectomy for stage I disease,
  141-142
Small cell lung cancer (SCLC), 255-397
  biomarkers in, 281-300
  cell biology in, 260-261
  cell lines of
    characteristics of, 36-37
    cloning of, in vitro soft agarose, 38-39
    DNA content of, flow cytometric analysis
      of, 39
  chemotherapy for, 307-320. See also
    Chemotherapy for small cell lung
    cancer
  classification of, 259-260
  clinical presentation of, 261-264
  conclusions on, 391-392
  creatine kinase in, 42-43
  cytoskeletal proteins in, 43
  deoxythymidine kinase in, 43
  etiology of, 257-259
  growth characteristics of, 260-261
  growth factors in, 41
  histologic diagnosis of, 259
  intrathoracic, radiologic presentation of,
    263-264
  monoclonal antibodies against, 44
  neuron-specific enolase in, 42
  and non-small cell lung interrelationship of,
    28
  pathogenesis, 257-259
  pathology of, 13-17, 259-260
    gross, 13-14
    microscopic, 14-16
    research efforts on, 16, 17
  peptide hormone production by, 41-42
  myc proto-oncogenes in, 16, 17, 40
  prognostic factors in, 270-272
  radiation therapy in, 329-350. See also
    Radiation therapy in small cell lung
    cancer

Small cell lung cancer *(continued)*
  relapse patterns in, 369–392. *See also*
      Relapse patterns in small cell lung
      cancer
  staging evaluation of, 264–270. *See also*
      Staging of small cell lung cancer
  surgical resection in management of,
      359–366. *See also* Surgical therapy of
      small cell lung cancer
  as systemic disease, 307–309
  therapeutic options and strategies for,
      309–311
Smokers, asymptomatic, screening of, 88–89
Smoking, lung cancer and, 9
  small cell, 257–258
Spinal cord
  compression of
      in small cell lung cancer, 388–389
      in stage III_{M_1} disease, management of,
          radiotherapy in, 250–252
  metastases to, diagnosis and management
      of, 427–428
Sputum cytology, diagnostic, 100, 102
Squamous cell carcinoma
  cell lines of, 38
  pathology of, 10–13
      gross, 10
      microscopic, 10–11
      research efforts on, 12–13
Stage I non-small cell lung cancer, 133–157
  clinical characteristics of, 135–137
  radiation therapy for, 149–156. *See also*
      Radiation therapy for stage I disease
  surgical therapy for, 135–146. *See also*
      Surgical therapy for stage I disease
Stage II non-small cell lung cancer, 159–182
  adjuvant therapy for
      chemotherapy, 179–180
      radiation, 176–179
      rationale for, 176
  modified, surgical therapy for, 161–164
  prognosis for, 174–175
  staging definitions from, 173
Stage III_{M_0} non-small cell lung cancer,
      183–229
  chest wall invasion in, 186–189
  extrapulmonary intrathoracic structure
      invasion by, 193–195
  locally advanced, radiation therapy
      for, 207–218. *See also* Radiation
      therapy for locally advanced stage III
      disease

main-stem bronchus involvement in, within
      2 cm of carina, 191–193
  management of, 185–196
      in chest wall invasion, 186–189
      in diaphragm invasion, 194
      in extrapulmonary intrathoracic structure
          invasion, 193–195
      in main-stem bronchus involvement
          within 2 cm of carina, 191–193
      with nodal involvement, 195
      in pericardial invasion, 194–195
      in phrenic nerve invasion, 194–195
      with pleural effusion, 195
      in pulmonary artery invasion, 194
      in superior sulcus tumors, 189–190
  mediastinal, 201–204. *See also*
      Mediastinal (N_2) disease
  superior sulcus tumors in, 189–190
  in superior vena cava invasion, 195
Stage III_{M_1}/Stage IV non-small cell lung
      cancer, 231–253
  chemotherapy of, 233–239. *See also*
      Chemotherapy of disseminated non-
      small cell lung cancer
  radiation therapy of, 243–253. *See also*
      Radiation therapy of stage III_{M_1} disease
Staging, 113–129
  AJC system for, 116–118
  Autopsy, 118–119
  clinical-diagnostic, 118
  definitions for, 113–119
  international system for, 119
  invasive techniques for, 126–128
  of N_2 disease
      invasive, 203–204
      noninvasive, 203
  noninvasive techniques for, 120–126. *See
      also* Noninvasive staging techniques
  plan for, optimal, 128–129
  postsurgical treatment pathologic, 118
  pretreatment, 118
  process of, 120–128
  retreatment, 118
  of small cell lung cancer, 264–270
      bone metastases in, 268–269
      intra-abdominal metastases in, 270
      CNS metastases in, 269–270
      hepatic metastases in, 269
      procedures for, 265–266, 267*t*
  surgical-evaluative, 118
  systems for, 119
Staging classification, 118–119

Statistics, 9-10

Subcutaneous fibrosis, radiation, 421

Sulcus, pulmonary, superior

    carcinoma of, diagnosis and management

      of, 211-213

    tumors of, management of, 189-190

Superficial radiation, 61

Superior pulmonary sulcus

    carcinoma of, diagnosis and management

      of, 211-213

    tumors of, management of, 189-190

Superior vena cava

    invasion of, by T_3 tumor, management of,

      195

    obstruction of

      by small cell lung cancer, palliative

        radiotherapy in, 349-350

      in stage III_{M_1} disease, management of,

        radiotherapy in, 244-245

Superior vena caval (SVC) syndrome

    diagnosis and management of, 412-414

    in small cell lung cancer, 262

Supportive care, 399-431

Supraclavicular node biopsy, diagnostic, 108

Supravoltage radiation, 61

Surgical oncology, 55-59

    diagnosis and, 55-56

    operative considerations in, 58-59

    physiologic evaluation and, 57-58

    postoperative considerations in, 59

    staging and, 56-57

Surgical therapy

    for mediastinal disease, 201-204

      prognosis in, 201-203

    for small cell lung cancer, 309, 359-366

      historical results of, 360-361

      limited-stage, relapse patterns after,

        370-371

      rationale for, 361-365

      results of recent studies on, 361-365

    for stage I disease

      adjuvant intrapleural therapy in,

        144-145

      evaluation before, 138-139

      mediastinoscopy prior to, 139

      procedure for, 139-142

      results of, 142-144

    for stage II disease, 161-164

      adjuvant chemotherapy after, 179-180

      adjuvant radiation therapy after,

        176-179

    for stage III_{M_0} disease

      chemotherapy as adjuvant to, 221-227.

        See also Chemotherapy, adjuvant, for

        stage III_{M_0} non-small cell lung cancer

      with chest wall invasion, 187-188

      of main-stem bronchus within 2 cm of

        carina, 191-193

      of superior sulcus, 190

    thoracic complications of, 417-418

Survival rate, 5-year, 9

Synchronous lung nodules, problems of, 138

Syndrome of inappropriate antidiuretic

      hormone secretion (SIADH) in small

      cell lung caner, 263, 285

Tenoposide, 81

    for small cell lung cancer, 312

6-Thioguanine, 79

Thoracentesis

    diagnostic, 108

    staging, 127

Thoracoscopy

    diagnostic, 108

    staging, 127

Thorax, complications involving, 411-421

    chemotherapy-induced pulmonary cardiac

      toxicity as, 420-421

    dermatitis as, 421

    esophageal compression as, 416-417

    esophagitis as, 421

    nerve entrapment as, 417

    pericardial disease as, 415-416

    pleural effusion as, 414-415

    postsurgical, 417-418

    after radiation therapy, 418-420, 421

    subcutaneous fibrosis as, 421

    superior vena cava syndrome as, 412-414

Three-dimensional dosimetry for

      radiotherapy in stage I disease,

      154-155

Thrombophlebitis, migratory, diagnosis and

      management of, 430

Tissue(s)

    reactions of, normal, to radiation, 68-70

    volume of, in radiotherapy

      of locally advanced stage III disease,

        213-216

      of small cell lung cancer, 338-339

      of stage II disease, 168-170

Tissue diagnosis

    bronchoscopy in, 102-103

    mediastinoscopy in, 107

    parasternal exploration in, 107-108

Tissue diagnosis *(continued)*
  thoracoscopy in, 108
  scalene and supraclavicular node biopsy in,
    108-109
TNM classification system, 113-114
Tobacco smoke, lung cancer and, 9
  small cell, 257-258
Tomography
  computed, diagnostic, 94-95, *96-97, 98.*
    See also Computed tomography (CT)
  conventional, diagnostic, 92-93, *94*
Trousseau's syndrome, diagnosis and
  management of, 430
Tumor(s)
  primary, in TNM system, 114, *115*
  reoxygenation of, in radiation oncology, 67
  T_3N_0-T_3N_1, 185-186. *See also* Stage III_{M_0}
    non-small cell lung cancer

Uranium miners, small cell lung cancer in,
  258

Vascular complications, diagnosis and
  management of, 431
Vena cava, superior
  invasion of, by T_3 tumor, management of,
    195
  obstruction of

    by small cell lung cancer, palliative
      radiotherapy in, 349-350
    in stage III_{M_1} disease, management of,
      radiotherapy in, 344-345
Vimentin in tumors, 43-44
Vinblastine, 80, 81
Vinca alkaloids, 80-81
Vincristine, 80, 81
  with cytoxan and adriamycin. *See* CAV
Virus(es) in cancer etiology, 72
Volume loss in consolidated lobe, 89, *91*
Vomiting, diagnosis and management of, 422

Water-clear phenomenon in large cell
  carcinomas, 23
Weight loss, 430
  as prognostic factor in small cell lung
    cancer, 271
Whole-body or hemibody irradiation for small
  cell lung cancer, 347-349
World Health Organization (WHO) Lung
  Cancer Classification, purpose of, 6

X-ray, chest. *See* Chest, x-ray of
X-ray beam arrangement in radiotherapy
  of locally advanced stage III disease,
    213-216
  of stage II disease, 168-170